T0200211

# MANUAL OF ORTHOPAEDICS

## Eighth Edition

Editor

**Marc F. Swiontkowski, MD**
Professor
Department of Orthopaedic Surgery
University of Minnesota
Minneapolis, Minnesota

Associate Editors

**Steven D. Stovitz, MD, MS**
Associate Professor
Department of Family Medicine and Community Health
Team Physician, Athletics Department
University of Minnesota
Minneapolis, Minnesota

**Dagan Cloutier, PA-C**
Physician Assistant
New Hampshire Orthopaedic Center
Bedford, New Hampshire

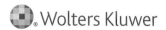. Wolters Kluwer

Philadelphia · Baltimore · New York · London
Buenos Aires · Hong Kong · Sydney · Tokyo

*Director, Medical Practice:* Brian Brown
*Senior Development Editor:* Stacey Sebring
*Editorial Coordinator:* Louis Manoharan
*Marketing Manager:* Kirsten Watrud
*Production Project Manager:* Sadie Buckallew
*Design Coordinator:* Stephen Druding
*Manufacturing Coordinator:* Beth Welsh
*Prepress Vendor:* S4Carlisle Publishing Services

Eighth edition

Copyright © 2022 Wolters Kluwer.

10  9  8  7  6  5  4  3  2  1

**Library of Congress Cataloging-in-Publication Data**

ISBN-13: 978-1-9751-4335-0
ISBN-10: 1-975143-35-3

Library of Congress Control Number: 2020947464

Shop.lww.com

MKO1120

# Preface

The eighth edition of the *Manual of Orthopaedics* further expands the conversion of the manual from one focused on medical students and orthopaedic surgery junior residents to adding the audience of emergency room providers, urgent care providers, primary care providers, and now physician assistants and nurse practitioners (PAs/NPs) practicing in musculoskeletal care centers. This is the fourth edition to use this title, which was changed from the original title of *Manual of Acute Orthopaedic Therapeutics*. The title change started the evolution toward the broader audience, which is now complete. This introduction will conclude with a list of new features in the eighth edition. It remains a worthwhile task to review the history of this useful "spiral notebook" to place the continuing changes within the context of the evolution of musculoskeletal care.

The *Manual of Acute Orthopaedic Therapeutics* was the creation of Dr. Larry Iversen, who worked out its basic framework and conceptualization with his orthopaedic mentor, Dr. D. Kay Clawson. Dr. Iversen was at the time a senior resident working closely with Dr. Clawson, who was the first professor and chairman of the Department of Orthopaedic Surgery at the University of Washington. The orthopaedic services at the University Hospital and King County Hospital (later renamed Harborview Medical Center) were active and focused mainly around the management of injured patients. Drs. Clawson and Iversen saw the need for a manual that would improve education and patient care in these institutions. Those were days when the management of long bone fractures was in transition from traction and casting to surgical techniques, and the University of Washington Orthopaedic department was at the forefront with wonderful, dedicated, and creative clinicians like Drs. Robert Smith and Sigvard Hansen. In those times, care was primarily delivered by junior house staff, interns, and medical students, and they needed information readily at hand. Therefore, the manual provided the "how-to's" for traction, casting, and pre- and postoperative care while explaining the rationale for treatment decisions and providing an excellent reference list for later review and in-depth study. This manual was a labor of love for Drs. Iversen and Clawson; the two would often work on the manuscripts for three straight weeks seated around the dining room table in Dr. Clawson's home. Little Brown publishers liked the concept of the book and added it to its growing list of subspecialty spiral manuals; the book enjoyed broad acceptance.

Each of the first three editions brought a review of the contents and reference list for each chapter as the field continued to evolve. In 1987, I returned to the University of Washington, where I had done my training (and used the second edition), to assume a position at Harborview Medical Center. In 1991, I was a new professor in the department and chief of the orthopaedic service, and Dr. Clawson asked me to assume his place with the manual. It was then Dr. Iversen and I who labored for 2 weeks in the medical school library revising the chapters, updating the reference lists, adding sections of historical references, changing several illustrations, and adding fresh chapters on infection and rheumatologic conditions. As such we began to broaden the scope of the manual to include conditions that were nonacute and nontrauma related in order to make the manual more useful for students and interns as well as to provide a more comprehensive tool for primary care physicians. The changes in care delivery moved strongly in favor of attending delivered/supervised care in academic centers where the manual was in widespread use. As such the chapters evolved drastically as the push toward surgical management of fractures had dramatically changed the way trauma patients were managed—for the better, we believe.

For the fifth edition, Dr. Iversen, with a mature, busy private practice in Bremerton, Washington, chose to step aside. I moved from the University of Washington to assume the chair of the Orthopaedic Surgery Department at the University of Minnesota in 1997 and brought the project along. This was the point where we made a major philosophical shift in the manual, changing its title to the *Manual of Orthopaedics*. It became a more comprehensive tool, covering nearly all areas of orthopaedic surgery in new chapters. Members of the Department of Orthopaedic Surgery at the University of Minnesota agreed to support the project by authoring new chapters on pediatric orthopaedics, nontraumatic hand and shoulder surgery, spine, and chronic and nonacute lower extremity orthopaedics. Treatment protocols preferred by the attending staff at Hennepin County Medical Center, where the University of Minnesota has a level 1 trauma rotation, were added. These were placed at the end of appropriate chapters, and the intent was to provide a set of principles for decision making, which serve as a starting point for developing individualized treatment plans for patients. The manual at that time moved from a two-author project to a multiauthor, single orthopaedic surgery department project in the evolution toward greater usefulness for students, house staff, and primary care physicians.

In the sixth edition, the trend continued. New chapters were added on injection techniques, and sections within each individual "nonacute" chapter provide guidelines for primary care and emergency room providers to evaluate presenting complaints from patients. In the era of increasing emphasis on cost containment, we tried to provide guidelines for primary care and emergent/urgent providers as to when expensive diagnostic tests should be offered and provided direction for how the use of physical and occupational/hand therapy should be utilized. Dr. Stovitz, a primary care physician with broad clinical experience in musculoskeletal conditions, was added as a coeditor. He reviewed all chapters in order to ensure that the entire manual had maximized usefulness for the primary care and emergent/urgent care provider.

In the seventh edition, chapters were updated with fresh reviews of the literature focusing on the inclusion of newer level I and level II data. New authors were included in greater than 50% of the chapters to gain a fresh perspective and to update the chapter outlines where indicated.

For this eighth edition, we have involved another editor, Dagan Cloutier, PA-C. We have attempted to make this edition a useful tool for the new PA/NP with a primary care–based training who has been recruited to work in a musculoskeletal care center. Dagan is the founding editor of the *Journal of Orthopaedics for Physician Assistants* (JOPA), now published by the *Journal of Bone & Joint Surgery* where I serve as editor in chief. He has vast practice experience treating a wide range of musculoskeletal conditions and has been heavily involved in preparing new PA/NP graduates for practice in orthopaedic care delivery. We have updated every chapter with high level of evidence references, provided new tables and illustrations, and added more than a half a dozen new authors from the Department of Orthopaedic Surgery at the University of Minnesota. All four editors have reviewed every chapter and added updates as treatment and diagnostic protocols have evolved through patient care research.

The discussion of individual musculoskeletal conditions and the reference lists are not meant be comprehensive, rather they are meant to provide a starting point in approaching an individual patient with a musculoskeletal problem. Every student, resident, and PA/NP is encouraged to delve more deeply into the study of the condition; both the reference list and historical references will be useful in gaining more information for personal gratification or for preparing for teaching conference discussions. Generally speaking, there is no single way to manage a musculoskeletal injury or condition; we have attempted to provide scholarly discussions that cover the gamut of approaches while informing the reader of what we think is the best current method. We have attempted to be clear about which conditions are appropriately managed by primary care and emergent/urgent care providers and which need orthopaedic subspecialist care.

No individual in the Department of Orthopaedic Surgery or Family Medicine at the University of Minnesota will receive personal remuneration for this project. The funds derived from the sale of this book will be utilized to further resident and student education and research. This principle rings true to the initial motivation of Drs. Clawson and Iversen in creating this manual. The eighth edition continues to be dedicated to these two fine surgeon educators as well as to the many students, residents, primary care, PA/NP, and emergent/urgent care providers who will benefit from the eighth edition of the *Manual of Orthopaedics*.

Marc F. Swiontkowski, MD
Steven D. Stovitz, MD, MS
Dagan Cloutier, PA-C

# Contributors

**Julie E. Adams, MD**
Professor
Department of Orthopedic Surgery
Erlanger Orthopaedics/UT College of
  Medicine
Chattanooga, Tennessee

**Jordan Barker, MD**
Adult Reconstruction Fellow
University of Minnesota/Regions
  Hospital
St. Paul, Minnesota

**Mohit Bhandari, MD, PhD**
Professor
Department of Orthopaedic Surgery
McMaster University
Hamilton, Canada

**Jonathan P. Braman, MD**
Professor
Department of Orthopedic Surgery
University of Minnesota
Minneapolis, Minnesota

**Timothy Carlson**
Medical Student, Class of 2021
University of Minnesota
Minneapolis, Minnesota

**Caitlin C. Chambers, MD**
Assistant Professor
Department of Orthopedic Surgery
University of Minnesota
Minneapolis, Minnesota

**Peter A. Cole, MD**
Professor
Department of Orthopedic Surgery
University of Minnesota/Regions
  Hospital
St. Paul, Minnesota

**Jessica M. Downes, MD**
Assistant Professor
Department of Orthopedic Surgery
University of Minnesota/Hennepin
  County Medical Center
Minneapolis, Minnesota

**Alicia K. Harrison, MD**
Associate Professor
Department of Orthopedic Surgery
University of Minnesota
Minneapolis, Minnesota

**Aaron Huser, DO**
Paley Orthopedic and Spine Institute
West Palm Beach, Florida

**Susan Kline, MD, MPH**
Professor of Medicine
Division of Infectious Diseases and
  International Medicine
University of Minnesota
Minneapolis, Minnesota

**David Eduard Lebel, MD, PhD**
Assistant Professor
Department of Surgery
University of Toronto/The Hospital for
  Sick Children
Toronto, Canada

**Thuan V. Ly, MD**
Associate Professor
Department of Orthopaedic Surgery
Ohio State University/Wexner Medical
  Center
Columbus, Ohio

**Scott B. Marston, MD**
Assistant Professor
Department of Orthopedic Surgery
University of Minnesota/Regions
  Hospital
St. Paul, Minnesota

**James W. Mazzuca, DPM**
Assistant Professor
Department of Orthopedic Surgery
University of Minnesota/TRIA
  Orthopaedic Center
Bloomington, Minnesota

**Robert A. Morgan, MD**
Associate Professor
Department of Orthopedic Surgery
St. Louis University
St. Louis, Missouri

**Bradley J. Nelson, MD**
Associate Professor
Department of Orthopedic Surgery
University of Minnesota
Minneapolis, Minnesota

**Christian M. Ogilvie, MD**
Associate Professor
Department of Orthopedic Surgery
University of Minnesota
Minneapolis, Minnesota

**Temi Ogunleye**
Medical Student, Class of 2021
Burrell College of Osteopathic Medicine
New Mexico State University
Las Cruces, New Mexico

**Fernando A. Pena, MD**
Assistant Professor
Department of Orthopedic Surgery
University of Minnesota
Minneapolis, Minnesota

**David Polly, MD**
Professor
Department of Orthopedic Surgery
University of Minnesota
Minneapolis, Minnesota

**Matthew D. Putnam, MD**
Professor
Department of Orthopedic Surgery
Erlanger Orthopaedics/UT College of
    Medicine
Chattanooga, Tennessee

**Steven D. Stovitz, MD, MS**
Associate Professor
Department of Family Medicine and
    Community Health
Team Physician, Athletics Department
University of Minnesota
Minneapolis, Minnesota

**Elizabeth Swanson, DO**
Assistant Professor
Department of Pediatrics
University of Minnesota
Minneapolis, Minnesota

**Marc F. Swiontkowski, MD**
Professor
Department of Orthopaedic Surgery
University of Minnesota
Minneapolis, Minnesota

**David C. Templeman, MD**
Professor
Department of Orthopedic Surgery
University of Minnesota/Hennepin
    County Medical Center
Minneapolis, Minnesota

**Walter H. Truong, MD**
Assistant Professor
Department of Orthopedic Surgery
University of Minnesota/Gillette
    Children's Specialty Healthcare
St. Paul, Minnesota

**Emily A. Wagstrom, MD**
Assistant Professor
Department of Orthopedic Surgery
University of Minnesota/Hennepin
    County Medical Center
St. Paul, Minnesota

**Ariel A. Williams, MD**
Assistant Professor
University of Minnesota
Minneapolis, Minnesota

# Contents

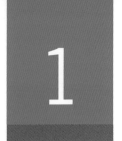

# General Approach to the Patient with Musculoskeletal Pain

Steven D. Stovitz

## I. General Approach

Medical training usually focuses on the prevention and treatment of life-shortening events, such as myocardial infarctions, stroke, and cancer. Consequently, when a patient comes in with a *mere* musculoskeletal complaint, clinicians are often unprepared. We find that students and young clinicians who see patients with musculoskeletal complaints downplay the patient's symptoms. A patient's complaint of "my knee bothers me when I run more than three miles" may be met with the clinician thinking, "Well then don't run more than three miles." Physician downplaying of musculoskeletal complaints may be especially frequent when a patient with knee pain also has an elevated risk for cardiovascular disease or diabetes mellitus.

However, patient-centered care asks us to listen to and assist patients with their concerns. Although musculoskeletal pain may not be immediately life-shortening, if it results in a sedentary lifestyle or a depressed mood, it may be a threat to long-term health. It is clear that higher levels of physical activity are associated with lower risk for cardiovascular morbidity and mortality.[1-4] If musculoskeletal pain is prohibiting the patient from maintaining his or her desirable amount of physical activity, it may be predisposing them to obesity, type 2 diabetes, hypertension, and hypercholesterolemia. In this manner, musculoskeletal pain may be considered a cause of cardiovascular disease. Given that we now live in an age of diseases of sedentary lifestyles, it is the clinician's job to help patients maintain a physically active lifestyle. If the knee pain worsens with running, then encourage other activities (i.e., help them to discover strategies to cross-train). Also, we need to be wary of using the term "overuse" when describing the cause of a patient's musculoskeletal pain. Although it is true that some repetitive motions in specific areas can cause soft-tissue stress, adults who are more active often have *less* musculoskeletal pain.[5,6] Our focus needs to be on making a proper diagnosis and encouraging the patient to remain active in ways that will not prolong the injury. Too much rest, in addition to putting patients at risk for cardiovascular disease, is often detrimental to injury healing (e.g., with tendinopathies).[7]

## II. The History

When gathering a history of the chief complaint from the patient with musculoskeletal pain, many of the principles are well ingrained in standard medical training programs: onset, duration, frequency, location, severity, character, radiation, precipitating, and relieving factors. The piece of the history that is unique in evaluating the patient with musculoskeletal pain is that of "function." It is important to understand the lifestyle of the patient and discover where, when, and how the pain uniquely impacts the lifestyle of each particular patient.

Regarding a patient's medical history, keep in mind associations of conditions. Patients with diabetes mellitus have a greater than average risk of developing adhesive capsulitis in the shoulder (i.e., a frozen shoulder). Patients who have a history of an anterior cruciate ligament (ACL) knee injury are more likely to develop meniscal tears. And, patients who have a history of stress fractures may have a composition of bone that puts them at risk for another stress fracture.

## III. Review of Systems

Clinicians should become familiar with pertinent areas of focus in the review of systems. Nowhere is this more important than in the evaluation of back pain. When evaluating a 35-year-old patient with back pain, often no imaging or laboratory tests are indicated. However, when the patient also reports concurrent fevers, night sweats, or unexplained weight changes, imaging and further diagnostic testing is certainly justified.[8] When patients have systemic complaints, it is necessary to consider rheumatologic causes of joint pains.

A focused review of systems for joint pains in the extremities may be as follows:

| Joint Complaint | Pertinent Review of Systems |
|---|---|
| Shoulder | Neck pain, hand pain, chest pain,[a] abdominal pain[b] |
| Elbow | Neck pain, shoulder pain, hand pain |
| Hand and digits | Neck pain, shoulder pain, elbow pain |
| Hip | Back pain, abdominal pain, pelvic pain |
| Knee | Back pain, hip pain |
| Lower leg, ankles, and feet | Back pain, hip pain, knee pain |

[a]Chest pain may radiate to either the left or the right shoulder.
[b]Diaphragmatic irritation can cause shoulder pain through irritation of the phrenic nerve.

## IV. The Physical Examination

As discussed extensively throughout this book, each joint has its own unique physical examination. Still, a few general principles remain.

- Proper exposure of the affected area is necessary to assess any overlying skin infections and to perform many of the musculoskeletal tests.
  - It is very difficult to perform a Lachman's test for an ACL injury if the patient is wearing long pants that do not pull up to the mid-thigh.
- Always seek permission from the patient prior to exposing any areas.
- In general, have the patient try active range of motion before you move the joint through passive range of motion. Certainly, there are exceptions to this rule, but it is a good general guideline.
- Consider approaching each joint through the following four steps: (1) observation, (2) palpation, (3) range of motion, and (4) special tests.
- Students and clinicians are often overwhelmed by the number of special tests in the musculoskeletal examination. Many conditions can be diagnosed simply from steps (1), (2), and (3). Knowing your anatomy helps!
- Medical and PA students are taught to fully examine patients prior to ordering tests. However, if you are ordering a test to evaluate for a possible fracture, you may want to avoid forcefully tugging on the joint (as required by some special tests) before viewing an X-ray. Consider X-ray radiography after a brief examination, but prior to fully completing your examination.
- Enjoy learning and using the musculoskeletal examination. It is one of the last remaining parts of medicine that can generally be done with the use of a clinician's eyes, ears, hands, and intellect.

## REFERENCES

1. Haskell WL, Lee IM, Pate RR, et al. Physical activity and public health: updated recommendation for adults from the American College of Sports Medicine and the American Heart Association. *Circulation*. 2007;116:1081-1093.

2. Blair SN, Morris JN. Healthy hearts—and the universal benefits of being physically active: physical activity and health. *Ann Epidemiol.* 2009;19:253-256. Accessed August 28, 2019. https://linkinghub.elsevier.com/retrieve/pii/S1047279709000350

3. Jakicic JM, Kraus WE, Powell KE, et al; for the 2018 Physical Activity Guidelines Advisory Committee. Association between bout duration of physical activity and health: systematic review. *Med Sci Sports Exerc.* 2019;51:1213-1219. Accessed August 28, 2019. http://www.ncbi.nlm.nih.gov/pubmed/31095078

4. Vasankari V, Husu P, Vähä-Ypyä H, et al. Association of objectively measured sedentary behaviour and physical activity with cardiovascular disease risk. *Eur J Prev Cardiol.* 2017;24:1311-1318. Accessed August 28, 2019. http://journals.sagepub.com/doi/10.1177/2047487317711048

5. Chakravarty EF, Hubert HB, Lingala VB, Fries JF. Reduced disability and mortality among aging runners. *Arch Intern Med.* 2008;168:1638. Accessed August 28, 2019. http://www.ncbi.nlm.nih.gov/pubmed/18695077

6. Stovitz SD, Johnson RJ. "Underuse" as a cause for musculoskeletal injuries: is it time that we started reframing our message? *Br J Sports Med.* 2006;40:738-739. Accessed August 28, 2019. http://www.pubmedcentral.nih.gov/articlerender.fcgi?artid=2564383&tool=pmcentrez&rendertype=abstract

7. Murtaugh B, Ihm JM. Eccentric training for the treatment of tendinopathies. *Curr Sports Med Rep.* 2013;12:175-182. Accessed August 28, 2019. https://insights.ovid.com/crossref?an=00149619-201305000-00013

8. Chou R, Fu R, Carrino JA, Deyo RA. Imaging strategies for low-back pain: systematic review and meta-analysis. *Lancet.* 2009;373:463-472. Accessed August 28, 2019. http://www.ncbi.nlm.nih.gov/pubmed/19200918

# 2

# The Diagnosis and Management of Musculoskeletal Trauma

Peter A. Cole and Timothy Carlson

## I. Introduction

A. **Relevance.** The relevancy of orthopaedic trauma as a discipline has increased greatly over the past decade both in North America and around the world. A main driver includes an awareness of the epidemic in fractures across the developing world as mechanized transport has entered their economies. In more developed countries, traumatology and fracture care has established itself as a well-established subspecialty discipline. The Orthopaedic Trauma Association in North America and the AO (Arbeitsgemeinschaft für Osteosynthesefragen) globally are powerful, well-endowed organizations who are committed to education and research in the treatment of fractures.

One of the greatest imperatives is the treatment of **aging baby boomers** who account for massive demands on the healthcare system. "The boomers" hit the 65-year-old age mark in 2011, and it is estimated that by 2040, there will be 35,000,000 more people over the age of 55 years than there are currently and that the number of hip fractures alone will increase from 250,000 to 500,000 on an annual basis. Many places in the world are already feeling the effects of this with a steady increase in hip fracture frequency of 1% to 3% annually.[1]

The upward sloping geriatric musculoskeletal trauma is due to the vulnerability of the skeletal system from the natural process of relative bone mineral loss manifesting in osteoporosis, with a coincident attrition of the muscular system called sarcopenia.[2] Compounding the number of injuries in this group is the increasingly active lifestyle of this aging population and increasing lifespan. To put it in perspective, it is estimated that one-third of all women reaching the age of 90 will sustain at least one hip fracture.[3]

Pushing the subspecialty of fracture care even further in the past 10 years, are new frontiers in fracture treatment inclusive of the chest wall, sternal, and scapula fractures? Furthermore, new approaches to problem injuries and continued enhancement to the tools of treatment in the implant and instrument domains have arisen. Interestingly, two areas in which there was significant enthusiasm in the past decade really have not had widespread acceptance: computer navigation and biologics in trauma.

B. **Definition of musculoskeletal trauma.** Musculoskeletal trauma includes any injury to the **bone, joint (including ligaments), or muscle (including tendons)**. Nearly always, such injuries occur in combination because the energy imparted to breaking a bone or tearing a ligament is also dissipated to impact structures nearby or even distant from the most obvious site. With greater experience, such injury combinations become more predictable for the diagnostician.

C. **Multiple injuries.** Common in high-energy fracture mechanisms that are responsible for pelvic, spine, shoulder girdle, or long bone fractures are frequently associated with injury to other organ systems. It is incumbent upon the trauma team to remain vigilant to the likelihood of injuries to other bones and organ systems. Often, the dramatic and salient injuries, the so-called distracting injuries, during the initial patient evaluation will attract the diagnostic and therapeutic attention, whereas occult and, possibly equally, grave injuries remain initially undetected.

For example, it is estimated that only 7% of patients who die from life-threatening high-energy pelvic fractures actually die from arterial exsanguination related to the pelvic fracture itself,[4] whereas the rest succumb due to injury involving other organ systems, with head injury representing the predominant cause.[5] Forty percent of patients with femur fractures have other associated fractures,[6] and 90% of patients with scapula fractures have other associated injuries. Heightened awareness when evaluating the trauma patient will keep the missed injury rate to a minimum.

D. **Missed injury rate.** The missed injury rate in the context of polytrauma has been reported to be 4% to 18%.[7,8] It is important to drive down this rate with appropriate protocols that underscore the importance of the secondary survey, as well as a rereview of the patient's physical examination each ensuing day after injury. A **secondary survey** is a head-to-toe review by a physician that occurs after the initial **primary survey**, which is defined as the evaluation of the patient's airway, breathing, circulation, disability, and exposure. This is followed by screening imaging of the cervical spine (spiral computed tomography [CT] scan, anteroposterior chest, and pelvic X-ray).

The main reasons cited for missing injuries include multisystem trauma with another more apparent orthopaedic injury, trauma victim being too unstable for a full orthopaedic evaluation, altered sensorium, hastily applied initial splints obscuring injuries, and inadequate radiographs.[9]

E. **Multiple patients.** It is not uncommon, particularly at a Level I trauma center, to require simultaneous evaluation of multiple patients, such as with poly-motor vehicle collisions, explosions, or catastrophic building failures. Doctors who have had some training on the fundamentals of trauma surgery and, in particular, **Advanced Trauma Life Support (ATLS)**, which includes strategies for triaging patients and resources during a mass casualty situation, must be available in order to effectively **"captain the ship."** Typically (but not exclusively), in North America, it is a general surgery trauma surgeon who is running the trauma room. It is beyond the scope of this orthopaedic text to delve into the specifics of ATLS management; however, we focus on some of the fundamentals and cover the triage process of multiple orthopaedic injuries that may present during such circumstances. To further master the details of ATLS management, refer to the *ATLS Manual* (10th edition) published in 2018.

It is imperative to understand what is an orthopaedic emergency and what is orthopaedically urgent. A review of the **"orthopaedic emergencies"** in a subsequent section of this chapter helps to understand how these injuries need to be prioritized for treatment. Furthermore, it is important to understand what measures can be taken to **stage orthopaedic treatment**. Not all broken bones need immediate definitive treatment, and the practitioner must understand how to **titrate the proposed treatment to the physiologic presentation** of the patient. For example, a patient with limited physiologic reserve, due to a great physiologic challenge from hemorrhagic shock and compromised ventilation from a hemothorax, should not spend excessive hours in the operating room getting several fractured bones stabilized. In such a case, it may be prudent to employ damage control orthopaedics (DCO) with the application of external fixation across fractured long bones or joints for immediate and provisional stability. These measures save a lot of time, blood loss, anesthesia, fluid challenge, and avoid the "second hit" during a potentially critical stage in postinjury, physiologic, inflammatory, and evolution. These

DCO measures also give the orthopaedist more time to solicit expertise, get to know the patient and family, plan the details of an operation, and understand the comorbidities and the likelihood of patient compliance. All these factors impact the ultimate treatment that the orthopaedic surgeon chooses to render and will influence positive outcomes.

## II. Evaluating the Trauma Patient from the Orthopaedic Perspective

The patient who presents from an accident scene should receive a much different type of workup than would be called for by a scheduled history and physical examination. The person taking primary responsibility for the orthopaedic injuries must heed the trauma surgeon's call and clearly communicate diagnostic or treatment priorities for the orthopaedic conditions and, ultimately, fit those into the context of overall priorities.

Trauma care is organized in three stages: primary survey, secondary survey, and definitive management, though even definitive management can have stages. The primary survey, trauma series of X-rays, blood draws and insertion of appropriate lines, endotracheal tube, and Foley catheter all are considerations depending on the condition of the patient.

A. **Primary survey.** The primary survey is concerned with the preservation of life. The first steps in managing the trauma patient follow the **ABCs**. These initial steps have generally been performed by the paramedic team, but the surgeon in charge should follow the established ABC sequence.

1. **Airway.** The most common cause of preventable death in accidents is airway obstruction, so the trauma leader must immediately check whether the patient's airway is adequate and patent. Any obstruction (e.g., vomitus, tongue, blood, dentures) must be removed, and the airway secured by a jaw thrust maneuver or tracheal intubation.

2. **Breathing.** After airway obstruction has been ruled out or controlled (i.e., intubation), the patient's ventilation should be assessed. The major life-threatening problems are tension pneumothorax, massive hemothorax, and flail chest. Again, this aspect of the physical examination requires the examiner to inspect, touch, and auscultate the patient because this is typically done before radiographic diagnosis is available. Recognize that very recent data that may redefine priorities and favor maintenance of circulation before breathing, such as during cardiopulmonary resuscitation. The theory is that the existing intravascular supply of oxygenated blood (approximately 5 L) in the bloodstream can be effective only if it circulates to key end organs.[9]

3. **Circulation.** After breathing has been addressed, cardiovascular status must be immediately evaluated and supported. Prompt determination of vital signs is essential. Control of **external bleeding** is accomplished by direct pressure. Temporary tourniquet should not be left beyond the transport period as this has become a more common field measure for stabilization. Simple elevation of the lower extremities helps prevent venous bleeding from the limbs and increases cardiac venous return and preload. The classic Trendelenburg (head down) position is not used for more than a few minutes because it can interfere with respiratory exchange. In the critically injured or hemodynamically labile patient, venous blood samples should be taken for immediate **type and cross matching**.

Until cross-matched blood is available, rapidly infuse 1 to 2 L of isotonic Ringer's lactate or normal saline solution. If **blood loss is minimal**, blood pressure should return to normal and remain that way with only maintenance intravenous (IV) balanced saline solution.

In general, hypotension in a trauma patient should not be assumed to come from a long bone fracture, and another source must be sought. The following gross **estimates of localized blood loss** (units) from adult closed fractures can be useful in establishing baseline blood replacement requirements:

| Pelvis | 1.5–4.5 |
|---|---|
| Hip, femur | 1.0–2.5 |
| Humerus, knee, tibia | 1.0–1.5 |
| Elbow, forearm, ankle | 0.5–1.0 |

4. **Disability.** A comprehensive neurologic evaluation should be performed, including evaluation of the level of consciousness using the Glasgow Coma Score, cranial and peripheral nerve function, and motor and sensory function. This should be repeated in the primary and secondary survey. Deterioration in serial examinations should prompt neurology or neurosurgical evaluation.

5. **Exposure.** The patient should be fully undressed to perform a thorough evaluation. They should subsequently be covered in warm blankets, and body temperature should be maintained with warm room temperature, warming blankets or pads, and by infusing warmed IV fluids.

B. **Trauma imaging.** Now that the primary survey has been performed and the most critical steps have been taken, even before a thorough history and physical examination, this trauma imaging series should be reviewed; the examiner is ruling in or out the next most critical clues to saving life and limb. The trauma series classically consisted of three X-rays: **lateral cervical spine,** an **anteroposterior chest,** and an **anteroposterior pelvic** view. However, spine and trauma surgeons have found greater utility in a **diagnostic CT scan of the cervical spine** because it affords better sensitivity and specificity than radiographs alone and eliminates the need for repeat imaging as often is necessary in the multitrauma patient.[10] Any patient who is involved in high-energy trauma, who has head injuries, is under chemical substance influence, or is otherwise deemed unable to provide reliable responses during the primary survey should have this imaging because physical examination can be unreliable.

In circumstances when the cervical spine radiograph is performed instead of the CT scan, such as in alert patients with isolated injury, the images must show the inferior endplate of cervical vertebrae 7 (C7), or it should be deemed inadequate and repeated. Both odontoid and C7–T1 pathology are frequently missed injuries even after the secondary survey. **If a spine fracture is detected**, then a complete spinal series including anteroposterior, lateral and odontoid cervical views, and thoracic plus lumbar spine view is mandatory in view of the increased possibility of segmental spinal injury. CT may be required to rule out upper cervical fractures. The documented incidence of multiple level spine fractures is 7% to 12%. A full spine series should be obtained in the unconscious trauma victim.

Care must be taken not to be misled by overlying backboards, over- and under-penetrated films, and equipment, clips, and buckles that are frequently left on the X-ray field. Examples abound of subtle femoral neck fractures that were obscured on the X-ray by a belt buckle, a pneumothorax in the upper lobe that was cut out of view because of positioning, or a critical sacral fracture masked by the opacity of a backboard. When these factors are present, radiographs should be repeated.

C. **History and physical examination.** The history should include a careful account of the accident, a description of the mechanism of injury, and a statement of the degree of violence involved. Concomitant medical disease, drug abuse, and alcoholism should be considered as contributing factors. The transporting paramedic team or member of the accompanying family should be interviewed for these details if the patient cannot reliably give an appropriate history. A useful mnemonic to guide the initial history is the word **AMPLE:**

| A: | **Allergies** |
|---|---|
| | The physician working up an orthopaedic patient should be particularly aware that open fractures should be treated with antibiotics to cover the spectrum of bacteria that are at risk for certain types of wounds (see the section on open fractures). Furthermore, every patient having an orthopaedic operation should receive perioperative antibiotics, making the question of allergies quite germane. A penicillin allergy is the most common. |
| M: | **Medications** |
| | Medications can influence surgical decision-making. They will also tip off the practitioner to important comorbidities and perhaps imply the need for a general medicine consultation prior to surgery. Patients on anticoagulants should have bleeding and clotting parameters checked because it may be prudent to stop such medicines or reverse a coagulopathy prior to surgery. |
| P: | **Past** illness |
| | Diabetes can influence outcomes of orthopaedic surgery, and heart disease can increase surgical risk. Steroids and the use of tobacco products increase orthopaedic surgical complications as well as outcomes as measured by healing time and healing rates. These risks should be discussed with patients and family members for proper prognostication. |
| L: | **Last** meal |
| | This is important when considering whether the patient needs to go to the operating room urgently, as the risk of aspiration of food or vomitus is higher postprandial. Most anesthesiologists opt to hold on the administration of anesthesia within 6 to 8 hours of food intake. This concern should not, however, override the emergent nature of certain life- or limb-threatening conditions, which are discussed below. |
| E: | **Events** of injury |
| | Injury circumstances such as height of fall, direction of impact, the presence or absence of restraints (seat belt/airbags), extrication time from vehicle, hours in the field, outside temperature, being trapped under heavy objects, smoke inhalation, and many other possibilities are warning flags to the experienced practitioner, which clue in certain medical or orthopaedic conditions and injury patterns. |

D. **Secondary survey.** The **secondary survey** is a complete **physical examination** from head to toe. By this juncture, the potentially life-threatening pathology of the ABCs has been addressed, and necessary resuscitation is underway. The patient should be completely undressed for the secondary survey for a most thorough examination.
  1. **Neurologic mental status.** The **level of consciousness** of the patient should first be noted. A brief **"disability examination"** in an awake patient is a rapid, organized neurologic examination, which documents mental orientation, verbal response to questioning, and response to stimuli. Furthermore, each extremity should be examined for motor and sensory function as well; accurate documentation is crucial because neurologic examinations can reveal progressive deficits. It is imperative that all four

extremities be examined and documented. It is good to develop a pattern of examination and stick with that pattern each time for consistency.

In an unconscious patient, a **Glasgow Coma Score** is rapidly conducted on the basis of pupil response to light, motor activity, and withdrawal from painful stimuli (Table 2-1). This information is initially obtained by the medics who perform the initial in-the-field evaluation. It is frustrating to the orthopaedic surgeon or neurosurgeon to be asked to evaluate a patient who has been sedated and chemically paralyzed (for intubation/airway control) in the trauma room, particularly when the initial neurologic examination was not properly documented. In general, the use of **maximal monitoring and minimal medication** is a useful trauma room principle.

2. **Head and neck.** Carefully palpate **skull and facial bones** and look for **lacerations** hidden in the hair. **Cranial trauma should raise an immediate suspicion for cervical spine injury**, given the sudden and violent force it takes to injure the face and cranium. Radiographs of facial bones are difficult to interpret, unless previous clinical examination suggests the presence of trauma. The **association between cervical spine and head injuries** must be emphasized. In a guided manner with cervical immobility, remove or loosen the C-collar to palpate the posterior cervical spine looking for tenderness or spasm. In a conscious patient, any neck pain or spasm is a cervical spine injury until proven otherwise. In an unconscious patient, the neck must be protected with a hard C-collar until bony injury

| TABLE 2-1 | Glasgow Coma Scale | |
|---|---|---|
| **Eye opening (E)** | | |
| Spontaneous | | 4 |
| To speech | | 3 |
| To pain | | 2 |
| None | | 1 |
| **Verbal response (V)** | | |
| Oriented | | 5 |
| Confused conversation | | 4 |
| Inappropriate words | | 3 |
| Incomprehensible sounds | | 2 |
| None | | 1 |
| **Motor response (M)** | | |
| Obeys command | | 6 |
| Localizes | | 5 |
| Withdraws from pain | | 4 |
| Abnormal flexion | | 3 |
| Extensor response | | 2 |
| None | | 1 |

(E + M + V) = Glasgow Coma Score between 3 and 15.

is ruled out by cervical imaging and physical examination. A benign physical examination by itself is unreliable if there are distracting injuries or if the patient is intoxicated. If a cervical spine injury is diagnosed, appropriate spine consultation should be obtained immediately, and the extremity neurologic examination should be reported and documented.

3. **Thorax and abdomen.** Although the thorax and abdomen are largely the domain of the general surgeon, the orthopaedic surgeon is taking an increasingly relevant role in the management of rib fractures, and specifically flail chest injuries. The examiner must inspect, palpate, and auscultate the abdomen and thorax to determine possible underlying injury. In high-energy trauma, rib fractures are common, and sternal fractures are not rare. Flail chest is an entity in which multiple adjacent ribs are fractured in two or more places. Accepted definitions of flail chest include:

   a. Three or more consecutive ribs fractured in two places.
   b. Three or more rib fractures with an associated sternal fracture and/or opposite rib fractures.[11]

   Examination should include sternal compression and compression of the thorax in the medial–lateral directions between the examiners' hand. **Crepitance or acute tenderness** should tip off the examiner to fractures that should be sought on a chest X-ray or CT scan of the chest.

   **Hemothorax** and **pneumothorax** often cause preventable death. Furthermore, this assessment helps the orthopaedist place musculoskeletal injuries in the broader context of the patient. Occasionally, subcutaneous crepitance, which feels like popcorn or a sponge in the soft tissues, represents escape of air from the lungs because of a pneumothorax in the context of displaced rib fractures. This phenomenon can involve the chest wall or neck where air is driven into the tissue planes.

4. **Abdominal injury** is also a common cause of preventable death. The imprint of clothes or a contusion of the abdominal wall from the seat belt suggests an intraabdominal injury. Airbags have altered patterns of injury in frontal collision.[12] Appropriate diagnostic studies should follow the suspicion of injury, and in many centers, the **spiral "whole-body" CT scan of the chest, abdomen, and pelvis** has supplanted selective CT scans, ultrasounds, and peritoneal lavage.

5. **Pelvis.** Low back pain, pubic tenderness, or pain with compression of the iliac crests can indicate a pelvic ring injury. Sequential anterior-to-posterior compression over the iliac wings can help discriminate gross pelvic motion. Abdominal injuries have been associated with severe pelvic fractures at a rate of 30% and may cause severe internal bleeding.[13] As stated earlier, a patient can lose four units of blood after a displaced pelvic fracture, even more if associated with major venous or arterial tears.

   A **rectal examination** must be done in all patients with a spine or pelvic injury, both to **check for bleeding and loss of sphincter tone**, indicative of neurologic injury. Furthermore, a **high-riding prostate** also indicates major urologic disruption common to high-energy pelvic fractures in men. An inspection of the **urethral meatus for hemorrhage** should also be performed, and such a finding is further an indication of a genitourinary system disruption. Bloody urine or the **inability to void** raises the suspicion of a urethral injury, so a retrograde urethrogram should be considered before a catheter is inserted.[14] In male patients, blood at the penile meatus or a "high-riding" prostate on rectal examination is a clear indication for obtaining a retrograde urethrogram before bladder catheterization. If the catheter does not pass easily, it should not be forced, and the urologist should be consulted. If a bladder injury is suspected, then it is essential to insert an indwelling catheter unless the patient is voiding clear urine.

A **bimanual pelvic examination** is appropriate in female patients to rule out open fractures that can penetrate the vaginal vault, if displaced rami fractures are noted on a scout pelvic X-ray. **Perineal inspection** for integument lacerations should be conducted and, in the setting of displaced pelvic fractures, should be assumed to represent an open pelvic fracture.

6. **Back and spine.** Carefully log roll the patient and **palpate the entire spine** to detect tenderness or defects of the interspinous ligaments. It is very important that a log roll be conducted properly with three assistants controlling simultaneous rotation of the entire body. A fourth assistant should be controlling the cervical spine (while in a hard collar) with gentle traction. An increase in the interspinous distance accompanied by local swelling and/or tenderness may signify injury. Occasionally, ecchymosis or kyphosis can be recognized, and their presence or absence should be documented.

7. **Upper and lower extremities examination.** When **gross deformity and crepitation** are present, further examination of the fracture site is not necessary. Otherwise, all four limbs should be palpated thoroughly, and each joint placed through a passive range of motion. Look specifically for point tenderness. Any obvious **fractures or deformities are splinted**, and any **open wounds covered** with sterile saline-moistened dressings. Dressings over open wounds, particularly over fractures, should not be taken down multiple times by multiple examiners. Such repeated exposures will only increase the rate of infection with each exposure to the contaminated environment.[15] A more detailed description of fracture wound management is given later in this chapter. Every diagnosed fracture should have properly centered X-rays of the joint above and below. Circulation of the limb distal to any fracture should be carefully evaluated and documented. A description and presence of all wounds after applying a sterile dressing should be recorded.

## III. Orthopaedic Emergencies and Urgencies

Surgical stabilization of fractures is generally not classified as emergent or urgent and typically can be done on a semielective basis. For example, an **isolated, closed fracture that is not threatening local blood supply may wait days to weeks**. There are many considerations, however, which go into the optimal timing of surgery, and **immediate consultation with an orthopaedist clarifies the issue of timing of surgery**.

All the **emergent entities, and most of the urgent injuries, ultimately have a common denominator: blood supply**. The lack of circulation affects adequacy of tissue oxygenation, and consequently, limb or life is threatened. This may occur on a macroscopic level, such as with a hemorrhaging pelvis in which a person's life is threatened, or on a microscopic basis, such as when end-organ perfusion is cut off, beginning with occlusion of the venules in a muscle bed resulting from increased interstitial pressure exceeding IV pressure during the condition of compartment syndrome. Threatened blood supply to local tissues can be a more subtle phenomenon that requires further understanding of the vasculature to certain bones. For example, a relatively benign appearing X-ray of a femoral neck fracture to the inexperienced eye may not gain much attention, but the experienced clinician knows that even a nondisplaced femoral neck fracture can threaten the hip joint forever through a process called **avascular necrosis (AVN)**. Certain other orthopaedic injuries may not accurately be classified as emergent because life or limb is not immediately at risk, but they still warrant heightened attention. Such injuries may be classified as urgent because they need prompt action by an orthopaedist and surgical timing in the range of 6 to 24 hours. In the next two sections on emergent and urgent orthopaedic injuries, the discussion addresses these in descending order from most to least acute.

A. **Orthopaedic emergencies**

 1. **Hemodynamically unstable patient with a pelvic fracture.** This is the one injury in which circulation can be compromised to an extent that a life is immediately at risk and in which an orthopaedic intervention can be life-saving. The pelvic ring can be disrupted in high-energy accidents (or low-energy falls in osteoporotic patients) and nearly always is disrupted in at **least two points around the ring**. The saying "it is impossible to break a ring at a single point" nearly always applies to the pelvis. Therefore, the examiner should look for a lesion posteriorly in the sacrum or the sacroiliac joint and anteriorly in the pelvic rami or the pubic symphysis.

    **When a pelvic fracture is recognized on the anteroposterior X-ray view obtained with the initial trauma series, two more radiographs should be obtained: a pelvic inlet view and pelvic outlet view.** These are orthogonal views of the pelvis, which help to critically evaluate all the pelvic bony landmarks as well as displacement of fractures. If there is significant displacement (more than 5 mm) at any one pelvic fracture line, a **pelvic CT scan** should be obtained. Many orthopaedists will prefer a CT scan with even lesser fracture displacements to more critically evaluate the injury or preoperatively plan. **If a fracture line enters the acetabulum, then Judet X-ray views should be obtained.** These are 45° angled X-ray views from the right and left sides of the patient centered on the pelvis, once again giving the examiner orthogonal views to critically assess the bony landmarks of each acetabulum. Note that **it is wasteful to obtain "five views of the pelvis" for every pelvic fracture** as the Judet views are not needed unless the acetabulum is involved. Likewise, inlet and outlet X-rays are not needed unless the pelvic ring is disrupted.

    The pelvis is like a cylinder or sphere of bone that contains many critical soft-tissue structures and organs such as the bladder, the iliac vessels, prostate or vaginal vault, and the rectum. All these organs are at risk, but the worrisome life-threatening hemorrhage is what must be diagnosed promptly and addressed. Bleeding typically continues until tamponade can occur and clotting factors take control. **A sheet or commercial binder around the pelvis of a patient, who is hemodynamically unstable until the anteroposterior radiograph of the pelvis rules in or out a displaced pelvic fracture, is an important measure.** The sheet must be clamped very snug at the level of the greater trochanters in order to close down the volume of the broken and separated sphere, thus leading to earlier tamponade of bleeding vessels.[16] There is nothing to lose because if the patient does not have such an injury, the binder is simply removed. Some pelvic slings now have pressure calibration to ensure adequate yet safe pressure application through the binder. There is essentially no role for the trauma room application of an external fixator because this maneuver has been obviated by the pelvic sling concept.

 2. **Extremity arterial injury.** Probably, the next most emergent condition that an orthopaedist faces is the extremity at risk for limb loss. This can occur due to a torn or lacerated artery or compartment syndrome. Arterial injury can be caused by blunt or penetrating trauma. There are **four "hard signs" of arterial injury that warrant immediate vascular exploration**, and time should not be wasted ordering and performing a diagnostic arteriogram. The rationale is that a vascular surgeon knows the proximity of the injury based on the wound or the X-ray that demonstrates the pathology. There is no sense in using precious minutes finding out what is already known when irreversible ischemic damage to nerve and muscle tissue occurs after 4 hours of warm ischemia time. A warm ischemia in excess of 6 hours is the generally accepted time interval within which arterial continuity must be restored in order to avoid loss of limb.

**The Four "Hard Signs" of Arterial Injury.** The best screening examination for an arterial injury should be quick, noninvasive, portable, and cost-effective, as well as reliable. Determination of the arterial pressure index (API) requires the use of a Doppler machine and a blood pressure cuff. It has been investigated as a screening tool for clinically significant arterial compromise.[17] The API has also been referred to in the literature as the ABI (ankle–brachial index) or AAI (ankle–arm index), and the terms are interchangeable. To conduct an API examination, a blood pressure cuff is placed just above the ankle or wrist in the injured limb so that a systolic pressure can be determined with a Doppler probe at the respective posterior tibial artery or radial artery. The dorsalis pedis or ulnar arteries may logically be used as well, as long as the blood pressure cuff is placed distal to the injury. The same measurement is determined on an uninjured upper or lower extremity limb (Fig. 2-1). **The API is simply the calculation of the systolic pressure of the injured limb divided by the systolic pressure of the uninjured limb:**

$$\text{API} = \frac{\text{Doppler Systolic Arterial Pressure in Injured Limb}}{\text{Doppler Systolic Arterial Pressure in Uninjured Extremity}}$$

As pulses have been reported to be palpable distal to major arterial lesions, including complete arterial disruption,[18] and perception of a pulse is subjective and impossible to quantify, physical examination alone or the detection of a palpable pulse is not appropriate for definitive diagnosis. The reason that pulses can be palpated distal to some arterial lesions is because of collateral circulation and retrograde pulsations.

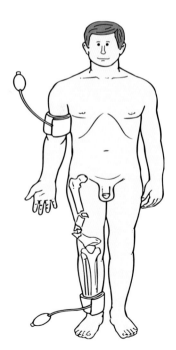

**Figure 2-1.** Placement of the pressure cuff and Doppler probe. One systolic pressure measurement is taken in an uninjured limb, and the other systolic pressure measurement is taken on the injured limb distal to the injury.

As it is impossible to spell out every clinical scenario that may be associated with an arterial injury, it should be reiterated that every case bears individual judgment, and given the absent morbidity of the API examination, a thorough approach to testing and documentation is the most prudent course. The clinician should approach the patient who has a high-risk vascular injury with a clear diagnostic algorithm (Fig. 2-2). Besides the patient with one of the four hard signs of vascular arterial injury who warrants immediate surgical exploration, a patient's API should dictate the next step. If the API is greater than 0.9, the patient may be followed clinically without any further workup. **If the API is less than 0.9, they should proceed to the next diagnostic step of either an arteriogram, a CT angiogram, or duplex ultrasound,** the results of which will dictate the final plan of action.

There are times when the API is unreliable, and this is when the major vessels to the extremity are calcified. This condition can cause spuriously high readings, or perhaps "normal" despite the presence of an arterial injury. The other circumstance, which is more common, is decreased API measurements because of poor fracture alignment, which can cause mechanical compression of the fracture. Another condition is compartment syndrome, in which elevated interstitial pressure can compress major vessels and cause spuriously low measurements.

a. **Pulsatile hemorrhage**
b. **Expanding hematoma**
c. **Audible bruit**
d. **Pulseless limb**

The only time an arteriogram would be warranted in such an acute circumstance is when there is multilevel injury (multiple fractures or shotgun wound) in which the vascular surgeon cannot be sure at what level the arterial damage has occurred.

The more difficult diagnostic problem occurs in the majority of patients who present with more subtle clues to vascular injury. Such "soft

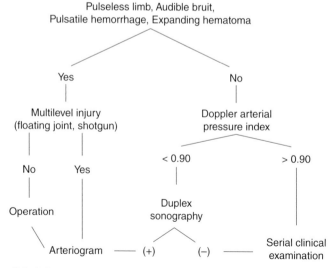

**Figure 2-2.** A diagnostic algorithm for a patient with a possible extremity arterial injury.

signs" might include a history of severe hemorrhage at the accident scene, subjectively decreased pulses, a deficit of an anatomically related nerve, or a nonpulsatile hematoma. Other soft signs include the orthopaedic **injury patterns that have been associated with a high incidence of arterial damage:**

a. **Knee dislocations**
b. **Highly displaced tibia plateau fractures**
c. **Medial tibia plateau fractures**
d. **Ipsilateral fractures on either side of a joint (floating joint)**
e. **Gunshot or knife wounds in proximity to neurovascular structures**
f. **The mangled extremity**

3. **Compartment syndrome.** Acute compartment syndrome is a condition in which there is increased pressure within a closed soft-tissue space, with the capacity to cause ischemic necrosis to the tissues. Therefore, it should be recognized that the condition can occur in any muscular compartment of the body, although it is most commonly encountered in the leg. It is perhaps the most common orthopaedic emergency and often difficult to diagnose. In the awake and alert patient, symptoms include the following:

a. **Pain out of proportion to the injury** (despite adequate narcotic analgesia)
b. **Pain with passive stretch** of the muscles within the compartment
c. **Paresthesias**

Furthermore, these symptoms should occur in the setting of swollen tissues. A diminished or absent pulse is such a late and subjective sign that its absence should never be relied upon to exclude the diagnosis of compartment syndrome. These clinical symptoms obviously cannot be used in the obtunded patient and should not even be relied upon in a patient with altered sensorium due to intoxication, for example. The clinician should have great suspicion for compartment syndrome in the setting of high-energy trauma or comminuted and displaced fractures, and if he/she encounters such a patient with very swollen tissues (often characterized as "tense"), a pressure measurement should be taken of the suspected compartments. It is important to note that compartment syndrome is well described in low-energy mechanisms and does not have to be associated with a fracture. Chart **documentation should be rigorous and periodic** when tracking the possibility of compartment syndrome; excellent patient examination should occur at intervals no more than 3 hours apart until compartment syndrome can be ruled out.

Most emergency and operating rooms have readily available pressure measuring devices such as the Stryker Quick Stick, which can be used to measure suspected compartments. An indwelling catheter rigged with a mercury manometer[19] or an arterial line attached to a pressure transducer can also be used. **If there is ever any doubt as to whether a patient has compartment syndrome, such measurements must be taken to confirm or rule out the diagnosis. Intracompartmental pressures exceeding the diastolic pressure by less than 30 mm Hg ($\delta P < 30$ mm Hg) warrant emergent fasciotomies.**[20] Fasciotomy incisions should extend to nearly the length of the compartment to ensure complete decompression and adequate visualization and assessment of tissues. A text should be reviewed prior to the operation to review recommended incisions that address each and every compartment of the suspected part of the extremity (thigh, leg, foot, hand, antebrachium, brachium, buttock, and more).

4. **Mangled extremity and traumatic amputations.** Another clinical entity that should warrant great concern for limb viability is the so-called mangled extremity. The mangled extremity is not clearly defined, but it represents the end of an injury spectrum that involves a magnitude of trauma that destroys soft tissue to the extent that limb survival is in question.

The principles of open fracture management, as discussed in the next section, should be heeded, and the algorithm for a vascular workup should be followed expeditiously (see III.A). Most importantly, several services should come to bear in assessment, workup, and coordination of care, including trauma surgery, orthopaedic surgery, plastic surgery, and, if necessary, vascular surgery. Communication around treatment considerations and timing should be open, clear, and decisive. Patients and loved ones should be included in the communication in order to understand the gravity of the injury and that amputation is a real and sometimes optimal solution.[21]

An accurate neurovascular examination should be performed and documented. **If an adult patient has a severed tibial nerve, amputation should be considered, given the expected associated functional deficit**, although absent tibial nerve sensation at presentation does not necessarily mean that neurodiscontinuity has occurred. Plantar sensation is, therefore, an unreliable measure of long-term tibial nerve dysfunction and should not be used as a criterion for early amputation.[22] A patient with a mangled extremity should be managed at a Level I trauma center where the appropriate expertise and experience are available.

There are several prognostic factors that influence outcome and, therefore, should be weighed in the consideration for limb salvage versus amputation. A number of scoring systems have been developed to account for these variables; however, none has proved reliable in predicting limb viability.

Early management includes skeletal stabilization versus amputation, wide and aggressive debridement of all devitalized tissue, abundant irrigation, reestablishing vascular continuity, and reoperations every couple of days for wound management until definitive coverage can be executed by a microvascular team if necessary. An antibiotic bead pouch or a vacuum-assisted closure system for open wounds is helpful in the interim between cases.

For the **complete traumatic amputation of a finger or entire extremity, a replantation should be considered when the mechanism does not involve crushing or traction.** The proximal stump is first dressed with Ringer's lactate-soaked dressing, and pressure is applied. A tourniquet is to be avoided. The **amputated part should be wrapped in a Ringer's lactate moistened sterile sponge and placed in a plastic bag. It should be cooled by placing it in a container with ice**, which delays autolysis and thus allows time for transport to a center with a replantation team. The **part must not be frozen or placed in direct contact or encased within ice**. It is best to simply lay the part on top of the ice with a layer of protective material between them. If the travel distance by car is less than 2 hours, then this form of transport can be used. If not, arrangements should be made for air evacuation. **Make no promises to the patient** regarding whether replantation can be attempted or what the outcome will be. **Absolute indications for attempts at replantation include multiple-digit amputations, thumb amputations, amputations at or proximal to the wrist, and pediatric amputations. Border digits are a relative indication. Prognosis is improved when an extremity has been amputated in a sharp cutting mechanism as opposed to a crushing or traction mechanism**.

5. **Femoral neck fracture in the nonelderly.** The age of the patient should be defined in physiologic terms with the idea that "saving" the femoral head is more prudent than a hip replacement. Because of the experience in the field of arthroplasty, it is now reasonable to begin considering joint replacement in individuals as young as 55 years. A femoral neck fracture in a young patient is considered an emergency because the blood supply to the femoral head is threatened. **The lateral epiphyseal arterial branch off the medial femoral circumflex artery is the dominant blood supply to the femoral head** (the artery of the ligamentum teres supplies

10%). There is a risk of **AVN** of the femoral head after a femoral neck fracture, which can lead to femoral head collapse, a catastrophic complication in a young active patient in whom a hip replacement or a hip fusion is a suboptimal salvage option.

The **risk of AVN exists in nondisplaced fractures**; therefore, all such femoral neck fractures in the younger patient are regarded as emergent. For the displaced variety, an open reduction is indicated to establish anatomic alignment followed by internal fixation. In the nondisplaced variety, percutaneous fixation may be appropriate, but the hip capsule should still be surgically decompressed.

The **possible mechanisms for arterial insufficiency include**[23] the following:

Intracapsular tamponade from bleeding into a closed space

Kinking of vessels from tenting bone fragments

Arterial disruption

When considering these mechanisms, one can understand that urgent decompression and stable realignment can be helpful in restoring blood flow. Although timing of surgery remains controversial and some studies have demonstrated a reduced rate of AVN with urgent reduction (within 8 hours), others have reported similar results even with reduction after 24 hours.[24] Until the results of randomized trials or very large cohort studies are available, urgent surgical intervention is prudent.[25]

6. **Hip dislocation.** For the same reason as for the femoral neck fracture, a dislocated hip is an emergent condition because prognosis and the rate of AVN are directly related to the amount of time the hip remains dislocated.[26] One or two attempts at a closed reduction in the emergency department is indicated, but, if unsuccessful, a trip to the operating room for anesthesia and muscular relaxation is appropriate.

7. **Threatened soft tissues.** Anytime a fracture or dislocated bone is tenting the skin, and the injury cannot be reduced, the patient should go to the operating room emergently so that a closed reduction with pharmacologic paralysis can be attempted. If that fails, an open reduction should be performed. This scenario commonly occurs with ankle and subtalar fractures or dislocations, wrist fractures, and even fractures and dislocations around the knee. **Leaving any joint dislocated does not make sense when considering the tissues at risk** (even if it is not compromising skin), venous obstruction, and pain.

B. **Orthopaedic urgencies**

1. **Open fractures**

a. **Emergency department management.** Early and careful treatment of wounds is necessary to decrease the chance of infection. Simple limb realignment should be performed for provisional splintage. **Wounds, large or small, should immediately be covered with a sterile dressing, and the temptation for multiple examiners to reexpose the wound must be avoided to decrease the likelihood of infection. Any laceration of the integument in the vicinity of a fracture should be assumed to represent an open fracture and, therefore, should be formally explored in the operating room. Cover the wound with a simple saline-moistened dressing. Do not probe or blindly use surgical hemostats in the wound.** Externalized material is contaminated and will contaminate deeper recesses if replacement into the wound is attempted outside the operating environment.

**Open fractures** are generally **classified** using the Gustilo system (Table 2-2). With increasing severity, the complications of deep infection, nonunion, and amputation increase. **A Type IIIB open fracture requires a muscle flap for wound closure. A Type IIIC fracture is**

| TABLE 2-2 | Gustilo and Anderson Classification of Open Fractures |
|---|---|
| Type I | Skin opening of 1 cm or less, quite clean; most likely inside out; minimal muscle contusion; simple transverse or short oblique fractures |
| Type II | Laceration >1 cm; extensive soft-tissue damage; minimal-to-moderate crushing component; simple transverse or short oblique fractures with minimal comminution |
| Type IIIA | Extensive soft-tissue laceration associated with muscle, skin, and/or neurovascular injury but with adequate coverage of bone; typically segmental or comminuted fractures |
| Type IIIB | Extensive soft-tissue injury with periosteal stripping and bone exposure; usually associated with severe contamination |
| Type IIIC | High-energy features of other Type IIIs but with arterial injury requiring repair |

From Gustilo RB, Mendoza RM, Williams DM. Problems in management of type III open fractures. A new classification of type III open fractures. *J Trauma*. 1984;24:742, with permission.

**one that requires a vascular repair for limb viability.** The Gustilo classification is useful, but because of its subjective criteria, such as the use of the terms "high energy," "comminution," and "contamination," there is poor intraobserver reliability.[27] That being stated, it has been cited as the most commonly referenced article and classification in the field of orthopaedic trauma.

b. **Operating room management. All large wounds, open fractures, nerve disruptions, and most tendon lacerations should be debrided and repaired in the operating room. Debridement** means removal of all foreign matter and devitalized tissue in or about a lesion. Irrigation with large quantities of saline does not replace the need for proper surgical debridement technique. Saline lavage is a useful adjunct to good debridement. There has been recent debate about the benefits of pulsatile lavage versus simple irrigation and also about the utility of emulsifying soaps and antibiotic-impregnated saline. Although high-pressure pulsatile lavage has been demonstrated to impair bone healing and force deeper penetration of bacteria into tissues, there is no clear advantage of either of the other methods.[28] Typically, we irrigate open fractures with 9 L of normal saline using low-pressure settings, yet the subject remains under investigation.[29,30]

The wound should be **debrided from the outside in**. The skin edges are sharply trimmed to viable margins. The debridement is then continued into the depth of the wound until the entire damaged area has been identified and resected. Muscle viability is evaluated on the basis of the criteria described by Artz et al.[31]: capacity to bleed, color, contractility, and consistency. These are helpful descriptors in determining whether or not to resect muscle.

With an open fracture, **all devitalized bone without soft-tissue attachments should be removed**. The exception is pieces with articular cartilage that should be saved to attempt to reconstruct a joint surface. Great care must be taken not to devitalize the bone further with surgical exposure. Initial internal fixation of open fractures is preferable if rigid stabilization is provided without significantly jeopardizing the blood supply.[32] Again, the soft-tissue coverage should not create enough tension to cause any devitalization from a lack of blood supply. **Use**

**monofilament sutures for skin closure**, not braided wire or multifilament synthetic, cotton, or silk sutures. A drain should be considered. Repeat "second-look" operations are mandatory when the suspicion for evolving myonecrosis is present. **The burden of proof rests with the surgeon electing to close the wound.** Cover all exposed tendons, nerves, and bone, but not at the expense of compromising blood supply to injured skin and subcutaneous tissues. Acute consultation with an orthopaedic or plastic surgeon skilled in myoplasty is indicated if adequate coverage over implants and bone cannot be accomplished. During the interval between debridement and definitive soft-tissue coverage, it is wise to cover the wound with an antibiotic bead pouch or a vacuum-assisted wound closure technique.[33,34] This aids in maintaining an aseptic environment during the waiting interval.[32]

c. **Antibiotic management.** It should be emphasized that **the primary management of an open fracture is surgical and that antibiotics play a strictly adjunctive role.** Furthermore, all patients with an open wound should be up to date with tetanus immunization or be treated with tetanus toxoid. Although there are numerous recommended tetanus prophylaxis schedules, the authors generally follow the recommendations of the American College of Surgeons (ACS). Table 2-3 lists the current guidelines. With any open fracture or major wound, start parenteral **bactericidal antibiotics** immediately in the emergency department.[35]

**Cephalosporins are the drug of choice for prophylaxis of Gustilo Type I and II injuries.** Patients who are allergic to penicillin (excluding history of anaphylaxis) usually may receive cephalosporins. A small test dose is recommended before giving the entire dose. If cephalosporins cannot be given safely, then vancomycin or clindamycin should be administered. To obtain an adequate concentration of antibiotics in the fracture hematoma, begin the antibiotic therapy as soon as an open fracture is diagnosed. To avoid many of the side effects of antibiotics, such as superinfections, limit the duration of prophylactic antibiotic to **48 hours postoperative.** The mindset should be that the primary treatment is surgical and that antibiotics are simply adjuvant treatment.

**Vancomycin** 1 g IV daily[36] should only be a fallback option because the isolates of resistant strains of bacteria have increased in number recently, and this drug is the mainstay of treatment for methicillin-resistant *Staphylococcus aureus*.

| TABLE 2-3 | Prophylactic Treatment of Tetanus | | | |
|---|---|---|---|---|
| Previous Doses of Tetanus Toxoid[a] | Non–Tetanus-Prone Wounds | | Tetanus-Prone Wounds | |
| | Tt[b] | TIG | Tt[b] | TIG |
| <3 doses or unknown | Yes | No | Yes | Yes |
| ≥3 doses | Only if last dose ≥10 y ago | No | Only if last dose ≥5 y ago | No |

[a] Tetanus toxoid may have been administered as DT, DTaP, Td, or Tdap.
[b] DPT or DT for children less than 7 years of age.
TIG, tetanus immune globulin; Tt, tetanus toxoid–containing vaccine.
Adapted from Liang JL, Tiwari T, Moro P, et al. Prevention of Pertussis, Tetanus, and Diphtheria with Vaccines in the United States: Recommendations of the Advisory Committee on Immunizations Practices (ACIP). MMWR *Recomm Rep* 2018; 67:1.

For Type III open wounds with marked contamination or large exposure, gram-negative coverage should be added to the antibiotic spectrum. **Aminoglycosides** have been used as an appropriate agent during this short-term period of treatment for gram-negative organisms, although broader coverage with combination drugs (i.e., piperacillin and tazobactam) has become mainstays in many hospitals. If there is a risk of contamination of **soil, or sewage, an agent that acts against clostridium species is important to add.** Although penicillin may be added to the regimen for this purpose, the antibiotic Zosyn is a good choice offering broad coverage and eliminates the need for administration of three different medications for infection.

d. **Gunshot wounds.** If possible, **identify** the caliber and type of **weapon**. This information helps determine whether the wound was caused by a high- or low-velocity weapon. The majority of civilian injuries are **low velocity and do not seem to be associated with higher infection rates, even when associated with a fracture**.[37] Decision-making regarding the fracture proceeds as with a closed fracture. If the bullet **enters a joint**, it is important to ensure there are no retained fragments and joint lavage should be considered.

The protocol for management of a low-velocity gunshot is as follows:

**High-velocity weapons** have a muzzle velocity greater than 610 m/second or an impact velocity of 2,000 to 2,500 ft/second. These weapons cause severe cavitation within the wound, which make debridement necessary. Big-game rifles, such as a 0.30 to 0.030 or a 0.30 to 0.06, can approach this high-velocity impact energy, and wounds from these must be treated accordingly with irrigation and debridement, possibly on a serial basis depending on the cavitation injury. Gunshot wounds of high-impact energy cause marked comminution of the fracture and leave a gaping exit. These are managed as an open fracture and certainly require appropriate vascular screening, as previously discussed.

i. **Tetanus prophylaxis**
ii. **One day of antibiotics** (first-generation cephalosporin)
iii. **Local cleansing**
iv. **Debridement of devitalized skin**
v. **Superficial irrigation**
vi. **Sterile dressing**

2. **Open joints.** Open joint injuries are also at risk for septic complications. **The surgeon should assume that lacerations over a joint extend into the joint until the contrary is proven in the operating room.** Air in the joint noted on radiographs is a sign that a laceration extends into the joint. It is a reasonable idea to inject the joint with saline or a methylene blue–enhanced saline to check for communication with the suspected laceration, which is confirmed by leakage of the injected fluid from the joint. A healthy volume of fluid under pressure must be used to enhance sensitivity of this test. Recent studies have demonstrated that 60 to 75 mL will identify only 46% to 50% of arthrotomies. To achieve 95% sensitivity, a minimum of 155 mL must be injected. Because most patients have some discomfort after injection of 60 mL, a negative test should be interpreted with caution.[38] An operative joint lavage, either open or arthroscopic technique, should be performed if an open joint is suspected. Certainly, if there are foreign bodies in the joint, such as missile fragments from gunshot wounds, these must be evacuated. A course of 48 hours of gram-positive and gram-negative coverage with parenteral antibiotics (as with a Gustilo Type IIIA fracture) is a reasonable and prudent adjunct to surgery.

3. **Talus fractures.** Although underpowered and inconclusive, recent studies seem to suggest that time to operative fixation does not matter, whereas talar neck comminution and open fractures do correlate with worse outcomes and a higher rate of AVN.[39,40] As the talus is at risk for AVN, collapse, and subsequent arthrosis, and as it is a weight-bearing joint, most orthopaedic traumatologists prefer to operate on this fracture urgently. Certainly, the highly displaced variety of talus fracture (pantalar or subtalar dislocation or body extrusion), in which soft-tissue tenting occurs, is an emergency because of the eventuality of full-thickness skin necrosis, which can lead to catastrophic complications. Waiting for the soft tissues to "calm down," complications related to wound slough and dehiscence may be avoided,[41] but this is a judgment call.

4. **Long bone fractures in the face of multisystem trauma.** Patients who present with a femur fracture and other injuries to critical organs such as the lung, brain, or abdomen, or who have extended periods of hypotension, are at risk for complications such as acute respiratory distress syndrome, fat embolism syndrome, extended intensive care unit (ICU) stays, and pneumonia. **Historically, patients with femoral fractures treated with a splint or skeletal traction were at increased risk for these sequelae. Early stabilization of femur fractures gained momentum in the 1980s and 1990s and helped to decrease such complications and allowed for earlier mobility and thus fewer consequent problems from extended recumbent periods** on a ventilator in the ICU. In the adequately resuscitated patient, aggressive stabilization for femur and pelvic fractures has a favorable effect on pulmonary function following blunt trauma.[42] In general, fixation of femur fractures with an interlocking nail is indicated in the multiply injured patient.[43,44] Evidence supports femur fixation within 24 hours of injury in the polytrauma patient.[45-47]

Timing and titration of orthopaedic procedures, however, is very important and requires thoughtful consideration. With widespread execution of "early total care," "at-risk" patients, those who are under-resuscitated or have concomitant chest trauma, experienced additional complications as a result of the "second hit" associated with intramedullary nailing of the femur. DCO is a philosophy that favors femur stabilization with an external fixator rather than an intramedullary nail in order to prevent this second physiologic insult that occurs from intramedullary reaming and manipulation.[48] It is thought that the intramedullary nailing should be delayed if a patient is physiologically challenged from multiple injuries; however, early (less than 24 hours) femur stabilization with an external fixator is still prudent.[49] With that being said, recent research has demonstrated no increased morbidity or mortality with early intramedullary nailing (<24 hours), in the setting of polytrauma and femur fracture.[50]

## IV. Pediatric Orthopaedic Considerations

A. **General principles of fracture care.** Pediatric orthopaedics is a separate discipline due to many nuances in diagnosis and management that are very different than adult orthopaedic fracture care. Obtaining a history is more difficult and takes significant patience, and often, family helps to solicit appropriate information. Children have injury patterns that are distinctive, and with an understanding of these recurring patterns, effective management can be learned and applied with greater confidence.

Reducing fractures is frequently more effective in a setting where general anesthesia can be administered as it is otherwise difficult to gain the cooperation of the child. The rule **"one doctor, one manipulation"** should be observed in the emergency department setting. With all types of injuries involving the epiphyseal plate, an accurate diagnosis as to the type of injury is important. Minor residual deformity in Salter–Harris I and II (see below) injuries correct themselves with subsequent growth, so open reduction is not indicated because the operation itself may cause more trauma. What the clinician can accept for angular deformity is more liberal in children because of their remarkable capacity to remodel deformity. For this reason, there are far fewer indications for surgical stabilization with internal fixation than in adults. Helpful treatment principles follow.

1. Up to **30° of angulation** in the plane of joint motion is **acceptable** in metaphyseal fractures in young children. The **younger** the patient, the **greater the angulation acceptable. The closer the fracture is to the dominant growth plate, the greater the capacity to remodel.** The dominant growth plate is
   a. **Femur—distal**
   b. **Tibia—proximal**
   c. **Humerus—proximal**
   d. **Radius—distal**
2. If a **fracture deformity** is obvious on inspection, the fracture should be **reduced**.
3. Fractured femurs in the 3- to 8-year-old group can be allowed to have **1.0 to 1.5 cm of overlap (Bayonet apposition) owing to the potential for overgrowth**.
4. **Children do not experience stiffness of otherwise normal joints, though elbows warrant early mobilization to prevent stiffness.**

B. **Growth plate injuries. The epiphyseal plate is weakest at the site of cell degeneration and provisional calcification (growth plate zones of calcification and hypertrophy).** Children who have undergone a rapid growth spurt, and in those who are excessively heavy for their skeletal maturity, are particularly vulnerable to such growth plate injuries. **Salter** classified traumatic epiphyseal separations into the following functional groups.[51]

1. **Class 1.** A fracture through the zone of provisional calcification without fracture of bone tissue. Such an injury does not involve a germinal layer unless associated with severe trauma either from the initial injury or from attempted reductions. Radiographic diagnosis is difficult because of the lack of bony injury. Growth disturbances are rare but do occur.
2. **Class 2.** An epiphyseal plate fracture with an associated fracture through the bony metaphysis. Growth disturbance (physeal arrest) is also rare in this category of injury but may depend on the bone, joint, and mechanism.
3. **Class 3.** An epiphyseal plate fracture associated with fractures through the epiphysis. These fractures involve the articular surface. Histologically, there is a fracture through the germinal layers. Accurate reduction is essential to prevent subsequent growth disturbance, but even so, alterations in growth are unpredictable. If the articular surface has more than 1 mm of "step-off," open reduction is indicated.
4. **Class 4.** A fracture through the epiphysis, epiphyseal plate, and metaphysis. Such an injury almost invariably results in significant growth disturbance unless it is anatomically reduced. Open reduction and internal fixation are indicated if there is any displacement.
5. **Class 5.** This is an axial load or "smash" injury that destroys all or part of the epiphyseal plate and results in growth arrest. Radiographic diagnosis can also be difficult as with the Type I injury. Close monitoring for remaining growth is essential. Surgical resection of the bone bridge and fat interposition are necessary if growth arrest results.

C. **Diagnostic and therapeutic pediatric pitfalls**
   1. Treating accessory ossicles as fractures

2. Missing an osteochondral fracture
3. Not following a child long enough to follow effect of growth arrest (valgus or varus deformity)
4. Missing a stress fracture
5. Confusing an epiphyseal fracture for a ligament injury ("kids generally do not sprain")
6. Missing a tibial spine fracture
7. Overdiagnosing instability of C2–C3 ("pseudosubluxation")
8. Overtreating an upper humeral fracture (tremendous remodeling capacity)
9. Failing to realize the instability of an apparently undisplaced lateral condylar fracture of the humerus
10. Overlooking radial head dislocation (should bisect the capitellum) on both the anteroposterior and lateral radiographs
11. Distal forearm fractures lose initial reduction frequently and deserve close follow-up
12. Overlooking abdominal injury in a child with a thoracolumbar flexion injury
13. Always obtain an opposite limb (joint) X-ray to aid interpretation of a physeal injury, particularly in the injured elbow.

## V. Principles of Radiographic Diagnosis

Accurate diagnosis and optimal orthopaedic treatment is dependent upon excellent radiologic execution and interpretation. **The clinician must, at the very least, demand two good quality, orthogonal, appropriately penetrated, X-ray views centered on the bone or joint of interest without overlying objects obscuring detail.** This basic principle is perhaps the most violated orthopaedic axiom, which leads to mismanagement, frustration, litigious outcomes, and compromised patient care.

A long bone has an **articular surface made up of hyaline cartilage** at each end. **This end of the bone is called the epiphysis in the skeletally immature patient.** In general, a goal of treatment is to ensure that a fracture heals with anatomic alignment of articular fragments. Therefore, **intraarticular fractures deserve a critical radiographic assessment typically with oblique views in addition to an anteroposterior and lateral view**. An alternative to oblique X-rays is the CT scan, but X-rays should never be omitted altogether. Just adjacent to the epiphysis is the metaphysis, which is made up of the broad funnel-shaped area of bone with thin cortices and dense trabecular bone. In between each metaphysis is the area of bone called the diaphysis. In general, the metaphyseal and diaphyseal fragments do not need to be reduced anatomically during treatment and healing. The treatment principle in these areas of bone is to restore length, alignment, and rotation of the bone. **Any diaphyseal fracture warrants orthogonal X-rays of the joint above and below the injury to look for associated fractures or luxations. Frequently, inexperienced clinicians or radiology technicians attempt to interpret views of a joint or long bone that is not centered on the radiographic cassette. In an effort to include an entire bone and its adjacent joints on a single film, an entire long bone may be "fit into" an angled cassette. Unfortunately, the detail needed to accurately discern articular or diaphyseal detail is lost owing to angulation of the X-ray projection. The clinician must, therefore, insist on dedicated views of joints in addition to views of the long bones with which they coincide.**

Providers may bypass the radiograph and go directly to a CT scan to interpret fractures. This practice is wrong. Most of the time, radiographs suffice for common orthopaedic injuries and, in fact, contain all the necessary detail the clinician needs for appropriate treatment. The ubiquitous ordering of CT scans is an expensive and wasteful strategy and simply bypasses appropriate diagnostic algorithms; furthermore, the risks of excess radiation load are substantial, especially in children. Furthermore, X-rays yield better information about the quality or density of bone and better information about displacement and spatial context of related bones.

The role of **computed axial tomography** and associated sagittal, coronal, and three-dimensional reconstructions might be necessary in complex fractures, particularly those that enter joints. It is also particularly useful for assessment of spine and pelvic injuries. The CT scan helps to assess greater bony detail and often provides a roadmap during preoperative planning. Critical CT findings to look for in certain injuries include the following:

A. **Spine—subluxation of vertebral elements**
B. **Pelvis—sacral fractures and sacroiliac involvement**
C. **Acetabulum—intraarticular fragments of the acetabulum or femoral head** (which suggests necessary axial traction)
D. **Impaction injury to the acetabulum**
E. **Glenoid Bankart injuries and humeral Hill–Sachs deformities after shoulder dislocations**
F. **Distal femur—coronal plane (Hoffa) fractures**
G. **Tibia plateau and pilon—fracture vector and comminution**
H. **Talus—talar dome and lateral process injuries** (often missed on X-ray)
I. **Calcaneus comminution at subtalar joint**
J. **Associated fractures in high-energy Chopart and Lisfranc midfoot fractures**

## VI. Principles of Fracture Healing

Factors generally reported with delayed union and nonunion fracture are as follows[52]:

A. **Too much motion** destroys the vascular budding into the fracture hematoma and interferes with revascularization. Adequate stabilization of the fracture, therefore, is mandatory.[52]
B. **Distraction** decreases the surrounding vascularity and increases the length of the bony bridge necessary to heal the fracture. This is especially critical with intramedullary nail treatment.
C. **Patient factors** include smoking, diabetes, steroid medications, and poor nutrition.

## VII. Stress Fractures

Normal bone might undergo fatigue or stress fractures when subjected to unaccustomed repetitive use. This condition can range from a stress fracture of a metatarsal in a runner who has recently increased his/her training distance or in an older person who is being mobilized after having been confined to a chair or bed. A **history** of having done something repetitively out of one's normal exercise routine, followed by pain, should raise the question of stress fracture in the mind of the physician. Common sites of stress fracture include the metatarsals after unusually long walks or running, the distal fibula in runners, the tibia in football players (frequently misdiagnosed as shin splints), and the femoral neck in both young and older patients. Stress fractures are common in military recruits.

The **physical examination** reveals tenderness to pressure on the bone at the site of the fracture. Occasionally, swelling and erythema are present. Radiographic examination can be negative in the first 10 to 14 days, after which a small, radiolucent line can usually be seen in association with increasing adjacent bone sclerosis. A bone scan shows radioactive uptake earlier and may be indicated in the competing athlete, particularly if the suspected fracture is in the tibia or femoral neck, both of which have a high incidence of complete fracture if the athlete continues competition. Magnetic resonance imaging (MRI) can definitively identify a stress fracture. Healing stress fractures have been mistaken for bone tumors.[53]

**Treatment** should be based on the relief of symptoms unless there is a danger of complete fracture under normal use. Under such circumstances, the injury should be treated like any nondisplaced fracture with relative rest. Generally, operation is reserved for recalcitrant injury.

VIII. **Soft-Tissue Injuries**

  A. **Tendon**

    1. **Diagnosis**[54,55]

      a. **First-degree strain** (mild)

        i. The **etiology** is trauma to a portion of the musculotendinous unit from excessive forcible stretch.

        ii. Symptoms include local pain that is aggravated by movement or tension.

        iii. Signs of injury include mild spasm, swelling, ecchymosis, local tenderness, and minor loss of function and strength.

        iv. Complications include recurrence of the strain, tendonitis, and periostitis at the tendinous insertion site.

        v. Pathologic changes cause a low-grade inflammation and some disruption of muscle–tendon fibers, but no appreciable hemorrhage.

      b. **Second-degree strain** (moderate).[54,55]

        i. The **etiology** is trauma to a portion of the musculotendinous unit from violent contraction or excessive forcible stretch.

        ii. **Symptoms and signs** include local pain that is aggravated by movement or tension of the muscle, moderate spasm, swelling, ecchymosis, local tenderness, and impaired muscle function.

        iii. **Complications** include a recurrence of the strain.

        iv. The **pathologic findings** consist of hemorrhage and the tearing of muscle–tendon junction fibers without complete disruption.

      c. **Third-degree strain** (severe).[54,55]

        i. **Symptoms and signs** include severe pain and disability, severe spasm, swelling, ecchymosis, hematoma, tenderness, loss of muscle function, and, usually, a palpable defect. An avulsion fracture at a tendinous insertion may mimic a severe strain.

        ii. A **complication** is prolonged disability.

        iii. **Radiographs** can demonstrate an avulsion fracture at the tendinous attachment as well as soft-tissue swelling.

        iv. The **pathology** consists of a ruptured muscle or tendon with the resultant separation of muscle from muscle, muscle from tendon, or tendon from bone.

    2. **Treatment.** Direct treatment toward limited immobilization, followed by eccentric exercises. In some clinical situations, this requires removal of devitalized tissue and repair by the sites and type of suture that will not cause further devitalization. When possible, sutures are placed in the surrounding fascia and not in the muscle itself.

    3. Tendons are relatively avascular structures and do not handle infection well. At sites where they course along long synovial tunnels, **blood supply** is via the long axis of the tendon or vincula. Trauma or sheath infections can jeopardize nutrition of the tendon.

    4. As a **general principle**, a lacerated or ruptured tendon should be repaired primarily with a nonreactive material and a suture technique to ensure continued approximation of the tendon ends. Even with prophylactic antibiotics, primary repair of tendons in wounds more than 12-hour-old carries considerable risk. A nonreactive synthetic suture or braided wire is the suture of choice. If the tendon is expected to glide subsequently, then handling the tendon with sponges and forceps is avoided because this causes further trauma and may be associated with dense adhesions.

5. Any involved **tendon sheath** should be opened in a longitudinal manner so that the tendon is unroofed for the entire excursion of a repaired laceration site to:
   a. **Prevent "triggering"** of the enlarged sutured site
   b. **Allow for revascularization** of the tendon at the suture site
   c. **Prevent fixation** on the relatively immobile sheath.
6. Only those with special training in hand surgery should repair **digital flexor tendons in the hand**.

**B. Ligaments**
1. **Types of injury**
   a. **First-degree sprain** (mild)
      i. **Signs** include mild point tenderness, no abnormal motion, little or no swelling, minimal hemorrhage, and minimal functional loss.
      ii. **Complications** include a tendency toward recurrence.
      iii. The **pathology** consists of minor tearing of the ligamentous fibers.
   b. **Second-degree sprain** (moderate)
      i. **Signs** include point tenderness, moderate loss of function, slight-to-moderate abnormal motion, swelling, and localized hemorrhage.
      ii. **Complications** can include a tendency toward recurrence, persistent instability, and traumatic arthritis.
      iii. The **pathology** is a partial tear of a ligament.
   c. **Third-degree sprain** (severe)
      i. **Signs** include a loss of function, marked abnormal motion, possible deformity, tenderness, swelling, and hemorrhage.
      ii. **Complications** can involve persistent instability and traumatic arthritis.
      iii. **Stress radiographs** demonstrate abnormal motion when pain is adequately relieved.
      iv. The **pathology** is a complete tear of a ligament.
2. Diagnosis of the extent of the ligamentous injury presents a challenge. Rupture may be suspected from the mechanism of injury or from physical examination, which reveals tenderness over the ligament. The injury might be fairly painless, especially if the ligament is completely disrupted. Once hemorrhage and swelling occur, this diagnostic possibility is limited. **Another diagnostic aid is a stress radiograph, but it must be compared with the opposite and normal side.** Such films should be made when the pain is inhibited by regional or general anesthesia. Arthroscopy or arthrography can provide pertinent information and a diagnosis, but a skilled arthroscopist should first be consulted. An MRI scan can be used to make the diagnosis.
3. **Treatment** of a complete ligamentous rupture is in essence the treatment of a dislocated joint after the dislocation has been reduced. In general, preserving motion is most important, and early mobilization is the treatment of choice. A temporary orthosis, however, during the acute period (i.e., 7 to 10 days) is certainly prudent, if not humane, when pain and swelling are excessive. Ligaments are relatively avascular, so healing is slow. The larger ligaments must be protected until the scar matures (8 to 16 weeks). The cruciate ligaments of the knee do not heal in-substance tears possibly related to the intraarticular physiologic milieu and often require bracing or surgical reconstruction when instability is limiting.

**C. Nerves**
1. Nerve injuries are of **three types**: contusion or **neuropraxia**, crush or **axonotmesis**, and complete division or **neurotmesis**. Blunt injuries and

those associated with fractures tend to be either neuropraxia or axonotmesis. For this reason, the fracture should be treated in its usual manner, and the nerve injury observed. If it is neuropraxia, recovery will be complete within 6 to 12 weeks. If it is an axonotmesis, recovery from the trauma site to the next muscle to be innervated should be followed, keeping in mind that the expected recovery rate is 1 mm/day or about 1 in/month. If reinnervation does not occur on time, exploration is indicated. When the distance from the site of trauma to the next innervated muscle that can be assessed causes a 6-month delay, early exploration is indicated. An electromyogram shows reinnervation approximately 1 month before it can be detected clinically, but one is dependent on the skill of the electromyographer for interpretation. A traction injury is usually a mixed lesion with a large element of neurotmesis of individual axons at various places along the nerve. A nerve injury associated with sharp trauma is usually neurotmesis, and surgical repair is indicated.

The **brachial plexus** presents a special diagnostic and treatment challenge. Injuries from lacerations, especially in children, should be repaired primarily. Most brachial plexus injuries, however, are caused by traction and are either an avulsion of the root from the cord or the typical tearing of the axons at multiple levels along the nerve. MRI is essential for differentiation. If the lesion is an avulsion injury, no recovery is possible, and the patient should be started early on rehabilitation. If the lesion is the typical traction injury, the patient should be followed up to document recovery. If no recovery appears at the appropriate time intervals, exploration and possible suture or nerve graft should be considered.

2. As a general principle, **secondary repair** (3 to 6 weeks after injury) is preferable to primary repair for the following reasons:
   a. The repair is done as an **elective procedure**.
   b. There is **less hesitancy in extending the incision** for proper mobilization of the nerve.
   c. It is easier to delineate the **extent of damage** along the nerve.
   d. The **epineurium** has some degree of scarring and hence holds the suture better.
   e. The **distal axon tubules** are open because Wallerian degeneration has occurred, and regeneration has a chance to proceed.
   f. There are synthetic neural conduits now commercially available to support the anastomoses and interpositions.
3. There are many **exceptions** to the preference for **secondary repair**, such as suturing.
   a. A **digital nerve**
   b. A **nerve in the brachial plexus**
   c. An isolated nerve injury **less than 8- to 12-hour-old** inflicted by a **razor** or sharp **knife**
4. **Nerve surgery should be performed by a surgeon experienced in microscopic techniques.**

### D. Hematomas

1. **Treatment** of large hematomas (large compared with the area of confinement) whether subcutaneous or in muscle usually should consist of evacuation as an elective procedure in the operating room. A hematoma is not absorbed but undergoes organization, fibrosis, and scarring. Aspiration of a clot is not possible, so a large hematoma is evacuated by open drainage. Before considering this, the surgeon must be sure that the hematoma is not expanding or is the cause of shock. If it is, vascular surgery consultation is mandatory to consider primary repair.

## IX. Frostbite

**A. Classification.** Frostbite[56] is a pathologic entity that occurs on a spectrum of severity depending on temperature and duration of exposure. **Frostnip** results in pallor and numbness, but no tissue damage after rewarming. **Chilblain** typically involves the patient's face, pretibial region, or dorsum of the hands and results from repeated exposure. **Trench foot** occurs during water immersion of an extremity in subfreezing conditions.

Frostbite occurs commonly in temperatures less than 2 °C and includes the following degrees of severity:

**1° = hyperemia and edema**

**2° = hyperemia and vesicle formation with partial-thickness necrosis**

**3° = full-thickness skin necrosis**

**4° = full-thickness skin and underlying structure necrosis**

**B. Treatment**

1. **Prehospital care.** Protection of the frostbitten part from mechanical trauma. Avoid rewarming until it can be done definitively.

2. **Rewarming.** Hypothermia of the patient should be treated first. Stimulation of the vagus nerve or myocardium with nasogastric tubes, Swan-Ganz catheter, or other methods should be avoided. If the patient is breathing, intubation is not appropriate. The patient should be rewarmed in a water bath with mild antibacterial soap at 40 °C to 42 °C (104 °F to 108 °F). A flushed appearance indicates reperfusion, and the patient should be removed from the bath.

3. **Definitive care.** The goals of definitive care are to preserve viable tissue and prevent infection. If possible, a burn center should be contacted for initiation of thrombolytic therapy to salvage threatened tissue and limbs. The injured limb should be elevated and protected from even mild trauma. Lambswool should be placed between the toes. Analgesics and ibuprofen 4 mg/kg should be administered three times a day. Tetanus prophylaxis is appropriate. Any source of nicotine should be strictly prohibited.

## X. Conclusion

The musculoskeletal system is an intricate and complex assembly of multiple organ systems presenting a massive array of presenting pathology that takes years and decades to master. In fact, over the past quarter century, the specialties that address this vast area of medicine not only include the ever-growing subspecialties in orthopaedic surgery, but growing sophistication of other disciplines such as nonoperative sports medicine, physical medicine and rehabilitation, occupational medicine, and other related fields outside the medical school pathway. This chapter provides a brief overview of many of the salient areas of diagnosis and treatment into which you can further delve in the chapters to follow.

## REFERENCES

1. Cummings SR, Melton LJ. Epidemiology and outcomes of osteoporotic fractures. *Lancet.* 2002;359:1761-1767.
2. Marzetti E, Calvani R, Tosato M, et al. Sarcopenia: an overview. *Aging Clin Exp Res.* 2017;29:11-17.
3. Lewiecki EM, Wright NC, Curtis JR, et al. Hip fracture trends in the United States, 2002-2015. *Osteoporos Int.* 2018;29:717-722.
4. Poole GV, Ward EF. Causes of mortality in patients with pelvic fractures. *Orthopaedics.* 1994;17:691-696.
5. Pfeifer R, Tarkin IS, Rocos B, Pape HC. Patterns of mortality and causes of death in polytrauma patients—has anything changed? *Injury.* 2009;40(9):907-911.

6. Court-Brown CM, Robinson CM. Femoral diaphysis fractures: epidemiology. In: Browner BD, Jupiter JB, Levine AM, et al, eds. *Skeletal Trauma*. Vol 2. 3rd ed. WB Saunders; 2003:1884-1924.

7. Ward WG, Nunley JA. Occult orthopaedic trauma in the multiply injured patient. *J Orthop Trauma*. 1991;5:308-312.

8. Keijzers GB, Campbell D, Hooper J, et al. A prospective evaluation of missed injuries in trauma patients, before and after formalizing the trauma tertiary survey. *World J Surg*. 2014;38:222-232.

9. American College of Surgeons' Committee on Trauma. *Advanced Trauma Life Support for Doctors® (ATLS®)*. 10th ed. American College of Surgeons; 2018.

10. Looby S, Flanders A. Spine trauma. *Radiol Clin North Am*. 2011;93(1):97-110.

11. Lafferty PM, Anavian J, Will RE, Cole PA. Operative treatment of chest wall injuries: indications, technique, and outcomes. *J Bone Joint Surg Am*. 2011;93(1):97-110.

12. Loo GT, Siegel JH, Dischinger PC, Alo K, Velmahos G, Chan L. Airbag protection versus compartmental intrusion effect determines the pattern of injuries in multiple trauma motor vehicle crashes. *J Trauma*. 1996;41:935-951.

13. Demetriades D, Karaiskakis M, Toutouzas K, et al. Pelvic fractures: epidemiology and predictors of associated abdominal injuries and outcomes. *J Am Coll Surg*. 2002;195(1):1-10.

14. Bone LB, McNamara K, Shine B, John B. Mortality in multiple trauma patients with fractures. *J Trauma*. 1994;37:262-264.

15. Tscherne H. Management of open fractures. In: Tscherne H, Gotzen L, eds. *Fractures with Soft Tissue Injuries*. Springer-Verlag; 1984:10-32.

16. Bottlang M, Krieg JC, Mohr M, Simpson TS, Madey SM. Emergent management of pelvic ring fractures with use of circumferential compression. *J Bone Joint Surg Am*. 2002;84(S2):43-47.

17. Lynch K, Johansen K. Can Doppler pressure measurement replace "exclusion" arteriography in the diagnosis of occult extremity trauma? *Ann Surg*. 1991;214:737-741.

18. Weaver FA, Yellin AE, Bauer M, et al. Is arterial proximity a valid indication for arteriography in penetrating extremity trauma? A prospective analysis. *Arch Surg*. 1990;125:1256-1260.

19. Whitesides TE Jr, Haney TC, Hirada H, Holmes HE, Morimoto K. A simple method for tissue pressure determination. *Arch Surg*. 1975;110:1311-1313.

20. McQueen MM, Court-Brown CM. Compartment monitoring in tibial fractures. *J Bone Joint Surg Br*. 1996;7:99-104.

21. Hansen ST Jr. Technology over reason. *J Bone Joint Surg Am*. 1987;69:799-800.

22. Bosse MJ, McCarthy ML, Jones AL, et al. The insensate foot following severe lower extremity trauma: an indication for amputation? *J Bone Joint Surg Am*. 2005;87(12):2601-2608.

23. Swiontkowski MF. Intracapsular hip fractures. In: Browner BD, Jupiter JB, Levine AM, et al, eds. *Skeletal Trauma*. Vol 2. 3rd ed. WB Saunders; 2003:1700-1775.

24. Swiontkowski MF, Winquist RA, Hansen ST. Fractures of the femoral neck in patients between the ages of twelve and forty-nine years. *J Bone Joint Surg Am*. 1984;66:837-846.

25. Ly TV, Swiontkowski MF. Treatment of femoral neck fractures in young adults. *Instr Course Lect*. 2009;58:69-81.

26. Epstein HC, Harvey JP. Traumatic anterior dislocations of the hip. Management and results. An analysis of fifty-five cases. *J Bone Joint Surg Am*. 1972;54:1561-1562.

27. Brumback R, Jones A. Interobserver agreement in the classification of open fractures of the tibia. *J Bone Joint Surg Am*. 1994;76:1162-1166.

28. Anglen JO. Comparison of soap and antibiotic solutions for irrigation of lower-limb open fracture wounds. A prospective, randomized study. *J Bone Joint Surg Am*. 2005;87(7):1415-1422.

29. FLOW Investigators, Petrisor B, Sun X, Bhandari M, et al. Fluid lavage of open wounds (FLOW): a multicenter, blinded, factorial pilot trial comparing alternative irrigating solutions and pressures in patients with open fractures. *J Trauma*. 2011;71(3):596-606.

30. Bhandari M, Jeray KJ, Petrisor BA, et al. A trial of wound irrigation in the initial management of open fracture wounds. *N Engl J Med*. 2015;373(27):2629-2641. doi: 10.1056/NEJMoa1508502

31. Artz CP, Sako Y, Scully RE. An evaluation of the surgeon's criteria for determining the viability of muscle during debridement. *AMA Arch Surg*. 1956;73:1031-1035.

32. Henry SL, Osterman PA, Seligson D. The antibiotic bead pouch technique: the management of severe compound fractures. *Clin Orthop*. 1993;295:54-62.

33. Argenta LC, Morykwas MJ. Vacuum assisted closure: a new method for wound control and treatment: clinical experience. *Ann Plast Surg*. 1997;38:563-577.

34. Joseph E, Hamori CA, Bergman S, Roaf E, Swann NF, Anastasi GW. A prospective randomized trial of vacuum assisted closure versus standard therapy of chronic nonhealing wounds. *Wounds*. 2000;12:60-67.

35. Patzakis MJ, Harvey JP, Ivler D. The role of antibiotics in the management of open fractures. *J Bone Joint Surg Am.* 1974;56:532-541.
36. Calhoun J. Use of antibiotic prophylaxis in primary TJA. Frontlines. *AAOS Bull.* 2004;52(4):15.
37. Gustilo RB, Anderson JT. Prevention of infection in the treatment of one thousand and twenty five fractures in long bones. *J Bone Joint Surg Am.* 1976;58:453-458.
38. Nord RM, Quach T, Walsh M, Pereira D, Tejwani NC. Detection of traumatic arthrotomy of the knee using the saline solution load test. *J Bone Joint Surg Am.* 2009;91(1):66-70.
39. Vallier HA, Nork SE, Barei DP, Benirschke SK, Sangeorzan BJ. Talar neck fractures: results and outcomes. *J Bone Joint Surg Am.* 2004;86-A(8):1616-1624.
40. Halvorson JJ, Winter SB, Teasdall RD, Scott AT. Talar neck fractures: a systematic review of the literature. *J Foot Ankle Surg.* 2013;52(1):56-61.
41. Lindvall E, Haidukewych G, DiPasquale T, Herscovici D Jr, Sanders R. Open reduction and stable fixation of isolated, displaced talar neck and body fractures. *J Bone Joint Surg Am.* 2004;86-A(10):2229-2234.
42. Routt MI, Simonian PT, DeFalco AJ, Miller J, Clarke T. Internal fixation in pelvic fractures and primary repairs of associated genitourinary disruptions: a team approach. *J Trauma.* 1996;40:784-790.
43. Bosse MJ, MacKenzie EJ, Reimer BL, et al. Adult respiratory distress syndrome, pneumonia, and mortality following thoracic injury and a femoral fracture treated either with intramedullary nailing with reaming or with a plate: a comparative study. *J Bone Joint Surg Am.* 1997;79:799-809.
44. Duwelius PJ, Huckfeldt R, Mullins RJ, et al. The effects of femoral intramedullary reaming on pulmonary function in a sheep lung model. *J Bone Joint Surg Am.* 1997;79:194-202.
45. Bone LB, Johnson KD, Weigelt J, Scheinberg R. Early vs. delayed stabilization of femoral fractures. *J Bone Joint Surg Am.* 1989;71:336-340.
46. Johnson KD, Cadambi BA, Seibert GB. Incidence of adult respiratory distress syndrome in patients with musculoskeletal injuries: effect of early operative stabilization of fractures. *J Trauma.* 1985;25:375-383.
47. Riska EB, Bonsdorff HV, Hakkinen S, et al. Primary operative fixation of long bone fractures in patients with multiple injuries. *J Trauma.* 1977;17:111-121.
48. Pape HC, Grimme K, Van Griensven M, et al. Impact of intramedullary instrumentation versus damage control for femoral fractures on immunoinflammatory parameters: prospective randomized analysis by the EPOFF study group. *J Trauma.* 2003;55:7-13.
49. Bone LB, Giannoudis P. Femoral shaft fracture fixation and chest injury after polytrauma. *J Bone Joint Surg Am.* 2011;93(3):311-317.
50. Liu XY, Jiang M, Yi CL, Bai XJ, Hak DJ. Early intramedullary nailing for femoral fractures in patients with severe thoracic trauma: a systemic review and meta-analysis. *Chin J Traumatol.* 2016;19:160-163.
51. Cepela DJ, Tartaglione JP, Dooley TP, Patel PN. Classifications in brief: Salter-Harris classification of pediatric physeal fractures. *Clin Orthop Relat Res.* 2016;474:2531-2537.
52. Weitzel PP, Esterhai JL. Jr. Delayed union, nonunion and synovial pseudarthrosis. In: Brighton CT, Friedlaender GE, Lane JM, eds. *Bone Formation and Repair.* American Academy of Orthopaedic Surgeons; 1994:505-527.
53. Eisele SA, Sammarco GJ. Fatigue fractures of the foot and ankle in the athlete. In: Heckman JD, ed. *Instructional Course Lectures.* Vol 42. American Academy of Orthopaedic Surgeons; 1993:175-183.
54. Taylor DC, Dalton JD Jr, Seaber AV, Garrett WE Jr. Experimental muscle strain injury: early functional and structural deficits and the increased risk for reinjury. *Am J Sports Med.* 1993;21:190-194.
55. Maffulli N, Wong J, Almekinders LC. Types and epidemiology of tendinopathy. *Clin Sports Med.* 2003;22(4):675–692. doi:10.1016/s0278-5919(03)00004-8
56. Shenaq DS, Gottlieb LJ. Cold injuries. *Hand Clin.* 2017;33(2):257-267. doi: 55.1016/j .hcl.2016.12.003

## SELECTED HISTORICAL READINGS

Godina M. Early microsurgical reconstruction of complex trauma of the extremities. *Plast Reconstr Surg.* 1986;78:285-292.
Gustilo RB, Mendoza RM, Williams DM. Problems in management of type III open fractures. A new classification of type III open fractures. *J Trauma.* 1984;24:742-746.

Nash G, Blennerhassett JB, Pontoppidan H. Pulmonary lesions associated with oxygen therapy and artificial ventilation. *N Engl J Med*. 1967;276:368-374.

Salter RB, Harris WR. Injuries involving the epiphyseal plate. *J Bone Joint Surg Am*. 1963;45:587-622.

Shackford SR, Hollingworth-Fridlund P, Cooper GF, Eastman AB. The effect of regionalization upon the quality of trauma care as assessed by concurrent audit before and after institution of a trauma system: a preliminary report. *J Trauma*. 1986;26:812-820.

Subcommittee on Classification of Sports Injuries. *Standard Nomenclature of Athletic Injuries*. American Medical Association; 1976.

Tibbs PA, Young AB, Bivins BA, Sachatello CR. Diagnosis of acute abdominal injuries in patients with spinal shock: value of diagnostic peritoneal lavage. *J Trauma*. 1980;20:55-57.

Traverso LW, Lee WP, Langford MJ. Fluid resuscitation after an otherwise fatal hemorrhage: I. Crystalloid solutions. *J Trauma*. 1986;26:168-175.

Urbaniak JR, Roth JH, Nunley JA, Goldner RD, Koman LA. The results of replantation after amputation of a single finger. *J Bone Joint Surg Am*. 1985;67:611-619.

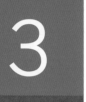

# 3 Complications of Musculoskeletal Trauma

Emily A. Wagstrom

Complications of musculoskeletal trauma are distressingly common. Some complications are a consequence of the injury itself and may be unavoidable, whereas others are iatrogenic and potentially preventable. Regardless of the etiology of the complication, prompt recognition and appropriate treatment lessen the impact of the complication and improve the outcome.

## I. Systemic Inflammatory Response Syndrome

A. Systemic inflammatory response syndrome (SIRS) is a condition occurring after trauma or sepsis that is characterized by multiple organ dysfunction (MOD) and is mediated by the acute inflammatory response to injury. The severity of SIRS is correlated with the overall burden of the injury as well as the magnitude of surgery performed within the first 2 days after injury.[1] Although the degree of the inflammatory response is generally proportionate to the amount of trauma, genetic susceptibility to an exaggerated response has been shown to be present in patients with a specific single nucleotide polymorphism.[2] SIRS has many manifestations ranging from occult hypoxemia due to mild pulmonary dysfunction to fatal MOD.[3] SIRS is diagnosed when two or more of the following four criteria are present (SIRS score)[4]:

1. *Body temperature* is below 36°C or greater than 38°C.
2. *Pulse* is greater than 90 beats/min.
3. Respiratory rate is greater than 20 breaths/min; or arterial *partial pressure* of *carbon dioxide* is less than 4.3 kPa (32 mm Hg).
4. *White blood cell count* is less than 4,000 cells/mm$^3$ ($4 \times 10^9$ cells/L) or greater than 12,000 cells/mm$^3$ ($12 \times 10^9$ cells/L); or the presence of greater than 10% *immature neutrophils* (band forms).

Fat embolism syndrome (FES) and acute respiratory distress syndrome (ARDS) are other clinical manifestations of similar phenomenon that are related to SIRS. FES may be one of the etiologic factors contributing to SIRS, whereas ARDS is now recognized as the "final common pathway" of the pulmonary consequences of SIRS. The diagnosis of ARDS is based on the Berlin definition[5]:

1. Timing: within 1 week of a known clinical insult or new/worsening respiratory symptoms
2. Chest imaging: bilateral opacities not fully explained by effusions, lobar/lung collapse, or nodules
3. Origin of edema: respiratory failure not fully explained by cardiac failure or fluid overload
4. Oxygenation:
   a. Mild: $PaO_2/FiO_2$ between 200 and 300 with PEEP or CPAP $\geq$ 5
   b. Moderate: $PaO_2/FiO_2$ between 100 and 200 with PEEP $\geq$ 5
   c. Severe: $PaO_2/FiO_2$ less than 100 with PEEP $\geq$ 5

FES is generally a self-limited pulmonary disease that usually occurs within 3 days of a facture. The **diagnosis** of FES is suspected if the following symptoms and signs are present in a patient with a fracture[6-8]:
1. Disturbances of consciousness (i.e., confusion, delirium, coma)
2. Tachycardia and dyspnea
3. History of hypovolemic shock
4. Petechial hemorrhages

Any combination of the above symptoms may be present in patients with isolated or multiple fractures. Patients with major long bone fractures are particularly at risk and should be monitored for occult hypoxemia with continuous, noninvasive pulse oximetry.[9] When hypoxia is documented, supplemental oxygen is provided. Patients with hypoxia should be evaluated for coagulopathy and monitored for pulmonary, renal, and hepatic dysfunction that may develop into full-blown SIRS.

Patients presenting with signs and symptoms of SIRS are generally not considered to be candidates for immediate stabilization of their orthopaedic injuries. Instead, in these circumstances, "damage-control" methods are employed to provide provisional stabilization of fractures, with a delay of definitive fixation until the patient is considered physiologically stable. A more detailed discussion of this topic is given in Chapter 2.

B. Laboratory findings
1. Thrombocytopenia (platelet count <150,000) and hypoxemia (arterial oxygen tension [$PaO_2$] <60 mm Hg) are the **most clinically useful signs.** Hypoxemia itself is very common in trauma patients and may or may not suggest pulmonary compromise.[9] Elevated interleukin 6 (IL-6) levels are associated with SIRS, and this is a useful marker to follow in patients with multiple injuries.[10] Patients with higher levels IL-6, as well as other inflammatory markers, are at an increase risk of organ dysfunction. IL-6 levels can be incorporated with other biomarkers and the patient's physiologic state to determine appropriate timing of surgical intervention.[11]
2. **Electrocardiographic changes** may be present and include tachycardia, a prominent S wave on lead I, a prominent Q wave on lead II, a shift **in** the transition zone to the left, arrhythmias, inverted T waves, depressed RST segments, and a right bundle branch block. Serial electrocardiograms are useful.
3. **Increased serum lipase** is indicative of FES, but is of little practical value because of the impact of blunt trauma on this laboratory parameter.
4. **Chest roentgenographic changes**, when present, are patchy pulmonary infiltrates. The clinical manifestations of fat embolism usually precede these changes. The pulmonary findings become more severe in patients who meet the criteria for ARDS.

C. Recommended treatment
1. **Respiratory support** is the cornerstone of the prevention and treatment of SIRS, ARDS, FES, and MOD. It is provided to keep the $PaO_2$ between 50 and 100 mm Hg. Patients with ARDS and MOD usually need prolonged ventilatory support with continuous positive airway pressure. Renal dialysis may be necessary in the MOD group. In patients with isolated fractures who are physiologically stable, early (within 24 hours) fixation of femur fractures helps limit the incidence of this complication.[8,12] In polytrauma patients, early appropriate care is recommended within 36 hours after the patient has been fully resuscitated.[13]
2. **Shock** is treated as outlined in Chapter 2, I.A.3.
3. Coagulopathy is monitored and treated with fresh frozen **plasma** and/ or cryoprecipitate. Platelet counts should ideally be maintained above 50,000/mL.

## II. Nerve Compression Syndromes

A. Acute carpal tunnel syndrome (CTS, median nerve entrapment at the wrist)

1. Acute CTS can occur following distal radial fracture or carpal fracture/dislocation. This is the result of compression of the median nerve from hematoma or bony displacement. When occurring as a complication of trauma, the condition may develop and progress rapidly. Acute CTS must be recognized and treated emergently, first with fracture or dislocation reduction, which often results in resolution of symptoms. If symptoms to not resolve, emergent carpal tunnel relese is indicated. (see Chapter 21).

B. **Ulnar nerve compression at the elbow** ("tardy" ulnar nerve palsy, acute ulnar palsy) is commonly associated with fractures and dislocations around the elbow in children as well as adults. Acute ulnar neuropathy following injury is most often the result of iatrogenic damage such as injury occurring during pinning of a supracondylar fracture in a child, or retraction during internal fixation of a distal humerus fracture in an adult.

1. An early **diagnostic sign** is the inability to separate the fingers (interosseous weakness). There is usually decreased sensation in the fourth and fifth fingers. Light pressure on the cubital tunnel may reproduce the pain. Nerve **conduction** studies show a slowing of the ulnar nerve conduction velocity as it crosses the elbow (see **Appendix F**). However, this test is not useful diagnostically until at least 3 weeks after injury.

2. If symptoms are minimal, ulnar nerve compression is managed with observation and passive range of motion of the fingers. **Surgical therapy** consists of exploration, neurolysis, and possible transposition of the ulnar nerve beneath the flexor muscle mass anterior to the medial epicondyle when the pattern of injury or fracture permits. This treatment usually stops any progressive neuropathy but does not guarantee complete regression of the neurologic symptoms or signs.

C. **Peroneal nerve palsy** may be due to the **compression of the common peroneal nerve** in the area of the fibular head or as the nerve enters the anterior **compartment**. Apparent peroneal palsy may also be a manifestation of more proximal **injury to the peroneal division of the sciatic nerve**. Thus, peroneal palsy may be a complication of hip or pelvic fracture/dislocation.

1. **Diagnosis** is often based on motor loss, which includes weakness of dorsiflexion of the ankle and toes as well as eversion of the foot. History of a hip, tibia, ankle, or foot injury is likely. Pain is usually on the lateral aspect of the leg and dorsal aspect of the foot. Pressure over the nerve trunk may cause local pain as well as radiation into the sensory distribution of the nerve. Pressure over the nerve as it courses around the proximal fibula results from patient positioning in the operating room or intensive care unit or from poorly applied splints.

2. **Treatment.** Associated hip, knee, or ankle dislocations are emergently reduced. If there is an operable cause, neurolysis is indicated. During the recovery stage, a lateral shoe wedge or plastic ankle-foot orthosis (AFO) maintains eversion of the foot. Tendon transfer may be appropriate for some patients with a permanent foot drop.

D. **Sciatic nerve** neuropraxia can accompany hip dislocation or fracture dislocation (acetabular fracture). Note that some sciatic palsies may present as an isolated peroneal palsy, as discussed above.

1. The main differentiating factor in the **diagnosis** of a sciatic neuropathy is an L5 or S1 root injury resulting from pelvic or spine fracture. A sciatic neuropathy must be suspected when multiple neurologic (L4–S3) segments are involved. A helpful differentiating test is straight-leg raising just short of discomfort; pain caused by a sciatic neuropathy is increased

by internal rotation and relieved by external rotation of the hips. This reaction is not seen with lumbar radiculopathies.

2. **Treatment** is aimed at the cause of the sciatic neuropathy, and the neuropathy itself is treated with observation. If the sciatic nerve is known to be damaged and is not improving, neurolysis may be indicated. In general, the tibial portion of the nerve recovers well, but the peroneal portion does not.[14] This may be related to the fact that it is the peroneal portion that lies against the pelvis as it exits through the greater sciatic foramen.

### III. Compartment Syndromes

A compartment syndrome is defined as "a condition in which increased pressure within a space compromises the circulation to the contents of that space."[15] Although most commonly applied to the osteomyofascial compartments of the extremities, compartment syndrome can occur in the abdomen and in major muscle groups about the spine and pelvis. Other terms that have been used to describe compartment syndrome are Volkmann's ischemia, local ischemia, traumatic tension in muscles, impending ischemic contracture, exercise ischemia, exercise myopathy, anterior tibial syndrome, medial tibial syndrome, rhabdomyolysis, and calf hypertension. Compartment syndrome following trauma is most common in men under the age of 35 with fractures of the tibia or forearm, and those participating in sporting activity when the injury occured.[16,17]

A. Locations

1. In the **upper extremity**, typical locations include the volar and dorsal compartments of the forearm (Fig. 3-1). There are also several intrinsic compartments of the hand.

2. In the **lower extremity**, typical locations include the anterior, lateral, superficial posterior (gastrocnemius, soleus), and deep **posterior** compartments of the leg (Figs. 3-2 and 3-3). Compartment syndromes are also seen in the thigh, gluteal, and foot compartments.[18]

B. Etiologies

1. **Decreased compartment volume,** for example, occurring following closure of fascial defects, application of tight circumferential dressings, and localized external pressure, can precipitate a compartment syndrome.[19]

2. **Increased compartment content** arises from the following:

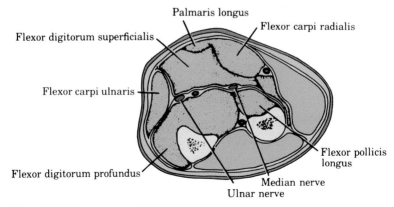

**Figure 3-1.** Volar compartment syndrome of the forearm. Symptoms and signs of weakness of finger and wrist flexion, pain on finger and wrist extension, hypesthesia of the volar aspect of the fingers, and tenseness of the volar forearm fascia.

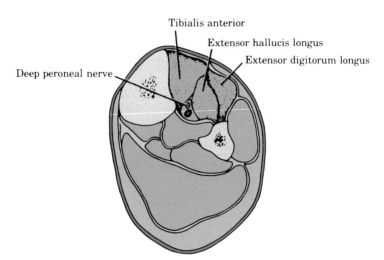

**Figure 3-2.** Anterior compartment syndrome of the leg. Symptoms and signs are weakness of toe extension and foot dorsiflexion, pain on passive toe flexion and foot plantar flexion, hypesthesia in the dorsal first web space, and tenseness of the anterior compartmental fascia.

    a. **Bleeding** caused by a major vascular injury, edema from massive tissue crushing, or a bleeding disorder

    b. **Increased capillary permeability** due to shock, postischemic swelling, exercise, direct trauma, burns, intraarterial drugs, or orthopaedic surgery

    c. **Increased capillary pressure** from exercise or venous obstruction

    d. **Muscle hypertrophy**

    e. **Direct infusion** (infiltrated intravenous [IV] line, injection gun)

    f. Application of excessive traction (Fig. 3-4)

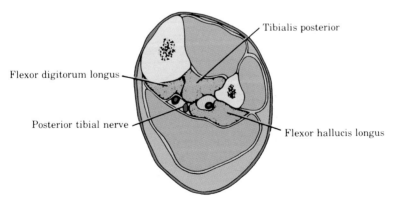

**Figure 3-3.** Deep posterior compartment syndrome of the leg. Symptoms and signs are weakness of toe flexion and foot inversion, pain on passive toe extension and foot eversion, hypesthesia of the plantar aspect of the foot and toes, and tenseness of the deep posterior compartmental fascia (between the tibia and the Achilles tendon).

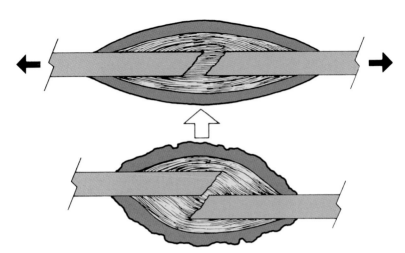

**Figure 3-4.** Distraction of fracture fragments (excessive traction) can increase compartmental tissue pressure and be a cause of a compartment syndrome.

    **C. Increased tissue pressure** is the key feature of compartment syndromes. Once the pressure is elevated, it can compromise the local circulation by at least three mechanisms: decreased perfusion pressure, arteriolar closure, and reflex vasospasm. Muscle cell death and nerve dysfunction begin approximately 6 hours after the pressure begins to approach 30 mm Hg lower than the patient's diastolic pressure.

    **D.** The clinical approach

        1. **Identify** the at-risk patients as early as possible and **examine them frequently**. Continuous real-time monitoring of intramuscular pressure should be done if the patient's mental status and/or the ability to examine the patient are compromised in any way.[20] If the risk is high and the patient is under anesthesia, consider **prophylactic decompression**. Hypotensive patients are at particular risk. Patients under anesthesia are frequently hypotensive; in a series of patients undergoing tibial nailing, the preoperative blood pressure was predictive of the postoperative blood pressure and may be used in this setting for calculation of perfusion pressure.[21]

        2. Carefully **document** the time and findings of each **examination**.

        3. The appearance of excess **pain, sensory deficits,** or **muscle weakness** demands a thorough examination to rule out a compartment syndrome (Table 3-1). Because the compartment syndrome is usually progressive, **frequent examination** (ideally by the same examiner) is indicated in questionable cases. Of the five "Ps" traditionally taught to be associated with compartment syndrome (pain, pulselessness, pallor, paresthesias, and paralysis), only pain and paresthesias are useful for the early diagnosis of compartment syndrome. Classically, pain with gentle passive motion is the first sign, and pulselessness is the last. Patients who are at risk for developing compartment syndrome of an injured extremity should not undergo neuraxial anesthesia.[20] Patient-controlled anesthesia techniques are also capable of masking the pain associated with compartment syndrome and should be used with caution in "at-risk" patients.

          a. Check each potentially involved nerve using **two-point discrimination** and **light touch** because both are more sensitive than the commonly

| TABLE 3-1 | Diagnostic Factors in Compartment Syndromes of the Lower Extremity | | | |
|---|---|---|---|---|
| Compartment | Distribution of Sensory Changes | Muscles Weakened | Painful Passive Movement | Location of Tenseness |
| Anterior | Deep peroneal (first web space) | Toe extensors and tibialis anterior | Toe flexion | Anteriorly between tibia and fibula |
| Lateral | Superficial and deep peroneal (dorsum of foot) | Peroneals | Inversion of foot | Laterally over fibula |
| Deep posterior | Posterior tibial (sole of foot) | Toe flexors and tibialis posterior | Toe extension in distal half | Posteromedially of leg between Achilles tendon and tibia |
| Superficial posterior | None | Gastrocnemius and soleus | Foot dorsiflexion | Over the bulk of the calf |

From Matsen FA III. Compartmental syndrome. *Clin Orthop*. 1976;113:8, with permission.

    used pin. Compare with the opposite extremity to better discern subtle changes.

  b. Grade the **strengths** of all potentially involved muscles (see **Appendix B**).

  c. The **passive muscle stretch** test causes severe pain if the muscle is ischemic.

  d. The **peripheral pulse** is frequently normal in the presence of a compartment syndrome. If it is abnormal, the diagnosis of a major arterial occlusion or compartment syndrome must be entertained.

  e. Laboratory findings are nonspecific, but myoglobinuria may be of some help in the diagnosis of acute compartment syndrome.[20]

4. The **tissue pressure** is typically measured with a handheld device such as the STIC (Critical Care Diagnostics, Schoolcraft, MI). Tissue pressures are normally higher in children (up to 17 mm Hg) than adults (up to 10 mm Hg).[22] Tissue pressure readings within 30 mm Hg of the patient's diastolic blood pressure (perfusion pressure <30 mm Hg) are strongly suggestive of evolving compartment syndrome.[23] It is important to measure along the entire length of the involved compartment and use the highest pressure reading to determine if compartment syndrome is present.[24] The anterior compartment of the lower leg is nearly always involved in patients with compartment syndrome and has been called the "sentinel" compartment. Continuous monitoring of the anterior compartment can be performed by connecting a saline-filled IV tube to an angiocatheter inserted into the muscle, which is connected to a standard pressure transducer.

5. If the examination suggests a compartment syndrome, decompression of the involved compartments should be performed emergently. It is very important to perform a longitudinal incision that spans the majority of the length of the involved compartment. Inadequate skin release does not provide adequate decompression[25] and is a common reason for continued tissue ischemia and poor outcome.

  a. If the decompression does not produce the expected improvement, one should consider the possibilities of inadequate decompression, compartment syndrome in another compartment that wasn't released, incorrect diagnosis, or secondary arterial occlusion. Careful **reexploration** and possibly arteriography are indicated.

6. Because myoglobinuria and renal failure can complicate compartment syndromes, adequate hydration and urinary output, with alkalinization of urine using IV sodium bicarbonate, should be ensured. Dark urine may usually be attributed to myoglobinuria in the absence of hematuria.

7. If the compartment syndrome is recognized more than 24 hours after the onset of symptoms, fasciotomy should not be performed. The risk of deep infection is high and often results in limb loss.[20,26]

**IV. Chronic Regional Pain Syndrome (CRPS, Also Known as Sympathetically Maintained Pain Syndrome, Sudeck Atrophy, Reflex Sympathetic Dystrophy)**
CRPS can be classified into two types: CRPS Type I and CRPS Type II and is differentiated by a direct injury to a nerve (Type II) or no injury to a specific nerve (Type I). Type I develops after an initiating noxious event, and the symptoms are disproportionate to this event. It is associated with edema, changes in skin blood flow, abnormal pseudomotor activity, allodynia, and hyperalgesia. It is not limited to a single nerve distribution. Type II results in burning pain, allodynia, and hyperpathia after injury of a nerve.[27] Suspect early CRPS in any patient with persistent complaints of pain, especially associated with hyperesthesia of the skin and/or abnormal pseudomotor response. For example, an excessively sweaty extremity that has severe pain with light touch (such as with bedding sheets or clothing) should be suspected as having CRPS. **For successful treatment, the diagnosis must be made before the classic signs** of thin shiny skin, excessive hair growth, attrition of nails, and diffuse osteoporosis occur. Whenever the diagnosis is suspected, institute treatment immediately. Treatment consists of regional sympathetic nerve blocks plus vigorous active physical therapy to mobilize any edema, as well as to increase the muscle activity and the range of joint motion. The condition can occur in the upper extremity as well as in the lower extremity from the knee distally.

**V. Venous Thromboembolism**
Deep vein thrombosis (DVT) is extremely common in trauma patients.[28] The risk is greatest in patients with spine, pelvis, and hip trauma but is sufficiently high to warrant prophylactic treatment in all injured patients. Goel et al.[29] found an 11% incidence in patients with fractures below the knee. Thomas and Van Kampen[30] found that 2% of outpatients in a cast following fracture developed symptomatic DVT, whereas 1% had pulmonary embolism (PE). Appropriately treated orthopaedic trauma patients have a 3% to 5% incidence of DVT.[31] The risk of DVT is further increased in patients with hereditary (often occult) thrombophilia, women who receive hormone replacement therapy, pregnant patients, and those who are obese, have cancer, or a history of DVT.

A. **Prophylactic treatment** to prevent DVT is initiated in every trauma patient upon admission. Pneumatic compression devices are placed immediately, and prophylaxis with low-molecular-weight heparin (LMWH) is started within 24 hours if there are no other contraindications.[31] Among patients with high risk for DVT and unable to be anticoagulated prophylactically, inferior vena cava filter (IVCF) should be considered.[31-33]

B. The **diagnosis** of DVT should be entertained in any patient with lymphedema and/or unusual pain in an injured extremity. PE is rarely the first manifestation of DVT. When the diagnosis of DVT is considered, screening the extremities with duplex Doppler venous ultrasound is usually done first. Contrast venography is not usually done except in the research setting because of its invasiveness and potential complications. Spiral CT has become the diagnostic method of choice when considering PE.[34]

C. When DVT is identified, patients are anticoagulated. The American College of Chest Physicians (CHEST) recent guidelines recommend treatment with direct oral anticoagulants (DOACs) such as dabigatran, rivaroxaban, apixaban, or edoxaban over medications such as warfarin or LMWH. The duration of therapy should be 3 months.[35]

## VI. Myositis Ossificans

A. Heterotopic bone formation often occurs after injury or surgery and can occur in any collagenous supportive tissue of skeletal muscles, tendons, ligaments, and fascia. There are **four clinical types**; three may be seen in injured patients:

1. **Myositis ossificans progressiva** is rare and can be genetic. It usually occurs between the ages of 5 and 10 years (younger than 20 years) and proceeds relentlessly to progressive ossification of skeletal muscles. It is often present in the shoulders and neck as firm subcutaneous masses, which can be hot and tender and can undergo ossification. Often associated are microdactyly of the great toes and thumbs, ankylosis of the interphalangeal and metatarsophalangeal joints, and bilateral hallux valgus. Minor trauma often causes exacerbations. Treatment may include diphosphonate combined with surgery for severe joint malpositioning and functional impairment.

2. **Myositis ossificans paralytica** occurs in proximal paralyzed muscles. The ossification occurs 1 to 10 months after a spinal cord injury. This process causes decreased passive range of motion. The three classic sites are in the vastus medialis, the quadratus femoris, and the hip abductors. Surgical treatment is indicated only if the position and function of the extremity are unacceptable and when the ossification has matured. After excision, the dead space created must be drained by closed suction and the wound carefully observed for a hematoma.

3. **Myositis ossificans circumscripta** can be idiopathic but is more commonly caused by focal trauma and is common as a sports injury in the contact setting. It is more common in teenage or young adult males. It presents as an uncomfortable, indistinct mass that shows local induration and a local increase in temperature. The lesion occurs 80% of the time in the arm (biceps brachialis) but also occurs in the thigh (abductors and quadratus femoris). Roentgenograms show fluffy calcification 2 to 4 weeks after injury. In 14 weeks, the calcification matures, and in 5 months, ossification occurs. The differential diagnosis includes osteosarcoma and periosteal osteogenic sarcoma. Treatment is by excision, only if the lesion is unusually large or painful and after ossification is mature. Postoperative nonsteroidal anti-inflammatory medication is generally recommended to limit recurrence.

4. **Myositis ossificans traumatica**, the most common type of heterotopic ossification, presents the same way as the circumscripta type except for a clear history of trauma and/or surgery, with localized ossification within the traumatized area.[36] Treatment is controversial but is generally aimed at the prevention of ossification by immediate application of cold compression to the area of muscle injury. Later, heat is applied. An operation is indicated only when the ossification causes permanent impairment and only after the process has stabilized, often as soon as 6 to 8 months after injury.

B. The precise pathophysiology of myositis ossificans is not known. Preventive treatment should be designed to stop the sequence of osteogenesis.

1. **Pharmacologic treatment** is generally prophylactic and has historically included bisphosphonates to inhibit hydroxyapatite crystallization, mithramycin to interfere with mobilization of calcium, and cortisone to decrease bone formation at the site of injury. None of these drugs, however, has proved to be an extremely beneficial therapeutic agent. Indomethacin and Naprosyn have been shown to help minimize posttraumatic heterotopic ossification associated with acetabular fractures and arthroplasty.[36-39] There remains controversy regarding the use of nonsteroidal anti-inflammatory drugs (NSAIDs) and fracture healing. Recent

meta-analysis suggests that these medications can result in delayed or nonunion.[40] The risk of nonunion and the risk of heterotopic ossification formation must be weighed before deciding on use of NSAIDs. Similarly, low-dose irradiation with 800 to 1,000 radians has been shown to be very effective at preventing heterotopic ossification.[41]

2. When **surgical treatment** is indicated, the traditional approach has been to wait until the ossification is mature—that is, when the bone scan is negative and the alkaline phosphatase level is decreasing. Many authors have recently advocated earlier resection before these tests have returned to normal.[42]

## REFERENCES

1. Pape HC, Griensven MV, Hildebrand FF, et al. Systemic inflammatory response after extremity or truncal fracture operations. *J Trauma*. 2008;65:1379-1384.
2. Hildebrand F, Pape HC, van Griensven M, et al. Genetic predisposition for a compromised immune system after multiple trauma. *Shock*. 2005;24:518-522.
3. Giannoudis PV, Pape HC, Cohen AP, et al. Review: systemic effects of femoral nailing: from Küntscher to the immune reactivity era. *Clin Orthop Relat Res*. 2002;404:378-386.
4. https://www.mdcalc.com/sirs-sepsis-septic-shock-criteria
5. Ferguson ND, Fan E, Camporota L, et al. The Berlin definition of ARDS: an expanded rationale, justification, and supplementary material. *Intensive Care Med*. 2012;38(10):1573-1582.
6. Ganong RB. Fat emboli syndrome in isolated fractures of the tibia and femur. *Clin Orthop Relat Res*. 1993;291:208-214.
7. Lindeque BG, Schoeman HS, Dommisse GF, et al. Fat embolism and the fat embolism syndrome. A double-blind therapeutic study. *J Bone Joint Surg Br*. 1987;69:128-131.
8. Müller C, Rahn BA, Pfister U, et al. The incidence, pathogenesis, diagnosis, and treatment of fat embolism. *Orthop Rev*. 1994;23:107-117.
9. Wong MW, Tsui HF, Yung SH, et al. Continuous pulse oximeter monitoring for inapparent hypoxemia after long bone fractures. *J Trauma*. 2004;56:356-362.
10. Giannoudis PV, Harwood PJ, Loughenbury P, et al. Correlation between IL-6 levels and the systemic inflammatory response score: can an IL-6 cut-off predict a SIRS state? *J Trauma*. 2008;65:646-652.
11. Gaski, GE, Metzger, C, McCarroll, T, et al. Early immunologic response in multiply injured patients with orthopaedic injuries is associated with organ dysfunction. *J Ortho Trauma*. 2019;33(5);220-228.
12. Turen CH, Dube MA, LeCroy MC. Approach to the polytraumatized patient with musculoskeletal injuries. *J Am Acad Orthop Surg*. 1999;7:154-165.
13. Vallier HA, Moore TA, Como JJ, et al. Complications are reduced with a protocol to standardize timing of fixation based on response to resuscitation. *J Orthop Surg Res*. 2015;10(1):155.
14. Fassler PR, Swiontkowski MF, Kilroy AW, et al. Injury of the sciatic nerve associated with acetabular fracture. *J Bone Joint Surg Am*. 1993;75:1157-1166.
15. Matsen FA III. *Compartmental Syndromes*. Grune & Stratton; 1980:162.
16. McQueen MM, Gaston P, Court-Brown CM. Acute compartment syndrome. Who is at risk? *J Bone Joint Surg Br*. 2000;82:200-203.
17. McQueen, MM, Duckworth, AD, Aitken, SA, et al. Predictors of compartment syndrome after tibial fracture. *J Ortho Trauma*. 2015;29(10);451-455.
18. Manoli A II, Fakhouri AJ, Weber TG. Concurrent compartment syndromes of the foot and leg. *Foot Ankle*. 1993;14:339.
19. Whitesides TE, Heckman MM. Acute compartment syndrome: update on diagnosis and treatment. *J Am Acad Orthop Surg*. 1996;4:209-218.
20. American Academy of Orthopaedic Surgery. Management of acute compartment syndrome: clinical practice guideline. Accessed April 14, 2019. https://www.aaos.org/uploadedFiles/PreProduction/Quality/Guidelines/Guidelines_and_Reviews/guidelines/ACSguideline.pdf
21. Kakar S, Firoozabadi R, McKean J, et al. Diastolic blood pressure in patients with tibia fractures under anesthesia: implications for the diagnosis of compartment syndrome. *J Orthop Trauma*. 2007;21:99-103.
22. Staudt JM, Smeulders MJ, van der Horst CM. Normal compartment pressures of the lower leg in children. *J Bone Joint Surg Br*. 2008;90:215-219.
23. McQueen MM, Court-Brown CM. Compartment monitoring in tibial fractures. The pressure threshold for decompression. *J Bone Joint Surg Br*. 1996;78:99-104.

24. Heckman MM, Whitesides TE, Greve SR, et al. Compartment pressure in association with closed tibia fractures—the relationship between tissue pressure, compartment and the distance from the site of fracture. *J Bone Joint Surg Am.* 1994;76:1285-1292.

25. Cohen MS, Garfin SR, Hargens AR, et al. Acute compartment syndrome. Effect of dermotomy on fascial decompression in the leg. *J Bone Joint Surg Br.* 1991;73(2):287-290.

26. Finkelstein JA, Hunter GA, Hu RW. Lower limb compartment syndrome: course after delayed fasciotomy. *J Trauma.* 1996;40:342-344.

27. Goh EL, Chidambaram S, Ma D. Complex regional pain syndrome: a recent update. *Burns Trauma.* 2017;5(1):2.

28. Abelseth G, Buckley RE, Pineo GE, et al. Incidence of deep-vein thrombosis in patients with fractures of the lower extremity distal to the hip. *J Orthop Trauma.* 1996;10:230-235.

29. Goel DP, Buckley R, deVries G, et al. Prophylaxis of deep-vein thrombosis in fractures below the knee: a prospective randomised controlled trial. *J Bone Joint Surg Br.* 2009;91:388-394.

30. Thomas S, Van Kampen M. Should orthopaedic outpatients with lower limb casts be given deep vein thrombosis prophylaxis? *Clin Appl Thromb Hemost.* 2010;17:405-407.

31. Sagi HC, Ahn J, Ciesla D, et al. Venous thromboembolism prophylaxis in orthopaedic trauma patients: a survey of OTA member practice patterns and OTA expert panel recommendations. *J Orthop Trauma.* 2015;29(10):e355-e362.

32. Toro JB, Gardner MJ, Hierholzer C, et al. Long-term consequences of pelvic trauma patients with thromboembolic disease treated with inferior vena caval filters. *J Trauma.* 2008;65:25-29.

33. Starr AJ, Shirley Z, Sutphin PD, et al. Significant reduction of pulmonary embolism in orthopaedic trauma patients. *J Orthop Trauma.* 2019;33(2):78-81.

34. van Strijen MJ, de Monyé W, Schiereck J, et al. Single-detector helical computed tomography as the primary diagnostic test in suspected pulmonary embolism: a multicenter clinical management study of 510 patients. *Ann Intern Med.* 2003;138(4):307-314.

35. Kearon C, Akl EA, Ornelas J, et al. Antithrombotic therapy for VTE disease: CHEST guideline and expert panel report. *Chest.* 2016;149(2):315-352.

36. Hyder N, Shaw DL, Bollen SR. Myositis ossification: calcification of the entire tibialis anterior after ischaemic injury (compartment syndrome). *J Bone Joint Surg Br.* 1995;78:318-319.

37. Matta JM, Siebenrock KA. Does indomethacin reduce heterotopic bone formation after operations for acetabular fractures? A prospective randomized study. *J Bone Joint Surg Br.* 1997;79:959-963.

38. Moed BR, Karges DE. Prophylactic indomethacin for the prevention of heterotopic ossification after acetabular fracture in high risk patients. *J Orthop Trauma.* 1993;7:33-38.

39. Schmidt SA, Kjaersgaard-Andersen P, Pedersen NW, et al. The use of indomethacin to prevent the formation of heterotopic bone after total hip replacement. A randomized, double-blind clinical trial. *J Bone Joint Surg Am.* 1988;70:834-838.

40. Wheatley, BM, Nappo, KE, Christensen, DL, et al. Effect of NSAIDs on bone healing rates: a meta-analysis. *J Am Academy Ortho Surg.* 2019;27(7):e330-e336.

41. Bosse MJ, Poka A, Reinert CM, et al. Heterotopic ossification as a complication of acetabular fracture. Prophylaxis with low-dose irradiation. *J Bone Joint Surg Am.* 1988;70:1231-1237.

42. Viola RW, Hanel DP. Early "simple" release of posttraumatic elbow contracture associated with heterotopic ossification. *J Hand Surg Am.* 1999;24:370-380.

## SELECTED HISTORICAL READINGS

Geerts WH, Code KI, Jay RM, et al. A prospective study of venous thromboembolism after major trauma. *N Engl J Med.* 1994;331:1601-1606.

Gelberman RH, Garfin SR, Hergenroeder PT, et al. Compartment syndromes of the forearm: diagnosis and treatment. *Clin Orthop Relat Res.* 1981;161:252-261.

Gossling HR, Pellegrini VD Jr. Fat embolism syndrome: a review of the pathophysiology and physiological basis of treatment. *Clin Orthop Relat Res.* 1982;165:68-82.

Matsen FA III, Winquist RA, Krugmire RB Jr. Diagnosis and management of compartmental syndromes. *J Bone Joint Surg Am.* 1980;62:286-291.

Paterson DC. Myositis ossificans circumscripta. Report of four cases without history of injury. *J Bone Joint Surg Br.* 1970;52:296-301.

Peltier LF. Fat embolism. An appraisal of the problem. *Clin Orthop Relat Res.* 1984;187:3-17.

Riska EB, von Bonsdorff H, Hakkinen S, et al. Prevention of fat embolism by early internal fixation of fractures in patients with multiple injuries. *Injury.* 1976;8:110-116.

Rorabeck CH, Bourne RB, Fowler PJ. The surgical treatment of exertional compartment syndrome in athletes. *J Bone Joint Surg Am.* 1983;65:1245-1251.

Ten Duis HJ, Nijsten MW, Klasen HJ, et al. Fat embolism in patients with an isolated fracture of the femoral shaft. *J Trauma.* 1988;28:383-390.

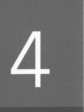

# Prevention and Management of Acute Musculoskeletal Infections

4

Susan Kline and Elizabeth Swanson

Prevention of infection is key to successful orthopaedic surgery. Meticulous attention to aseptic technique in the operating room, proper skin preparation and surgical scrub, the use of modern gown and mask techniques, planning the operation to shorten the time the tissues are exposed to air, laminar flow air, and prophylactic antibiotics are all important in the prevention of infection. However, none is as critical as meticulous debridement of contaminated wounds and any devitalized tissues and careful handling of tissues to prevent cell death. When infection does occur following an operation or from hematogenous origin, early diagnosis and prompt effective treatment can prevent disastrous complications.

## I. Prevention of Postoperative Musculoskeletal Infections

**A. Perioperative care.** Refer to Chapters 2, III, and 11, I, for techniques described for the prevention of operative and posttraumatic infections.

**B. Early diagnosis of postoperative wound infection**

1. Whenever a patient's postoperative or postinjury status does not follow the normal or expected course, the surgeon should be alert to the possibility of infection. A respiratory problem such as mild atelectasis may be a cause of persistent postoperative temperature elevation (this is especially common in patients who smoke), but such a potential diagnosis should not lull the surgeon into complacency. Wound infection may be the cause, or the two could be concurrent. Large hematomas can themselves be the cause of fever, but hematomas also represent the best culture media for bacteria and should be avoided if possible or evacuated if present. Always obtain a culture of any evacuated hematoma.

2. When there is a concern for a developing wound infection, inspect the wound and document the findings at least daily, using sterile techniques. Inspect the wound for tense skin, erythema, abnormal tenderness or swelling, and purulent drainage. These are frequent signs of inflammation and infection. Culture any drainage.

3. If the patient does not respond promptly to antibiotic treatment or if the wound remains indurated, aspiration should be carried out using aseptic technique with a large needle inserted into the wound area but away from the suture line.

4. A low-grade fever in patients with wound infections who have had antibiotics is not uncommon. In such instances, the temperature rarely exceeds 37.8°C (100°F) and may show a mild afternoon elevation.

5. In summary, be alert to the possibility of infection. Establish the diagnosis through cultures whenever possible, and treat the infection aggressively. If in doubt, the best course is generally to return the patient to the operating room and open the wound, irrigate hematoma and debride it to remove hematoma and necrotic wound tissue, and reclose the wound using the most "tissue friendly" suture technique (see Chapter 11). If a low-grade inflammatory process involves a joint, or the patient complains of pain from passive motion of the joint, this should alert the surgeon to the possibility of a septic joint. Consultation with another experienced surgeon can be helpful.

C. **Treatment of postoperative wound infection.** The principles of treatment include removal of all dead tissue and any hematoma along with appropriate antibiotic therapy. The wound is nearly always left open for secondary closure except when the infection involves a joint. If the wound is closed, a suction drain is mandatory. Once the diagnosis of a surgical wound infection or deep musculoskeletal infection has been established, antibiotic treatment proceeds, according to the established diagnosis, such as for wound infection, acute osteomyelitis, or septic arthritis.

II. **Bone and Joint Infections**

A. Bones and joints represent special problems for the host defense mechanisms. Normal bone has an excellent blood supply; however, once pus forms in the marrow, the increased intramedullary pressure leads to loss of the vascular supply to bone because of its rigid structure, resulting in areas of infected, devitalized bone. Septic emboli in bone or vascular thrombosis are other mechanisms leading to devascularization. Local phagocytic activity can be deficient (such as in metaphysis where there is lack of phagocytic cells lining the capillaries), and delivery of humoral factors (antibodies, opsonins, complement) may also be inadequate. Ligaments and tendons are relatively avascular structures and do not handle infection well. Joints pose a particular problem, with decreasing vascularity of the cartilage and menisci over time in children and avascularity in adults. In addition to the direct destructive effect of cell breakdown on cartilage, the pus under pressure interferes with cartilage nutrition and blood supply to the periarticular structures. At particular risk is the epiphyseal blood supply, resulting in avascular necrosis. Antibiotics can inhibit or cure an infection only when they can reach the infecting organism in bacteriostatic or bactericidal concentrations. Because bones and joints are relatively avascular during infection, tissue penetration of antibiotics may be limited.

B. Osteomyelitis can be caused by hematogenous inoculation, spread from adjacent tissues, or direct inoculation. Acute hematogenous osteomyelitis is the predominant mechanism of bone infection in prepubertal children, and is common in elderly adults, patients with central venous catheters, and intravenous (IV) drug users. Long bones are usually affected. The metaphyseal region is particularly susceptible to infection in children given the area's slowed circulation through dilated sinusoids, leading to an increased risk of bacterial deposition and proliferation. *Staphylococcus aureus* is the most common bacterial etiology of hematogenous osteomyelitis in all ages. In its earliest phase, acute hematogenous osteomyelitis can often be cured by prompt, appropriate antibiotic therapy. If effective treatment is delayed and devascularization of the involved tissues results, surgical treatment is a necessary adjunct to the antibiotic therapy.

C. In joint infections, even under the best of circumstances, late treatment (perhaps as early as 3 days [see https://www.ncbi.nlm.nih.gov/pmc/articles/PMC126863/] after the infection starts) may result in the loss of, or abnormal function of, the joint. Thus, appropriate antibiotic therapy must be initiated as early as possible. Appropriate therapy requires knowledge of the etiologic agent and its sensitivities.

D. **Diagnosis**

1. For both joint infections and osteomyelitis, every effort should be made to obtain a bacterial culture prior to starting antibiotics, whenever possible, which improves the chances of identifying the involved pathogen, and determine sensitivity to antibiotics. Once the culture specimen is obtained and while awaiting pathogen identification, it is important to initiate appropriate empirical antibiotic therapy based on suspected pathogens considering prevalence and susceptibilities of organisms in the community, the patient's age, underlying medical conditions, clinical features, severity of infection, as well as antibiotic pharmacodynamics, safety, and efficacy.

2. The earliest symptom or sign that may help differentiate a bone or joint infection is usually pain or localized tenderness in the periarticular region.

In infants and young children, refusal to move or use an extremity may be noted first. The cardinal signs of infection—redness, heat, and swelling—may appear later than pain and tenderness, or not at all. When examining a child with a fever of unknown origin, note any pain or alteration of the normal range of motions of a joint and carefully palpate all metaphyseal areas to determine local tenderness. Roentgenograms are of little value in making a diagnosis in the very early stages of osteomyelitis, although careful comparison with the opposite side may show abnormal soft-tissue shadows. Abnormalities can usually be seen on roentgenograms by 2 weeks after the onset of osteomyelitis, and bone or joint destruction is seen during the chronic phase of the disease. CT is sensitive for early bony erosions and later sequestra, given its excellent bony resolution; however a normal CT does not exclude early osteomyelitis because of its poorer soft tissue resolution and inability to detect bone marrow edema. MRI is considered most sensitive and specific, and is the imaging study of choice for the diagnosis of osteomyelitis.[1-4] Clinical context is of paramount importance in the evaluation of any abnormal imaging findings. Osteomyelitis should always be included in the differential diagnosis for a patient with the radiographic appearance of a bone tumor.[5] Radioisotopic bone scanning, especially indium imaging, is helpful in early localization of bone infection.[6-12]

3. Erythrocyte sedimentation rate (ESR) and C-reactive protein (CRP) serum levels are useful in laboratory evaluations.[13-16]

4. Identification of the infecting organism is essential. Pathogen yield is the highest when multiple specimens are sampled, including blood, bone, and joint fluid. In the early stages of the disease, particularly if there is a spiking temperature, blood cultures can identify the organism and should be drawn on all patients suspected to have osteomyelitis. Bone biopsy or needle aspiration is best for organism identification and should be obtained whenever possible (may provide the only microbiological diagnosis in up to 50% of pediatric patients). Bone biopsy may be considered prior to antibiotics to increase pathogen recovery if the patient is stable, without systemic signs of illness, and if the sampling can be performed urgently. If acute metaphyseal tenderness is present, the organism can frequently be obtained by inserting a needle into the site of maximum tenderness. A serrated biopsy needle is useful if subperiosteal pus is not encountered. If a joint is involved, the effusion should be aspirated before joint lavage. Processing the aspirates should include the following:

a. Immediate Gram stain.

b. Culture for aerobic and anaerobic bacteria. Swabs for culture are less sensitive; tissue or fluid is preferred.

c. For children less than 4 years of age: inoculate pus or joint fluid into aerobic blood culture bottles to enhance recovery of *Kingella kingae*.[17]

d. White blood cell count and differential.

e. Fungal and mycobacterial stains and cultures should be considered for patients with specific risk factors (foreign travel, TB exposure risk), as well as culture-negative cases of osteomyelitis unresponsive to empiric antibiotic therapy.[4]

f. Molecular studies such as broad-range 16S rDNA PCR or specific pathogen PCRs (e.g., *Staphylococcus*, *Lyme*, *Kingella*) may be considered in appropriate cases (e.g., patients pretreated with antibiotics or those with suspected pathogens that are difficult to grow on culture such as *Bartonella* or *Kingella*).

g. If a bone biopsy was done, tissue samples should be sent for histology to confirm a diagnosis of osteomyelitis.

**E. Differential diagnosis.** Care must be taken to differentiate soft-tissue infection, or cellulitis, from an infection involving a bone or joint. This is a particularly important precaution when the infection overlies a joint because any aspiration of a reactive sterile effusion by passing a needle through the soft-tissue infection may create a pyarthrosis. Tenderness and swelling from unrecognized trauma over a bone, particularly with some periosteal reaction, can present a confusing picture; however, the absence of fever and systemic signs is helpful. Nonbacterial inflammatory arthritis, including viral and toxic synovitis and autoimmune arthritis, must be included in a differential diagnosis, but until proven otherwise, think first of septic arthritis. The differentiation between a mild, well-localized infection and a localized bone tumor can sometimes require a surgical biopsy.[5] Spontaneous hemorrhages in patients with hemophilia and fractures in paraplegic patients, particularly patients with meningomyelocele, are special situations that can confuse the picture.

**F. Bacterial considerations**[14,18,19]

1. In acute hematogenous osteomyelitis, *S. aureus* is the most common etiologic agent in all age groups. An increasing number of isolated *S. aureus* strains are methicillin resistant. Other common causes of osteomyelitis in adults are coagulase-negative staphylococci, streptococci, enterococci, and gram-negative bacteria (such as *Pseudomonas aeruginosa*, *Enterobacter*, *Proteus*, *Escherichia coli*, and *Serratia*), anaerobic organisms, and *Mycobacterium tuberculosis*.

   In pediatric patients beyond the neonatal period, the most common organisms, after *S. aureus*, are *K. kingae*, which is very common in patients between 3 months and 3 years of age,[17,20,21] *Streptococcus pyogenes*, and *Streptococcus pneumoniae* (typically <3 years of age, and relatively infrequent due to widespread streptococcal conjugate vaccine).[22] Coagulase-negative staphylococcus osteomyelitis may occur in association with medical devices and central lines. Enteric gram negatives and anaerobes are uncommon causes of acute hematogenous osteomyelitis in children.

   Other uncommon causes of osteomyelitis in both adults and children include nontuberculous mycobacteria, endemic mycoses, *Candida*, *Aspergillus*, *Bartonella*, and atypical bacteria. Bacterial identification and antibiotic susceptibility testing is key to choosing the best antibiotic, not only for *S. aureus* but for other potentially antibiotic-resistant organisms. Contaminated open fractures can cause osteomyelitis of the fractured bone, typically at the fracture site. Staphylococci and aerobic gram-negative rods are the most common causes of osteomyelitis after open fractures. Osteomyelitis in this setting can present as nonunion of the bone or poor wound healing.[2]

   Bacterial causes of septic arthritis are similar to those of osteomyelitis, with *S. aureus* and *Streptococci* leading as pathogens in adults and children. Other causes in adults include gram-negative rods and miscellaneous bacteria, including anaerobes and polymicrobial infections.[23] Other pathogens in children beyond the neonatal period include *K. kingae*, which is common between 3 months and 3 years of age. Group A streptococcus and *S. pneumoniae* may also occur in this age group and through adolescence. *Haemophilus influenza* type b (Hib) has become uncommon, occurring mostly in incompletely immunized children in areas with low Hib vaccination rates. *Neisseria gonorrhoeae* must be considered among sexually active persons, particularly with single (especially the knee joint) or multiple joint findings. If there has been a preceding infection or if there is a concurrent infection in another organ system, one may suspect that the etiologic agent is the same as that from the initiating focus. However, because this is not always the case, direct culture from the bone or joint infection is advised.

2. In infants younger than 1 month, *S. aureus* remains the predominant agent of osteomyelitis and septic arthritis, but a range of other bacteria must also be considered. Group B streptococcus and enteric gram-negative organisms (e.g., *E. coli*, *Proteus* species, *Klebsiella pneumoniae*, *Serratia*) are also common in this population. Infants in the neonatal intensive care unit and/or those with indwelling venous catheters, surgeries, or prior antibiotic therapy may have musculoskeletal infections due to coagulase-negative staphylococci. Nonenteric gram-negative organisms such as *Pseudomonas aeruginosa* or other opportunistic organisms may lead to healthcare-associated osteoarticular infections in these infants.[24] Rarely, anaerobic organisms such as *Bacteroides fragilis* and fungal agents such as *Candida albicans* lead to bone or joint infections in neonates.

**G. Special considerations**

1. Osteomyelitis of the vertebral bodies and associated diskitis: Vertebral osteomyelitis usually presents with infection in two adjoining vertebral bodies and the adjacent "sandwiched" intervertebral disc. In adults, *S. aureus* and coagulase-negative staphylococci are the most common microorganisms identified, followed by streptococci. Vertebral osteomyelitis in children occurs mostly in adolescents and is most often caused by *S. aureus*, and less frequently by streptococci, coagulase-negative staphylococcus, and *Bartonella henselae*.[25,26] Tuberculosis can be a common cause in endemic areas or in immigrants from endemic areas. Brucellosis is also seen in endemic areas. Gram-negative rods and *Candida* can be causes of spinal osteomyelitis in postoperative patients, immunocompromised patients, and IVDUs.[27,28] Spinal osteomyelitis is usually hematogenous in origin. It can be associated with an epidural abscess or psoas muscle abscess. Patients usually present with pain and tenderness in the spine with or without fever. In addition, the patient may have neurologic compromise, and ESR is usually high. MRI is the most effective modality for diagnosing osteomyelitis of the spine. Imaging-guided percutaneous biopsy or aspirate is the preferred method to obtain the causative organism. A minimum of 6 weeks of IV antibiotics is standard and may need to be extended. Surgical intervention is not always needed. But surgical drainage should be considered when there is an epidural abscess, when there is a large paravertebral abscess, when medical management alone is not effective, when the spine needs to be stabilized, or if there is neurologic compromise.

2. Infections of the intervertebral discs, or acute discitis, may be encountered in young children typically <5 years of age without antecedent infection or surgery.[25,29] When organisms are recovered, they are usually *Staphylococcus aureus*. Others have included *Kingella kingae* (considered in some series as the most common etiology of spondylodiscitis) in patients 6–48 months of age,[25,26] coagulase-negative staphylococcus, and others. Toddlers may merely refuse to stand or walk, whereas older children complain of pain in the back or lower extremity. The infection is usually low grade without fevers and gradual onset of symptoms. Roentgenograms reveal that the involved disc narrows rapidly over the first 2 to 3 weeks. A bone scan shows increased activity in the adjacent vertebrae. The difficulty in obtaining a bacterial diagnosis, even with needle biopsy, combined with the benign course of this condition, has led many clinicians to ignore efforts at establishing a bacterial diagnosis. However, the condition must be differentiated from vertebral osteomyelitis with secondary disc destruction; in the latter condition, it is essential to obtain the bacterial diagnosis as an integral part of treatment of what can be a severe disease. The same precaution applies to disc infections following laminectomy. In

these cases, an infection should be suspected when a postsurgical patient complains of increasing back pain starting 1 to 2 weeks postoperatively.

3. Patients with hemolytic disorders, particularly those with sickle cell disease, are prone to the development of a subacute form of osteomyelitis. *Salmonella* infections are frequent, but other types of bacterial osteomyelitis are not uncommon.[19] Because the diagnosis is usually made late, treatment is difficult and may require extensive surgical debridement and prolonged antibiotic therapy.

4. Open contaminated fractures are especially at risk for developing infections at the fracture site (3%–25%). The most common causative organisms are staphylococci and aerobic gram-negative bacilli. Unusual bone infections due to fungi and nontuberculous mycobacteria can also occur due to the direct inoculation of the wound with these environmental organisms. Surgical debridement, irrigation of the wound, and stabilization of the bone is very important; fixation of the fracture is generally required. IV antibiotics are also indicated for highly contaminated wounds. If an open fracture results in osteomyelitis, successful management requires surgical debridement, establishing the causative organism, and initiating effective antibiotic therapy, which is guided by cultures and antibiotic susceptibility testing. Once the patient has been stabilized, the infection diagnosed, and appropriate therapy begun and tolerated, the IV course can be completed as an outpatient through home infusion therapy to complete a total of 4- to 6-week course. Oral therapy has been shown recently to be equally efficacious.

5. Another special problem is presented by the patient who sustains a puncture wound in the sole of the foot. Despite initial cleansing and debridement, cellulitis, arthritis, or osteomyelitis involving the foot develops in many patients.[13] This is most commonly caused by *P. aeruginosa*. Early surgical debridement of the infected foot, including the plantar fascia, combined with preoperative and postoperative anti-*P. aeruginosa* antibiotics, has been the most effective method of management. For a serious infection, antibiotic therapy with an aminoglycoside (e.g., tobramycin), or an antipseudomonal beta-lactam (e.g., cefepime, ceftazidime, imipenem, or meropenem), or a quinolone (ciprofloxacin or levofloxacin) should be administered[18]; however, quinolones are relatively contraindicated for use in prepubertal children. In addition, it is best to avoid fluoroquinolones in fractures because of its potential effects of decreased bone healing. Quinolones can impede bone fracture healing in experimental models, and therefore, should be avoided when possible if fracture healing is needed.[30] Appropriate sensitivities guide antibiotic selection. Duration of therapy is empirical and may be guided by the clinical appearance and the CRP or ESR.[13,29] Aminoglycoside doses need to be adjusted according to peak and trough serum levels, and monitoring must include weekly serum creatinine (Cr) measurements and regular audiologist evaluation. Patients with human immunodeficiency virus or acquired immunodeficiency syndrome can have septic joints, which may frequently be missed because of the relatively weak immune response to the infectious agent. Joint aspiration should be performed in this setting.[31]

6. **Lyme arthritis.** Lyme arthritis, the most common vector-borne infection in the United States, is caused by the spirochete *Borrelia burgdorferi*, which is transmitted to humans primarily via the *Ixodes scapularis* tick from its natural hosts, deer and white-footed mice.[32] Arthritis, the most common form of late Lyme disease (other forms being encephalopathy and polyneuropathy), can occur from weeks to months after the original infection. Approximately 60% of patients with untreated primary disease

develop arthritis.[33] Clinical presentation includes fever and joint effusion, which may be confused with acute septic arthritis, especially in children.[34] Treatment with oral antibiotics such as doxycycline for 4 weeks or the parenteral agent ceftriaxone for 2 weeks usually results in lasting cure. However, a small percentage of patients experience ongoing symptoms despite antibiotic therapy. Possible reasons include persistent infection, residual joint damage, or a chronic autoimmune synovitis.[35]

**H. Antibiotic treatment of bone and joint infections**[18,19,36]

1. For initial treatment of bone or joint infection, choose an antibiotic effective against the suspected organism and a route of administration that ensures delivery of therapeutic levels to the infected site. The IV route is generally preferred for initial treatment, although some antibiotics achieve comparable blood concentrations when given orally.

2. The duration of parenteral treatment is 3 to 4 weeks for septic arthritis and 4 to 6 weeks for osteomyelitis (the longer duration for infections caused by *S. aureus*). In adults with infections, the treatment may be completed, for select susceptible organisms using oral quinolones after the initial pain, swelling, and fever have resolved with IV antibiotics. Quinolone antibiotics (ciprofloxacin, levofloxacin) have allowed oral therapy against a broad spectrum of bacteria including *Pseudomonas*.[18,37] Moxifloxacin can be helpful, especially if anaerobic oral bacteria are involved, for example, jaw osteomyelitis in penicillin allergic patients. But moxifloxacin has no antipseudomonas activity. In treating children with osteomyelitis, treatment may be initiated with an IV agent, such as nafcillin or cefazolin, and the 4- to 6-week treatment course may be completed with oral antibiotics once fevers, pain, and signs of local inflammation have resolved, and CRP is consistently decreasing. Recent studies show similar success rates with early transition to oral therapy compared to longer IV courses.[38-40,43] Oral therapy should be discussed with an infectious diseases consultant and tailored to the isolated organism. If no organism is isolated, the oral agent should have similar spectrum as the IV therapy on which the patient improved and should be given in high doses for good bone penetration. A common IV to oral antibiotic transition in children is from cefazolin to high-dose cephalexin. For all ages, the dosage of antibiotics (oral or parenteral) is at the upper therapeutic level. When possible, adequate drug levels for both oral and parenteral agents should be documented. Many antibiotics need to be dose adjusted for renal insufficiency based on the estimated GFR or CrCl. Providing outpatient parenteral antibiotics greatly reduces the cost of treatment. The CRP or ESR is also a helpful guideline to determine the duration of treatment.[13] A summary of antimicrobial agents commonly used in acute bone and joint infections is presented in Table 4-1. These agents are known to enter bone and joint sites readily when given in adequate doses.

3. In an acute infection in which the organism is not immediately identified, the choice of therapy is determined by the organisms most commonly expected in the various age groups, along with the other factors previously listed. General guidelines are presented in Table 4-2.

4. A local instillation or continuous irrigation with an antibiotic solution is almost never indicated. Systemic antibiotics when properly administered achieve adequate levels in viable tissues.[18,19] In many posttraumatic conditions, delivery of local antibiotics in methyl methacrylate beads is worthwhile.[36] This treatment is indicated especially when a delayed bone graft or soft-tissue muscle flap is planned. Continue antibiotics until the infection has been eliminated. A normal or declining ESR or CRP is one of the most helpful laboratory tests to indicate control of infection.

**TABLE 4-1** Antimicrobial Agents Commonly Used Initially in Acute Bone and Joint Infection

| Antibiotics | Usual Susceptible Organisms | Daily Dosage (IV Route) | Comments |
|---|---|---|---|
| Cefazolin (cephalosporins) | Methicillin-sensitive *S. aureus* and coagulase-negative staphylococci; will also treat streptococci, pneumococci, and *K. pneumoniae* | Neonatal[a] (≤1 mo postnatal age):<br><br>≤2 kg body weight:<br><br>≤7 d postnatal age: 50 mg/kg/d divided q12h<br><br>8–28 d: 75 mg/kg/d divided q8h<br><br>> 2 kg body weight:<br><br>≤7 d postnatal age: 100 mg/kg/d divided q12h<br><br>8–28 d: 150 mg/kg/d divided q8h<br><br>Pediatric (>1 mo of age):<br>100–150 mg/kg/d divided q6h–q8h; maximum 12 g/d<br><br>Adult: 3–6 g divided doses of 8 h | A drug of choice; IV route preferred, but may be given intramuscularly (IM). Adjust dosage according to blood urea nitrogen or, preferably, Cr clearance |

| Nafcillin | Methicillin-sensitive S. aureus and coagulase-negative staphylococci | Neonatal (≤1 mo postnatal age)[a]: | A drug of choice |
|---|---|---|---|
| | | <1 kg body weight: | |
| | | ≤14 d postnatal age: 50 mg/kg/d divided q12h | |
| | | 15–28 d: 75 mg/kg/d divided q8h | |
| | | 1–2 kg body weight: | |
| | | ≤7 d: 50 mg/kg/d divided q12h | |
| | | 8–28 d: 50–75 mg/kg/d divided q8h–12h | |
| | | >2kg body weight: | |
| | | ≤7 d: 75 mg/kg/d divided q8h | |
| | | 8–28 d: 100 mg/kg/d divided q6h | |
| | | Pediatric (>1 mo): 150–200 mg/kg/d divided q6h; max 12 g/d | |
| | | Adult: 2–12 g divided doses of 4–6 h | |
| Clindamycin | S. aureus, pneumococci, streptococci (not enterococci), and many B. fragilis strains | Pediatric[a,b] (full-term neonates, infants, children, adolescents): 40 mg/kg/d PO or IV or IM divided q6–8h; max dose 2.7 g/d | Considered an excellent agent for B. fragilis infections if isolate is susceptible |
| | | Adult: 600–900 mg divided doses of 6–8 h | |

*(continued)*

## TABLE 4-1    Antimicrobial Agents Commonly Used Initially in Acute Bone and Joint Infection (*continued*)

| Antibiotics | Usual Susceptible Organisms | Daily Dosage (IV Route) | Comments |
|---|---|---|---|
| Vancomycin | Methicillin-resistant staphylococci | Neonatal[a]: <br><br> Term infants >7 d: 5 mg/kg/dose IV q6h <br><br> Pediatric (>1 mo)[b]: 5 mg/kg/dose IV q6h <br><br> Adult: 15 mg/kg IV q12h | Preferred for Methicillin resistant Staphylococcus aureus (MRSA). Also an alternative for streptococci and enterococci in case of Penicillin (PCN) allergy or resistance |
| Daptomycin | Methicillin-resistant staphylococci and vancomycin-resistant enterococci | Neonatal[c]: N/A <br><br> Pediatric[c]: 6 mg/kg/d IV q24h <br><br> Adult: 6 mg/kg IV q24h | Alternative treatment for resistant organisms when vancomycin cannot be used |
| Penicillin G (aqueous) | Streptococci, PCN-susceptible pneumococci, gonococci, staphylococci, and enterococci | Neonatal[a] (≥1 kg body weight): <br><br> ≤7 d: 25,000–50,000 units/kg/dose q8h IV/IM <br><br> 8–28 d of age: 25,000–50,000 units/kg/dose q8h IV/IM <br><br> Pediatric (>1 mo of age): 250,000–400,000 units/kg/d divided q4–6h; maximum dose 24 million units per d <br><br> Adult: 12–24 million units of 4–6 h | Useful for open fractures contaminated with barnyard waste and for treatment of clostridia infection <br><br> (Consider adding gentamicin 1 mg/mg q8h for synergy for enterococci and streptococci with PCN MIC >0.5 μg/mL) |

| Ampicillin | Same as penicillin G; also *H. influenzae*, some strains of *E. coli*, *Proteus*, and *Salmonella* | Neonatal[a]: | *H. influenzae* now shows >20% ampicillin resistance in many areas. Therefore, empiric therapy must be with ceftriaxone or cefuroxime |
| | | ≤2 kg body weight: | |
| | | 8–28 d: 150 mg/kg/d divided q12h | |
| | | 29–60 d: 200 mg/kg/d divided q6h | |
| | | >2 kg body weight: | |
| | | ≤28 d: 150 mg/kg/d divided q8h | |
| | | 29–60 d: 200 mg/kg/d divided q6h | |
| | | Pediatric (>2 mo): 200–400 mg/kg/d divided q4–6h; maximum dose 12 g/d | |
| | | Adult: 8–12 g daily divided doses q4–6h | |
| Ceftriaxone | Select gram-negative organisms or mixed infections | Neonatal (≤1 mo)[a]: use cefotaxime if bilirubin is high or receiving calcium-containing IV solution | Generally reserved for resistant or mixed infections |
| | | Pediatric (>1 mo): 75–100 mg/kg/d divided q12–24h; max dose 4 g/d | |
| | | Adult: 2 g q24h | |

(continued)

| TABLE 4-1 | Antimicrobial Agents Commonly Used Initially in Acute Bone and Joint Infection (*continued*) | | |
|---|---|---|---|
| **Antibiotics** | **Usual Susceptible Organisms** | **Daily Dosage (IV Route)** | **Comments** |
| Cefepime | Gram-negative infections including *Pseudomonas aeruginosa* | Neonatal (≤1 mo)[a]: 60–100 mg/kg/d divided q12h<br><br>Pediatric (>1 mo): 100–150 mg/kg/d IV divided q8h; max dose 6 g/d<br><br>Adult: 2 g IV q12h | |
| Meropenem | Gram-negative infections including ESBL-producing *Pseudomonas aeruginosa* | Neonatal (≤1 mo)[a]:<br>≤7 d: 40 mg/kg/d IV divided q12h<br>>8–28 d: 60 mg/kg/d IV divided q8h<br><br>Pediatric (>1 mo): 60 mg/kg/d IV divided q8h<br><br>Adult: 1 g IV q8h | |
| Imipenem | Select gram-positive and gram-negative infections including *Pseudomonas aeruginosa* | Neonatal (≤1 mo)[a]:<br>≤7 d: 50 mg/kg/d IV divided q12h<br>8–28 d: 75 mg/kg/d IV divided q8h<br><br>Pediatric (>1 mo): 60–100 mg/kg/d divided q6h; max daily dose: 4000 mg/d<br><br>Adult: 500 mg IV q6h | |

| | | |
|---|---|---|
| Ceftazidime | Select gram-negative organisms including *Pseudomonas* or mixed infections | Neonatal (≤1 mo)[a]: <br><br> ≤7 d: 100 mg/kg/d divided q12h <br><br> 8–28 d: 150 mg/kg/d divided q8h <br><br> Pediatric: 125–150 mg/kg/d divided q8h; max 6 g/d <br><br> Adult: 1–2 g q8–12h | |
| Gentamicin | Empirical in combination regimen for gram negatives (neonates) or synergy for gram positives | Neonatal (≤1 mo)[a]: <br><br> ≤2 kg body weight <br><br> 0–28 d: 5 mg/kg/dose IV q36–48 h <br><br> >2 kg body weight: <br><br> ≤7 d: 4 mg/kg/dose IV q24h <br><br> 8–28 d: 4–5 mg/kg/dose IV q24h <br><br> Pediatric (>1 mo of age): 7.5 mg/kg/d IV divided q8h <br><br> Adults: Gentamicin can also be used at a lower dose (1 mg/kg IV q8h) for synergy with gram-positive bacterial infections, enterococci, and some streptococci | Usually not used for gram-negative infections in adults, only used for synergy for gram-positive infections |

(continued)

**TABLE 4-1  Antimicrobial Agents Commonly Used Initially in Acute Bone and Joint Infection (continued)**

| Antibiotics | Usual Susceptible Organisms | Daily Dosage (IV Route) | Comments |
|---|---|---|---|
| Tobramycin | | Neonatal (≤1 mo)[a]:<br><br>≤2 kg body weight<br><br>0–28 d: 5 mg/kg/dose IV q36–48 h<br><br>>2 kg body weight:<br><br>≤7 d: 4 mg/kg/dose IV q24h<br><br>8–28 d: 4–5 mg/kg/dose IV q24h<br><br>Pediatric (>1 mo of age): 6–7.5 mg/kg/d IV divided q8h<br><br>Adult: 3–7.5 mg/kg/d in three equal doses (dose adjusted based on peak and trough levels) can be given as a single daily dose | May be given either IV or IM. Renal function must be carefully checked, and therapy beyond 10 d must be administered cautiously because of potential nephrotoxicity and ototoxicity. May be synergistic with piperacillin against some strains of *P. aeruginosa*; also usually synergistic with penicillin against enterococci. Reduce dosage to 3 mg/kg/d as soon as clinically indicated. Follow with peak and trough serum levels if available |

[a]Neonatal and pediatric dosing in this table is taken from AAP Redbook 2018[41] and Nelson's Pediatric Antimicrobial Therapy 2019[42] and refers to non-CNS dosing. Complete workup must be done to rule out CNS infection in neonates with bone/joint infection with sepsis presentation. Please consult with a neonatologist, pediatric infectious diseases specialist, or pediatric pharmacist for neonatal dosing specific to each patient, as multiple factors including gestational age, birth weight, underlying conditions, risk assessment for CNS infection, and renal and hepatic function may affect optimal dosing. There is also inconsistency among the major published reference guidelines for dosages in newborns, and new pharmacokinetic-pharmacodynamic studies are emerging in neonates.[43]

[b]Dosing is from Liu et al. IDSA 2011 MRSA guideline.[44]

[c]Use only if there is no other option in children and with infectious diseases consultation; daptomycin is potentially neurotoxic in neonates, should not be used in patients <1 year of age, and is still under investigation in children for pharmacokinetics, safety, and efficacy.[38,41] Dosing listed is per IDSA 2011 MRSA guideline for alternative to vancomycin and clindamycin.

Adapted and modified from Hansen ST Jr, Ray CG. Antibiotics in orthopaedics. In: Kagan BM, ed. *Antimicrobial Therapy*. 3rd ed. WB Saunders; 1980, with permission.

**TABLE 4-2    Tentative Selection of Therapy When Organisms Are Not Immediately Identified**

| Situation | Organisms Suspected | Suggested Antibiotic Choice |
|---|---|---|
| **<3 mo** | | |
| Osteomyelitis and septic arthritis | S. aureus | Nafcillin or vancomycin, |
| | Group B streptococcus | plus |
| | Gram-negative enterics (E. coli, Serratia, K. pneumoniae, Proteus) | gentamicin or cefotaxime (for gram-negative enterics) |
| | Nosocomial: | or |
| | Coagulase-negative staphylococcus, | Vancomycin plus third- or fourth-generation cephalosporin if signs of sepsis or hospitalized in NICU for >1 week |
| | Pseudomonas (less common) | If concern for Pseudomonas, include cefepime or ceftazidime |
| **3 mo to 3 y** | | |
| Osteomyelitis and septic arthritis | S. aureus | Cefazolin (covers Methicillin sensitive Staphylococcus aureus (MSSA), streptococci; and Kingella) |
| | Kingella kingae | or |
| | Group A streptococcus | Clindamycin or Nafcillin (for MSSA, streptococci) |
| | S. pneumoniae and | plus |
| | H. influenzae (if incompletely immunized) | addition of a cephalosporin if not improving (for Kingella) |
| | | If incompletely immunized against Hib, include a third-generation cephalosporin |
| | | If MRSA risk factors are present, begin with vancomycin (or clindamycin if resistance is <10% in community and patient has signs of sepsis on presentation), plus a cephalosporin if not improving to cover Kingella |

*(continued)*

**TABLE 4-2    Tentative Selection of Therapy When Organisms Are Not Immediately Identified (continued)**

| | | |
|---|---|---|
| **>3 y** | | |
| Osteomyelitis and septic arthritis | S. aureus | Cefazolin or nafcillin or clindamycin (if coverage for MSSA is high in community) |
| | Group A streptococcus | |
| | S. pneumoniae (if incompletely immunized) | If MRSA risk factors are present, begin with vancomycin until susceptibility is known, or clindamycin if resistance is <10% in community and patient is not septic on presentation |
| **Adult** | | |
| Osteomyelitis | S. aureus | A cephalosporin (first- or third-generation agent) or nafcillin |
| | | Vancomycin if high risk for methicillin-resistant S. aureus (MRSA) |
| Septic arthritis | S. aureus | A cephalosporin or nafcillin (ceftriaxone if gonococcus is strongly suspected) |
| | | Vancomycin if high risk for MRSA |
| **Special considerations** | | |
| Chronic hemolytic disorders | | |
| Osteoarthritis | S. aureus | A cephalosporin (third generation if Salmonella is suspected) or vancomycin until sensitivity results are available |
| Septic arthritis | Pneumococci | |
| | Salmonella group[a] | |
| Infections following puncture wounds of the foot | P. aeruginosa | Cefepime or ceftazidime actually achieve better drug levels than aminoglycosides (gentamicin or tobramycin) |
| Infections following trauma or surgery | S. aureus | Broad-spectrum beta-lactam and vancomycin |
| | Streptococci | |
| | Gram-negative organisms | |

[a]Infections caused by Salmonella should be documented by culture and sensitivity testing before empirical treatment with agents such as ampicillin (or chloramphenicol) is initiated.

Adapted and modified from Hansen ST Jr, Ray CG. Antibiotics in orthopaedics. In: Kagan BM, ed. Antimicrobial Therapy. 3rd ed. WB Saunders; 1980, with permission.

I. **Adjunctive treatment.** Most orthopaedists believe that the healing process is aided by immobilizing the infected area. There is disagreement over casting or splinting. Undoubtedly, patients are more comfortable when the infected area is immobilized. If damage to the bone is significant, cast immobilization may be important to prevent a pathologic fracture. If damage to articular cartilage is suspected, motion of the involved joint is recommended after a brief 1- to 2-day period of immobilization.

J. **Surgical intervention.** Appropriate antibiotic treatment initiated within the first 48 hours of acute osteomyelitis or septic arthritis is usually satisfactory. However, early diagnosis is rarely the case. If treatment is initiated over 48 hours after onset, it is important to determine whether medical treatment alone is adequate. Err on the side of more aggressive operative drainage. If the patient has been on an appropriate antibiotic for more than 24 hours without significant resolution of pain and temperature, surgical intervention is indicated. Surgical principles in osteomyelitis include adequate drainage of infected and necrotic bone.[45] Debridement and removal of all hardware and flap soft-tissue closure and achieving stability of the bone are all important.

1. In a bone infection, metaphyseal or subperiosteal abscesses must be drained. If metaphyseal point tenderness is present, and there is doubt whether this represents significant metaphyseal or subperiosteal pus, it is safer to err on the side of a small surgical exploration or aspiration with a biopsy needle. If pus is encountered, open surgical drainage is indicated.

2. **Joints**

   a. In joint infections, satisfactory evacuation of pus can be achieved by needle aspiration. When the joint is easily visible and palpable, such as with the knee joint, repeated needle aspiration is usually adequate to keep the joint decompressed. Aspiration should be done with a 16–18G needle. Irrigation of the joint to ensure removal of as much cellular debris as possible is helpful.[14] The hip joint presents special problems.[14] The blood supply to the femoral head is intraarticular; hence, any increase in intracapsular pressure can deprive the femoral head of its circulation. Because hip joint effusions are not readily palpable, it is difficult to be certain that repeated aspirations will decompress the joint. For this reason, most authorities believe that immediate surgical drainage of a septic hip is indicated, and some believe that the shoulder should be treated similarly. The hip joint can be drained anteriorly between muscle planes or posteriorly with a muscle-splitting incision. The capsule and synovium are opened and drains are inserted.

   Arthroscopic lavage is an effective alternate for shoulder or knee infections. The possible exception to surgical drainage is in gonococcal arthritis because of differential virulence of the rapidly treated joint infection.[46]

   b. At times, the fibrin entering the joint as a transudate forms clots and isolates segments of the joint from decompression. Hypertrophy of synovium and adhesions may also affect the ability of the surgeon to decompress the joint adequately. Under these circumstances, it is advisable to debride the joint arthroscopically or with an open procedure. Joints most easily amenable to arthroscopic lavage are the knee, shoulder, and ankle.

K. Chronic osteomyelitis presents a different problem from acute infection. Acute infection in the earliest phase is primarily a medical disease, with surgical techniques used as an adjunct. In chronic infection, the primary treatment is surgical removal of all dead and poorly vascularized tissue. If this removal is properly done along with appropriate antibiotic therapy, it is possible to eradicate most sites of chronic osteomyelitis. The operation must be carefully planned because it often involves significant removal of bone and surrounding tissues. In the case of chronic joint infections, it may mean complete resection of the joint with the creation of a pseudarthrosis or an arthrodesis. Rotational muscle flaps or free-tissue transfer may be required to cover areas of viable but poorly covered bone. IV and oral antibiotics serve as valuable adjuncts, and consultation with an infectious diseases specialist is recommended early in the course. Patient quality of life can be profoundly impacted by chronic osteomyelitis[46]; treatment leading to resolution of the infection does improve this impact.

**L.** Gas gangrene

1. Gas gangrene can be a fatal process and can be prevented by thorough debridement and removal of all devitalized tissue, delayed wound closure when in doubt, and antibiotic treatment as recommended previously.

2. *Clostridium perfringens* infections carry a 65% overall mortality rate, which increases to 75% in infants and elderly patients. The diagnosis should be suspected when the patient is pale, weak, perspiring, and more tachycardic than the degree of fever warrants. The patient frequently complains of severe pain. Mental confusion and gas in the tissues are late signs, as are the characteristic mousy odor, jaundice, oliguria, and shock.

3. Other gas-producing species in addition to *C. perfringens* (10 isolated toxins) include *E. coli, Enterobacter aerogenes,* anaerobic streptococci, *B. fragilis,* and *K. pneumoniae.* Antitoxin does not appear to help much because it is neutralized as rapidly as it reaches muscle. Treatment consists of debridement and high doses of antibiotics. Penicillin is usually the best for the *C. perfringens* group; it should be given in amounts of 20–24 million units per day. Clindamycin or metronidazole is a good alternative antibiotic in patients who are allergic to penicillin. Some clostridia are resistant to clindamycin, making it necessary to check sensitivities carefully. Hyperbaric oxygen is only an adjunct to surgery. Its use allows the surgeon to save more tissue than might otherwise be possible, and it lowers the mortality rate slightly.

   Although exceedingly uncommon, group A streptococcal myonecrosis can have a similar course and result in death in a high percentage of cases. It must be treated with aggressive surgical debridement or amputation in addition to appropriate antibiotic therapy. Toxic shock syndrome has also been noted in orthopaedic patients and is caused by unique staphylococcal and streptococcal strains. Although toxic shock syndrome is also a surgical condition, it carries a more favorable prognosis. Necrotizing fasciitis can be caused by several bacterial types (most commonly group A streptococcus) and often requires debridement combined with appropriate antibiotic therapy. Infectious disease consultation is indicated for each of these infectious conditions.

**III. Summary**

**A.** Infections in the musculoskeletal system present special problems for treatment with antibiotics alone. Cartilage becomes avascular with age, tendon and ligaments are relatively hypovascular, and bone is vulnerable to situations that render it avascular. Because antibiotics can be effective only if they are delivered to the site of infection, every effort must be made to preserve a normal blood supply and normal joint fluid dynamics. The essentials of treatment are as follows:

1. Prompt diagnosis with identification of the bacteria through culture and with sensitivity for determining the appropriate antibiotic

2. Rapid initial treatment with the most effective bactericidal antibiotic

3. Constant evaluation to assess the need for surgical drainage of pus or removal of devitalized tissue

4. Antibiotic therapy by a route that ensures adequate blood levels and administration until the signs of infection, as manifested usually by a decreasing ESR and/or CRP, resolve completely

5. Judicious use of immobilization and traction to improve patient comfort and provide the best possible environment for primary healing
6. Adequate soft-tissue coverage of underlying bone and joint infections

**B.** The greatest benefit of antibiotics in musculoskeletal infection is in preventing the mortality and morbidity that result from chronic osteomyelitis and joint destruction from pyarthrosis. Even chronic infection can be controlled, and a satisfactory functional result is obtained in most patients by the use of surgery and appropriate antibiotics.

## REFERENCES

1. Lee YJ, Sadigh S, Mankad K, Kapse N, Rajeswaran G. The imaging of osteomyelitis. *Quant Imaging Med Surg.* 2016;6(2):184-198.
2. Pineda C, Vargas A, Rodríguez AV. Imaging of osteomyelitis: current concepts. *Infect Dis Clin North Am.* 2006;20(4):789-825.
3. Pineda C, Espinosa R, Pena A. Radiographic imaging in osteomyelitis: the role of plain radiography, computed tomography, ultrasonography, magnetic resonance imaging, and scintigraphy. *Semin Plast Surg.* 2009;23(2):80-89.
4. Harik NS, Smeltzer MS. Management of acute hematogenous osteomyelitis in children. *Expert Rev Anti Infect Ther.* 2010;8(2):175-181.
5. Cottias P, Tomeno B, Anract P, et al. Subacute osteomyelitis presenting as a bone tumor. A review of 21 cases. *Int Orthop.* 1997;21:243-248.
6. Schauwecker DS. The scintigraphic diagnosis of osteomyelitis. *AJR Am J Roentgenol.* 1992;158:9-18.
7. Restrepo S, Vargas D, Riascos R, et al. Musculoskeletal infection imaging: past, present, and future. *Curr Infect Dis Rep.* 2005;7(5):365-372.
8. Tang JS, Gold RH, Bassett LW, et al. Musculoskeletal infection of the extremities: evaluation with MR imaging. *Radiology.* 1988;166:205-209.
9. Tehranzadeh J, Wang F, Mesgarzadeh M. Magnetic resonance imaging of osteomyelitis. *Crit Rev Diagn Imaging.* 1992;33:495-534.
10. Unger E, Moldofsky P, Gatenby R, et al. Diagnosis of osteomyelitis by MR imaging. *AJR Am J Roentgenol.* 1988;150:605-610.
11. Pineda C, Vargas A, Rodríguez AV. Imaging of osteomyelitis: current concepts. *Infect Dis Clin North Am.* 2006;20(4):789-825.
12. Palestro CJ, Love C, Miller TT. Infection and musculoskeletal conditions: imaging of musculoskeletal infections. *Best Res Clin Rheumatol.* 2006;20(6):1197-1218.
13. Crosby LA, Powell DA. The potential value of the sedimentation rate in monitoring treatment outcome in puncture wound-related *Pseudomonas* osteomyelitis. *Clin Orthop Relat Res.* 1984;188:168-172.
14. Dagan R. Management of acute hematogenous osteomyelitis and septic arthritis in the pediatric patient. *Pediatr Infect Dis J.* 1993;12:88-92.
15. Frederiksen B, Christiansen P, Knudsen FU. Acute osteomyelitis and septic arthritis in the neonate, risk factors and outcome. *Eur J Pediatr.* 1993;152:577-580.
16. Unkila-Kallio L, Kallio MJ, Eskola J, et al. Serum C-reactive protein, erythrocyte sedimentation rate and white blood cell count in acute hematogenous osteomyelitis of children. *Pediatrics.* 1994;93:59-62.
17. Principi N, Esposito S. Kingella kingae infections in children. *BMC Infect Dis.* 2015;15:260.
18. Greenberg RN, Kennedy DJ, Reilly PM, et al. Treatment of bone, joint, and soft-tissue infections with oral ciprofloxacin. *Antimicrob Agents Chemother.* 1987;31:151-155.
19. Mader JT, Landon GC, Calhoun J. Antimicrobial treatment of osteomyelitis. *Clin Orthop Relat Res.* 1993;295:87-95.
20. Yagupsky P, Ben-Ami Y, Trefler R, Porat N. Outbreaks of invasive *Kingella kingae* infections in closed communities. *J Pediatr.* 2016;169:135-139.e1.
21. Chometon S, Benito Y, Chaker M, et al. Specific real-time polymerase chain reaction places *Kingella kingae* as the most common cause of osteoarticular infections in young children. *Pediatr Infect Dis J.* 2007;26(5):377-381.
22. Dartnell J, Ramachandran M, Katchburian M. Haematogenous acute and subacute paediatric osteomyelitis: a systematic review of the literature. *J Bone Joint Surg Br.* 2012;94(5):584-595.
23. Ross JJ, Saltzman CL, Carling P, et al. Pneumococcal septic arthritis: review of 190 cases. *Clin Infect Dis.* 2003;36:319-327.

24. Jefferies JM, Cooper T, Yam T, Clarke SC. *Pseudomonas aeruginosa* outbreaks in the neonatal intensive care unit—a systematic review of risk factors and environmental sources. *J Med Microbiol.* 2012;61(Pt 8):1052-1061.
25. Fernandez M, Carrol CL, Baker CJ. Discitis and vertebral osteomyelitis in children: an 18-year review. *Pediatrics.* 2000;105:1299-1304.
26. Fucs PM, Meves R, Yamada HH. Spinal infections in children: a review. *Int Orthop.* 2012;36(2):387-395. doi:10.1007/s00264-011-1388-2
27. Weissman S, Parker RD, Siddiqui W, et al. Vertebral osteomyelitis: retrospective review of 11 years experience. *Scan J Infect Dis.* 2014;46:193-199.
28. McHenry MC, Easley KA, Locker GA. Vertebral osteomyelitis: long-term outcome for 253 patients from 7 Cleveland-area hospitals. *Clin Infect Dis.* 2002;34:1342-1350.
29. Cushing AH. Diskitis in children. *Clin Infect Dis.* 1995;17:1-6.
30. Huddleston PM, Steckelberg JM, Hanssen AD, et al. Ciprofloxacin inhibition of experimental fracture healing. *J Bone Joint Surg Am.* 2000;82:161-173.
31. Malin JK, Patel NJ. Arthropathy and HIV infection. A muddle of mimicry. *Postgrad Med.* 1993;93:143-146, 149-150.
32. Shapiro ED, Gerber MA. Lyme disease. *Clin Infect Dis.* 2000;31:533-542.
33. Steere AC. Lyme disease. *N Engl J Med.* 2001;345:115-125.
34. Willis AA, Widmann RF, Flynn JM, et al. Lyme arthritis presenting as acute septic arthritis in children. *J Pediatr Orthop.* 2003;23:114-118.
35. Weinstein A, Britchkov M. Lyme arthritis and post-Lyme disease syndrome. *Curr Opin Rheumatol.* 2002;14:383-387.
36. Ostermann PA, Seligson D, Henry SL. Local antibiotic therapy for severe open fractures. A review of 1085 consecutive cases. *J Bone Joint Surg Br.* 1995;77:93-97.
37. Spellberg B, Lipsky BA. Systemic antibiotic therapy for chronic osteomyelitis in adults. *Clin Infect Dis.* 2012;54(3):393-407.
38. Castellazzi L, Mantero M, Esposito S. Update on the management of pediatric acute osteomyelitis and septic arthritis. *Int J Mol Sci.* 2016;17:E855.
39. Zaoutis T, Localio AR, Leckerman K, Saddlemire S, Bertoch D, Keren R. Prolonged intravenous therapy versus early transition to oral antimicrobial therapy for acute osteomyelitis in children. *Pediatrics.* 2009;123:636-642. doi:10.1542/peds.2008-0596
40. Keren R, Shah SS, Srivastava R, et al. Pediatric research in inpatient settings network. Comparative effectiveness of intravenous vs oral antibiotics for postdischarge treatment of acute osteomyelitis in children. *JAMA Pediatr.* 2015;169(2):120-128.
41. Kimberlin DW, Brady MT, Jackson MA. *Red Book: Report of the Committee on Infectious Diseases.* 31st ed. AAP Committee on Infectious Diseases; 2018.
42. Bradley JS, Nelson JD, Barnett E, et al. *Nelson's Pediatric Antimicrobial Therapy.* 25th ed. American Academy of Pediatrics; 2019.
43. Li HK, Rombach R, Zambellas R, et al. Oral versus intravenous antibiotics for bone and joint infection. *NEJM.* 2019;380:425-436.
44. Liem TBY, Slob EMA, Termote JUM, Wolfs TFW, Egberts ACG, Rademaker CMA. Comparison of antibiotic dosing recommendations for neonatal sepsis from established reference sources. *Int J Clin Pharm.* 2018;40(2):436-443.
45. Liu C, Bayer A, Cosgrove S, et al. Clinical practice guidelines by the Infectious Diseases Society of America for the treatment of methicillin-resistant *Staphylococcus aureus* infections in adults and children: executive summary. *Clin Infect Dis.* 2011;52(3):285-292.
46. Maffulli N, Papalia R, Zampogna B, Torre G, Albo E. The management of osteomyelitis in the adult. *The Surgeon.* 2016;14:345-360.
47. Lerner RK, Esterhai JL Jr, Polomano RC, et al. Quality of life assessment of patients with posttraumatic fracture nonunion, chronic refractory osteomyelitis and lower extremity amputation. *Clin Orthop Relat Res.* 1993;295:28-36.

# 5

# Acute Nontraumatic Joint Conditions

Christian M. Ogilvie

## I. History

Document the onset of the symptoms: Did the joint pain begin days, weeks, or months ago? Morning stiffness is important to differentiate inflammatory forms (rheumatoid arthritis [RA] and ankylosing spondylitis) from noninflammatory forms (degenerative joint disease) of arthritis. The character and duration of the pain are more important. Is the pain only associated with activity or is it present even at rest? Is only one joint involved or are multiple joints affected? Are they symmetrically involved? In the hands, the proximal finger joints are often involved in RA and the distal finger joints are more often involved in osteoarthritis[1] (Table 5-1). A thorough history of medical problems and social issues and a current review of systems are essential. One must consider possible exposure to infectious diseases and current systemic symptoms of illness when differentiating the possibilities.

## II. Examination

Check for fever because the temperature may be elevated with septic arthritis. Muscle wasting occurs more often with RA. Tenderness about the joint and

| TABLE 5-1 | History and Examination | | |
|---|---|---|---|
| History | Rheumatoid Arthritis | Septic Arthritis | Degenerative Joint Disease |
| Onset | Weeks | Day(s) | Months |
| Morning stiffness | ++ | — | — |
| Pain duration | Hours | Constant | Minutes |
| Pain with activity | ++ | +++ | ± |
| Number of joints involved | Multiple, symmetric | One (occasionally more) | Variable |
| Finger joint | Proximal | — | Distal |
| Examination | | | |
| Febrile | ± | ++ | 0 |
| Muscle wasting | ++ | 0 | + |
| Synovial tenderness | + | ++ | ± |
| Increased warmth | ± | ++ | 0 |
| Effusion | + | ++ | ± |
| Joint range of motion | ↓ | ↓↓↓ | ↓ |

+++, extremely important symptom or sign; ++, very important symptom or sign; +, important symptom or sign; ±, symptom or sign might or might not be present; 0, symptom or sign is not present; ↓, decreased; ↓↓↓, markedly decreased.

increased warmth are more indicative of inflammatory conditions. The examination should determine the presence of an effusion (fluid in the joint). Severe guarding against joint motion associated with pain is usually indicative of a septic condition (Table 5-1).

### III. Radiologic and Laboratory Data

**A. Radiologic findings.** Look for evidence of periarticular soft-tissue swelling, joint effusion, osteopenia, joint space narrowing, periarticular erosions, joint subluxation, and articular cartilage or bone destruction.[1] All of these findings are evidence of inflammatory (rheumatoid or septic) arthritis. In contrast, marginal osteophytes, subchondral cysts, joint space narrowing, and subchondral sclerosis are associated with osteoarthritis (Table 5-2). In the lower extremity, weight-bearing radiographs show joint space narrowing best, increasing the diagnostic value of the study.

**B. Laboratory data** (Table 5-3)

1. **Synovial fluid analysis involves assessing the following:**
   a. **Appearance (color)**
   b. **Clot (presence or absence)**
   c. **Viscosity**
   d. **Glucose** (compare with simultaneous serum glucose)
   e. **Cell count per cubic millimeter**
   f. **Differential cell count**
   g. The type of **crystals** that might be present in the joint fluid aspirate as evaluated under a polarizing light microscope
   h. **Gram stain and synovial fluid culture:** aerobic, anaerobic, fungal, acid-fast bacillus

2. Helpful **blood tests** include a complete blood count, erythrocyte sedimentation rate (ESR), C-reactive protein (CRP), uric acid, rheumatoid factor (RF), and anticitrullinated protein antibody (ACPA).

### IV. Differential Diagnosis of Acute Nontraumatic Joint Conditions (Table 5-4)[1-3]

**A. Rheumatoid arthritis** (Table 5-5)[4]

1. **History** reveals joint and tendon involvement that becomes more symmetric as the disease progresses. Females predominate at 2.5 to 1.[5]
2. **Examination** shows synovial thickening, joint tenderness, subcutaneous nodules, weakness associated with muscle wasting, and, often, systemic disease.

| TABLE 5-2 | Radiologic Findings | |
|---|---|---|
| **Rheumatoid Arthritis** | **Septic Arthritis** | **Degenerative Joint Disease** |
| *Early* | | |
| Periarticular soft-tissue swelling | Joint effusion | Joint space narrowing |
| Periarticular osteoporosis | — | Marginal osteophytes |
| *Late* | | |
| Joint space narrowing | Articular cartilage and bone destruction | Subchondral sclerosis |
| Periarticular erosions | — | Subcortical cysts |
| Articular cartilage and bone destruction | — | Marginal osteophytes |
| Joint subluxation secondary to ligamentous involvement | — | — |

| TABLE 5-3 | **Synovial Fluid Analysis** | | | |
| --- | --- | --- | --- | --- |
| Finding | Normal | Rheumatoid Arthritis | Septic Arthritis | Degenerative Joint Disease |
| Appearance | Clear | Cloudy | Turbid | Clear |
| Clinical viscosity test | High (fluid remains intact when slowly pulled between thumb and index finger) | Watery (fluid breaks into droplets easily) | Very watery | High |
| Glucose | Within 60% or more of serum glucose | Low | Very low | Normal |
| Cell count/mm$^3$ | 200 | 2,000–50,000 | Usually >50,000 | 2,000 |
| Differential cell count | Monos | 50/50 | Polys | Monos |

| TABLE 5-4 | **Differential Diagnosis of Inflammatory Polyarthritis** |
| --- | --- |

**A. RA**

**1.** Seropositive—female, symmetric joint and tendon involvement, synovial thickening, joint inflammation in phase, nodules, weakness, systemic reaction, erosions on radiogram, rheumatoid factor present, CH$_{50}$ level depressed in joint fluid that has 5,000–30,000 WBCs/mm$^3$, approximately 50%–80% polymorphs

**2.** Seronegative—either sex, symmetric joint and tendon involvement, joint inflammation in phase, little or no systemic reaction, usually no erosions radiographically, rheumatoid factor absent, CH$_{50}$ not depressed in joint fluid that has 3,000–20,000 WBCs/mm$^3$, approximately 20%–60% polymorphs

**B. Collagen–vascular**

**1.** SLE—female, symmetric joint distribution identical to RA, no erosions radiographically, noninflammatory joint fluid with good viscosity and mucin clot and 1,000–2,000 WBCs/mm$^3$, mostly small lymphocytes, mucosal lesions, rash, systemic reaction, renal involvement, neurologic disorders, blood disorders (e.g., leukopenia), immunologic phenomenon (false-positive serologic test for syphilis, anti-dsDNA antibody), antinuclear antibody (ANA), photosensitivity, serositis (pleurisy, pericarditis). Hochberg MC. Updating the American College of Rheumatology revised criteria for the classification of SLE. Hochberg MC. Updating the American College of Rheumatology revised criteria for the classification of systemic lupus erythematosus. *Arthritis Rheum.* 1997;40(9):1725.

**2.** Scleroderma—tight skin; Raynaud's phenomenon; resorption of digits; dysphagia; constipation; lung, heart, or kidney involvement; symmetric tendon contractures; little or no synovial thickening; radiographic calcinosis circumscripta; positive ANA with speckled or nucleolar pattern

**3.** Polymyositis (dermatomyositis)—proximal muscle weakness, pelvic and pectoral girdles, tender muscles, skin changes, typical nail and knuckle pad erythema, symmetric joint involvement, electromyographic evidence of combined myopathic and denervation pattern, abnormal muscle biopsy, elevated creatine phosphokinase

**4.** Mixed connective tissue disease—swollen hands, Raynaud's phenomenon, tight skin, symmetric joint and tendon involvement, possible joint erosions radiographically, positive ANA speckled pattern, antiribonucleoprotein antibody increased, good response to corticosteroid therapy given in anti-inflammatory doses

(continued)

| TABLE 5-4 | Differential Diagnosis of Inflammatory Polyarthritis (*continued*) |
|---|---|

**5.** Polyarteritis nodosa—symmetric involvement, diverse clinical picture of systemic disease, histologic diagnosis

### C. Rheumatic fever

Young (2–40 y), sore throat, group A streptococci, migratory arthritis, rash, heart or pericardial involvement, elevated antistreptolysin O titers. Migratory joint inflammation responds dramatically to aspirin treatment.

### D. Juvenile RA

Symmetric joint involvement, rash, fever, no rheumatoid factor, radiographic periostitis, erosions late, can recur in adults

### E. Psoriatic arthritis

Asymmetric boggy joint and tendon swelling, skin or nail lesions may not be prominent or may follow arthritis, DIP joints might be prominently involved, radiologic periostitis or erosions, no rheumatoid factor. $CH_{50}$ usually not depressed in inflammatory joint fluid with polymorph predominance

### F. Reiter's syndrome

Male, urethritis, iritis, conjunctivitis, asymmetric joints, lower extremity, nonpainful mucous membrane ulcerative lesion, balanitis circinata, keratosis blennorrhagica, weight loss. $CH_{50}$ increased in serum and in joint fluid with 5,000–30,000 leukocytes/mm³. Macrophages in joint fluid with 3–5 phagocytosed polymorphs (Reiter's cell)

### G. Gonorrheal arthritis

Migratory arthritis or tenosynovitis fully settling in one or more joints or tendons, either sex, primary focus urethra, female genitourinary tract, rectum, oropharynx, skin lesions, vesicles, gram-negative diplococci on smear but not on culture of vesicular fluid, positive culture at primary site, blood, or joint fluid

### H. Polymyalgia rheumatic

Elderly patient (>50 y), symmetric pelvic or pectoral girdle complaints without loss of strength, morning stiffness of long duration, fatigue prominent, weight loss, joints can be involved, especially shoulders, sternoclavicular joints, knees, sedimentation rate markedly elevated, fibrinogen always elevated, alpha 2 and gamma globulin elevation, anemia, response to low-dose (10–20 mg) prednisone, serum creatine phosphokinase normal, elevated alkaline phosphatase (liver)

### I. Crystal induced

**1.** Gout—symmetric arthritis, flexion contractures, prior history of acute attacks, tophi, joint inflammation out of phase, systemic corticosteroid treatment for RA, hyperuricemia, monosodium urate monohydrate crystals in joint fluid

**2.** Pseudogout—symmetric arthritis; flexion contractures; metacarpophalangeal, wrist, elbow, shoulder, hips, knees, and ankles; prior acute attacks (sometimes); joint inflammation out of phase; calcium pyrophosphate dihydrate crystals in joint fluid

### J. Other

Amyloid arthropathy, peripheral arthritis of inflammatory bowel disease, tuberculosis, subacute bacterial endocarditis, viral arthritis

DIP, distal interphalangeal; RA, rheumatoid arthritis; SLE, systemic lupus erythematosus; WBC, white blood cell. Modified from McCarty DJ. Differential diagnosis of arthritis: analysis of signs and symptoms. In: McCarty DJ, ed. *Arthritis and Allied Conditions*. 10th ed. Lea & Febiger; 1985:51-52.

| TABLE 5-5 | 2010 American College of Rheumatology/European League Against Rheumatism Classification for RA | |
|---|---|---|
| For newly presenting patients: | | |
| 1. Who have at least one joint with definite clinical synovitis (swelling) | | |
| 2. With the synovitis not better explained by another disease | | |
| Criteria for definite RA is a score of >6/10 after adding categories A–D | | Score |
| A. *Joint involvement* | | |
| 1 Large joint | | 0 |
| 2–10 Large joints | | 1 |
| 1–3 Small joints (with or without involvement of large joints) | | 2 |
| 4–10 Small joints (with or without involvement of large joints) | | 3 |
| >10 Joints (at least 1 small joint) | | 5 |
| B. *Serology (at least 1 test is needed for classification)* | | |
| Negative RF and negative ACPA | | 0 |
| Low-positive RF or low-positive ACPA | | 2 |
| High-positive RF or high-positive ACPA | | 3 |
| C. *Acute-phase reactants* | | |
| Normal CRP and normal ESR | | 0 |
| Abnormal CRP or abnormal ESR | | 1 |
| D. *Duration of symptoms* | | |
| <6 wk | | 0 |
| ≥6 wk | | 1 |

ACPA, anticitrullinated protein antibody; CRP, C-reactive protein; ESR, erythrocyte sedimentation rate; RA, rheumatoid arthritis; RF, rheumatoid factor.
From Alehata D, Neogi T, Silman AJ, et al. 2010 Rheumatoid arthritis classification criteria: an American College of Rheumatology/European League Against Rheumatism collaborative initiative. *Ann Rheum Dis*. 2010;69:1580-1588, with permission.

3. **Radiographs and laboratory data show that erosions are usually present, but RF is present in only 75% of patients.** Radiographs are often normal in acute forms of RA except for signs of swelling or periarticular osteopenia. Joint fluid contains 2,000 to 50,000 white blood cells (WBCs) per mm, approximately 40% to 80% of which are polymorphonuclear leukocytes. ACPA is more likely to be positive than RF in early disease.

B. **Osteoarthritis** (nonerosive degenerative joint disease)
1. **History** reveals a middle-aged or elderly patient unless the condition follows trauma.
2. **Examination** reveals that angulatory deformities and osteophytes are frequently present in the later stages of the disease.
3. **Radiographs** show narrowing of the cartilage space associated with marginal osteophytes. There is often subchondral bone sclerosis and occasionally subchondral cysts, which accompany these findings in the weight-bearing joints.

**C. Crystal-induced arthritis** (Table 5-6)
  1. **Gouty arthritis**
     a. The patient may report a history of similar attacks.
     b. **Examination** can show redness and warmth over the affected joint, typically the first metatarsophalangeal joint. Later, symmetric arthritis with contractures and tophi (subcutaneous crystal deposits) may develop.
     c. **Laboratory findings** include hyperuricemia and synovial fluid containing monosodium urate monohydrate crystals. The crystals, which are seen by compensated polarized light microscopy (sometimes by ordinary light microscopy), are negatively birefringent, needle-shaped rods.
  2. **Pseudogout**
     a. **History** sometimes reveals previous acute attacks.
     b. **Examination** discloses a symmetric arthritis with frequent contractures of the metacarpophalangeal, wrist, elbow, shoulder, hip, knee, and ankle joints. Radiographs may reveal the presence of calcium deposits in cartilage or, less often, in ligaments, meniscus, and joint capsules (chondrocalcinosis). The knee is the most common site. Although chondrocalcinosis has been classically associated with pseudogout, this condition is also seen with a high frequency in hyperparathyroidism, hemochromatosis, hemosiderosis, hypophosphatasia, hypomagnesemia, hypothyroidism, gout, neuropathic joints, and aging.[5]
     c. **Laboratory** analysis of the synovial fluid reveals calcium pyrophosphate dihydrate crystals that are regularly shaped and weakly positively birefringent but have a different extinction angle compared with that of urate crystals.
**D. Inflammatory polyarthritis** other than RA (Table 5-4)
  1. **Systemic lupus erythematosus** (SLE)
     a. **History** most commonly reveals symmetric joint distribution identical to that of RA in a female patient. Hair loss and Raynaud's symptoms (vasospasm of digital arteries) are common.
     b. **Examination** may disclose rash (facial erythema), mucosal lesions, serositis, and renal (hypertension and hematuria or edema) and brain (altered mental status, focal neurologic deficits) involvement. Joint involvement of the hands and wrists is most common followed by the knee.
     c. **Laboratory evaluation** with a CBC commonly shows anemia (40%), leukopenia (20%), and thrombocytopenia (30%). A depressed serum C3 and C4 and elevated antinuclear antibody (95% sensitive), anti-dsDNA antibody (70% sensitive), and anti-Sm antibody (30% sensitive, highly specific) are found. Antiphospholipid antibodies present in 50% of lupus cases. Test should also be done to check kidney function.[6] Joint fluid is noninflammatory with normal viscosity and mucin, and 1,000 to 2,000 WBCs per mm, which are mostly lymphocytes. The clinical viscosity test is considered normal or high if the fluid remains intact when slowly stretched between the examiner's thumb and index finger. A good mucin clot is one that occurs after a few drops of glacial acetic acid are added to a supernatant of centrifuged joint fluid and a dense, white precipitate forms.
  2. **Juvenile rheumatoid arthritis** (JRA)
     a. **History** shows symmetric joint involvement. The illness can recur in the adult. Short stature and limb length irregularity generally accompany the most severe forms because the physes are affected by the inflammatory process. Patients with systemic onset (10%) have intermittent

**TABLE 5-6    Differential Diagnosis of Inflammatory Monoarthritis**

**A. Crystal induced**

1. **Gout**—male, lower extremity, previous attack, nocturnal onset, precipitated by medical illness or surgery, response to colchicine, hyperuricemia, sodium urate crystals in joint fluid with polymorphs predominating, and WBCs 10,000–60,000/mm$^3$

2. **Pseudogout**—elderly, knee or other large joint, previous attack, precipitated by medical illness or surgery, flexion contractures, chondrocalcinosis on radiography, calcium pyrophosphate dihydrate crystals in joint fluid with polymorphs predominating, and WBCs 5,000–60,000/mm$^3$

3. **Calcific tendonitis or equivalent**—extraarticular, tendon or capsule of larger joints, previous attack same or another area, calcification on radiography, chalky or milky material aspirated from area, polymorphs with phagocytosed ovoid bodies microscopically

**B. Palindromic rheumatism**

Middle-aged or elderly male, very sudden onset, little systemic reaction, previous attacks, positive rheumatoid factors, little or no residual chronic joint inflammation, olecranon bursal enlargement

**C. Infectious arthritis**

1. **Septic**—severe inflammation, primary septic focus, drug or alcohol abuse, joint fluid with polymorphs predominating, WBCs 50,000–300,000/mm$^3$ (pus), infectious agents identified on smear and culture, or bacterial antigens identified in joint fluid. Lyme disease must be considered in the differential where exposure to tick vector is possible

2. **Tubercular**—primary focus, drug or alcohol abuse, marked joint swelling for long period, joint fluid with polymorphs predominating, acid-fast organisms on smear and culture

3. **Fungal**—similar to tuberculosis

4. **Viral**—antecedent or concomitant systemic viral illness, joint fluid can be of inflammatory or noninflammatory type, either mononuclear or polymorphonuclear leukocytes may predominate

**D. Other**

1. **Tendonitis**—as in **A.3** but without radiologic calcification, antecedent trauma, including repetitive motion

2. **Bursitis**—as above, but inflamed area more diffuse, antecedent trauma

3. **JRA**—one or both knees swollen in preteenager or teenager without systemic reaction, no erosions, mildly inflammatory joint fluid with some polymorphs

JRA, juvenile rheumatoid arthritis; WBC, white blood cell.
From McCarty DJ. Differential diagnosis of arthritis: analysis of symptoms. In: McCarty DJ, ed. *Arthritis and Allied Conditions*. 10th ed. Lea & Febiger; 1985:50, with permission.

fever of at least 3 days and a rash. Polyarticular onset (five or more joints) comprises 40% of patients.[7] There is a very high proportion of cervical spine involvement in patients with JRA. The prevalence of JRA has been estimated to be between 57 and 113 per 100,000 children younger than 16 years in the United States.[7]

b. **Examination** may reveal a rash and fever. Cardiac, renal, and ocular abnormalities may be present. Eye involvement occurs in 30% to 50% of early-onset JRA patients,[7] with anterior uveitis in 20% of those with pauciarticular disease (one to four joints involved in the first 6 months).[7]

c. **Laboratory tests** show radiologic periostitis with erosions later in the course of disease. RF, ACPA, and/or antinuclear antibody may be present. Other causes of arthritis in the child or adolescent must be excluded.

**E. Septic arthritis**

1. **Bacterial**

a. **History** may indicate drug or alcohol abuse and systemic illness (e.g., diabetes, chronic renal failure, or poor nutrition).

b. **Examination** can reveal severe inflammation and often a primary septic focus. Severe splinting (autoprotection by muscle spasm) of the joint is present, and pain is associated with passive motion.

c. **Laboratory tests** show a purulent joint fluid with polymorphonuclear leukocytes predominating (WBCs: 50,000 to 300,000 per mm$^3$). The infectious agent may be identified on smear or culture. Synovial glucose is less than 60% of a concurrent serum glucose. The ESR and CRP are elevated. Serial blood cultures obtained before antibiotic therapy often grow the infecting organism.

2. **Tubercular and fungal**

a. **History** may reveal a focus, chronic immunodeficiency (human immunodeficiency virus [HIV] or acquired immunodeficiency syndrome [AIDS]), drug or alcohol abuse, or poor nutrition.

b. **Examination** shows marked chronic joint swelling.

c. **Laboratory tests** reveal predominating polymorphonuclear leukocytes with acid-fast organisms present on smear and culture.

3. **Viral**

a. **History** often indicates antecedent or concomitant systemic viral illness.

b. **Laboratory analysis** of joint fluid can mimic inflammatory or noninflammatory conditions. Either mononuclear or polymorphonuclear leukocytes can predominate.

**F. Arthritis associated with infectious agents**

1. **Reiter syndrome**

a. **History** often reveals a sexually active man (chlamydia is the most common organism identified), with urethritis and conjunctivitis accompanying the arthritis. Patients have an equivocal response to anti-inflammatory drugs.

b. **Examination** often reveals urethritis, iritis, conjunctivitis, and nonpainful mucous membrane ulcerative lesions, with asymmetric arthritis of the joints in the lower extremities or back. Radiographs may show an asymmetric sacroiliitis as well as isolated involvement of the spine ("skip" areas). Heel pain is a commonly associated feature of the presentation.

c. **Laboratory data.** The joint fluid has 5,000 to 30,000 leukocytes per mm with macrophages that contain three to five phagocytosed polymorphonuclear leukocytes (so-called Reiter cell). Measurement of HLA-B27 antigen is not very useful.[7]

2. **Rheumatic fever**
   a. **History** reveals a sore throat, fever, rash, and migratory joint pain that responds dramatically to aspirin treatment in younger individuals (that are beyond the ages of Reye's syndrome).
   b. **Examination** shows a rash as well as heart (murmur) or pericardial (friction rub) involvement.
   c. **Laboratory tests** result in group A streptococci isolated on throat cultures and an elevated antistreptolysin O titer.
3. **HIV infection.** Migratory arthralgia and myalgia with accompanying muscle weakness are features of this disease. Radiographic changes are nonspecific.

G. **Inflammatory spondyloarthropathy** (Table 5-7)
   1. **Ankylosing spondylitis**
      a. **History** usually reveals clinical sacroiliitis in a young adult or adolescent male patient. A positive family history is often present. A good response to anti-inflammatory agents is common.
      b. **Examination** reveals limitation of spinal motion, uveitis, and diminished chest expansion. A positive Patrick's test indicative of sacroiliac involvement is typically present.
      c. **Laboratory evidence** of radiologic sacroiliitis and smooth, symmetric spinal ligamentous calcification is present, often with complete ankylosis (the "bamboo spine") and no skip areas. The HLA-B27 antigen should be present.[5]
   2. **Psoriatic arthritis**
      a. **Examination** shows asymmetric boggy joint and tendon sheath swelling. Skin or nail (pitting) lesions are generally present. The distal interphalangeal (DIP) joints of the hand are frequently involved.
      b. **Radiologic** periostitis, cortical erosions, or both can be seen along with spinal asymmetric sacroiliitis and isolated vertebral ankylosis (skip areas). The "pencil-in-cup" deformity is typically seen in the DIP joints of the hand. No RF is found. There is polymorphonuclear leukocytic predominance in the joint field.

| TABLE 5-7 | Differential Diagnosis of Inflammatory Spondyloarthropathy |
|---|---|
| **A. Ankylosing spondylitis**—male, symmetric sacroiliitis clinically and radiologically, limitation of spinal motion, uveitis, smooth symmetric spinal ligamentous calcification, ankylosis often complete, no skip areas, family history, HLA-B27 antigen often present, good response to anti-inflammatory drugs | |
| **B. Reiter's syndrome**—male with urethritis, skin-eye-heel, asymmetric peripheral joint involvement, sacroiliitis often asymmetric and skip areas of involvement in the spine, coarse asymmetric syndesmophytes in the spine, ankylosis incomplete and asymmetric, HLA-B27 often positive, equivocal response to anti-inflammatory drugs | |
| **C. Psoriatic spondylitis**—skin or peripheral joints involved, asymmetric sacroiliitis, skip areas, may be ankylosing, HLA-B27 often present | |
| **D. Inflammatory bowel disease**—sacroiliitis, often symmetric, ankylosing, bowel disease may be silent, spinal inflammation, does not vary with and is not responsive to treatment directed at bowel inflammation unlike peripheral arthritis, HLA-B27 often present | |
| **E. Other**—infection (bacterial tuberculous, fungal), osteochondritis, multiple epiphysitis in young adult | |

From McCarty DJ. Differential diagnosis of arthritis: analysis of symptoms. In: McCarty DJ, ed. *Arthritis and Allied Conditions.* 10th ed. Lea & Febiger; 1985:52, with permission.

3. **Spondyloarthropathy secondary to inflammatory bowel disease**
   a. **History** may not reveal bowel disease as a prominent feature, which can be subclinical.
   b. Bowel disease is found on **diagnostic evaluation**.
   c. **Laboratory tests** show radiologic evidence of sacroiliitis that is often symmetric and ankylosing.

## V. Treatment (Table 5-8)

### A. Rheumatoid arthritis[8]

1. **Nonsteroidal anti-inflammatory drugs** (NSAIDs) vary in cost but none is clearly superior in efficacy. Some patients simply cannot tolerate the side effects of certain NSAIDs and may find that only certain others are efficacious. Physicians should educate their patients as to the potential adverse effects of any medication. The treating physician may need to experiment with various anti-inflammatory medications before finding which preparation is best suited for the individual patient.

| TABLE 5-8 | Treatment | |
|---|---|---|
| **Rheumatoid Arthritis** | **Septic Arthritis** | **Degenerative Joint Disease** |
| 1. Drugs<br>  a. NSAIDs<br>  b. Methotrexate<br>  c. Hydroxychloroquine<br>  d. Sulfasalazine<br>  e. Steroids<br>  f. TNFi or non-TNF biologics<br>  g. Synthetic small molecule | 1. Antibiotics. Cefazolin (Kefzol) or nafcillin (Nafcil or Unipen) with gentamicin (Garamycin) or tobramycin (Nebcin) until the culture and sensitivity results are obtained, followed by specific antibiotic therapy | 1. Acetaminophen, anti-inflammatory agents<br>2. Support by bracing and other means<br>3. Physical therapy<br>  a. Heat<br>  b. Exercises |
| 2. Prophylactic synovectomy. If done, usually should follow 6 mo of medical management (Do not do if there is radiologic evidence of joint destruction manifested by a severe loss of cartilaginous space) | 2. Surgery. Operative debridement and irrigation of the joint, followed by appropriate drainage | 4. Injection treatments<br>  a. Steroids<br>  b. Lubrication: hyaluronic acid compounds |
| 3. Joint debridement and synovectomy (for pain relief only) | | 5. Surgery<br>  a. Debridement<br>  b. Osteotomy<br>  c. Partial or complete joint replacement<br>  d. Occasionally, arthrodesis |
| 4. Partial or complete joint replacement | | |
| 5. Arthrodesis | | |

NSAID, nonsteroidal anti-inflammatory drug; TNF, tumor necrosis factor.

    a. **Aspirin** is inexpensive but more gastrointestinal (GI) side effects may be seen than in other NSAIDs. Enteric-coated preparations may limit the dyspepsia but do not alter the risk of GI bleeding. A usual dose of enteric-coated aspirin is 975 mg QID. Tinnitus must be monitored in all patients receiving aspirin-containing compounds; it is an early sign of salicylate toxicity.

    b. **Other nonsteroidal, nonaspirin anti-inflammatory medications** are more convenient, but more expensive. Patients who take these medications long term should have biannual laboratory work to look for adverse hepatic, renal, hematopoietic, and other reactions. Physicians prescribing these medications should know their cost. For example, a 30-day supply (60 tablets) of generic naproxen, 500 mg (prescription or over the counter) costs at little as $7, whereas a 30-day supply of an over-the-counter brand name form of the same drug (Naprosyn) costs the patient about $190. The dosage of any anti-inflammatory drug should be the lowest possible that is effective in relieving symptoms. There are several classes of these drugs, including cyclooxygenase (COX-2) inhibitors, which have a decreased incidence of GI ulceration and are equally effective.[9] NSAID therapy is sufficient only for mild arthritis.

2. **Nonbiologic Disease-Modifying Antirheumatic Drugs (DMARDs)** may be used alone but are commonly used in combination with other DMARDs without an increase in toxicity in many cases.

    a. **Methotrexate (MTX)** is the first-line DMARD with results noticeable as early as 1 month after starting. Common side effects include stomatitis, anorexia, nausea, and cramps. Marrow suppression occurs at even small doses, and so blood counts must be checked regularly. Renal elimination requires creatinine clearance >30 mL per min.

    b. **Leflunomide (Arava)** can be used in place of MTX or in patients who did not tolerate or respond to MTX.

    c. **Sulfasalazine.** Effective but not well tolerated secondary to nausea, anorexia, and rash.

    d. **Hydroxychloroquine** (Plaquenil) is used in mild RA often with other medications. It may take up to 6 months to achieve a result. Rare retinal toxicity can be avoided if the drug stopped upon noticing visual disturbance or a question of eye toxicity, and if doses are kept under 6.5 mg/kg/day. Have an ophthalmologist follow the patient. Other effects are GI upset, skin rash, weight loss, peripheral neuritis, and convulsions.

    e. **Gold** is often effective for the treatment of rheumatoid and psoriatic arthritis; however, it is no longer considered to be the first-line therapy. The injectable forms are by far the most effective. The most common toxic reactions to injectable gold are stomatitis, dermatitis, and proteinuria. Less common side effects include leukopenia, thrombocytopenia, and, rarely, enterocolitis, pneumonitis, and aplastic anemia.[8]

    f. **Azathioprine**, a purine analog with immunosuppressive activity, has been shown to be effective in RA; it should be prescribed by rheumatologists.

3. **Biologic DMARDs**

    a. **Tumor necrosis factor (TNF) inhibitors** etanercept (Enbrel), infliximab (Remicade), adalimumab (Humira), golimumab (Simponi), and certolizumab (Cimzia) bind TNF, blocking its activity. They act more quickly and may be more effective at protecting joints from damage than the nonbiologic DMARDs. Rarely, there have been cases of serious infections, and the cost (tens of thousands of US dollars per year) must be considered. They have also been shown to be useful in combination therapy with MTX.[8]

b. **Non-TNF biologics** are often used with MTX but not with a second biologic DMARD. Rituximab (Rituxan) is an antibody against the B-cell surface antigen CD20. Abatacept (Orencia) is an engineered protein that blocks T-cell activation. Tocilizumab (Actemra) binds interleukin-6 receptors.[8]

4. **Corticosteroids** taken orally are frequently used in short courses and are used chronically in some patients. They are not considered to be DMARDs by most rheumatologists and have significant complications with extended use.

   a. **Usage**
      i. **Establish a specific diagnosis before treatment** with steroids.
      ii. **Adjust the dosage** to the situation. For RA, start with 10 to 20 mg to control symptoms, then taper over 2 to 4 weeks to the **lowest** tolerated dose (usually no more than 510 mg per day), and try not to exceed 10 mg per 24 hours. For SLE crisis, one might start with 60 mg in a 24-hour period.
      iii. Although more than 20 generic glucocorticosteroids are available, most rheumatologists have settled on **prednisone as the standard**.
      iv. **Monitor serum electrolytes and glucose** because steroids **cause** increased excretion of sodium and potassium and worsening blood glucose control in diabetics.
      v. **Administer** the steroid **once each morning** to minimize the effect on the pituitary–adrenal axis. If there is good control of the **inflammatory** process, use alternate-day therapy.
      vi. Obtain a **baseline eye examination** before starting long-term **therapy**. Steroids can cause cataracts and increased intraocular pressure.
      vii. Beware of **suppressed reaction to infection** as a complicating factor, especially if the patient's general condition is deteriorating while he or she is taking steroids.
      viii. With long-term therapy, be sure to recognize and manage complications of the systemic rheumatic disease as opposed to the **iatrogenic complications** of long-term steroid use, which are managed differently.
      ix. Patients should always **carry information** that they are on steroids.
      x. **Supplemental increased doses** are necessary when stress occurs, even minor stress such as a tooth extraction.

   b. **Undesirable effects**
      i. **Steroid diabetes** that is insulin resistant, but without ketosis or acidosis
      ii. **Muscle wasting** secondary to a negative nitrogen **balance**
      iii. **Buffalo hump** and **round face**
      iv. Sodium retention that results in **edema** (especially important for patients with heart disease)
      v. **Hirsutism** and occasional **alterations in menstrual function** in women secondary to adrenal atrophy
      vi. **Peptic ulcer disease** with possible **perforation** and abscess
      vii. **Suppressed wound healing**
      viii. **Osteoporosis** and avascular necrosis of the femoral or humeral head. Pathologic fractures are often associated. Calcium and vitamin D supplementation are recommended. Secondary osteoporosis may be prevented by bisphosphonates or teriparatide.[8]
      ix. **Lymphocytosis** and occasionally a **leukemoid** reaction

x. **Subcutaneous hemorrhages and acne**
xi. **Central nervous system changes** such as psychosis, seizures, and insomnia at higher dose
xii. **Immunosuppression** with **increased** risk of infections, candida, herpes zoster, and so on

5. **Surgical treatment**
   a. **Synovectomy**, if done, should follow at least 6 months of nonoperative management. This prophylactic procedure should not be performed if radiologic evidence of joint destruction manifested by a severe loss of cartilaginous space exists.
   b. There is still a place for **joint debridement** and synovectomy (open or arthroscopic) in patients with significant joint pain, but not enough joint destruction to justify surgical joint knee replacement. Arthroscopic synovectomy has been shown to be effective in various joints.
   c. **Joint replacement** may be necessary. The most common joints replaced in the patient with inflammatory arthritis are knee and hip, followed by shoulder, metacarpophalangeal, elbow, wrist, and ankle.
   d. Very rarely, **arthrodesis** is indicated, especially with ankle involvement.
   e. **Forefoot surgery** is frequently required and most commonly consists of first metatarsophalangeal joint arthrodesis combined with lesser metatarsophalangeal joint resection with claw toe release.

**B. Osteoarthritis**
1. Medical treatment consists of acetaminophen or **NSAID preparations**. Because of safety concerns with NSAIDs, acetaminophen is considered the first-line agent.[2] Dietary supplements may help pain in the short term pain but the quality of evidence is poor.[10] See V.A.1 for a more complete discussion.
2. Various **braces** are available to offer joint support (see also **Chapter 7**). Simple neoprene sleeves for the knee or elbow are useful. For unicompartmental knee arthritis, braces that "unload" the diseased compartment may be effective.[11]
3. **Physical therapy** can be helpful, especially in providing exercises to maintain muscle tone. Deep heat treatments provide symptomatic relief. The most effective therapy is patient-directed home therapy, which emphasizes maintaining strength and motion with low-impact exercise routines. Prolonged outpatient therapy is expensive and of limited value.
4. **Weight loss** is extremely useful for overweight patients with osteoarthritis. This may seem obvious in the weight-bearing joints of the lower extremity because of excessive force on the joints. Still, it is often neglected. In addition, there is increasing evidence that obesity is associated with an increase in osteoarthritis of the upper extremity, suggesting a systemic effect such as through inflammatory mediators.
5. Intraarticular steroid injections are helpful. The options available are listed in **V.C.2.b.** (pseudogout treatment). Injection of hyaluronic acid compounds (Euflexxa, Hyalgan, Orthovisc, Supartz, Synvisc) has been proven to be efficacious. This typically requires serial injections given 1 week apart over either 3 or 5 weeks, although a single-dose injection is available. The therapy has the same effectiveness as oral anti-inflammatory therapy.[12]
6. Various **surgical procedures** offer relief of joint pain and improved function. These include the following:
   a. **Debridement**, generally arthroscopic
   b. **Osteotomy** for varus malalignment of the knee to move the weight-bearing axis into the lateral, more normal compartment
   c. Partial or complete **joint resurfacing or replacement**

    d. Occasionally, **joint arthrodesis**. This is generally reserved for use in the previously septic joint.

    e. Autologous chondrocyte transplantation is a technique that may be used selectively for the management of focal traumatic articular cartilage defects. It is not indicated for diffuse osteoarthritis of the knee.[13]

## C. Crystal-induced arthritis

  1. **Gouty arthritis**[14]

    a. **Acute attacks** may be provoked by surgery or trauma or other systemic illnesses. They generally respond to the following agents:

      i. **Anti-inflammatory drugs** (NSAIDs or corticosteroids) should be started quickly and tapered when symptoms resolve.

      ii. **Colchicine**, one 0.5-mg tablet two to four times a day with a maximum dose per episode of 6 mg. Intravenous colchicine has a 2% mortality rate and should be avoided in elderly patients and patients with renal disease.

    b. **Prophylactic treatment** with colchicine, NSAID, or prednisolone for **3 to 6 months** after starting urate-lowering therapy. Consultation with a rheumatologist is advised.

    c. A xanthine oxidase inhibitor such as **allopurinol** (Zyloprim) works by lowering the uric acid pool of the body. Doses of 100 to 300 mg per day PO is common, with a maximum dose of 900 mg. The physician should be aware of the serious and possibly fatal adverse reactions to allopurinol, including agranulocytosis, exfoliative dermatitis, acute vasculitis, and hepatotoxicity. It is generally recommended that these agents be initiated only after resolution of an attack of gout.

    d. **Uricosuric agents:** Probenecid and sulfinpyrazone. These agents increase the amount of uric acid excreted in the urine, so their use can be associated with uric acid renal calculi. As with allopurinol, the therapy should be initiated after resolution of the acute attack.

      i. **Probenecid** (Benemid), 0.5 mg PO QID up to 2 g per day

      ii. **Sulfinpyrazone** (Anturane), 100 mg PO BID up to QID.

    e. Recommendations for **managing hyperuricemia**.

      i. **Confirm** the elevated serum uric acid by repeating the test.

      ii. **Determine** whether the condition is **secondary** to drugs or **blood** dyscrasia. One should rule out renal disease with a serum creatinine and 24-hour serum uric acid excretion test. If uric acid excretion is greater than 1 g per 24 hours, treat the hyperuricemia if symptomatic. If renal disease is present, allopurinol is first line therapy.

      iii. **Discuss dietary recommendation** to limit foods rich in purines, such as certain beef and fish.

      iv. **Generally withhold therapy** unless there has been one acute attack of gouty arthritis.

      v. **Rule out** hyperuricemia secondary to a lymphoproliferative or myeloproliferative disease.

      vi. Do not treat hyperuricemia secondary to **thiazide diuretics**.

  2. **Pseudogout**

    a. **Differentiate** pseudogout from acute gouty arthritis by joint fluid examination for specific crystals.

    b. Consider **aspirating** the joint fluid or **injecting** insoluble steroids intraarticularly using 0.1 mL for small joints and up to 1 to 2 mL for most large joints. The types of steroids useful for this application are as follows:

      i. **Hydrocortisone** acetate, 25 to 50 mg per mL

      ii. **Prednisolone** tertiary butyl acetate, 20 mg per mL

      iii. **Triamcinolone** hexacetonide (Aristospan), 5 and 20 mg per mL

        iv. **Betamethasone** acetate and sodium phosphate (Celestone), 6 mg per mL

        v. **Methylprednisolone** acetate (Depo-Medrol), 20 and 40 mg per mL

    c. **Colchicine** may provide dramatic relief.

    d. Many patients respond to **anti-inflammatory agents**.

**D. Inflammatory polyarthritis** (assuming no coexisting chlamydia infection)

  1. **Systemic lupus erythematosus**

    a. **Do not treat until the diagnosis is established.**

    b. **Do not overtreat.** Mild cases can be handled with reassurance, aspirin, indomethacin, or one of the many NSAID drugs that are available.

    c. An **occult infection** sometimes is difficult to diagnose and **differentiate** from an exacerbation of SLE. In these situations, be sure to rule out infections of the genitourinary tract, heart, and lungs.

    d. Advise the patient to **rest** as necessary.

    e. Avoid excessive exposure to the **sun**.

    f. **Antimalarial drugs (hydroxychloroquine** 400 mg per day)

    g. **Prednisone,** less than 10 mg per day PO, may be added to the regimen if the patient does not respond to the preceding measures.

    h. **Immunosuppressive agents** are indicated as steroid-**sparing** agents for treatment for SLE.

      i. The treatment of this disease is empirical and must be individualized and monitored by the rheumatologist. There are no absolutes.

  2. **Juvenile rheumatoid arthritis**[1,7]

    a. **NSAIDs** are the mainstay of therapy; one-third of patients can be managed with these drugs alone.[5] No NSAID has been proven more effective than any other.

    b. **Nonbiologic DMARDs** may be used earlier in the disease under new recommendations under an emphasis on better control.

      i. **MTX** is effective in 70% to 80% of patients with JRA.

      ii. **Leflunomide (Arava)** is less effective that MTX with similar side effects.

      iii. **Gold** is used in its injectable form, but infrequently. See **V.A.2** for a discussion of gold therapy. Oral gold therapy is ineffective.

      iv. **Antimalarial drugs** such as hydroxychloroquine may lack a clear advantage over placebo.

      v. **D-Penicillamine** is not recommended for routine use in JRA.

    c. **Biologic DMARDs** approved for use include etanercept, adalimumab, and abatacept. See **V.A.3.a–b.**

    d. **Corticosteroids** are typically only given systemically while waiting for DMARDs to take effect. Steroid injections into troublesome joints for synovitis are often helpful, but try to avoid multiple injections into the same joint.

    e. **Physical and occupational therapy** are helpful to maintain function, prevent contracture, and optimize motion and muscle strength. Therapeutic maneuvers should be performed twice daily at home. Night splints to prevent deformity are usually essential.

    f. **Orthopaedic surgery**

      i. **Synovectomy plays a limited role** in the early treatment of JRA.

      ii. **Reconstructive surgery** (e.g., soft-tissue releases, osteotomies, and total joint replacement) can be indicated.

    g. **Ophthalmologic evaluation** is necessary for early diagnostic treatment of any iridocyclitis.

    h. **Amyloidosis** is seen in 5% of patients and can be fatal if kidneys fail.

    i. **Do not forget the whole child, the effects of this disease on other organ systems, and the child's mental health.**

### E. Septic arthritis

1. **Antibiotics** (see **Chapter 4,** Table 4-2). Proper cultures are ideally obtained before initiating antibiotic therapy. These are obtained either as an aspirate or intraoperatively.
2. **Drainage** of the joint is usually necessary.
   a. **Needle aspiration and irrigation** are sometimes sufficient if the joint can be easily inspected for an effusion. The joint may need decompression more than once daily. The hip joint always requires open drainage. A knee joint infection can be handled by needle decompression if the exudate is not loculated and if aspiration clearly decompresses the joint. If marked improvement is not noted within 48 hours, the open (or arthroscopic) irrigation and debridement should be performed.
   b. **Operative irrigation and drainage** of the joint are often necessary with or without debridement. Postoperatively, wounds are usually closed over drains and judicious immobilization is used. Arthroscopic lavage is commonly used for knee and shoulder joint involvement.

### F. Arthritis associated with infectious agents

1. **Reiter's syndrome** treatment is symptomatic. The prognosis is guarded because chronic arthritis develops in many people. Sulfasalazine and MTX may be considered for chronic moderate-to-severe disease.
2. **Rheumatic fever**
   a. **Penicillin** is indicated for the initial treatment as well as continued prophylaxis.
   b. **Aspirin** is used for mild arthritis.
   c. **Prednisone** has been used for patients with carditis, but it may not prevent heart damage.[15]
   d. **Diuretics and digitalis** are often needed.
   e. **Rest** is recommended according to the degree of cardiac involvement.
   f. Obtain throat culture from family contacts.

### G. Inflammatory spondyloarthropathy

1. **Ankylosing spondylitis**
   a. **The most important part of the initial therapy** is an **educational effort** by the physician or physical therapist that should cover proper sleeping position, gait, posture, breathing exercises, and "measuring up" every morning (i.e., straightening the spine every day to reach a mark placed on the wall to help prevent kyphosis or at least identify its development).
   b. **NSAIDs** are the drugs of choice for milder cases. As with treatment for osteoarthritis, trial and error to identify the optimum drug is the rule. After relief is obtained, decrease the dose to the lowest possible effective dose.
   c. **Ophthalmologic evaluation** is indicated because anterior uveitis occurs in 10% to 60% of patients.
   d. **Sulfasalazine or MTX** may be useful in aggressive cases.
   e. **Radiation therapy** has been abandoned because of late malignancy reports.
2. **Psoriatic arthritis. Immunosuppressive drugs**, such as MTX, are useful when administered in doses of 7.5 to 25.0 mg PO or intramuscular (IM) once weekly.[5]

## REFERENCES

1. Singh JA, Saag KG, Bridges SL Jr, et al. 2015 American College of Rheumatology guidelines for the treatment of rheumatoid arthritis. *Arthritis Rheumatol.* 2016;68(1):1-26.
2. Zhang W, Moskowitz RW, Nuki G, et al. OARSI recommendations for the management of hip and knee osteoarthritis, Part II: OARSI evidence-based, expert consensus guidelines. *Osteoarthritis Cartilage.* 2008;16(2):137-162. doi:10.1016/j.joca.2007.12.013

3. McCarty DJ, Koopman WJ. *Arthritis and Allied Conditions: A Textbook of Rheumatology.* 12th ed. Vol 2. Lea & Febiger; 1993.

4. Aletaha D, Neogi T, Silman AJ, et al. 2010 Rheumatoid arthritis classification criteria: an American College of Rheumatology/European League Against Rheumatism collaborative initiative. *Ann Rheum Dis.* 2010;69(9):1580-1588.

5. Roberts MH, Erdei E. Comparative United States autoimmune disease rates for 2010-2016 by sex, geographic region, and race. *Autoimmun Rev.* 2020;19(1):102423.

6. Freeman J, Brown Rogers A, eds. *Lupus: A Patient Care Guide for Nurses and Other Health Professionals.* 3rd ed. National Institute of Arthritis and Musculoskeletal and Skin Diseases; 2006.

7. Prince FH, Otten MH, van Suijlekom-Smit LW. Diagnosis and management of juvenile idiopathic arthritis. *BMJ.* 2010;341:c6434.

8. Drugs for rheumatoid arthritis. *Treat Guidel Med Lett.* 2009;7(81):37-46; quiz 47-48.

9. Drugs for osteoarthritis. *Med Lett Drugs Ther.* 2020;62(1596):57-62.

10. Liu X, Machado GC, Eyles JP, Ravi V, Hunter DJ. Dietary supplements for treating osteoarthritis: a systematic review and meta-analysis. *Br J Sports Med.* 2018;52(3):167-175.

11. Kirkley A, Webster-Bogaert S, Litchfield R, et al. The effect of bracing on varus gonarthrosis. *J Bone Joint Surg Am.* 1999;81(4):539-548.

12. Miller LE, Fredericson M, Altman RD. Hyaluronic Acid Injections or Oral Nonsteroidal Anti-inflammatory Drugs for Knee Osteoarthritis: Systematic Review and Meta-analysis of Randomized Trials. *Orthop J Sports Med.* 2020;8(1):2325967119897909.

13. Farr J, Cole B, Dhawan A, et al. Clinical cartilage restoration: evolution and overview. *Clin Orthop Relat Res.* 2011;469(10):2696-2705.

14. Jansen TL, Janssen M. Lessons and pitfalls from the 2020 Gout Clinical Practice Guideline presented in Atlanta at the ACR 2019. *Clin Rheumatol.* 2020;39(6):2011-2016.

15. Cilliers AM, Manyemba J, Saloojee H. Anti-inflammatory treatment for carditis in acute rheumatic fever. *Cochrane Database Syst Rev.* 2003;(2):CD003176.

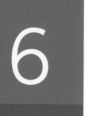

# 6 Pediatric Orthopaedic Conditions

Walter H. Truong, David Eduard Lebel, and Aaron Huser

## I. The Limping Child

The limping child is frequently referred to a primary physician's office or to an urgent/emergency care center and includes infants that have decreased motion in their limbs. There is a long list of possible causes to be considered. Important components of the evaluation include age at presentation, a thorough history, and a careful physical examination.[1,2]

**A. History of present illness.** History of trauma or injury, acuteness of onset of symptoms, presence of pain, constitutional symptoms (such as fever, malaise, chills), ability to bear any weight, early morning stiffness

**B. Review of systems.** Recent illnesses (upper respiratory tract illnesses [viral or streptococcal], gastrointestinal illness, etc.), rashes, joint swelling; additionally, recent exposure such as camping in wooded areas as well as a history of tick bites; international travel to less developed countries

**C. Past medical history.** This should include birth history (prematurity, time in the intensive care unit) and major motor milestone development history, as well as any previous surgeries, injuries, obesity, hormonal issues, and hospitalizations for any reason; previous infection with resistant bacteria.

**D. Family history.** Developmental dysplasia of the hip (DDH), autoimmune conditions (such as rheumatoid arthritis or lupus), short stature indicative of skeletal dysplasias, connective tissue disorders.

**E. Physical examination.** The physical examination should be tailored to each patient depending on the symptoms at presentation. The physical examination of a child with a recent or sudden onset of a painful limp or refusal to walk in the emergency department will be very different from an examination of a child with a chronic, painless limp in the outpatient clinic, but there are some broad tips to consider.

1. **Inspection.** If able, watch them walk. An antalgic gait is characterized by a decreased stance duration on the affected limb as compared to a stiff hip gait where this is not decreased. Check skin for signs of trauma or infection and look for rashes. Look for leg length differences by supine knee heights (Galeazzi sign) or anterior superior iliac spine (ASIS) to lateral malleolus length. If able to stand, iliac crest or posterior superior iliac spine (PSIS) comparisons can be helpful.[3]

2. **Palpation.** Palpate the entire length of the limb. Particular attention should be paid to any erythema, warmth, joint effusion, or focal tenderness.

3. **Range of motion (ROM).** Evaluate the ROM of the affected area and the joint above and below.

4. **Neurovascular.** A thorough neurovascular examination should also be completed, including motor strength, sensation, reflexes, pulses, and perfusion.

**F. Differential diagnosis** for a limping child encompasses a broad range of conditions and depends on many factors, including age, presence of pain, acuteness of onset, and clinical findings on physical examination.[1,2,4] Many conditions are present at birth or shortly after birth, but are not noticed until the child is walking. **Referred pain** describes pain attributed to one site or location by the patient but, in actuality, the source of the pain is at a different source (e.g., knee pain in a patient with a slipped capital femoral epiphysis [SCFE] involving the hip joint, lumbar discitis referred to the hip joint). As referred pain is frequently seen with some childhood conditions, joints above and below the apparent joint of interest should be examined thoroughly in isolation and worked up if indicated. This list of possible conditions is a guide and is not exhaustive.

1. **All ages**
   - Septic arthritis (peak 0 to 3 years), osteomyelitis (peak 0 to 4 years), pyomyositis, discitis
   - Tumor, pseudotumors
   - Metabolic diseases
   - Inguinal hernia, bowel obstruction, appendicitis, testicular torsion
2. **0 to 11 months (infant)**
   - DDH
   - "Nonaccidental injury" (child abuse) (peak before walking age)
3. **1 to 3 years (toddler)**
   - Toddler's fracture (nondisplaced tibia fracture) (low-energy trauma)
   - "Nonaccidental injury" (child abuse) (peak before walking age)
   - Transient hip synovitis (peak 4 to 8 years)
   - DDH
   - Neurologic disorders (cerebral palsy, Duchenne muscular dystrophy)
   - Juvenile idiopathic arthritis (JIA) (increased prevalence with age)
   - Congenital limb deficiency (femur, fibula, tibia)
4. **4 to 10 years (Juvenile)**
   - Trauma
   - Transient hip synovitis (peak 4 to 8 years)
   - Osteochondroses (Legg–Calvé–Perthes [peak 4 to 8 years], Köhler, and Osgood–Schlatter)
   - JIA
   - Discoid meniscus
5. **11 to 16 years (Adolescent)**
   - Trauma
   - SCFE (peak 11 to 13 years)
   - Osteochondroses (Legg–Calvé–Perthes [peak 4 to 8 years], Köhler, and Osgood–Schlatter)
   - Patellofemoral pain syndrome
   - Osteochondritis dissecans (OCD)
   - Late hip dysplasia
   - JIA
   - Idiopathic chondrolysis

**G. Imaging.** Further diagnostic testing depends on the differential diagnosis, and algorithms may be useful to guide the next steps.[2] Imaging and laboratory tests may be expensive, may represent radiation exposure, and may cause distress to the child; therefore, understanding the strengths and weaknesses of each modality is essential.[5]

1. **Radiography.** X-rays are often the first-line test in the setting of trauma and is widely available. Though sensitive to bony changes from fracture or tumors, it is less helpful in the setting of acute infection or soft-tissue pathology.
2. **Ultrasound (U/S).** U/S is useful for differentiating fluid from solid masses and to quantify and localize joint effusions, subperiosteal abscesses, or soft-tissue abscesses.[6] It is also useful to evaluate epiphyses in infants (DDH before 6 months of age, transphyseal fractures about the elbow in infants) when cartilage predominates, making X-rays less sensitive than U/S.

3. **Magnetic resonance imaging (MRI).** MRI is very sensitive and specific for areas of abnormal signal in soft tissues, as well as within the bone itself, and has no radiation risk. It is able to identify areas of bone marrow edema, soft-tissue edema, or fluid collections such as abscesses or joint effusions. In younger children (less than about 8 years), MRI will require the help of the anesthesia team for sedation or general anesthetic. It is also one of the most costly and time-consuming imaging modalities, and bony detail is better depicted by computerized tomography (CT) scan.

4. **Computerized tomography.** CT scans can cover a large area quickly and are extremely sensitive at diagnosing occult fractures, fluid collections, and thickening of visceral walls. However, they do represent a significant dose of radiation, are insensitive to edema within bone, and are poor at visualization of soft tissue.

5. **Bone scans.** These can look for increased metabolic activity over the entire body when pain is not localized well. Bone scans are no longer done routinely because of the large amount of radiation required and the lack of the specificity of the test.

H. **Laboratory studies.** Consider for a patient with no history of trauma and/or concern for inflammation or infection.
1. Complete blood count (CBC) with differential
2. Erythrocyte sedimentation rate (ESR)
3. C-reactive protein (CRP)
4. Blood cultures, if febrile
5. Joint aspirations should be sent for cell count and cultures.
6. If rheumatologic conditions or spondyloarthropathies are suspected, consider rheumatoid factor, antinuclear antibody, antistreptolysin titer, and HLA B-27.
7. In endemic areas for Lyme disease and for patients with a large knee effusion, yet a surprising ability to range the knee, also include Lyme serology and consider Lyme polymerase chain reaction (PCR) of joint aspirations.

II. **Lower Extremity Alignment Conditions**
A. **General**
1. Deformities of the lower limbs may occur in coronal, sagittal, and axial planes.
2. Coronal plane deformities are described as varus (commonly called bow legs) and valgus (commonly called knock knees).
3. Sagittal plane deformities are described as procurvatum (flexion deformity) or recurvatum (extension deformity).
4. Axial plane deformities are rotational in nature and are described by parents as in-toeing or out-toeing. Surgeons describe hip axial deformities as anteversion (rotated anteriorly relative to knee axis often causing increased hip internal rotation) or retroversion (rotated posteriorly relative to knee axis often causing increased hip external rotation) in the femur. In the tibia, we describe them as internal torsion (axis of the ankle internal relative to the knee causing internal foot progression angle (FPA)) and external torsion (axis of the ankle external relative to the knee causing external FPA).
5. The cause of these deformities may be related to the bones or soft tissues and it is through physical examination and imaging that we can determine the cause.

B. **Physical examination**
1. The patient should be dressed to adequately visualize the lower extremities. In young children, adolescents, and teens, we recommend providing them a pair of shorts for the examination. It is important to allow them privacy to change into these clothes prior to the examination.
2. *Gait examination.* Have the patient walk in a hallway. Observe position of their feet. This is called foot progression angle (FPA) (Fig. 6-1). FPA gives you an idea of the overall rotation of their lower limb. It is noted

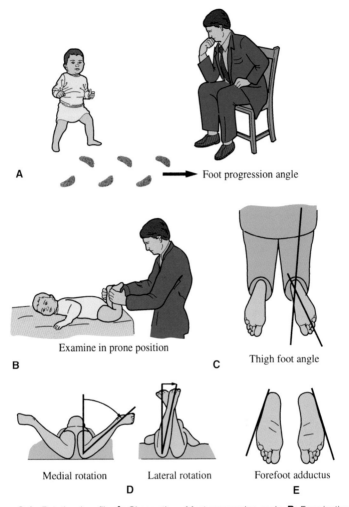

**Figure 6-1.** Rotational profile. **A:** Observation of foot progression angle. **B:** Examination of child in prone position to evaluate torsional deformity of the lower extremities. **C:** Thigh-foot angle. **D:** Hip internal (medial) and external (lateral) rotation. **E:** Forefoot (metatarsus) adductus.

to be positive if the foot externally rotates relative to a straight line or negative if the foot internally rotates. We also record the amount of degrees. For example, +10° would indicate that the foot is externally rotated approximately 10° to the straight, forward line. Also observe their heel striking the ground and toes pushing off the ground and whether they are able to achieve full knee extension and any sort of limp.

3. *Static standing.* Observe the child in static stance. View the patient from the front, the back, and both sides. Take note of the position of the knees relative to the feet. For instance, are the patellas pointing inward and the feet forward? Are the knees touching but the ankles far apart? Are the

ankles touching but knees far apart? Do the thighs appear angled relative to the lower legs? Is one leg bent while the other is fully extended? These will give you clues to making the right diagnosis. This is also a good time to observe the foot and look for the presence of arch and the relationship of the heel to the back of the leg. Frequently, we have the patient stand on their toes to demonstrate the heel (calcaneus) move from a lateral position (valgus) to a medial position (varus): called the Root sign.

4. *Prone examination.* We next move to the prone examination. This is ideally performed with a goniometer. The patient is lying on their stomach on a table facing the floor. Note whether the hips are able to achieve full extension on the table. This position also allows for a rotational examination with the hips in full extension.

   a. *Hip rotation* (see Fig. 6-1D). With the patient prone and knees flexed to 90°, rotate hip internally (foot moves laterally) and externally (foot moves medially) and note their maximal range. Make sure you stabilize the patient's pelvis while assessing rotation. Next, rotate the hip while palpating the greater trochanter. When you can feel the greater trochanter is most prominent, estimate the angle between the tibia and a vertical line. This is the approximate degree of *femoral neck anteversion.*

   b. *Ely test.* The next portion of the examination is called the *Ely test.* The leg is flexed maximally until resistance is felt. This test can be used to determine maximum flexion of the knee and rectus femoris spasticity/tightness/shortening.

   c. *Thigh-foot axis* and *bimalleolar axis. Thigh-foot axis* (see Fig. 6-1C): Angle formed by a line down the middle of the foot relative to the line down the length of thigh and is about 0-10 deg external. *Bimalleolar axis:* Angle formed by a line passing through the center of the lateral malleolus and medial malleolus relative to the line perpendicular to the long axis of thigh and is approximately 0-15 deg internal.

   d. Examine the plantar surface of the foot with the patient still in the prone position. Note the lateral curvature of the foot (see Fig. 6-1E). Is it straight or does it curve around (adductus)? Flatfeet will have shortened lateral column and collapse of the medial arch. In addition, the *heel bisector* is an imaginary line drawn that bisects the heel and is carried distally toward the toes and should intersect with the second or third toe.

5. *Supine examination.* Finally, have the patient turn over on the table so that he or she is facing the ceiling and lying on their back. Again, measurements obtained *during* this examination should ideally be done with a goniometer.

   a. *Hips.* Again, note the position of the hips at rest. Are they at full extension or is there a hip flexion deformity? To test hip flexion, gently place your fingers on the ASISs to stabilize the pelvis. This ensures that lumbosacral flexion is not confused with hip flexion. Start to flex the hip and note when you feel the ASISs start to move. This is the maximum amount of flexion. Test hip abduction and adduction similarly with your hands on the pelvis noting that when the pelvis starts to move the patient has reached that respective hip motion limit.

   b. *Knees.* Measure the knee in maximal extension. Also assess varus and valgus stability in maximal extension, noting the Q-angle (angle between the thigh and shin; 15-25 deg is normal with females having slightly higher angles). Anterior and posterior stability may also be tested using the anterior and posterior drawer test and *Lachman* test.

   c. *Ankles.* Finally, assess the ankles for maximum dorsiflexion and plantarflexion. During this examination, it is important to ensure that the subtalar joint is in a neutral position (lined up with the lower leg/tibia). Ankle DF should be 10 deg with knees extended and over 20 deg with knees flexed. Silverskiold test is positive if there is normal range with knees flexed but limited with an extended knee; this identifies isolated gastrocnemius contractures.

**C. Imaging**

1. Historically, an anteroposterior (AP), full-length radiograph of both lower extremities centered at the knees with the patellas facing forward was preferable for assessing coronal/frontal plane alignment. The downside of this modality is the parallax at the hips and ankles, as well as the radiation exposure (reference). Currently, we are using slot x-ray imaging technology to obtain these images because of the decreased radiation and essentially no distortion of the hips and ankles.

2. If you suspect deformity at the ankle or hips, additional, dedicated views of those areas should be obtained.

3. CT or MRI is still the gold standard to analyze rotational malalignments in the femurs and tibias, however, we are also using simultaneous biplanar x-ray slot images for with 3D reconstructions for this purpose.

4. **Radiographic analysis**

   a. *Mechanical axis.* The mechanical axis of a limb or bone is defined as the line passing through the center of the joint above to the center of the joint below. In the lower limb, this line is drawn from the center of the hip to the ankle and should pass through the center of the knee. If the line is medial to the knee, the patient has overall varus alignment, and if the line is lateral to the knee, the patient has overall valgus alignment.[7]

   b. *Lateral distal femoral angle.* This angle is formed using the mechanical axis of the femur (center of the hip to the center of the knee) and a line tangential to the distal femoral condyles. The lateral angle is measured and 87° is considered normal.[7,8]

   c. *Medial proximal tibial angle.* This angle is formed using the mechanical axis of the tibia (center of the knee to center of the ankle) and a line parallel to the tibial plateau. The medial angle is measured and 87° is considered normal.[7]

   d. *Femoral-tibial angle.* This is the angle formed from the intersection of the femoral mechanical axis and the tibia mechanical axis. Normal range is between 0° and 3° of valgus.

   e. *Joint-line congruence angle.* This angle is formed using the line tangential to the distal femoral condyles and the line parallel to the tibial plateau. The normal angle is 0° to 2°. Measurements outside this range are indicative of joint instability or intraarticular deformity.[7,8]

   f. Additional measurements can be performed on these images, depending on the deformity of interest.[7,8]

**D. Conditions/complaints**

1. **In-toeing**

   a. **Definition.** The feet turn in relative to the line of forward progression during walking. In-toeing is a frequent cause for parental concern. An important part of the evaluation should be listening to the concerns expressed by the parents and answering their questions.

   b. **Causes**

      i. **Increased femoral anteversion.** An internal rotation deformity of the femur. Femoral anteversion in a newborn is 40° to 45°. For most children, this gradually remodels with growth over time and will have improved by the age of 6 to 8. At skeletal maturity, normal femoral anteversion is approximately 10° to 15°.[9] Increased femoral anteversion seen in children, under the age of 8 or 9, is physiologically normal and should be observed for improvement over time. In children older than 9 years, it has been recommended that indications for surgery include anteversion greater than 50° or functional disability associated with it such as tripping, hip pain with forced external rotation of the hip to prevent tripping, or patellofemoral symptoms related to combined external torsion of the tibia.[10] In our practice, most of the children who have surgery for femoral anteversion also have cerebral palsy and treatment of the femoral anteversion is part of a global reconstruction.

ii. **Internal tibial torsion** is an internal rotation deformity of the tibia. Internal tibial torsion corrects with time and should be **resolved** by the age of 3 to 4.[11] The majority of patients are usually treated with observation. We do not recommend special shoes or bracing for internal tibial torsion. Isolated internal tibial torsion rarely requires operative management. Indications include age greater than 8 years and functional limitation or pain in the knee or ankle related to the torsional deformity such as frequent tripping or injury.

iii. **Metatarsus adductus.** Refers to a curvature of foot with the toes/forefoot turned inward. The diagnosis can be made when the heel bisector line intersects lateral to the second/third toe webspace, and the lateral border of the foot is rounded. This is a frequent finding in newborns/children and is often flexible. Simple massage and stretching can be performed by the parents for the first 6 months of life; however, recent literature suggests this may produce no different results than pure observation.[12] If the foot does not appear flexible, a course of serial casting may be considered. Persistent deformity may require workup for other neuromuscular conditions or neural axis abnormalities.

2. **Bowed legs/genu varum**

a. **Definition.** Clinically, the patient's knees will appear bowed, and the patient's ankles will be closer to midline than their knees. The **mechanical** axis on the full-length film falls medial to the center of the knee. The medial proximal tibial angle will be less than 85° and/or the lateral distal femoral angle will be greater than 90°.

b. **Causes**

i. "Physiologic." Part of the normal development. Most children who are referred for evaluation have a physiologic form of bowing. The lower extremity alignment evolves in children during the first 6 years of life. For genu varum, bowing after the age of 3 is considered abnormal.

ii. **Tibia vara** is an abnormal varus alignment of the knee because of altered growth of the medial portion of the proximal tibial physis. The **infantile form** (**Blount's disease**) occurs in children between the ages of 1 and 4. **Late-onset tibia vara** is seen in children older than 5 years. Both types have been associated with obesity.[13]

iii. **Further differential diagnoses**

(a) **Focal fibrocartilaginous dysplasia**. A focal cartilaginous deformity of the distal femur or proximal tibia in young children leading to bowing.

(b) **Coxa vara**. A congenital varus deformity of the proximal femur.

(c) One of the various forms of **skeletal dysplasias**. To help evaluate this, obtain additional radiographs of the hands, shoulders, and spine.

(d) One of the forms of **rickets** (e.g., familial hypophosphatemic rickets). To evaluate this further, consider obtaining **laboratory** studies, including vitamin D; parathyroid hormone; alkaline phosphatase; calcium, magnesium, and phosphorus levels. Also consider obtaining an endocrinology consultation.

c. **Treatment**

i. For children under the age of 3, treatment usually consists of observation. Inform the patient's parents of the expected course and communicate the findings and recommendations to the patient's primary physician. Continued observation can be performed during routine well-child checks. If the child's alignment varies from what is expected, the child can return for reevaluation.

ii. Children with conditions that do not fit the typical "physiologic" pattern may have pain or instability and should be referred for further evaluation. Further treatment consists of establishing the underlying cause and developing an appropriate treatment plan. After the diagnosis has been determined, treatment may consist of the following[13,14]:

(a) Guided growth/growth modulation with plates and screws or staples

(b) Bar resection

(c) Tibial/femoral osteotomy

3. **Knock knees/genu valgum**

a. **Definition.** Clinically, the patient may have an appearance of knock knees, with the knees closer to the midline than the angles (genu valgus). Radiographically, the lower limb mechanical axis will fall lateral to the middle of the knee. The lateral distal femoral angle will be less than 85° and/or the medial proximal tibial angle with be greater than 90°.

b. **Causes**

i. "Physiologic." Much like genu varum, there is a period during a child's life where genu valgus/knock knees is part of skeletal development. In general, after the age of 2 years, the knees will develop a more valgus appearance. Maximum valgus is around ages 4 and 5 years, and this will start spontaneously correcting toward adult alignment. After the age of 8 years, valgus alignment is considered abnormal.[15]

ii. Limb deficiency. Children with fibular hemimelia or congenital femoral deficiency frequently have lateral femoral condyle hypoplasia and develop genu valgum.[16]

iii. Posttraumatic/Cozen phenomenon. Genu valgus may be noted after a proximal tibial fracture in a child. This is called Cozen phenomenon and should correct spontaneously by 18 months from injury.[17]

iv. Idiopathic. After the age of 8 years, continued valgus is considered abnormal. If the patient does not have a known, underlying etiology, the genu valgum would be considered idiopathic.

v. Skeletal dysplasia/bone mineral disease. Skeletal dysplasias or diseases affecting bone mineral health such as rickets may also have genu valgum.

c. **Treatment**

i. For patients who are within the physiologic age group without an underlying etiology or who have a Cozen phenomenon, the mainstay for treatment is observation until the age of 8 years.

ii. Patients older than 8 years with genu valgum are usually treated with hemiepiphysiodesis using plate/screw constructs or stapling.

iii. Patients with closed physes with progressive genu valgum may require osteotomy of the femur or tibia.

## III. Common Childhood Foot Conditions

### A. Clubfoot (talipes equinovarus)

1. **Description.** A congenital deformity of the foot comprises ankle equinus, hindfoot varus, midfoot cavus, and forefoot adduction and supination. The foot "turns in" and "curves under" compared with the normal appearance.

2. **Incidence.** Approximately 1 in 1,000 live births, unilateral in 60% of the patients, and the ratio of boys to girls is 2:1. There may be a positive family history.

3. **Etiology.** Multiple theories exist, with the most likely cause being **multifactorial**. Theories include arrested fetal development, abnormal intrauterine forces, abnormal muscle fiber type, abnormal neuromuscular function, and germ plasm defects.

4. **Prenatal considerations.** The diagnosis of clubfeet for the unborn child is often made on a prenatal U/S. If consulted by an expectant mother or primary physician, reassurances should be made that the diagnosis of clubfoot/clubfeet is a very treatable condition. Other prenatal factors associated with clubfeet include breech position, large birth weight, and oligohydramnios.

5. **Associated conditions** include arthrogryposis, myelodysplasia, congenital limb anomalies, and various syndromes.

6. **Physical examination.** Please see the physical examination Section III.B. The typical deformities seen in club foot are midfoot cavus (C), forefoot adductus (A), hindfoot varus (V), and ankle equinus (E); (C.A.V.E.). Additionally, deep posterior and medial creases are frequently present in patients with clubfoot.

7. **Radiographic evaluation.** Radiographs in the newborn period are not useful because the tarsal bones are not well ossified. As treatment for patients with clubfeet has shifted to largely nonoperative methods, the role or need for radiographs has decreased. When an X-ray is deemed necessary, an AP and a lateral radiograph of the foot in maximum dorsiflexion are ordered for infants and children younger than 1 year. In children of walking age, a standing AP and lateral radiograph of the foot are requested and may show flattening of the talar dome and adduction of the talar head and neck with decreased calcaneal pitch.

8. **Treatment.** The goals of treatment are to achieve a plantigrade, flexible, painless foot. Currently, a method of casting developed by Ignacio Ponseti is the method of choice for clubfoot.[18] After completion of casting, patients typically require an Achilles tenotomy, followed by bracing until the age of 4. Surgical treatment is reserved for those patients whose feet do not respond to nonoperative treatment.

**B. Congenital vertical talus (CVT)**

1. **Definition.** A congenital condition in which the foot has a rigid flat foot appearance because of an irreducible dorsal dislocation of the navicular on the talus. Often referred to as a "rocker bottom" foot deformity.

2. **Incidence.** Much less common than clubfoot; the incidence is approximately 1 per 10,000 live births.

3. **Associated conditions.** Approximately 50% of CVT cases are associated with underlying disorders such as arthrogryposis, myelomeningocele, tethered spinal cord, or chromosomal abnormalities.

4. **Physical examination.** When evaluating the child's feet, assess the flexibility of the ankle and hindfoot as well as the posture of the midfoot and forefoot. Also remember to examine the child for other associated conditions involving their upper extremities, the spine, the hips, and their neurologic function.

5. **Radiographic evaluation.** In contrast to children with clubfeet, for young children with suspected CVT, radiographs may be helpful in confirming the diagnosis. An AP and lateral X-ray of the foot in *maximum plantarflexion* should be obtained. For children with a CVT, the talus will remain plantarflexed on the lateral X-ray and will not align with the forefoot. Also, despite dorsiflexion of the forefoot, the heel is almost always in equinus. The term **oblique talus** is sometimes used to describe the child with a flat or rounded appearing foot at birth but for whom the talus does line up with the first metatarsal or forefoot on the lateral plantarflexion X-ray. In patients with a **calcaneovalgus** foot at birth, the foot appears

very dorsiflexed at birth and may have a rounded appearance, but it has excellent flexibility of the ankle as well as of the midfoot and hindfoot.

6. **Treatment.** Similar to clubfoot, a casting method has been developed for CVT. However, at the completion of casting, the child is taken to the operating room and a pin is used to temporarily hold the navicular reduced to the talus and usually the Achilles tendon is lengthened.[19] Occasionally, an open reduction of the talar navicular may need to be performed.[19] For cases resistant to pinning/casting, a more aggressive release may need to be performed.

**C. Flat feet (pes planus)**

1. **Definition.** Feet in which the medial longitudinal arch is absent, resulting in hindfoot valgus and forefoot supination.

2. **Presentation**
   a. Parental concerns regarding the appearance and shape of the foot
   b. Pain often along talar head medially due to impact with the ground or lateral ankle due to calcaneofibular impingement.
   c. Difficulties with shoe wear

3. **Patient history.** It is important to note when the foot position was first noticed, whether the foot condition causes problems with function or pain, and any family history of ligamentous laxity/hypermobility or flat feet.

4. **Physical examination**
   a. See Section III.B for a general physical examination. During gait, note the presence or absence of medial longitudinal arch.
   b. Inspect the foot for calluses and pressure areas over bony prominences.
   c. Have the patient stand on tiptoe to assess mobility of the hindfoot. If the hindfoot moves from valgus when plantigrade to varus with standing on tiptoe and the foot forms an arch when on tiptoe, the foot is "**flexible**." If it does not correct, it is considered "**rigid**."
   d. Assess the length of the Achilles tendon by examining the range of ankle dorsiflexion.

5. **Radiographic examination.** For young children with a painless, flexible flat foot, no radiographs are indicated. If the flat foot is painful or rigid, standing AP, lateral, and oblique radiographs of the foot should be obtained.

6. **Flexible flat feet.** The flexible flat foot is a relatively common condition, although the true incidence is unknown. Most young children start with a flexible flat foot before developing a medial longitudinal arch during the first decade of life. Most children are symptom free, and no treatment is warranted. For the older child or adolescent with a flexible flat foot who experiences aching or discomfort associated with particular activities, one may wish to use an orthotic to support the arch. If the foot is flexible but there is a contracture of the Achilles tendon, one should prescribe a course of physical therapy for a heel cord stretching program. If the patient with an Achilles tendon contracture remains symptomatic despite physical therapy, one may consider injection of Botox into the calf muscle, possibly in conjunction with a stretching cast. For patients who fail conservative therapy, some authors support surgical correction of the hindfoot valgus deformity in conjunction with lengthening the tight gastrocnemius.[20] This is rarely necessary in a growing child with a flexible flat foot deformity.

7. **Rigid flat feet.** The most common cause for a rigid flat foot is a **tarsal coalition**. This is an incomplete separation of the tarsal bones during fetal development. The two most common types are the **calcaneonavicular** and the **talocalcaneal coalition**. The calcaneonavicular coalition may be best seen on the oblique foot radiograph. The talocalcaneal coalition is difficult to see with plain radiographs. If further radiographic imaging is required when plain radiographs are nondiagnostic, a CT scan of both feet is the study of choice.

8. If tarsal coalition has been excluded as the cause for the rigid flat foot, other possible causes include the following:
   a. **CVT**
   b. **JRA** or other sources of inflammation/irritability involving the subtalar joint
   c. **Neuromuscular** conditions
9. **Treatment** of the rigid flat foot. The goal of treatment is to achieve a pain-free, asymptomatic foot.
   a. Tarsal coalitions
      i. Nonoperative treatment. Many patients with tarsal coalitions are asymptomatic. If they become symptomatic, the first line of treatment is a short-leg walking cast for 6 weeks or arch supports.[21]
      ii. For patients with a calcaneonavicular coalition, operative treatment usually consists of excision of the coalition along with interposition of fat, muscle, or tendon to prevent recurrence. For patients with a talocalcaneal coalition, good results have been obtained with resection when the coalition comprises less than one-third of the total subtalar joint surface.[21,22] For patients with severe degenerative arthrosis of the subtalar joint or persistent pain following previous resection, a triple arthrodesis may be considered.
   b. Other causes of rigid flat foot may require osteotomies or fusion for treatment.

## D. Bunions (hallux valgus)

1. **Definition.** An abnormal bony prominence of the medial eminence of the first metatarsal associated with a hallux valgus deformity of the great toe. It is frequently associated with a medial deviation of the first metatarsal (**metatarsus primus varus**).
2. **Patient history.** These patients are most often adolescent girls with complaints of pain over the medial eminence, difficulty with shoe wear, or concerns regarding appearance. Pes planus, long first metatarsal, and positive family history are associated with the development of a bunion deformity in adolescents.
3. **Physical examination.** Assess the presence of hindfoot valgus and a coexisting flat foot in addition to the presence and severity of hallux valgus deformity. Evaluate the degree of angulation as well as the rotation of the great toe.
4. **Radiographic evaluation.** Standing AP and lateral radiographs of the foot are recommended. On the AP radiograph, one can assess the following parameters:
   a. First-second intermetatarsal angle (normal is <9°)
   b. Hallux valgus angle (normal is <15°)
   c. Hallux valgus interphalangeus angle (normal is <10°)
   d. Distal metatarsal articular angle (normal is <10°)
5. **Treatment.** It is important to distinguish the **functional** problems that the patient is experiencing as well as the patients' and their parents' concerns. In the adolescent patient in whom the primary concern is the appearance of the foot, every effort should be made to educate and counsel the family. For symptomatic patients with an underlying flexible flat foot condition, initial treatment should consist of a custom-molded, flexible medial-arch supporting foot orthotic. This will frequently correct the flat foot deformity, improve the hallux valgus deformity, and improve the patient's symptoms. For patients with a symptomatic hallux valgus deformity that fails conservative treatment, any surgical treatment should be postponed until skeletal maturity is reached because there is a high recurrence rate of bunions in adolescent patients.[23] If surgery is considered, careful examination of the foot is necessary to correct all the underlying

deformities, thus decreasing the risk of recurrence and increasing the likelihood of patient satisfaction.

6. **Surgical options.** There are numerous surgical options.
   a. **Soft-tissue procedures**
      i. Medial capsule advancement of first metatarsophalangeal (MTP) joint
      ii. Excision of the medial eminence of the metatarsal head
      iii. Adductor hallucis release
   b. **Bony procedures**
      i. Distal first metatarsal osteotomy
      ii. Proximal first metatarsal osteotomy
      iii. Double-level metatarsal osteotomy

## IV. Childhood Knee Disorders

Evaluation of the patient with knee pain

### A. History

1. Location of pain
2. Trauma/injury
3. Swelling of joint
4. Locking/buckling of knees
5. Association of pain with specific activities (running, descending stairs, sitting)

### B. Physical evaluation

1. **Inspection.** If able, watch them walk. Look for antalgic or stiff knee gait. Bent knee or hyperextended? Varus or valgus thrust? Erythema, induration, or effusion? Have them point to the area of pain.
2. **Palpation.** First palpate specific landmarks away from the area of pain but cover all pertinent structures. Anteriorly: patellar poles and facets, tibial tubercle, pes anserinus. Medially and laterally: joint line, collateral ligament attachments, femoral condyle, tibial plateau, anteromedial/anterolateral joint line in deep flexion. Posteriorly: hamstring attachments, posterior capsule and popliteus, heads of the gastrocnemius. Always compare to the other side. Feel for fluid; is it in the joint or superficial to it?
3. **ROM and stress examination.** Evaluate the ROM of the affected area and the joint above and below. Roll the hip with knee extended to isolate the hip. Stress in varus, valgus, Lachman, and posterior drawer.
4. **Neurovascular.** Check skin perfusion and sensation.

### C. Imaging

1. **Radiographs.** Obtain AP/lateral radiographs of knee to evaluate for any bony abnormalities. For evaluation of patella alignment or patella-related pain, add "merchant" or "sunrise" view. If concerned about a loose body or OCD lesion, include "notch" or "tunnel" view.
2. **MRI.** MRIs are very useful when concerned about meniscal pathology, including a discoid meniscus. They are also helpful for defining the extent of OCD lesions. Ligament tears are rare in young children but they are prevalent in adolescents.
3. **CT.** CT scans are reserved for ruling out occult fractures. Tibial plateau fractures and intercondylar femur fractures may be missed on X-rays and better defined by CT scan than MRI. Tibial spine fractures can also be visualized well by CT but it may not pick up concomitant meniscal tears or interposed intermeniscal ligament. The use of CT should generally be limited due to the radiation exposure in children, and most often a suspected fracture should be treated as such without advanced imaging.

### D. Differential diagnosis

1. **Anterior knee pain**[24,25]
   a. **Patellofemoral pain syndrome**

 i. **Presentation.** Symptoms may occur gradually or after previous knee injury; usually not associated with specific trauma. There are usually no symptoms of locking or buckling. Pain is frequently associated with activities such as walking, running, descending stairs, and sitting for prolonged periods (the movie theater sign).

 ii. **Physical examination.** One should include a thorough examination of the knee, paying particular attention to evaluate tracking of the patella, patella mobility medially and laterally, and genu valgum as defined by Q-angle (alignment of extensor mechanism measured by angle of line from ASIS to patella and line from patella to tibial tubercle). Also assess the lower extremity rotational profile (see Section D.1).

 iii. **Imaging.** AP, lateral, and patella views should be obtained to evaluate for evidence of patellar tilt as well as to rule out other potential sources of knee symptoms such as OCD (best assessed with a "Notch view") and other bony lesions.

 iv. **Pathophysiology.** Adolescent girls are affected more often than boys. Previously termed "chondromalacia patellae" or "anterior knee pain syndrome," it describes a condition in which the pain is attributed to the patellofemoral joint.

 v. **Treatment.** Most patients with patellofemoral knee pain respond to a course of physical therapy consisting of hamstring stretching and strengthening of the hip abductors and the quadriceps (specifically the vastus medialis obliquus [VMO]). This may be augmented by the use of a patellar-taping program or a patella-stabilizing knee brace for some patients with symptoms of patella hypermobility.

b. **Osgood–Schlatter disease**

 i. **Presentation.** Anterior knee pain over the tibial tubercle. Painful to jump, go up and down stairs. Can't kneel on knees.

 ii. **Physical examination.** Pinpoint tenderness over tubercle. May have swelling and bony prominence that is tender. Painful to straight leg raise or actively extend.

 iii. **Imaging.** X-rays may show ossicles in the epiphysis of the tubercle. May look like a fracture. If able to run and jump still and no history of a single event, unlikely to be an acute fracture.

 iv. **Pathophysiology.** One in the family of conditions known as "osteochondroses," this represents inflammation at the junction of the patellar tendon to the tibial tubercle. It most often occurs in girls aged 10 to 12 and boys aged 12 to 14. The patient usually complains of painful swelling over the area of the tibial tubercle, as well as pain associated with activities such as running or jumping sports. **Sinding–Larsen–Johansson syndrome** is a related condition arising at the proximal aspect of the patellar tendon, just distal to the inferior aspect of the patella.

 v. **Treatment.** Consists of hamstring and quadriceps stretching, nonsteroidal anti-inflammatory drugs (NSAIDs), periodic ice to the area, and modification of activities. It is self-limiting and resolves, but bony prominence over the tibial tubercle may persist and cause discomfort with kneeling.

c. **Acute patella dislocation**

 i. **Presentation.** A sudden event with pain and swelling. The patella usually dislocates laterally. Ask whether patella needed to be relocated by the patient or a provider. Detailed history of any previous instability events.

    ii. **Physical examination.** The patient may be tender over the medial retinaculum and femoral or tibial attachments of the medial patellofemoral ligament (MPFL), and a joint effusion may be present. Deep flexion is often painful, but full extension is achieved.

    iii. **Imaging.** AP/lateral/patella views of the knee should be closely evaluated for any evidence of osteochondral loose bodies in the joint. The patella may knock off an osteochondral fragment from the lateral femoral condyle with the process of dislocating or relocating. MRI is indicated if a loose body is suspected on X-ray or with "locking or catching" sensation at any point during recovery. An MRI may be appropriate for a large effusion in the face of a negative radiograph. This will allow for the evaluation of the retinaculum and MPFL as well as any cartilage injury.

    iv. **Pathophysiology.** Hypermobility, genu valgum, patella alta, and torsional issues are all risk factors. Any previous events could stretch out the MPFL, the primary soft-tissue constraint of the knee, and predispose to instability events.

    v. **Treatment.** If osteochondral fragments are present, the knee should be evaluated arthroscopically. Very large fragments may need to be repaired and internally fixed, and smaller fragments may be simply removed. If no osteochondral fracture is identified, treatment may consist of a short period (3 to 4 weeks) of immobilization to allow healing of the MPFL with a soft-sided knee immobilizer followed by a program of quadriceps strengthening exercises.

    vi. About 36% to 54% of patients have recurrent patella subluxation/dislocation episodes, even after rehabilitation. Surgical stabilization with soft-tissue MPFL reconstruction may be indicated with an even greater chance of recurrence with younger age and trochlea dysplasia.[26,27]

  **d. Patella sleeve fracture**

    i. **Presentation.** Acute event with jumping or landing. May be unable to extend knee. Large swelling anteriorly.

    ii. **Physical examination.** Large joint effusion and anterior swelling may be present. Extensor lag and weak or absent knee extension. Could still have some because of retinacular tissue. May feel a defect in extensor mechanism with palpation.

    iii. **Imaging.** X-rays may show patella alta with a small fleck of bone attached to slack patella tendon. Fracture is less obvious than adult patella fractures, especially if not displaced and patella alta not present. If the extensor mechanism is disrupted clinically with a negative radiograph, an MRI should be obtained.

    iv. **Pathophysiology.** Bone near the distal pole is often the weak point. Equivalent to adult patella fracture and will disrupt extensor mechanism. The patella's peripheral margins have a delay in ossification until adolescence. This un-ossified peripheral cartilage is prone to breaking off with an avulsed patella fragment, creating a sleeve fracture.[28]

    v. **Treatment.** Open repair is necessary for any displacement and extensor lag. Screws, sutures, and/or wires may be used to execute the tension band technique.

**2. Joint-line pain**

  **a. Discoid meniscus**

    i. **Presentation.** Patients may have complaints of snapping or popping of the knee. ROM may be blocked after a tear or subluxation of the meniscus. Susceptible to an acute tear mid-substance or capsular attachments, causing acute pain and swelling. Can present as chronic knee pain with a sudden block in motion but able to bear weight and actively move the knee. Most discoid menisci are asymptomatic and discovered on an MRI.

    ii. **Physical examination.** Little to no joint effusion. Joint line is tender to palpation. Examination of the knee may reveal snapping with flexion of the knee. Unstable menisci may snap or pop in extension.

    iii. **Imaging.** X-rays may show widening of the joint line with blunting of the condyle. MRI shows meniscal tissue, often thicker than normal, across the entire plateau with a possible tear.

    iv. **Pathophysiology.** Congenital abnormality and may have knee pain as early as age 4. Most patients are first seen between ages 6 and 12 or older. The incidence varies and is estimated to be from 3% to 5% in Anglo Saxons and as much as 20% in Japanese. Most cases involve the lateral meniscus.

    v. **Classification.** There are three principal types. Type I is stable, complete. Type II is stable, incomplete. Type III is unstable because of the absence of the meniscotibial ligament.

    vi. **Treatment.** Asymptomatic discoid menisci discovered incidentally do not need surgical treatment. For a stable discoid lateral meniscus, arthroscopic sculpting (saucerization) of the meniscus to a normal configuration is indicated. If it is unstable, stabilization with a capsular suture is recommended.[29]

  b. **Osteochondritis dissecans**

    i. **Presentation.** Atraumatic subacute knee pain. Often started after running or sports. Can be the cause for recurrent minor joint effusions. Locking or catching, and decreased ROM only if loose body is present.

    ii. **Physical examination.** Mild swelling may be present but rare, tenderness over femoral condyle, medial or lateral joint line, anteromedial/ antero lateral joint line in deep flexion.

    iii. **Radiographic examination.** AP/lateral/notch views of knee; notch (or tunnel) view may show lesion most effectively. Lateral view may also show lesion on the posterior aspect of the femoral condyle.

    iv. **MRI.** Assesses "stability" of fragment based on continuity of articular cartilage and subchondral bone. Can see surrounding edema and quantify size of the lesion.

    v. **Pathophysiology.** This is a condition of unknown etiology that results in vascular changes of the subchondral bone in the femoral condyle (typically the posterior-lateral aspect of the medial femoral condyle - a known watershed area for capillary blood supply), which may lead to fragmentation or separation of the fragment along with the overlying cartilage. It most often occurs in adolescents and more often in boys than in girls.

    vi. **Treatment.** Depends on the age of the patient and the stability of the fragment. Skeletally immature patients with stable lesion may respond to restriction of activities such as no running or impact. This may take 6 to 18 months to resolve. Patient near or at skeletal maturity or unstable lesion or those showing no clinical improvement after 6 months consider arthroscopic evaluation, possible drilling and/or grafting, and internal stabilization.

3. **Posterior knee pain/swelling**

  a. **Baker's cyst**[30,31]

    i. **Presentation.** Mass in popliteal fossa. Usually painless and does not block motion. No history of trauma.

    ii. **Physical examination.** Fullness, sometimes painful to palpation. Rarely blocks motion. Will transilluminate as it is cystic.

    iii. **Radiographic examination.** X-rays usually not helpful.

    iv. **U/S.** Can definitively diagnose by ensuring that it is completely cystic and can quantify the size of the lesion and origins of the stalk. However, **MRI** is the gold standard for characterizing the lesion and has the advantage of evaluating for any associated intraarticular pathology.

    v. **Pathophysiology.** Expansion of a bursa that communicates with the joint. Often from the gastrocnemio-semimembranosus or the subgastrocnemius bursa. May be enlarged because of intraarticular pathology. Occurs around 3 to 9 years, averaging at 5 years.

    vi. **Treatment.** Because almost all resolve spontaneously, they rarely need treatment. Most decrease in size or resolve over a few years. Some may rupture and cause significant pain and swelling into the gastrocnemius muscle. Symptomatic treatment is all that is required.

  4. **Miscellaneous**

    a. **Tumors/neoplasms.** Pigmented villonodular synovitis presents as pain and swelling of the knee. There may be block in motion. This is a benign but locally aggressive tumor. Patients with leukemia or bone tumors often present with bone or joint pain. If history and physical examination are not consistent with other causes of pain, consider possible malignancies including Ewing's sarcoma, osteogenic sarcoma, leukemia, lymphoma, and neuroblastoma.

## V. Common Childhood Hip Disorders

### A. Developmental dysplasia of the hip (DDH)

  1. **Definition.** DDH is a spectrum of disorders ranging from complete dislocation of the hip to a reduced hip joint with acetabular dysplasia. It is a common cause of hip pain and early arthritis in adults.

  2. **Incidence.** Approximately 1 in 1,000 live births.

  3. **Risk factors.** Include first born, female, breech position in utero, oligohydramnios, and a positive family history. It has also been associated with other congenital conditions, including congenital muscular torticollis, metatarsus adductus, and clubfeet.

  4. **Physical examination.** In the newborn child or young infant, physical examination should start with a careful evaluation of the parts of the child other than the hips, including the spine, neck, and upper and lower extremities. Then, focus examination on the hips, trying to detect any evidence of instability. The clinical tests performed include the Barlow, Ortolani, and Galeazzi tests. The **Barlow** and **Ortolani** tests are performed with the clinician stabilizing the pelvis with one hand and grasping the child's femur with the other, placing the thumb over the medial femoral condyle and the long finger over the greater trochanter. The hip is flexed to 90° and held in neutral abduction. The Ortolani maneuver consists of abducting the hip and trying to detect the "clunking" sensation of the dislocated femoral head relocating into the acetabulum. Likewise, the Barlow test consists of two maneuvers. The first consists of adducting the hip with gentle longitudinal pressure to provoke the hip to dislocate or subluxate. The second maneuver is the same as that described for the Ortolani maneuver to achieve reduction of the dislocated hip. The **Galeazzi** test consists of comparing the height of the knees with the hips flexed to discern any apparent femoral shortening. One should also check for symmetric degrees of hip abduction bilaterally as well as for asymmetry of the perineal skin folds. Finally, DDH can be bilateral, which can be easily missed clinically because there is no apparent asymmetry. These children may first come to the attention of the primary care provider after walking age, with increased lumbar lordosis, a limb length difference, or a "waddling gait."

5. **Radiographic evaluation.** In a young infant, U/S is the modality of choice to detect any evidence of hip abnormality. The U/S allows a static assessment of acetabular development (alpha and beta angles) and percentage of femoral head coverage, as well as a dynamic assessment of femoral head stability with stress maneuvers. In children older than 6 months, a plain AP radiograph of the pelvis is appropriate. Evaluation of the AP radiograph should include evaluation of ossific nucleus of the femoral head relative to Hilgenreiner's line (ossific nucleus should be inferior) and Perkin's line (ossific nucleus should be medial). It should also include assessment of Shenton's arc (Figure 6-2). The ossific nucleus of the involved size is usually smaller than the uninvolved side.

6. **Treatment**
   a. **Age 0 to 6 months.** In the newborn child up to 6 months of age, treatment consists of abduction bracing, usually performed with a **Pavlik harness**.[32] This is usually applied at the time the instability is noted. It is most successful when applied within the first 7 weeks after the child is born. As the child gets older, the success of the Pavlik harness decreases. It may also be used for children with a clinically stable hip but who have significant acetabular dysplasia noted on U/S. Moreover, the adequacy of the reduction or positioning of the hip in the Pavlik harness can be evaluated with U/S. Complications with use of the harness are avascular necrosis of the femoral head, femoral nerve palsy,

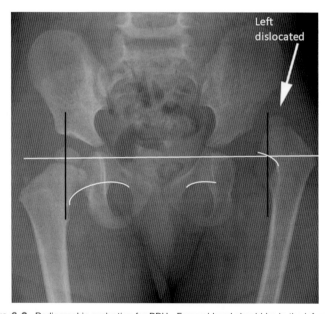

**Figure 6-2.** Radiographic evaluation for DDH. Femoral head should be in the inferomedial quadrant. Hilgenreiner's line (white line) is a horizontal line from lateral edge of the triradiate cartilage of one hip to the other. Perkin's line (black line) is a line perpendicular to Hilgenreiner's line and at the lateral edge of the acetabulum. Note the discontinuity of Shenton's arc (white arch) on the left.

and "Pavlik harness disease." Pavlik harness disease occurs when the femoral head was not adequately reduced in the acetabulum when the patient is in the harness, leading to progressive deformation of the posterior wall of the acetabulum and exacerbation of the dysplasia. If an adequate, concentric reduction of the femoral head cannot be achieved by 4 weeks after the harness has been applied, treatment with the Pavlik harness should be abandoned.[33,34]

  b. **Age 6 to 18 months or the child who fails Pavlik harness treatment.** Treatment for this group is aimed at achieving a satisfactory, congruent, stable reduction of the hip (i.e., get the femoral head reduced into the hip socket or "acetabulum"). This is achieved by performing either a **closed** (nonsurgical) or an **open** (surgical) reduction. Under anesthesia, an arthrogram is frequently performed at the time of the closed reduction and the child is placed in a spica cast. If the hip is noted to have a narrow "stable zone," a limited adductor release may be performed to improve stability. If a concentric closed reduction is not achievable or if excessive force is required to maintain the reduction, an open reduction may be performed. Popular methods for performing the open reduction include an anterior approach or the medial approach depending on the age of the child.[35]

  c. **Age from 18 months to 8 years.** Open reduction is required, and femoral shortening may also be required to reduce soft-tissue tension and thereby decrease the risk of avascular necrosis. If significant acetabular dysplasia is present, a pelvic osteotomy may also be performed.[35]

  d. **Children older than 8 years.** Children with persistent acetabular dysplasia or persistent hip subluxation may require secondary procedures such as femoral or pelvic osteotomies. Adolescents or young adults may present with hip pain from previously undiagnosed dysplasia. They may be candidates for periacetabular osteotomies.[36]

**B. Legg–Calvé–Perthes disease**
  1. **Definition.** Idiopathic avascular necrosis of the femoral head in children.
  2. **Presentation.** Most often affects children of ages 4 to 8; however, it may affect children as young as 2 or as old as 12 years; boys to girls ratio is 4:1; bilateral in 10% of the patients. Patients frequently have younger skeletal age than cohorts. Frequently, the disease presents as a painless limp (Fig. 6-3).
  3. **Etiology: idiopathic.** It has been associated with abnormalities of thrombolysis as well as deficiencies of protein C, protein S, or thrombolysin.
  4. **Differential diagnosis.** If bilateral hip involvement is present on radiograph, other possible etiologies should be excluded, including renal disease, hypothyroidism, multiple epiphyseal dysplasia or spondyloepiphyseal dysplasia, systemic corticosteroid use, storage disorders, and hemoglobinopathies.
  5. **Stages.** Waldenström originally described evolutionary stages that the disease course follows. These have been modified from the original description to include the following:
     a. **Initial stage.** Femoral head appears sclerotic early in the course of the disease.
     b. **Fragmentation stage.** Presence of subchondral fracture (crescent sign) is the hallmark of onset. The femoral head develops a "fragmented" appearance on radiograph as necrotic bone undergoes resorption.
     c. **Reossification stage.** There is evidence of healing; coalescence of femoral head fragmentation begins to occur.
     d. **Healed stage.** Reossification is complete. Femoral head returns to predisease density. Any remaining deformity is permanent.

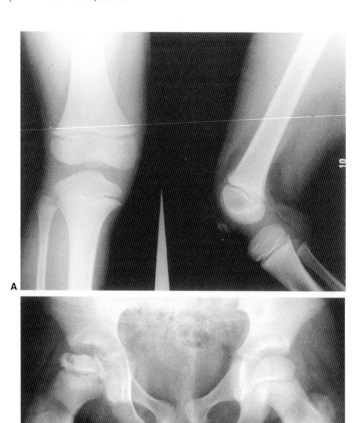

**Figure 6-3.** A 6-year-old boy with a 1- to 2-month history of limping and right knee pain. **A:** Radiographs of the knee are normal. **B:** An anteroposterior pelvis radiograph reveals changes in the right hip consistent with Legg–Calvé–Perthes disease.

6. **Classification systems.** To describe and compare outcomes and to study prognosis, various classification systems have been described.
   a. **Catterall.** Four-part system (I to IV) based on the amount of femoral head involvement.
   b. **Salter–Thompson.** Two-part system (A, B) simplified to less than 50% or greater than 50% involvement of femoral head.
   c. **Herring.** Recently revised to a four-part system (A, B, BC, and C) based on the height of lateral "pillar" (lateral one-third of femoral epiphysis).[37]

7. **Treatment.** For patients with Legg–Calvé–Perthes disease, it is important to determine who will benefit from treatment as well as how to treat them
   i. **Risk factors**
      (a) Older age at presentation (>8 years)
      (b) Greater degree of involvement of the femoral using the Herring classification
   ii. **Goals**
      (a) Maintaining hip ROM
      (b) "Containment" of the femoral head in the acetabulum
      (c) Ultimate goal of a congruent femoral head and acetabulum following the course of the disease
   iii. **Options**
      (a) Proximal femoral osteotomy
      (b) Adductor tenotomy and bracing
      (c) Arthrodiastasis
      (d) Triple osteotomy of the pelvis
      (e) Physical therapy
   iv. **Discussion.** For younger patients or patients with less involvement of the femoral head, treatment may consist primarily of NSAIDs, physical therapy, and restriction of activities to maintain hip ROM. For patients older than 8 or those with >50% femoral head involvement, treatment may consist of surgical containment from one of the options listed above. Unfortunately, for children with the most severe form of the disease, Herring C, treatment does not appear to change the natural history.

C. **Slipped capital femoral epiphysis**
   1. **Definition.** A disorder of the upper femur in which there is a separation (acutely or chronically) of the femoral epiphysis from the femoral neck through the region of the physis (growth plate). The femoral head becomes positioned posterior and inferior relative to the femoral neck.
   2. **Incidence.** Approximately 3 in 100,000; boys more frequently than girls. Bilateral involvement occurs in 20% to 60% of the cases. SCFE is seen most frequently in boys aged 12 to 16 and in girls aged 10 to 14. SCFE is associated with obesity, with more than half of the affected individuals weighing greater than the 95th percentile. (Note: not all patients with SCFE are obese.) Patients with an underlying hormonal or endocrine disorder have an associated increased risk for the development of SCFE. For patients with an unusual presentation such as atypical age (before age 10), bilateral involvement at presentation, or with other signs of possible endocrine abnormalities, a careful evaluation for endocrine disorders including hypothyroidism, hypopituitarism, or hypogonadism should be conducted.
   3. **Classification**
      a. **Temporal.** One method of classification is based on the duration of symptoms: acute: less than 3 weeks; chronic: greater than 3 weeks; and acute-on-chronic: a sudden exacerbation of the subclinical symptoms of long-standing duration.
      b. **Stability.** A patient with a **stable SCFE** is able to walk with or without assistance, with mild-to-moderate pain, or a slight limp. Patients with an **unstable SCFE** are unable to walk or to bear weight; their symptoms are similar to those of patients with a femoral neck fracture. Patients with an unstable SCFE are associated with a higher rate of complications.[38]
   4. **Treatment.** The most widely recommended form of treatment is surgical stabilization with **percutaneous pinning in situ**. For a stable SCFE, this

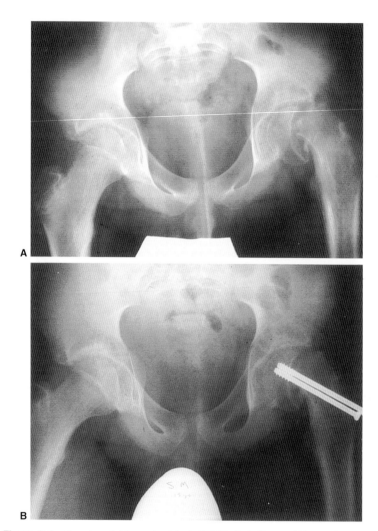

**Figure 6-4.** Slipped capital femoral epiphysis (SCFE). **A:** A 13-year-old boy with a severe, unstable left SCFE. **B:** Two cannulated screws were inserted for stabilization.

can usually be accomplished with a single, cannulated screw inserted under fluoroscopic control. The aim of the procedure is to insert the screw perpendicular to the femoral head in both the AP and lateral planes with close attention to avoid penetrating the femoral head and entering the hip joint. In cases of an unstable SCFE, a second screw may be inserted to further stabilize the femoral head (Fig. 6-4).

5. **Complications.** The primary complications associated with SCFE are **avascular necrosis** and **chondrolysis**. Avascular necrosis is the most

serious complication associated with patients with an SCFE. It is the interruption of the blood supply to the femoral head resulting in bone necrosis and subsequent destruction of the hip joint. It is uncommon with stable SCFE treated with pinning in situ. There is a greater incidence of avascular necrosis associated with an unstable SCFE.[38] Recent research supports the use of intraoperative monitoring of the vascular supply through an intraosseous pressure sensor.[39] Treatment options for unstable SCFE include gentle manipulation and fixation with two screws and possible capsulotomy or surgical hip dislocation with acute femoral head repositioning and femoral neck shortening.[40] However, there is still concern for avascular necrosis in unstable SCFE even after treatment. **Chondrolysis** is another complication of SCFE. It is a gradual loss of the joint ROM following stabilization of the SCFE. On postoperative radiographs, it appears as a gradual loss of the joint space over time.

## VI. Infectious and Inflammatory Conditions
### A. Osteomyelitis
1. **Definition.** A bacterial infection of the bone.
2. **Etiology.** Bacterial seeding can occur through several methods: direct inoculation (open fractures, penetrating wounds), local extension from adjacent sites, or hematogenous spread from distant sites. Children are skeletally immature and have physes (growth plates) at the ends of their long bones. The metaphyseal region of the bone just below the physis is a frequent location for osteomyelitis to occur due to capillary sludging adjacent to the physis.
3. **Presentation.** Patients may present with fever, pain, limping, and refusal to walk or bear weight on the affected lower extremity. Other symptoms of malaise or flu-like symptoms may or may not be present. One should inquire about immunization status as well as history of recent illnesses (e.g., otitis media, chicken pox, strep pharyngitis, URTI).
4. **Physical examination.** Site of involvement may or may not be easy to identify, particularly in younger patients. Careful palpation of entire extremity and the metaphyseal regions in particular is important. All joints should be placed through a ROM. Inspect for areas of redness, swelling, or warmth.
5. **Laboratory studies**
   a. CBC with differential
   b. ESR
   c. CRP
   d. Blood cultures (aerobic and anaerobic)
      The CRP has been recognized as a more rapidly responsive test than the ESR, increasing more quickly early in the evolution of the condition and declining more rapidly in response to treatment. If the diagnosis remains unclear, consider other diagnostic possibilities such as toxic synovitis, JRA, Lyme arthritis, and poststreptococcal arthritis.
6. **Radiographic studies.** Plain radiographs of the affected area should be obtained. In osteomyelitis, they may be frequently normal for the first 7 to 14 days. However, the radiographs may also be useful to rule out other diagnostic possibilities. MRI is very sensitive for osteomyelitis and allows assessment of bone involvement, soft-tissue inflammation or abscess formation, and the presence of a joint effusion. However, an MRI may require significant sedation or anesthesia for younger patients.
7. **Aspiration.** In patients with an identified focus of infection, an attempt at aspiration is recommended by many authors to identify the organism and

guide antibiotic therapy. This may be done with sedation in the emergency department or the fluoroscopic suite or, alternatively, under anesthesia in the operating room.

8. **Organisms.** On the basis of patient age:
   a. **Younger than 1 year**
      i. *Staphylococcus aureus*
      ii. Group B *Streptococcus*
      iii. *Escherichia coli*
   b. **1 to 4 years old**
      i. *Kingella kingae*
      ii. *S. aureus*
      iii. *Haemophilus influenzae*
   c. **Older than 4 years**
      i. *S. aureus*
   d. **Adolescent**
      i. *S. aureus*
      ii. *Neisseria gonorrhoeae*

9. **Treatment.** Appropriate intravenous antibiotic based on culture or most likely organism. Duration of antibiotic coverage is a matter of debate. Recent evidence and consensus suggest that a period of 5 days of intravenous (IV) treatment followed by oral antibiotics if the following criteria are met: (i) Clinical improvement; (ii) afebrile for 48 hours; (iii) child will take the oral antibiotic; and (iv) significant drop in the CRP compared to the diagnosis.[41]

10. **Surgical treatment.** If the patient does not respond to antibiotic treatment after the first 24 to 48 hours, consider the possibility of a subperiosteal or intraosseous abscess as well as other diagnostic possibilities. Consider surgical drainage of abscess or intramedullary canal if necessary.[42]

**B. Septic arthritis**[43]
1. **Definition.** An infectious arthritis of a joint, usually bacterial in nature.
2. **Etiology.** Most frequently, it occurs from adjacent osteomyelitis in which the metaphyseal portion of the bone is intraarticular (e.g., hip, shoulder, elbow, and ankle). When pus from metaphysis decompresses itself through cortex, joints can become infected. Infection is also possible through hematogenous spread or direct inoculation.
3. **Joints most commonly involved:** knee (41%), hip (23%), ankle (14%), elbow (12%), wrist (4%), and shoulder (4%).
4. **Presentation.** Young children usually refuse to walk or to bear weight on the lower extremity or to use their upper extremity. The child usually will be febrile (temperature $>38.5°C$) and may even show signs of sepsis. Septic arthritis may also occur in the newborn child; babies in the neonatal intensive care unit may present with pseudoparalysis of the affected limb with failure or refusal to move it.
5. **Physical examination.** If the joint involved is superficial, classic signs of joint redness, swelling, and warmth are sometimes present. However, if the joint is not superficial (hip, shoulder), no visible abnormality may be detectable. However, the patient will hold the affected limb in a position of maximum comfort (e.g., the hip in flexion and external rotation to allow the most space for intracapsular swelling). Any attempt at passive ROM is very painful and restricted because of guarding.
6. **Laboratory studies**
   a. CBC with differential
   b. ESR
   c. CRP
   d. Blood cultures

The CRP and ESR will become significantly elevated. The CBC may remain normal.

7. **Radiographic studies.** Plain radiographs of the affected joint should be obtained to look for any evidence of bony destruction or erosions. For patients with suspected hip pain, an U/S of the hip may confirm the presence of a hip joint effusion. In some institutions, aspiration is performed under U/S guidance.

8. **Joint aspiration** is performed to confirm the diagnosis. Joint fluid should be sent for white blood cell (WBC) count with differential, Gram stain, and culture (if quantity permits, glucose and total protein as well). If the patient is a teenager who is sexually active and for whom gonococcal infection is a possibility, the laboratory should be notified to perform cultures on chocolate agar in addition to the routine media. The Gram stain may be positive for bacteria in only approximately 50% of the patients. The cell count most often has greater than 50,000 WBCs and/or greater than 90% polymorphonuclear neutrophils (PMNs). If cultures are negative, a PCR should be considered to confirm the diagnosis.

9. **Organisms.** On the basis of patient age:
   a. **Younger than 1 year**
      i. *S. aureus*
      ii. Group B *Streptococcus*
      iii. *E. coli*
   b. **1 to 4 years**
      i. *S. aureus* and *K. kingae*
      ii. *H. influenzae* (less common now with *H. influenzae* B vaccination)
      iii. Group A *Streptococcus*
      iv. *Streptococcus pneumoniae*
   c. **Older than 4 years**
      i. *S. aureus*
      ii. Group A *Streptococcus*
   d. **Adolescent**
      i. *S. aureus*
      ii. *N. gonorrhoeae*
   e. **Less common** organisms include *Salmonella* and *Neisseria meningitidis*

10. **Treatment.** Using clinical predictors of fever, elevated ESR, refusal to bear weight, and elevated WBC, when a patient has three of the four predictors, there is a 93% probability of septic arthritis; with four predictors, the probability is 99%.[44] When CRP is added as an additional predictor, if a patient has all five predictors, the probability is equally high at 98%.[45,46] In patients suspected of septic arthritis, treatment consists of emergent aspiration of the joint. If aspiration confirms the diagnosis of septic arthritis, treatment proceeds to immediate surgical incision and drainage of the affected joint. Surgical decompression of the adjacent bone may also be indicated if there is evidence of an intraosseous abscess or bony involvement. Intravenous antibiotics should be administered once joint fluid cultures have been obtained. Empiric coverage should be started initially based on the most likely organism involved. Once culture and sensitivities have been identified, antibiotic coverage can be tailored accordingly. The duration of antibiotics is usually 4 to 6 weeks, although a switch from IV to oral follows the same criteria as for osteomyelitis.[41] Recently, the general concept of joint irrigation is being challenged. Other treatment options include periodic joint aspiration under U/S guidance or with antibiotic treatment without intervention unless no clinical improvement occurs.[47,48]

### C. Transient synovitis

1. **Definition.** An inflammatory, postviral process resulting in joint swelling and pain.

2. **Presentation.** Transient synovitis most frequently occurs in young children aged 3 to 8. Patients often may have had a recent URTI or other viral illness in the 2 to 3 weeks prior to the onset of symptoms. Patients are usually afebrile with a history of several days of pain or limping. The physician must differentiate between transient synovitis and a truly infectious process such as septic arthritis or osteomyelitis.

3. **Laboratory studies.** CBC with differential, ESR, and CRP are usually within the normal range. CRP elevation is the most predictable laboratory value to diagnose septic arthritis. Transient synovitis of the hip often presents with little to no WBC elevation and a mildly elevated ESR or CRP; a CRP of >20 is highly predictive of septic arthritis.[43]

4. **Radiographic studies.** Plain radiographs are usually normal or may show evidence of a joint effusion. U/S is helpful if deemed necessary for confirming the presence of a joint effusion.

5. **Aspiration.** Because the clinician is often confronted with having to exclude septic arthritis, joint aspiration can be helpful to examine the joint fluid. Gram stain, cell count, and culture should be obtained. The Gram stain should be negative, and the cell count should be between 5,000 and 15,000 WBCs with less than 25% PMNs.

6. **Treatment.** The primary treatment objective in the treatment of transient synovitis is to ensure that septic arthritis has been excluded. Once septic arthritis is excluded, the condition can be treated expectantly with reduction in activity, NSAIDs, and careful observation.[47]

### D. Lyme arthritis

1. **Definition.** A large joint effusion resulting from an infection caused by the tick-born spirochete organism *Borrelia burgdorferi*. This condition is especially prevalent in the New England states and in the Upper Midwestern states of Minnesota and Wisconsin.

2. **Presentation.** Patients often present with a large, atraumatic joint effusion, most often involving the knee joint. Patient is usually afebrile and has a mild limp but relatively painless joint ROM.

3. **Laboratory tests.** Blood tests include CBC with differential, CRP, ESR, and serum Lyme antibody titers. CRP and ESR may be elevated. Serum Lyme antibody titer results may take 24 to 48 hours to be available.

4. **Treatment.** When evaluating the patient, it is important to distinguish between septic arthritis and Lyme arthritis. Both patients may have a large joint effusion. The refusal to bear weight is the strongest predictor of the diagnosis of septic arthritis over Lyme arthritis. However, if the patient appears to have septic arthritis, aspiration of the joint may be necessary to exclude bacterial septic arthritis. When the diagnosis of Lyme arthritis can be confirmed by serum Lyme antibody test or joint fluid PCR tests for *B. burgdorferi*, treatment consists of 30 days of oral antibiotics.

## VII. Back Pain and Spine-Related Conditions

### A. Evaluation of the pediatric patient with back pain

1. **History**
   a. Location of pain (neck/thoracic/lumbar)
   b. Radiation of pain into lower extremities
   c. Associated symptoms such as numbness, tingling, weakness, change in bowel or bladder function, and pain at night
   d. Onset of pain (acute/gradual)
   e. Frequency and duration of symptoms

f. Any improvement with NSAIDs/aspirin

g. Is patient involved in athletic activities that are associated with repetitive hyperextension of back (e.g., figure skating, gymnastics, dance, football [particularly lineman], or hockey)?

2. **Physical examination.** Have patient dressed in examination gown or other appropriate clothing.

a. Back ROM: flexion/extension/side bending/rotation

b. Pain with palpation along spine

c. Radicular pain associated with straight leg test

d. Complete neurologic examination including the following:

  i. Motor strength

  ii. Sensation

  iii. Deep tendon reflexes

  iv. Signs of upper motor neuron abnormalities: clonus, Babinski, etc.

  v. Abdominal reflexes

e. Hip ROM: possible referred pain from hip pathology

**B. Radiologic tests.** If pediatric patients describe significant back pain that limits activities and/or any abnormal findings are present on physical examination, it is appropriate to obtain plain radiographs.

1. **AP and lateral radiograph** of thoracic and lumbar spine if pain is localized to thoracic or thoracolumbar region or any findings to suggest scoliosis.

2. Evaluate radiographs for signs of:

a. Scoliosis

b. Spondylolysis/spondylolisthesis

c. Loss of disc space

d. Vertebral end-plate changes (erosions, Schmorl nodes)

e. Other bony changes (absent pedicle, curvature without rotation, etc.)

3. **Additional imaging tests.** If neurologic abnormalities are identified on physical examination, consider MRI of spinal canal. If no neurologic findings are present but pain presentation is worrisome for underlying bony abnormality such as stress fracture or tumor or structural, consider either **MRI or three-phase nuclear medicine bone scan/single-photon emission computed tomography (SPECT) scan.**

4. **Differential diagnosis**

a. Mechanical low back pain

b. Spondylolysis/spondylolisthesis

c. Discitis

d. Lumbar Scheuermann disease

e. Herniated intervertebral disc or apophyseal ring fracture

f. Spine-related bone tumors

**C. Mechanical low back pain**

1. **Definition.** Back pain usually localized to the lower back without radiation to lower extremities and without neurologic findings on physical examination or radiographic abnormalities. Previously thought to be rare in children, it remains less common in children than in adults but can be a source of back pain if other causes have been definitively excluded. Symptoms most often occur after sitting for long periods, tend to be vague or nonspecific, and occur sporadically.

2. **Physical examination.** Notable for lack of abnormal findings.

3. **Radiographic examination.** Plain radiographs are normal. No specialized radiographic studies are recommended at the time of the initial evaluation.

4. **Treatment.**

  i. Referral to physical therapy for home-based exercise program of back strengthening and posture retraining.

    ii. Prescription for a short course (5 to 7 days) of NSAIDs.

    iii. Return to clinic in 1 to 2 months for follow-up. If symptoms do not improve or have changed, reconsider diagnosis.

**D. Spondylolysis/spondylolisthesis**

    1. **Spondylolysis.** A structural defect in the bone in the posterior elements of the spine. Most often in the "pars interarticularis" region of the L5 vertebra. Associated with hyperextension activities such as dance, gymnastics, and figure skating; presents as low lumbar back pain without radiation into the lower extremities but exacerbated by hyperextension activities. Oblique X-rays are not very sensitive for detecting pars defects, thus definitive diagnosis is by MRI when suspected.[49] Treatment: limitation of activities, bracing, and physical therapy.

    2. **Spondylolisthesis.** A translation or slippage of one vertebra on the **next** lower vertebra. The most common cause in children is an "isthmic spondylolisthesis," in which a lesion or defect in the pars interarticularis permits forward slippage of the superior vertebra. Treatment: If mild, consider observation. If severe (>50%) or refractory to therapy, recommend referral to orthopaedic surgeon for evaluation of possible surgical stabilization.

**E. Discitis.** A condition in which children develop back pain that arises from a presumed bacterial infection of the intervertebral disc. Patients may present with gradual onset of pain, loss of lumbar lordosis, and progressive decline in activity level potentially to the point of refusing to walk. The child may remain afebrile. Current theories of etiology suggest that it may start as a vertebral osteomyelitis that spreads to the adjacent disc space. If suspected, laboratory tests should be obtained, including CBC with differential, ESR, CRP, and blood cultures. The CBC may be normal but some elevation of the ESR and CRP is frequently present. Initial radiographs may be normal or show vertebral end-plate irregularities. Later radiographs may show a narrowing of the disc space involved. The diagnosis can be confirmed with specialized imaging tests such as nuclear medicine bone scan, CT, or MRI. Treatment consists of antibiotic therapy and, when appropriate, back immobilization with a removable spinal orthosis for symptomatic support.

**F. Lumbar Scheuermann disease.** A condition in which patients present with lumbar back pain without radicular symptoms. There are end-plate changes termed "Schmorl nodes" in the lumbar vertebra on plain radiographs. In contrast to Scheuermann disease of the thoracic spine (see below), which is associated with significant thoracic kyphosis and vertebral wedging, these changes are not found in the lumbar spine.

**G. Herniated intervertebral disc.** A herniation of the central portion of the disc, the "nucleus pulposus," into the spinal canal. Occurs in adolescent and teenage patients. Symptoms usually have an acute, specific onset and are associated with radicular symptoms of pain radiating down into the lower extremity. Neurologic examination is helpful to look for signs of motor weakness. Children and adolescents may also sustain an **avulsion fracture of the vertebral ring apophysis**. This may present with sudden onset of back pain with radicular-type symptoms radiating into the lower extremities. It is a separation of the end plate of the vertebra from the vertebral body through the growth plate. This may be visible on plain films as a small triangular fragment of bone displaced from the lower end plate of the vertebra. If a herniated disc or a vertebral ring apophysis avulsion-type fracture is suspected, an MRI scan can help confirm diagnosis.

**H. Bone tumors involving the spine.** There are several bone tumors that arise from the vertebral body or the posterior elements of the spine. They may present with pain, particularly night pain, deformity, or other associated symptoms.

Physical examination may reveal findings of scoliosis; however, radiographs may reveal a curvature of the spine without any rotational component present. This suggests that the curvature is postural and because of the painful process rather than a structural, scoliosis-type curve. Benign tumors that arise in the spine most frequently include osteoid osteoma, osteoblastoma, and hemangioma. Primary malignant tumors of the bone that arise in the spine are relatively rare.

I. **Idiopathic adolescent scoliosis**
   1. **Definition.** A deformity of the spine consisting of a lateral curvature measuring greater than 10° on a spine radiograph that also has a rotational component. The word "idiopathic" suggests no identifiable, underlying cause. There is probably a genetic component.
   2. **Presentation.** Most often patients are adolescent girls who have been detected either on school screening examination or by an observant primary physician. Boys have a lower incidence of progressive curves. The deformity may occasionally be seen in younger children. Family history is frequently positive. Idiopathic scoliosis is *painless* in most cases, *occasional mechanical pain could be associated with the deformity in up to 25% of patients.* The examiner should inquire about any neurologic symptoms, including weakness, numbness, radicular symptoms, or bowel or bladder changes.
   3. **Incidence.** For curves greater than 10°, the overall prevalence is approximately 2%. However, for curves measuring greater than 20° and requiring treatment, the prevalence is about 0.2%.
   4. **Physical examination.** All patients should be examined in a gown so that the back can be well visualized. Inspect pelvic height for evidence of limb length difference. Examine shoulder height and trunk position for evidence of asymmetry or truncal imbalance. With the patient standing, have the patient bend forward at the waist. Observe the patient's back for evidence of rib hump deformity (**Adam's forward bending test**). Finally, complete a thorough neurologic examination, including abdominal reflexes and tests for long tract or upper motor neuron lesions.
   5. **Radiographic evaluation.** Standing posteroanterior (PA) and lateral spine radiographs on a long cassette to include the thoracic, lumbar, and sacral regions of the spine. The curvature of the spine can be measured using the Cobb method which measures the angle between the most tilted endplate above the apex of the curve to the most tilted endplate below the apex of the curve, in the other direction.
   6. **Characteristics.** For true idiopathic scoliosis, the curve is most often:
      a. Convex to the right in the thoracic spine.
      b. Not associated with any neurologic changes.
      c. Without any signs or findings to suggest other medical conditions.
      If a curve does not fit this pattern, one must exclude other possible causes. If the curve is convex to the left, painful, has associated neurologic changes, or is rapidly progressive, one should consider obtaining an MRI scan to rule out possible underlying spinal cord abnormalities, such as syringomyelia, tethered cord, diastematomyelia, or spinal cord tumor.
   7. **Risk factors for progression** include young age, female gender, prepubertal status, and curve greater than 20°. The spine curve is at greatest risk for progression during periods of accelerated skeletal growth.
   8. The **goal of treatment** is to prevent further progression of the curve to a point that surgery is recommended.
   9. **Treatment** of idiopathic scoliosis depends on the size of the curve, the age of the patient, and its developmental status at the time of detection. Typically, for curves between 11° and 20°, only **observation** is needed with repeated spine radiographs as needed. The younger the child at the time of

curve detection, the greater the risk for future progression of the curve. If the curve is greater than 20° to 25° in a skeletally immature patient, **brace treatment** is indicated. Brace treatment is most effective in moderate-sized curves in growing adolescent patients. The goal of brace treatment is to arrest any further progression of the curve. For patients in whom a large curve of greater than 45° is already present or for whom the curve progresses despite brace treatment, the patient should be referred for consideration of surgical treatment. There are treatments that show some short term efficacy but are not currently standard of care such as nighttime bracing, spine specific exercises, and growth modulation of the spine.

**J. Kyphosis**
1. **Definition.** An increased curvature of the thoracic spine in the sagittal plane producing a rounded-back appearance.
2. **Characteristics.** Normal thoracic kyphosis is 15° to 45°. **Scheuermann disease** is a condition in which the thoracic curve on the lateral radiograph is greater than 45° to 50° and associated with wedging of three adjacent central vertebral bodies of 5° or more. It may be associated with end-plate changes of the vertebral bodies such as Schmorl nodes. It should be distinguished from postural kyphosis, in which the vertebral bodies do not exhibit changes and the curvature resolves with improvement of the patient's posture.
3. **Presentation.** Patients usually have mild back pain or concerns regarding appearance.
4. **Physical examination.** Careful examination of the back with the patient standing, on forward bending, and with hyperextension in the prone position can help determine the flexibility of the kyphosis. Increased thoracic kyphosis is frequently associated with increased lumbar lordosis. The possibility of hip flexion contractures should be assessed. A careful neurologic examination should also be performed.
5. **Radiographs.** Standing PA and lateral thoracolumbar spine radiographs should be obtained.
6. **Treatment.** Options include observation, bracing, and surgery. For patients who are asymptomatic with a relatively small curve, one may consider continued observation. For symptomatic patients who are skeletally immature with curves greater than 45° to 50°, one may consider brace treatment. Currently, there are no clear indications for surgical treatment. In general, severe deformities above 70°, significant pain, progressive deformity, and concerns regarding patient appearance in the setting of significant deformity are all indications for surgical treatment.[50]

**K. Lordosis**
1. **Definition.** An increase in "swayback" appearance of the lower lumbar spine.
2. **Presentation.** The patient may complain of low back pain, concern regarding appearance, or both.
3. **Etiology.** Possible causes include posture (especially in younger patients), bilateral congenital dislocation of the hip, hip flexion contracture, hamstring weakness, increased thoracic kyphosis, spondylolysis/spondylolisthesis, and congenital spinal deformity.
4. **Physical examination** should include careful evaluation of the back, hips, and lower extremities, as well as a thorough neurologic evaluation.
5. **Radiographs.** PA and lateral thoracolumbar spine radiographs should be obtained.
6. **Treatment.** Careful exclusion of underlying abnormalities should be undertaken. If other underlying causes have been excluded and the cause is thought to be postural, treatment may consist of further observation or therapy for pain.

## VIII. Neuromuscular Disorders

### A. Cerebral palsy[51,52]

1. **Definition.** A nonprogressive disorder resulting from an injury to the brain, usually within the first year of life, and resulting in impaired motor function.

2. **Classification.** Geographic (part of body most affected), type of motor dysfunction, or functional.

   a. **Geographic**
      i. **Hemiplegia.** Arm and leg on one side only affected
      ii. **Diplegia.** Major spasticity in lower limbs, less in upper
      iii. **Triplegia.** Three-limb involvement
      iv. **Quadriplegia.** All four limbs, "total body involved"

   b. **Motor type**
      i. **Spastic.** Increased stretch reflexes (pyramidal)
      ii. **Athetoid.** Fluctuating motor tone, often with spontaneous, involuntary rhythmic motor movements (extrapyramidal)
      iii. **Dystonia.** Similar to athetoid; intermittent or inconsistent tone
      iv. **Mixed.** A combination of spasticity and dystonia

   c. **Functional**: Gross Motor Function Classification System (GMFCS)[53]
      **Level I:** Ambulatory, difficulty with balance and speed. Able to hold a box going up stairs
      **Level II:** Ambulatory, difficulty with running or jumping. Uses rail when going up stairs
      **Level III:** Ambulatory in the community but with an assistive device
      **Level IV:** Nonambulatory in the community, mobile with wheelchair but has head control and may walk in therapy with a gait trainer
      **Level V:** Nonambulatory, even in therapy, poor head control, limited motor function

3. **Causes**
   a. **Prenatal.** Intrauterine infection, for example, TORCH (toxoplasmosis, rubella, cytomegalovirus, and herpes simplex), genetic, or chromosomal abnormalities
   b. **Perinatal.** Premature birth, low birth weight, asphyxia, erythroblastosis fetalis
   c. **Postnatal.** Infection, stroke, cardiac arrest, near drowning, nonaccidental trauma

4. **Hierarchical approach to problems**
   a. **Primary problems** include abnormal muscle tone, poor selective muscle control, and poor balance.
   b. **Secondary problems** include muscle and joint contractures and bony deformities (increased femoral anteversion, tibial torsion, and foot deformities).
   c. **Tertiary problems** include compensatory mechanisms for primary and secondary problems.

5. **Treatment**
   a. **Physical therapy**
   b. **Orthotics**
   c. **Assistive devices:** wheelchair, walker, crutches
   d. **Tone-reducing agents or medications:** oral (e.g., baclofen, Valium, dantrolene) or focal (e.g., Botox, phenol)
   e. **Neurosurgical options:** selective dorsal rhizotomy, intrathecal baclofen pump, ventral-dorsal rhizotomy.
   f. **Orthopaedic surgery:** soft-tissue lengthening procedures, bony realignment procedures.

**Ambulatory patients.** If children have independent sitting balance by age 2, there is approximately a 95% chance that they will eventually be able to ambulate. Children with cerebral palsy who can ambulate usually have difficulty because of increased motor tone, poor selective motor control, and poor balance. Frequently, muscle contractures and bony deformities develop over time. Three-dimensional gait analysis is useful to assess walking in these children to identify a problem list of orthopaedic issues or deformities that are contributing to the patient's difficulty in walking. Orthopaedic surgery usually consists of muscle lengthening or transfer procedures combined with bony realignment procedures for the underlying torsional deformities of the lower extremities. Most often, these are combined in one surgical setting to minimize recovery time and to speed the child's return to activities. The **selective dorsal rhizotomy** is a procedure to decrease lower extremity tone by cutting approximately 30% to 40% of the dorsal afferent sensory nerve rootlets. It is indicated for children with spastic diplegia who have pure spasticity, no contractures, and good balance. It is usually performed in children between the ages of 4 and 8. For children with cerebral palsy, optimum treatment consists of a combined approach involving the physical medicine and rehabilitation specialist, the neurosurgeon, the orthopaedic surgeon, the physical and occupational therapists, and the orthotist.

**Nonambulatory patients.** The principal difficulties that affect patients with total body involvement are hip subluxation or dislocation and neuromuscular scoliosis. These are important issues for these patients because they are wheelchair bound and often severely delayed. Painful sitting or difficulty with sitting balance resulting from scoliosis or pelvic obliquity can interfere significantly with their activities of daily living or personal care and can become painful. Patients should be monitored regularly for early detection of either hip dislocation or scoliosis.

**B. Spina bifida**[54]

1. **Definition.** A malformation of the spine, resulting from incomplete closure of the posterior elements of the spine as well as of the neural tube in which the meninges and neural elements are exposed at birth.

2. **Etiology** is multifactorial. There is a genetic component in that there is increased risk for first-degree relatives of patients with spina bifida. There is also an environmental role linked to insufficient dietary folic acid for women of childbearing age.

3. **Classification:** Defined by the lowest intact motor level and is often asymmetric; thoracic, thoracolumbar, mid-lumbar, low lumbar, lumbosacral.

4. **Associated disorders** include hydrocephalus requiring ventriculoperitoneal shunting, tethered spinal cord, Arnold–Chiari malformations, syringomyelia, and urologic problems.

5. **Ambulatory function** is determined primarily by the level of deficit. Patients who ambulate are usually who maintain active control of knee flexion and extension. Many children ambulate when young, but as they get older, it takes greater energy and oxygen consumption, and many resort to using a wheelchair.

6. **Orthopaedic conditions** depend on the level of involvement and often include lumbar scoliosis and kyphosis, hip dislocations, and foot deformities. Depending on ambulatory status, goals of treatment may vary. Often hip dislocations are painless and do not change function in nonambulatory patients, but spine abnormalities may affect sitting balance and cause skin issues. Ambulatory children with low lumbar or lumbosacral involvement do benefit from located hips, correction of crouch gait, and plantigrade feet. Braceable feet are key to maintaining skin integrity.

## REFERENCES

1. Flynn JM, Widmann RF. The limping child: evaluation and diagnosis. *J Am Acad Orthop Surg.* 2001;9(2):89-98.
2. Bartoloni A, Aparisi Gomez MP, Cirillo M, et al. Imaging of the limping child. *Eur J Radiol.* 2018;109:155-170.
3. Gurney B. Leg length discrepancy. *Gait Posture.* 2002;15(2):195-206
4. Phillips WA. The child with a limp. *Orthop Clin North Am.* 1987;18(4):489-501.
5. Wyers MR. Evaluation of pediatric bone lesions. *Pediatr Radiol.* 2010;40(4):468-473.
6. Hryhorczuk AL, Restrepo R, Lee EY. Pediatric musculoskeletal ultrasound: practical imaging approach. *AJR Am J Roentgenol.* 2016;206(5):W62-W72.
7. Paley D, Tetsworth K. Mechanical axis deviation of the lower limbs. Preoperative planning of uniapical angular deformities of the tibia or femur. *Clin Orthop Relat Res.* 1992;280:48-64.
8. Paley D. *Principles of Deformity Correction.* 1st ed. Springer; 2002.
9. Crane L. Femoral torsion and its relation to toeing-in and toeing-out. *J Bone Joint Surg Am.* 1959;41-A(3):421-428.
10. Staheli LT. Torsion—treatment indications. *Clin Orthop Relat Res.* 1989;247:61-66.
11. Staheli LT. Rotational problems in children. *Instr Course Lect.* 1994;43:199-209.
12. Eamsobhana P, Rojjananukulpong K, Ariyawatkul T, Chotigavanichaya C, Kaewpornsawan K. Does the parental stretching programs improve metatarsus adductus in newborns? *J Orthop Surg (Hong Kong).* 2017;25(1). doi:10.1177/2309499017690320.
13. Sabharwal S, Sabharwal S. Treatment of infantile blount disease: an update. *J Pediatr Orthop.* 2017;37(Suppl 2):S26-S31.
14. Birch JG. Blount disease. *J Am Acad Orthop Surg.* 2013;21(7):408-418.
15. Salenius P, Vankka E. The development of the tibiofemoral angle in children. *J Bone Joint Surg Am.* 1975;57(2):259-261.
16. Manner HM, Radler C, Ganger R, Grill F. Knee deformity in congenital longitudinal deficiencies of the lower extremity. *Clin Orthop Relat Res.* 2006;448:185-192.
17. Cozen L. Fracture of the proximal portion of the tibia in children followed by valgus deformity. *Surg Gynecol Obstet.* 1953;97(2):183-188.
18. Bor N, Coplan JA, Herzenberg JE. Ponseti treatment for idiopathic clubfoot: minimum 5-year followup. *Clin Orthop Relat Res.* 2009;467(5):1263-1270.
19. Miller M, Dobbs MB. Congenital vertical talus: etiology and management. *J Am Acad Orthop Surg.* 2015;23(10):604-611.
20. Oh I, Williams BR, Ellis SJ, Kwon DJ, Deland JT. Reconstruction of the symptomatic idiopathic flatfoot in adolescents and young adults. *Foot Ankle Int.* 2011;32(3):225-232.
21. Zhou B, Tang K, Hardy M. Talocalcaneal coalition combined with flatfoot in children: diagnosis and treatment: a review. *J Orthop Surg Res.* 2014;9:129.
22. Docquier PL, Maldaque P, Bouchard M. Tarsal coalition in paediatric patients. *Orthop Traumatol Surg Res.* 2019;105(1S):S123-S131.
23. George HL, Casaletto J, Unnikrishnan PN, et al. Outcome of the scarf osteotomy in adolescent hallux valgus. *J Child Orthop.* 2009;3(3):185-190.
24. Kodali P, Islam A, Andrish J. Anterior knee pain in the young athlete: diagnosis and treatment. *Sports Med Arthrosc Rev.* 2011;19(1):27-33.
25. Yen YM. Assessment and treatment of knee pain in the child and adolescent athlete. *Pediatr Clin North Am.* 2014;61(6):1155-1173.
26. Seitlinger G, Ladenhauf HN, Wierer G. What is the chance that a patella dislocation will happen a second time: update on the natural history of a first time patella dislocation in the adolescent. *Curr Opin Pediatr.* 2018;30(1):65-70.
27. Fulkerson JP, Shea KP. Disorders of patellofemoral alignment. *J Bone Joint Surg Am.* 1990;72(9):1424-1429.
28. Gao GX, Mahadev A, Lee EH. Sleeve fracture of the patella in children. *J Orthop Surg (Hong Kong).* 2008;16(1):43-46.
29. Stanitski CL. *Meniscal Lesions. Pediatric and Adolescent Sports Medicine.* WB Saunders; 1994:382-384.
30. Akagi R, Saisu T, Segawa Y, et al. Natural history of popliteal cysts in the pediatric population. *J Pediatr Orthop.* 2013;33(3):262-268.
31. Harcke HT, Niedzielski A, Thacker MM. Popliteal cysts in children: another look. *J Pediatr Orthop B.* 2016;25(6):539-542.
32. Omeroglu H. Treatment of developmental dysplasia of the hip with the Pavlik harness in children under six months of age: indications, results and failures. *J Child Orthop.* 2018;12(4):308-316.

33. Viere RG, Birch JG, Herring JA, Roach JW, Johnston CE. Use of the Pavlik harness in congenital dislocation of the hip. An analysis of failures of treatment. *J Bone Joint Surg Am.* 1990;72(2):238-244.

34. Weinstein SL, Mubarak SJ, Wenger DR. Developmental hip dysplasia and dislocation: Part I. *Instr Course Lect.* 2004;53:523-530.

35. Weinstein SL, Mubarak SJ, Wenger DR. Developmental hip dysplasia and dislocation: Part II. *Instr Course Lect.* 2004;53:531-542.

36. Bittersohl B, Hosalkar HS, Wenger DR. Surgical treatment of hip dysplasia in children and adolescents. *Orthop Clin North Am.* 2012;43(3):301-315.

37. Herring JA, Kim HT, Browne R. Legg-Calve-Perthes disease. Part I: Classification of radiographs with use of the modified lateral pillar and Stulberg classifications. *J Bone Joint Surg Am.* 2004;86-A(10):2103-2120.

38. Loder RT, Richards BS, Shapiro PS, Reznick LR, Aronson DD. Acute slipped capital femoral epiphysis: the importance of physeal stability. *J Bone Joint Surg Am.* 1993;75(8):1134-1140.

39. Schrader T, Jones CR, Kaufman AM, Herzog MM. Intraoperative monitoring of epiphyseal perfusion in slipped capital femoral epiphysis. *J Bone Joint Surg Am.* 2016;98(12):1030-1040.

40. Zaltz I, Baca G, Clohisy JC. Unstable SCFE: review of treatment modalities and prevalence of osteonecrosis. *Clin Orthop Relat Res.* 2013;471(7):2192-2198.

41. Quick RD, Williams J, Fernandez M, et al. Improved diagnosis and treatment of bone and joint infections using an evidence-based treatment guideline. *J Pediatr Orthop.* 2018;38(6): e354-e359.

42. Morrissy RT, Haynes DW. Acute hematogenous osteomyelitis: a model with trauma as an etiology. *J Pediatr Orthop.* 1989;9(4):447-456.

43. Kocher MS, Mandiga R, Murphy JM, et al. A clinical practice guideline for treatment of septic arthritis in children: efficacy in improving process of care and effect on outcome of septic arthritis of the hip. *J Bone Joint Surg Am.* 2003;85-A(6):994-999.

44. Kocher MS, Mandiga R, Zurakowski D, Barnewolt C, Kasser JR. Validation of a clinical prediction rule for the differentiation between septic arthritis and transient synovitis of the hip in children. *J Bone Joint Surg Am.* 2004;86-A(8):1629-1635.

45. Caird MS, Flynn JM, Leung YL, Millman JE, D'Italia JG, Dormans JP. Factors distinguishing septic arthritis from transient synovitis of the hip in children. A prospective study. *J Bone Joint Surg Am.* 2006;88(6):1251-1257.

46. Givon U, Liberman B, Schindler A, Blankstein A, Ganel A. Treatment of septic arthritis of the hip joint by repeated ultrasound-guided aspirations. *J Pediatr Orthop.* 2004;24(3):266-270.

47. Haueisen DC, Weiner DS, Weiner SD. The characterization of "transient synovitis of the hip" in children. *J Pediatr Orthop.* 1986;6(1):11-17.

48. Tornero E, De Bergua-Domingo JM, Domenech P, et al. Knee arthritis in children: when can it be safely treated with needle joint aspiration? A large children's tertiary hospital study. *J Pediatr Orthop.* 2019;39(3):130-135.

49. Dhouib A, Tabard-Fougere A, Hanquinet S, Dayer R. Diagnostic accuracy of MR imaging for direct visualization of lumbar pars defect in children and young adults: a systematic review and meta-analysis. *Eur Spine J.* 2018;27(5):1058-1066.

50. Polly DW Jr, Ledonio CGT, Diamond B, et al. What are the indications for spinal fusion surgery in Scheuermann kyphosis? *J Pediatr Orthop.* 2019;39(5):217-221.

51. Bleck EE. *Orthopaedic Management in Cerebral Palsy.* JB Lippincott; 1987.

52. Gage JR. *Gait Analysis in Cerebral Palsy. Clinics in Developmental Medicine.* Mac Keith Press; 1991.

53. Palisano R, Rosenbaum P, Walter S, Russell D, Wood E, Galuppi B. Development and reliability of a system to classify gross motor function in children with cerebral palsy. *Dev Med Child Neurol.* 1997;39(4):214-223.

54. Broughton NS, Menelaus MB. Orthopaedic management of spina bifida. In: Menelaus MB, ed. *Menalaus' Orthopaedic Management of Spina Bifida.* WB Saunders; 1998.

# 7

# Common Types of Emergency Splints

Marc F. Swiontkowski

## I. Emergency Splinting of the Spine

A. Patients with spinal injuries should be splinted with a **backboard** before they are moved, as shown in Fig. 7-1. Immobilize patients with suspected cervical spine injuries by placing sandbags, rolled towels, or rolled blankets on each side of the head. Then put a cravat through or around the backboard (or 3″ tape) or use the Velcro straps attached to the backboard and over the forehead. **In this way, the patient's head, neck, and backboard can be moved as one unit.** Commercial foam as well as plastic neck collars are available in different sizes and are carried by emergency medical technician (EMT) units. One can also make an adequate neck collar by placing foam or felt of the appropriate width, thickness, and length inside a tubular stockinet and then fastening the stockinet about the patient's neck. This method is particularly useful for immobilizing the neck of injured children where correct sizing is critical to immobilize the neck without extension or flexion. The only emergency indication for moving the neck of an individual with a suspected injured cervical spine is to improve an inadequate airway by aligning the neck with the torso and opening the airway with a jaw lift.

B. Be aware of possible **neurogenic shock**, which is treated by elevating the lower end of the backboard to improve venous return to the heart in the reverse Trendelenburg position.

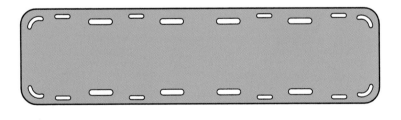

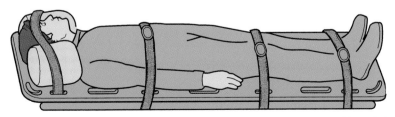

**Figure 7-1.** A backboard may be used in an emergency to transport a patient with a spinal injury.

**C.** If complete evaluation identifies a cervical spine fracture, the patient is usually placed in **traction** or hard collar immobilization. The direction of traction depends on the injury. If there is no dislocation, a neutral or slightly extended position is preferred (see Chapter 10).

## II. Upper Extremity Splinting

**A. Remember to remove rings from an involved hand!** Swelling can make them impossible to remove without cutting them off and they obscure X-rays. Petroleum jelly or ultrasound jell can be useful for ring removal.

**B.** Figure-of-8 splint

1. The **principal use** is for **clavicular fractures** (see Chapter 14).
2. **Application**. The factory-made figure-of-8 clavicular strap is recommended because it is a webbed fabric and does not stretch. If a properly fitting factory-made strap is not available for children younger than 10 years, make a figure-of-8 strap with a tubular stockinet filled with felt or cotton padding, as shown in Fig. 7-2. These should be used only if they make the patient more comfortable. A sling is generally more effective for patient comfort in this regard. Generally, the figure-of-8 splint does not improve fracture reduction.
3. **Precautions**
   a. **Prevent skin maceration** with a **powdered pad** in the axilla.
   b. In adults, restrict the use of the sling and encourage glenohumeral motion after 2 weeks to **prevent shoulder stiffness**.
   c. Do not tighten the figure-of-8 strap to the point that the **axillary artery or brachial plexus is compressed as manifested by arm swelling and paresthesias**.

**C. Velpeau and sling-and-swathe bandages**

1. These bandages are **used for shoulder dislocations, proximal humerus fractures, and humeral fractures**.

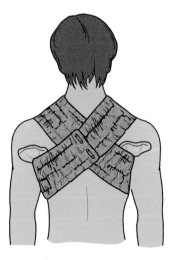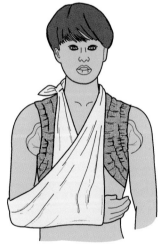

**Figure 7-2.** Typical figure-of-8 splint made for a child younger than 10 years with a fractured clavicle. In adults, use a factory-made splint when possible.

2. One **application** of Velpeau bandage using bias-cut stockinet is shown in Fig. 7-3. The common application of the typical sling-and-swathe bandage is shown in Fig. 7-4. Either type of bandage can be covered with a light layer of fiberglass or plaster to prevent unraveling of the material.
3. **Precautions**
   a. **Prevent skin maceration** with a **powdered pad** in the axilla and between the arm and chest.
   b. **Prevent wrist and finger stiffness** with active exercise.
4. A number of commercial **shoulder immobilizers** are available. Although they provide less secure immobilization than the Velpeau and sling-and-swathe bandages, these ready-made items have proved

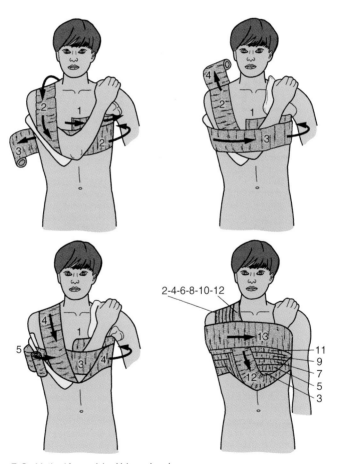

**Figure 7-3.** Method for applying Velpeau bandage.

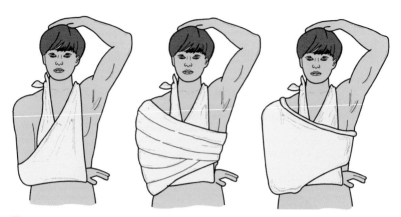

**Figure 7-4.** Sling-and-swathe bandage, covered by a single layer of plaster to help prevent unraveling of the material.

satisfactory. Commercial straps for acromioclavicular (AC) separations are also available; they have straps that go over the distal one-third of the clavicle and lift up on the elbow to reduce the AC separation or distal clavicle fracture. They are generally not used because they may cause skin necrosis if enough pressure is applied to improve alignment of the joint or fracture.

**D.** Use **air splints** in emergency situations for the distal extremity. Reduction of dislocated joints and improving limb alignment before splinting is indicated. The air splint is closed over the extremity by its zipper and inflated by flowing air into the mouth tube. High pressure from mechanical pumps can produce circulatory embarrassment and should not be used. Skin maceration occurs if air splints are used for any extended period. Cardboard or magazines can be used with tape of any sort to achieve temporary immobilization.

**III. Lower Extremity Splinting**

**A.** Thomas splint

1. Use for **femoral shaft fractures** and, **occasionally, knee injuries.** The following description is for the emergency situation. The Thomas splint may also be used as fixed skeletal traction, as described in Chapter 10, **VII.F.3.**

2. The ideal Thomas splint **application** uses a full-ring splint that measures 2 in greater than the circumference of the proximal thigh. If a full-ring splint is not available, use a half-ring splint with a strap placed anteriorly. The ring engages the ischial tuberosity for countertraction, and traction is applied to the end of the splint with an ankle hitch, as shown in Fig. 7-5. A Spanish windlass is made by taping several tongue blades together. These twist the material used to secure the ankle hitch to the end of the splint, producing a traction force. The half-ring splint still engages the ischial tuberosity, and the strap buckles down across the anterior thigh. Towels or a tubular stockinet placed on the Thomas splint with safety pins support the leg, as shown in Fig. 7-6.

3. **Hare splints and Roller splints** are also commercially available. They differ from the Thomas splint only by the foot attachments and leg supports. They are in widespread use by EMTs.

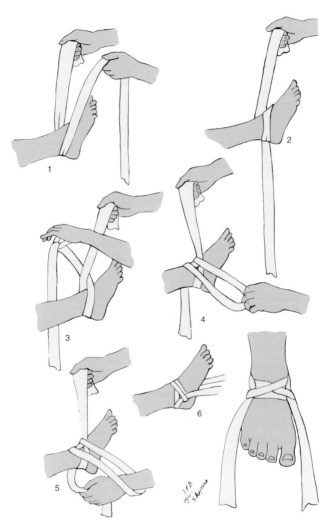

**Figure 7-5.** A Collins hitch is a means of applying traction from the ankle to the end of the Thomas splint, but it is used only in emergency situations.

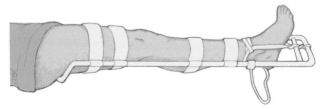

**Figure 7-6.** A Thomas splint may be used at the scene of the accident for a fracture of the femur.

4. Most **precautions** relate to the complications of fixed skeletal traction and are discussed in Chapter 10, **VII**. Do not leave the temporary splint on for more than 2 hours, whenever possible, because the ankle hitch places significant pressure on the skin and may produce necrosis.

**B. Jones compression splint**

1. Use in **acute knee trauma** (patellar, knee, and some tibial fractures) and **acute ankle injuries**.

2. Apply by wrapping the injured leg from the toes to the groin in rolled cotton. Next, add a single layer of elastic bandage. Apply 5- × 30-in plaster splints posteriorly, medially, and laterally to keep the ankle in a neutral position. Medial and lateral splints support the knee in the desired degree of flexion. Do not overlap the splints, or a circumferential plaster will be created about the extremity. The splints are then overwrapped with bias-cut stockinet or ACE wraps in a herringbone manner. If a fiberglass splint is used, a U-stirrup and posterior splint should be placed to stabilize the ankle against anterior/posterior and varus/valgus forces. This is particularly important when holding the ankle in a neutral position after a closed reduction.

3. **Precautions**
   a. Do not apply **wraps too tightly**.
   b. Do not make **upper wraps tighter than lower wraps** or venous return will be impeded, causing swelling and circulatory problems in the distal limb.

4. Although they provide less **satisfactory** compression, commercial **knee immobilizers** are acceptable in most cases.

**C. Short leg or modified Jones compression splint**

1. Use in **acute ankle and foot trauma** such as ankle sprains, calcaneal fractures, and other foot injuries.

2. The splint is **applied** in a manner similar to that described for the Jones splint except that it does not extend above the tibial tubercle.

3. **Precautions** are the same as those for the Jones compression splint.

**D. Commercial leg and ankle braces**

1. **Short leg walkers** or pneumatic walking boots—constructed of a rigid foot piece and double uprights and secured with Velcro fasteners—are available for conditions not requiring more rigid cast immobilization.

2. **Lace-up canvas ankle supports** with removable aluminum stays are also often convenient and useful for ankle sprains and instability.

3. **Air splints** with inflatable medial and lateral supports have recently proven extremely useful as supports for ankle sprains and stable fractures that are well along in the healing process.

**E. Other emergency splints**

1. **Make-do splints** may be used as a temporary measure. One may apply a pillow splint, rigid cardboard, magazine, or a wooden splint to the upper or lower extremity. A pillow splint for the ankle is shown in Fig. 7-7A.

2. **Precautions**
   a. **Avoid circulatory embarrassment** by applying splint straps or wraps in such a way as to prevent pressure on the skin over a bony prominence or a tourniquet effect to the extremity.
   b. **Splint**
      i. For **closed fractures**, restore gross limb angulation into better alignment before the splint is applied using gentle traction first in the direction of the angulation and then in the long axis of the limb.

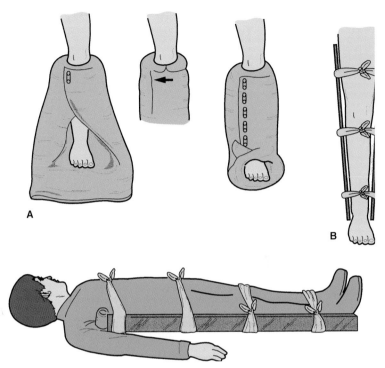

**Figure 7-7. A:** A pillow splint may be applied to a leg with a distal injury as a temporary measure. **B:** Board splints may be used for lower extremity fractures in emergency situations.

  ii. Restore alignment in the same manner if there is **tenting of the skin** over the injury.

  iii. For **open fractures**, gross limb alignment should be restored, the wound inspected and dressed with sterile technique, and a splint applied.

 c. Cover **exposed bone** with a saline- or betadine-moistened sterile dressing as first aid treatment.

# 8 Cast and Bandaging Techniques

Marc F. Swiontkowski

## I. Materials and Equipment

### A. Plaster

1. Plaster bandages and splints are made by **impregnating crinoline with plaster of Paris** [$(CaSO_4)_2H_2O$].[1,2] When this material is dipped into water, the powdery plaster of Paris is transformed into a solid crystalline form of gypsum, and heat is given off:

$$(CaSO_4)_2H_2O + 3H_2O \longleftrightarrow 2(CaSO_4 \times 2H_2O) + heat$$

   Anhydrous calcium sulfate:    Hydrated calcium sulfate:
   plaster of Parisgypsum

2. The amount of heat given off is determined by the amount of plaster applied and the temperature of the water.[3,4] The more plaster and the hotter the water, the more heat is generated. The interlocking of the crystals formed is essential to the strength and rigidity of the cast. Motion during the **critical setting period** interferes with this interlocking process and reduces the ultimate strength by as much as 77%. The interlocking of crystals (the critical setting period) begins, when the plaster reaches the thick creamy stage, becomes a little rubbery, and starts losing its wet, shiny appearance. Cast drying occurs by the evaporation of the water not required for crystallization. The evaporation from the cast surface is influenced by air temperature, humidity, and circulation about the cast. Thick casts take longer to dry than thin ones. Strength increases as drying occurs.

3. Plaster is available as bandage **rolls** in widths of 8, 6, 3, and 2 in and **splints** in 5-in × 45-in, 5-in × 30-in, 4-in × 15-in, and 3-in × 15-in sizes. Additives are used to alter the setting time; three variations are available: (1) Extra fast setting takes 2 to 4 minutes, (2) fast setting takes 5 to 6 minutes, and (3) slow setting takes 10 to 18 minutes.

### B. Fiberglass cast.
Three decades ago, a number of companies developed materials to replace plaster of Paris as a cast material. Most of these are a fiberglass fabric impregnated with polyurethane resin. The prepolymer is methylene bisphenyl diisocyanate, which is converted to a nontoxic polymeric urea substitute. The exothermic reaction does not place the patient's skin at risk for thermal injury.[2,5,6] These materials are preferred for most orthopaedic applications, except in acute fractures in which reduction maintenance is critical. Fiberglass casts provide lower skin pressure than plaster casts when properly applied.[7]

1. **Advantages.** These materials are strong and lightweight and resist breakdown in water; they are also available in multiple colors and patterns.

2. **Disadvantages.** They are harder to contour than plaster of Paris, and the polyurethane may irritate the skin. Fiberglass is harder to apply, although the more recently introduced bias stretch material shows an improvement. Review in detail the instructions from each manufacturer before using the casting materials. Patients are commonly under the impression that fiberglass casts can be gotten wet. This is incorrect; if submerged, they need

to be changed to avoid significant skin maceration. Gore-Tex padding material is available to aid in drying of the material, but submersion of a cast is still to be discouraged.

**C. The water.** Warm water causes more heat to be given off and affords faster setting. Cold water allows for less heat and for slower setting. Plaster of Paris in the water bucket from previously dipped plaster accelerates the setting time of the next plaster cast or splint. The water used for dipping should be deep enough to cover the material rolls standing on end.

**D. Cast padding**

1. **Webril** has a smooth surface and less tendency for motion within the thickness of the padding than some of the other padding materials. It requires the most practice to achieve a smooth application, however.

2. **Specialist** is softer than Webril and contains wood fiber. It has a corrugated appearance, and there is more tendency for sliding to occur within the material. It is easier to apply without wrinkles than Webril, but it becomes very hard if caked with blood.

3. **Sof-Roll** is a soft padding similar in appearance to Webril but slightly thicker. It has greater tear resistance and is, therefore, easier to stretch.

4. **Stockinet**
   a. **Bias-cut** stockinet may be used under a cast as a single layer. It is easy to apply without wrinkles and is better than tubular stockinet if there is a large difference in the maximum and minimum diameters of the extremity. Bias-cut stockinet can be made snug throughout, in contrast to tubular stockinet, which can be snug in the large diameter of the extremity but very loose in the narrow diameter. Plaster sticks to the stockinet, so there is no sliding between the cast and the stockinet padding.
   b. **Tubular** stockinet is made of the same material as the bias-cut type and is available in varying tube sizes ranging from 2 to 12 in.

5. **Felt or Reston** should be used to pad bony prominences and for cast margins. When padding over bony prominences, such as the anterior superior iliac spine, make a cruciate incision in the felt for better contouring.

6. **Moleskin adhesive** can be used to trim cast margins.

**E. Adherent materials.** Adherent substances (such as Dow Corning medical adhesive B) are applied to prevent slipping and chafing between the skin and the padding. They can contribute, however, to an increased amount of itching inside the cast. Tincture of benzoin compound should not be used in this situation because of fairly frequent skin reactions. Commercial adhesive removers are available.

**F. Equipment**

1. Use a clean **bucket**. Plaster residue and other particles in the water can alter the setting time.

2. **Gloves** keep hands clean and prevent dry skin if one applies many casts. They also make a smoother finish than is achieved by bare hands. They are mandatory for working with fiberglass materials.

3. **Shoe covers and aprons or gowns** keep shoes and clothes clean to prevent one from appearing sloppy in plaster-covered attire.

4. Use appropriate **draping** to maintain the dignity of the patient as well as to keep plaster off all areas not casted.

5. **Cast cutters**
   a. **The cast-cutting electric saw** has an oscillating circular blade that cuts firm rigid surfaces, such as casts or bony prominences. When lightly touched, the skin vibrates with the blade, but the blade does not cut. If the blade is firmly pressed against the skin or dragged along

it, then it will cut. The saw is noisy and causes considerable anxiety, especially in children. Therefore, it is wise to show younger patients that cast saws are safe by touching the blade to the palm of the hand. Playing music in the cast room has been shown to decrease anxiety in children having casts removed.[8] The cast saw causes dust to fly; consequently, the use of this tool is best avoided in clean operating rooms. In addition, cast saws can cut skin if applied with excessive force, so it is best to avoid using them on anesthetized patients.

    b. **Hand cutters** are useful when a saw is not available or to avoid frightening a child with the noise of the saw, to lessen the amount of plaster dust in the operating room, and to remove damp plaster.

6. **Cast spreaders** are used to open the cut edges of a cast for access to underlying cast padding, which is then cut with scissors. Spreaders come in various sizes for large and small casts.

7. **Cast knives** have sharp blades and preferably have large handles for better control. Sharp blades are essential; therefore, most practitioners prefer to use no. 22 disposable surgical blades.

8. **Cast benders** adjust cast edges to relieve skin binding and pressure.

9. **Cast dryers** blow warm to hot air around a plaster cast. They are generally not necessary. An exposed cast and a fan work just as well and are safer. Cast dryers can burn skin and tend to hasten the drying time of the outer layers only.

## II. Basic Principles of Cast Application

### A. Casts are used for the following purposes:

1. **To immobilize** fractures, dislocations, injured ligaments, and joints; to provide relief from pain caused by infections and inflammatory processes; and to facilitate healing

2. **To allow earlier ambulation** by stabilizing fractures of the spine or lower extremities

3. **To improve function** by stabilizing or positioning a joint, such as for wrist drop after a radial nerve injury, which also allows more useful hand function

4. **To correct deformities,** as in serial casting for clubfoot (see Chapter 6 for the Ponseti technique) or joint contractures

5. **To prevent deformity** resulting from a neuromuscular imbalance or from scoliosis

### B. Principles.

Although plaster of Paris has been used extensively in the treatment of fractures for more than 100 years, there is no unanimity of opinion as to the best technique for application. It can be safely concluded that even the tightest of skintight casts allows some motion at the fracture site, whereas a loosely fitted, well-padded cast with proper three-point fixation can provide satisfactory immobilization. Three points of force are produced by the practitioner, who molds the cast firmly against the proximal and distal portions of the extremity (two of the points) and locates the third point directly opposite the apex of the cast, as shown in Fig. 8-1. Periosteal or other soft-tissue attachments are usually required on the convex side of the cast to provide stability. In this way, a curved cast can provide a straight alignment of the extremity within it. Charnley has stated, "If a fracture slips in a well-applied plaster, then the fracture was mechanically unsuitable for treatment by plaster, and another mechanical principle should have been chosen." Another method for providing immobilization by plaster is based on hydraulics. Fractures of the tibia do not shorten significantly when placed in a "total contact" cast. The leg is a cylinder containing mostly fluid, and when this water column is encased in rigid plaster, the cylinder does not shorten in height because tissue fluid is not compressible.

**Figure 8-1. A:** Three-point plaster fixation will stabilize a fracture when the soft-tissue bridging the fracture acts as a hinge under tension. **B:** If the three forces are applied in the wrong direction, the fracture displaces.

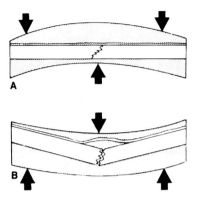

**C.** The following **application techniques** have been satisfactory in our hands:
1. The patient is **informed** of the procedure and instructed in whatever co-operation is necessary.
2. The surgeon or cast technician must have clearly in mind **what to do and what will be required** (the position of the patient and assistants, how many rolls of plaster will be needed, tools to trim the cast edges, etc.). All materials and equipment required to do the job properly should be assembled. (Once cast application starts, it is difficult to stop and obtain something that was forgotten.) The patient's position must be comfortable and must allow the surgeon and assistant to apply the cast expeditiously. Special maneuvers required to perform and hold the re-duction are rehearsed.
3. **A circular cast should not be used in fresh trauma or postopera-tively** when one anticipates swelling, **unless** the cast is bivalved or split initially and provisions are made for adequate patient monitoring.
   a. **Adequate observation** means an examination by a competent ob-server at least once hourly until any swelling begins to recede. Signs of compartmental syndrome, in order of importance, are increas-ing pain and discomfort in the extremity, increasing tenseness or tenderness in the involved compartment, pain with passive range of motion of the muscle in the involved compartment, decreasing sensation—especially to two-point discrimination and light touch—in the distribution of the nerves that travel through the involved compartment, increasing peripheral edema, and, finally, decreasing capillary filling. **Good peripheral circulation with distal arterial pulses is no assurance that a compartment syndrome is not developing (see Chapter 3, III).**
   b. An excellent alternative to plaster casts in this situation is a Jones com-pression splint, as described in **Chapter 7, III.B and C.**
4. **If unexpected swelling occurs** in a circular cast, **bivalve or split** the cast immediately all the way to the patient's skin (see **IV.B and C).**
5. Unless specifically contraindicated, **clean** the part to be casted with soap and water, then dry it with alcohol. Apply the cast over a single layer of cast padding with edges of the material minimally overlapping. Protect unusual bony prominences with a ¼-in felt or foam rubber padding.
6. **Dip the plaster or fiberglass rolls in water** by placing them on end, and this allows air to escape and results in complete soaking of the plaster. The

bandages are sufficiently soaked when the bubbling stops. They can be left in the water up to 4 minutes without decreasing the strength of the cast, but the setting time decreases with the length of time they are immersed. Therefore, for maximum working time, remove bandages soon after the bubbling stops. Lightly crimping the ends of the plaster bandages helps prevent telescoping of the roll.

7. Except for very large casts (e.g., body casts and spicas), **all plaster bandages should be dipped and removed from the water at the same time**. Thus, all the plaster in the cast is at the same point in the setting process. This scheme maximizes the interlocking of the crystals between the layers of plaster, thereby maximizing the strength of the cast. In addition, delamination between the bandages is decreased.

8. Use **cool water** for larger casts when more time is needed to apply all the plaster or fiberglass, and use **warm water** for smaller casts or splints. **Never use hot water** because enough heat can be generated to burn the patient.[9] Similarly, do not place limbs with fresh casts onto plastic-covered pillows; these tend to hamper heat dispersion significantly and may result in burning. If the patient complains of burning, it is prudent to remove the cast immediately and reapply using cooler water.

9. Keep the plaster bandage on the cast padding, lifting it off only to tuck and change directions—that is, to push the plaster roll around the patient's body or extremity. Use the largest bandages, usually 4- and 6-in bandage rolls, that are consistent with smooth, easy applications. Using large bandages allows the fastest application of plaster and provides sufficient time for molding before the critical setting period. **Six or seven layers of plaster** or two to three layers of fiberglass casting material are usually sufficient, except in patients who are particularly hard on casts. The cast should be of uniform thickness (seven layers or ¼ in). Avoid concentrating the plaster about the fracture or the middle of the cast. Avoid placing two circumferential rolls directly on top of each other while wrapping the plaster on the patient's extremity. Reinforce casts where they cross joints by incorporating plaster or fiberglass splints longitudinally. Incorporate reinforcing plaster splints into body and spica casts (see **III.B** and **C**).

10. During application of the cast, **turn the padding back at the edges of the cast and incorporate it.** Another method of finishing the edges is to turn back the padding after the cast has set and to hold the padding down with a single, narrow plaster splint; a row of ordinary staples; or moleskin.

11. **Apply all the material rapidly** so that there is time to work and mold it before the critical setting period. The cast should have a sculptured look, not only for cosmetic reasons but also for comfort. If the fracture is to be stabilized by the three-point fixation principle, it is more important to maintain the three forces of pressure on the cast during the critical setting period than to have a perfectly smooth surface on the cast. This step is more difficult for fiberglass casts.

12. Once the critical period of interlocking of crystals begins, **molding and all motion should stop** until the material becomes rigid. Otherwise, the cast is weakened considerably.

13. After the cast sets and becomes rigid, **trim the edges** using a plaster knife or cast saw. Use the knife by supporting the cutting hand on the cast and pulling the portion of the plaster to be trimmed up against the knife blade rather than blindly cutting through the plaster and possibly cutting the patient. If the cast is too thick or hard, an oscillating cast saw is preferred.

14. Apply **forearm casts** to allow full 90° flexion of all metacarpophalangeal joints and opposition of the thumb to the index and little fingers.

15. Extend **leg casts** to support the metatarsal heads, but not to interfere with flexion and extension of the toes. This rule is invalid when the toes need support (as with fractures of the great toe or metatarsals) or when there is a motor or sensory deficit. In these situations, the cast is extended as a platform to support and protect the toes. Place a ½-in piece of sponge rubber beneath the toes and incorporate it into the plaster for walking casts, or supply the patient with a commercial cast shoe.

16. Immobilize as few joints as possible, but as a general rule, one **immobilizes the joint above and below a fresh fracture**.

17. Instruct the patient regarding
    a. **Signs and symptoms of compression** from swelling within the cast
    b. **Elevation** of the injured part above the level of the heart for 2 to 3 days after the injury
    c. **How soon to walk** on the cast (if appropriate and generally never sooner than 24 hours)
    d. **Instructions for weight bearing and ambulation**; this should include crutch or walker training
    e. **How to exercise** joints not incorporated in plaster
    f. **Date of the next appointment**
    g. **Person to call** in case of cast problems or evidence of a compression syndrome

### III. Special Casting/Splinting Techniques

A. **Use plaster splints** when rigid immobilization is not required or when significant swelling of the extremity is anticipated.

1. **Upper extremity**
   a. Usually, splint the **wrist** dorsally by applying a 3-in-wide plaster splint over cast padding from the metacarpophalangeal joints to the proximal forearm. While the plaster is still wet, wrap the arm with bias-cut stockinet or a single layer of an elastic bandage so that the plaster conforms to the extremity as it hardens. A dorsal splint may be preferable to a volar splint because it allows easier finger and hand function. Combined dorsal and volar splints are frequently used together; this is preferred and gives better support of the limbs. Commercial splints are just as effective in managing distal radius fractures in children.[5]
   b. Splint the **elbow** with 5-in × 30-in plaster wraps applied posteriorly with enough distal extension to support the wrist. The splint should not go further distally than the distal palmar crease to facilitate metacarpophalangeal motion. Apply 3-in plaster strips medially and laterally across the elbow for reinforcement. Wrap the arm and plaster splint with bias-cut stockinet or a single layer of an elastic bandage while the plaster is wet.

2. **Lower extremity.** Usually make posterior plaster splints in the lower extremity by applying a standard cast (knee cylinder, short-leg, or long-leg cast, as described in **III.D, E, F**) and then bivalving the cast and retaining only the posterior shell. Hold the posterior splint to the leg with bias-cut stockinet or an elastic bandage wrap. Alternatively, use 5-in × 30-in posterior and medial/lateral splints, leaving the anterior aspect of the leg covered only by soft roll.

B. **Body casts**

1. Apply the **basic body jacket** over large tubular stockinet. Place ⅛- to ½-in felt pads over the shoulders (if suspenders are used), costal margins, iliac crests including anterior iliac spine, and the dorsal spine. Make a cruciate cut in the felt placed over the crests to distribute pressure uniformly over the bony prominence. Apply a single layer of plaster snugly over the padding. Splints may be used, as shown in Fig. 8-2. If suspenders

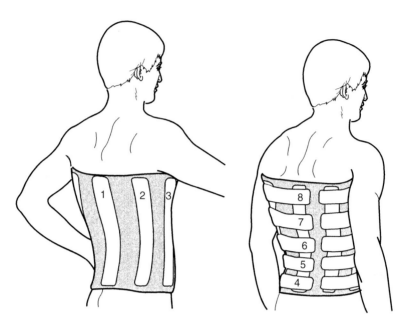

**Figure 8-2.** Typical application of plaster splints for a body jacket. The splints are placed closer together in the lower aspect of the body jacket. The splints are numbered in order of application.

are required, make a "V" with 5-in × 30-in splints. Place the point of the "V" between the scapulae and bring the ends over the shoulders. Snugly apply rolled plaster over the splints and mold. Usually extend the jacket posteriorly from the top of the sacrum to the inferior angle of the scapulae and anteriorly from the symphysis pubis to the sternal notch. Body jackets may be applied with the lumbar spine in flexion or extension as well as the neutral position. For hyperextension body jackets, often used in thoracolumbar fractures, use the Goldthwaite iron apparatus for positioning, as in Fig. 8-3.

2. The **Minerva body jacket** is named after the goddess Minerva, who sprang forth from Jupiter's head when it was cleaved by Vulcan in an attempt to relieve Jupiter's headaches. Minerva appeared chanting a triumphant song and wearing a large metal headdress. The Minerva body jacket incorporates the skull and is used to immobilize the cervical spine; its most frequent application is in children. This type of jacket is applied in the same manner as the body jacket, but also calls for the following steps: Place a fluted felt pad around the entire neck, with the neck halter traction over the padding. Tie the halter straps at the ear level to prevent the halter's slipping off the head. Place another felt pad along the length of the spine and the occiput. Wrap the rest of the head with 3-in sheet cotton padding. At least two operators are necessary for even application of the plaster, one for the head and one for the body. Roll 3-in plaster bandages about the head and neck. Apply narrow splints around the chin, neck, occiput, and forehead. Use wide splints all the way from the sacrum to the occiput, with another wide splint extending from the chest to the chin. Incorporate these splints into the cast by snugly wrapping plaster bandages

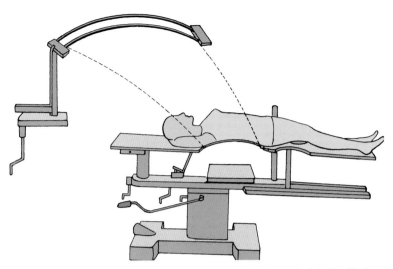

**Figure 8-3.** Goldthwaite irons, used to make a hyperextension plaster body jacket. The irons are removed after the cast is set.

over them. Then mold together the plaster about the head, neck, and body at the same time. Carefully mold beneath the mandible. Cut the plaster in a "V" to release the chin and also cut out about the ears and face (Fig. 8-4, inset). Trim the plaster above the jaw line and leave the eyebrows exposed. A Minerva body jacket is useful in children and when cervical or halo vests (Fig. 8-4) orthoses are not appropriate or available.

3. **Other types of body jackets**
   a. A **Risser localizer cast** is occasionally used for scoliotic spines or for patients with thoracolumbar fractures. Apply a pelvic plaster mold first, then attach pelvic and head halter traction. Make a pressure pad with felt backed by four to six layers of plaster. Produce or hold correction of the scoliosis by applying this pad against the apical ribs and incorporating it into the body jacket that incorporates the jaw, neck, and occiput, but not the head. Make the surface of the pressure area large enough to avoid local necrosis of the skin.
   b. **Halo traction** can be incorporated into a plaster or fiberglass body jacket with suspenders, and it provides continuous or fixed cervical traction (Fig. 8-5). The halo traction is more commonly incorporated into a sheepskin-lined plastic body jacket, which is more lightweight and comfortable (Fig. 8-6).

C. **Spica** is a Latin word that means "ear of wheat" because a spica wrap was used to wrap sheaves of wheat in the fields. The same type of wrap is used to immobilize proximal joints with the **spica cast**. Various types of spica casts are described as follows:

1. Pad a **bilateral short-leg** (panty) **spica** in much the same way as for the body jacket, but include the legs. These casts are generally applied on fracture tables (adults) or spica boards (children). Use tubular or bias-cut stockinet. Pad bony prominences with $1/8$- to $1/2$-in felt with cruciate incisions. Apply plaster or fiberglass to the upper portion of the cast as is done with the body jacket. Reinforce the hips with splints as shown in Fig. 8-7.

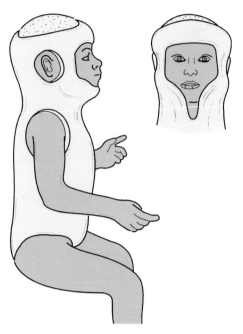

**Figure 8-4.** Completed Minerva body jacket.

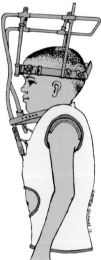

**Figure 8-5.** Halo traction cast. (From Bleck EE, Duckworth L, Hunter N. *Atlas of Plaster Cast Techniques*. 2nd ed. Year Book; 1978, with permission.)

Apply plaster or fiberglass well next to the perineal post under the sacrum to avoid weakness in the area (the intern's triangle). Snugly tie the splints in with plaster or fiberglass bandage rolls extending to the supracondylar portion of the femurs. Mold the material well over the iliac crests. The patient may be lifted from the table with the sacral rest still in the plaster.

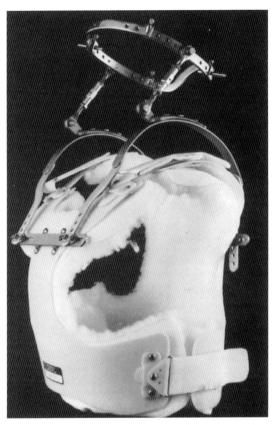

**Figure 8-6.** A commercially available malleable polyethylene jacket may be substituted for the plaster cast for use with the halo apparatus. Patients report this is significantly more comfortable than the plaster jacket.

Turn the patient on his or her abdomen and cut out the sacral rest. Trim the edges of the cast in the usual manner.

2. Examples of long-leg hip spicas are shown in Fig. 8-8. Apply the leg portion of the cast like any other long-leg cast, using the special splints about the hips as described for the short-leg spica. Support the casted extremities with struts, which are usually made of wooden stakes (¼ in × 2 in or ¾ in × ½ in) or dowels. Cover with plaster or fiberglass and attach them to the casted extremity by wrapping a bandage in a cordlike figure-of-eight fashion about the strut and cast and then roll the bandage around the strut and cast to create a well-molded cast. Sedate or anesthetize infants and small children before spica cast application; they are generally applied in the operating suite.

3. Apply the **shoulder spica** with the patient standing or supine on a spica table that has a metallic backrest. The arm may be supported with finger traps, or with a cooperative patient in the sitting or standing position,

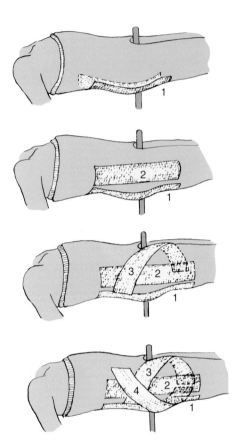

**Figure 8-7.** Plaster splints to reinforce hip spicas, in addition to those used in the body jackets.

the cast may be applied while an assistant holds the arm. The principles of padding and cast application for body jackets and long-arm casts are combined to produce a shoulder spica. In addition to the splints normally used for body and long-arm casts, apply a wide splint from the lateral chest, up under the axilla, to the medial side of the arm. Place other splints across the posterior aspect of the arm, over the shoulder, to the opposite side. Tie in the splints with rolled plaster or fiberglass and place a strut between the arm and the trunk.

D. **Knee cylinder casts.** Remove all hair from the medial and lateral aspects of the lower leg. Spray the leg with a nonallergenic adhesive. Place medial and lateral strips of self-adhering foam, moleskin adhesive, or adhesive tape on the skin with 6 to 12 in of the material extending distal to the ankle. Then place a cuff of ¼-in sponge rubber or felt padding measuring 1 in in width over the strips just above the malleoli. When the strips are turned back and incorporated into the fiberglass or plaster, they suspend the cast, and with the thick padding, they prevent pressure on the malleoli. Wrap the leg with a single layer of cast padding and apply the plaster with the knee flexed 5°. Extend the cast proximally as far as possible and distally to just above the flare of the malleoli; the length of the cast provides for lateral and medial stability. Mold the plaster

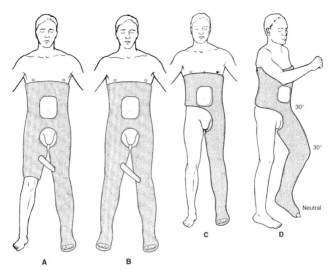

**Figure 8-8.** Long-leg hip spicas. **A:** One and one-half spica. **B:** Double spica. **C:** Single spica. For all long-leg spica casts, it is important to keep the hip and knee gently flexed for patient comfort and ease of positioning. The ankle must be kept in neutral dorsiflexion **(D).** In children, it is often advisable to stop the cast at the malleoli distally, leaving the foot free.

or fiberglass medially and laterally above the femoral condyles to help prevent the cast from sliding distally.

**E. Short-leg casts**

1. Apply the **short-leg cast** with the patient sitting on the end of a table with the knee flexed 90°. Alternatively, apply it with the patient supine, the hip and knee flexed 90°, and the leg supported by an assistant. The type of padding matters little, except that Webril and stockinet tend to shear less and, therefore, may allow for a tighter cast over a longer period of time. Use only one-two layers of padding, except over the malleoli, where extra padding is required frequently. For most casts, have the ankle in a neutral position. Two plaster bandages are usually required, and the width selected (3, 4, or 6 in) varies with the size of the patient. Fold 4-in splints longitudinally in half, and place one splint on all four sides of the ankle for reinforcement before applying the second plaster bandage. Extend the cast distally from the metatarsophalangeal joints and proximally to one finger breadth below the tibial tubercle. Trim the edges and pad as previously described.

2. If desired, a **walking cast** may be made with either a rubber rocker walker or a stirrup walker. Place either one in the midportion of the longitudinal arch of the foot in line with the anterior border of the tibia. With a rocker walker, the medial longitudinal arch is filled with plaster splints to make a flat base. Then, the walker is secured with a third plaster bandage. Commercially available walking shoes (or boots), which fit over the casted foot, are more widely used. A flat plaster base on the plantar aspect of the cast is required for these shoes (or cast boots). If the ankle must be held in equinus (such as required for cast treatment of an Achilles tendon rupture), a stirrup walker is advantageous, and the patient's opposite shoe should be adjusted to the appropriate height for walking. All walking casts should dry for at least 24 hours before weight bearing.

### F. Long-leg casts

1. First apply a **short-leg cast** as described earlier (see **III.E.1**). Then extend the knee to the position desired and continue the cast padding to the groin. Two 6-in plasters or fiberglass bandages are usually required for the upper portion of this cast, except in patients with heavy thighs. After the first bandage is applied, fold 4- or 5-in splints longitudinally and place them medially and laterally across the knee joint for reinforcement. After the second plaster or fiberglass bandage is applied, mold the cast medially and laterally in the supracondylar area to help prevent the cast from slipping distally when the patient begins to stand.

2. The long-leg **walking cast** is made as described in **III.E.2**, but the knee must be flexed no more than 5°.

3. **Casting techniques of Dehne and Sarmiento**

   a. The cast treatment programs made popular by Dehne and Sarmiento (see Selected Historical Reading) are designed to allow early weight bearing of a fractured tibia. The affected leg is placed in a very snug cast that maintains the tissue and fluids of the leg within a rigid container. Shortening is prevented by the **hydraulic principle** that fluids are not compressible. Thus, the patient can bear weight soon after a fracture without excessive further shortening, and fracture healing is benefitted by the improved vascularity derived from ambulation. The advocates of these casting techniques describe a "total contact cast." The authors believe, however, that all casts to the lower extremities should be total contact casts. Rolling scooters have become a common alternative to crutch ambulation.

   b. The **long-leg total contact cast** as described by Dehne is applied like a long-leg walking cast with only minor modifications.

      i. **Cast the knee in extension.** Some patients, however, find this position uncomfortable and may require a position with 3° to 5° of flexion.

      ii. This cast may need to be **wedged** to correct angular deformities of the fracture site. For this reason, apply one or two extra layers of the Webril at the fracture site.

   c. The **below-the-knee total contact**, or patellar tendon-bearing, **cast** is applied much as a regular short-leg walking cast is, with the following modifications (Fig. 8-9):

      i. Keep the affected limb in a long-leg cast or a Jones compression splint until the **swelling subsides** (2 to 4 weeks).

      ii. Apply the **cast padding to the lower leg and extend** to 2 in proximal to the superior pole of the patella.

      iii. First apply a short-leg cast and extend it to just inferior to the tibial tubercle. Sarmiento suggests molding the cast into a **triangular shape**, with the sides of the triangle formed by the anterior tibial surface, the lateral peroneal muscle mass, and the posterior aspect of the leg.

      iv. Then have the assistant position the knee in 40° to 45° of flexion. The quadriceps muscles must be completely relaxed. Use a 4-in bandage of plaster to extend the cast to the superior pole of the patella. Mold carefully over the medial tibial flare as well as into the patellar tendon and the popliteal fossa. The lateral wings should be as high as possible. Trim the posterior portion of the cast to one fingerbreadth or ½ in below the level of the cast indentation that was made anteriorly into the patellar tendon. The posterior wall of the cast should be low enough to allow 90° of knee flexion without having the cast edge rub on the hamstring tendons. These casts generally require the use of plaster because of the critical molding involved, which is difficult with fiberglass.

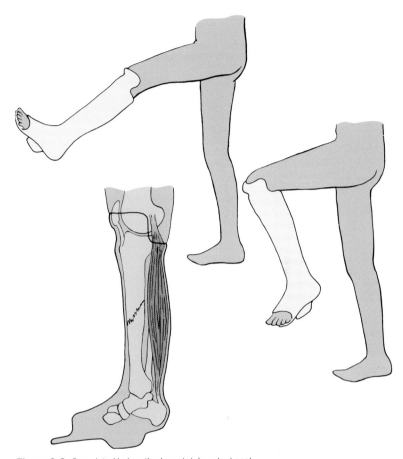

**Figure 8-9.** Completed below-the-knee total contact cast.

    v. If **angulation** occurs at the fracture site with this cast, replace rather than wedge the cast. If the patient ambulates well enough to maintain muscle bulk, the original cast may not need to be replaced.

    vi. **Do not switch from a below-the-knee total contact cast to a regular short-leg cast** at some point midway in the healing phase of the fracture because a regular short-leg cast offers no rotational stability. Evidence has shown that this type of cast is no more effective in immobilizing tibia fractures than a standard short-leg cast.[10]

4. **The authors believe that a long-leg weight-bearing cast is easier and safer (in regard to skin and fracture complications) for most individuals to apply than the below-the-knee total contact cast.** Comparing the treatment results published in the literature provides no evidence that one technique is superior to the other. The theoretic advantage of providing knee motion with the Sarmiento technique is offset by the expertise required to apply this cast properly.

5. Begin **weight bearing** at 24 to 36 hours after plaster cast application when the patient can tolerate it; patients with fiberglass casts can be encouraged to weight bear 3 to 6 hours after casting.

## IV. Cutting, Bivalving, Splitting, and Removing Casts
### A. General techniques

1. In removing or splitting casts, use the **oscillating saw**. Reassure the patient by giving a cast saw demonstration before actually cutting the cast. Stabilize the hand holding the electric saw on the cast, and push the blade through just the plaster or fiberglass with short repetitive strokes, as shown in Fig. 8-10. Avoid bony prominences as the cast saw can cut into the skin over them. Fiberglass casts with thin padding are at the highest risk for thermal injury of the skin during removal, whereas plaster casts with thicker padding are at the lowest risk.[11]

2. **Windows** may be cut from the cast to expose wounds. The windows must be replaced, however, and rewrapped with either a new plaster or an elastic bandage to prevent local edema.

**B.** Should unexpected swelling occur, **bivalve the cast. Bivalving is superior to simply splitting the cast.** The technique consists of cutting the plaster as well as the cast padding on both sides of the extremity. The anterior and posterior parts of the cast can be held in place with bias-cut stockinet or an elastic bandage. Advantages of this technique are that the anterior half of the cast may be removed to inspect the compartments and that complete anterior, posterior, and circumferential compression is relieved.

**C. Splitting** a cast requires cutting a ½-in strip of plaster from the full length of the cast; otherwise, the proximal aspect of the plaster may act as a circumferential tourniquet.[2] Again, divide the plaster and padding down to the skin because soft dressing might also cause constriction. In the case of the lower extremity, the cast is split anteriorly with a diamond-shaped section of plaster removed from the anterior aspect of the ankle. Spread the cast for relief of the symptoms. Pad the area with felt where the strip of plaster was removed and overwrap with a rubber elastic bandage to avoid local edema. **This technique is not as satisfactory as bivalving a cast, but is sometimes appropriate for managing postoperative swelling.**

## V. Adhesive Strapping and Bandaging
### A. Terminology

1. Use **adhesive strapping** (taping) for the possible prevention and treatment of athletic injuries. Use strips of adhesive tape instead of one continuous winding.

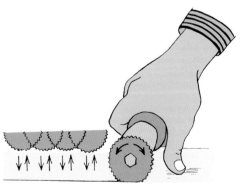

**Figure 8-10.** Saw-cutting technique that avoids skin laceration.

2. **Bandaging** (wrapping) uses nonadhesive materials (gauze, cotton cloth, and elastic wrapping) in the treatment of athletic injuries. Employ one continuous unwinding of material.

**B. Adhesive strapping**

1. **Purposes of strapping**
   a. **To protect and secure protective devices**
   b. **To hold dressings in place**
   c. **To limit motion**
   d. **To support and stabilize**

2. **Construction factors**
   a. **Tape grade** (backing material). Heavy backing materials have 85 longitudinal fibers per square inch and 65 vertical fibers per square inch. Lighter grades have 65 longitudinal fibers per square inch and 45 vertical fibers per square inch. **Store** the tape in a cool, dry place. Keep the tape standing on end and not on its side to prevent deformation of the roll.
   b. **Adhesives.** Use a rubber-based spray-on adhesive primarily with athletes because strength of backing, superior adhesion, and economy are needed. Use acrylic adhesives in surgical dressing applications because a high degree of backing and superior adhesion are not the primary requirements.

3. **Application and removal**
   a. **Preparation**
      i. **Clean the skin** with soap and water, and dry.
      ii. **Remove all hair** to prevent irritation.
      iii. **Treat** all cuts and wounds.
      iv. **Apply** a nonallergic **skin adherent.**
      v. **Position** properly.
   b. **Size of tape**
      i. Use ¼- to 1-in tape on **fingers, hands,** and **toes.**
      ii. Use 1¼- or 1½-in tape on **ankles, lower legs, forearms,** and **elbows.**
      iii. Use 2- or 3-in tape on **large areas, knees,** and **thighs.**
   c. **Rules of application**
      i. **Avoid continuous strapping** because this causes constriction. Use one turn at a time and tear after overlapping the starting end of the tape by 1 in.
      ii. **Smooth and mold the tape** as it is laid on the skin.
      iii. **Overlap** the tape at least one half its width over the tape below.
      iv. Allow the tape to **fit the natural contour** of the skin—that is, let it fall naturally and avoid bending around acute angles.
      v. Keep the tape roll in one hand and **tear** it with the fingers.
      vi. Keep constant and even **unwinding tension**.
      vii. For **best support**, strap directly over the skin.
   d. **Techniques for removal**
      i. **Remove** the tape along the longitudinal axis rather than across it. If near a wound, **pull toward the wound,** not away from it.
      ii. **Peel** the tape back by holding the skin taut and pushing the skin away from the tape rather than by pulling the tape from the skin.

4. **Skin reactions. Most tape reactions are mechanical,** not allergic. Allergic reactions are characterized by erythema, edema, papules, and vesicles. Test for an allergic reaction by patch testing. Consult a dermatologist for assistance in doing this testing. If the test is positive, the above signs manifest themselves within 24 to 48 hours.
   a. **Mechanical irritation** is produced when tape is removed from the skin. It frequently occurs as a result of shearing the skin when the tape is applied

in tension or used for maintaining traction. Such application induces vasodilation and an intense reddening of the skin, which disappears shortly after tape removal. The reaction is due to simple skin stripping—that is, direct trauma to the outer skin layers resulting in loss of cells.

b. **Chemical irritation** occurs when components in adhesive mass or the backing of the tape permeate the underlying tissues. This irritation has been largely eliminated through tape manufacturing processes.

c. **Another irritative effect** is localized inhibition of sweating, and this is corrected by the use of nonocclusive (porous) tape.

**C. Bandaging**

1. **Purposes of bandaging**

   a. **To hold dressing in place** over external wounds

   b. **To apply compression pressure** over injuries and thus control hemorrhage

   c. **To secure splints** in place

   d. **To immobilize** or limit motion of injured parts

2. **Materials**

   a. **Gauze,** which holds dressings in place over wounds or acts as a protective layer for strapping

   b. **Cotton cloth** for support wrapping or dressing

   c. **Elastic wrapping** for compression wrapping or dressing

**D. Medicated bandage**

1. The medicated bandage (Unna boot) **contains** zinc oxide, calamine, glycerine, and gelatin, and it **is usually indicated** for lower extremity areas of skin loss that require protection and support. This type of support dressing prevents edema and allows ambulation in patients with known venous conditions at the time of cast removal.

2. **Application**

   a. **Cleanse** the area and position the ankle at an appropriate angle.

   b. **Make a circular turn** with the medicated bandage **around the foot** and direct the bandage **obliquely over the heel**. Then cut the bandage. This procedure ensures a flat surface.

   c. **Repeat** until the heel is adequately covered. Make the first layer snug and apply the roll in a pressure-gradient manner; that is, apply the greatest pressure distally with progressively diminishing pressure over the upper leg.

   d. **Do not reverse any turns** because the ridges formed may cause discomfort as the bandage hardens. Ensure that each turn overlaps one half of a preceding turn. Avoid winding the bandage on too tightly.

   e. **Cover the leg** approximately three times and extend the bandage 1 to 2 in below the knee; otherwise, the bandage may slip toward the ankle. Allow the bandage to harden. Prevent soiling of clothing with gauze or stockinet over the medicated bandage. Leave the bandage on for 3 to 7 days, and repeat treatment if necessary.

**VI. Joint Mobilization**

**A. Following cast removal**

1. **While the cast is still on,** range of motion exercises of the adjacent joints not immobilized and isometric exercises for the immobilized muscles (e.g., weight bearing in a cast) serve both to improve nutrition and to decrease atrophy of the articular cartilage, bone, and muscle. Edema and the rehabilitation required after cast removal are also minimized.

2. **Warn the patient that after removal of any cast from a lower extremity, some swelling is normal.**

3. **Once the cast is removed,** an elastic compression stocking or ACE bandage is desirable for support.

a. Prescribe a **specific exercise program** to increase the range of motion. Moist heat, such as a bath or whirlpool, may help mobilize the joint. Referral to a physical therapist is often advisable.

b. If swelling appears to be a problem, **contrast baths** may be indicated (the 3-3-3 treatment): rest 3 minutes in cool water, exercise 3 minutes in warm water, repeat 3 times; follow up with 30 minutes of elevation. Repeat the entire process three times daily.

c. **Active exercise** is the key to success. Passive range of motion exercise too frequently becomes a repeated manipulation. Manipulation under anesthesia is occasionally necessary, but this should be followed with an aggressive inpatient therapy program.

**B.** It is not always true that the sooner **the joints adjacent to a fracture** are mobilized, the better the range of motion obtained. The following factors must be considered:

1. **Fractures not involving articular surfaces**

   a. Joint movement is slow to return and poor in range if attempted movement produces **pain**, associated muscle spasm, and involuntary splinting.

   b. **Early joint movement can delay fracture healing if fixation is not rigid.**

   c. **A normal joint tolerates longer periods of immobilization.** The "safe" period of immobilization coincides well with the normal time necessary for adjacent fracture healing. Only in the older patient with degenerative changes in the joint, there is a likelihood of intraarticular adhesions and periarticular stiffening, even with short periods of immobilization.

   d. **Some joints may tolerate immobilization better than others,** but this presumption is not well documented.

   e. Postinjury or postcasting **edema is "glue."** The area is soon infiltrated with young fibroblasts. Excessive formation of collagen causes early and frequent permanent stiffness, especially when collateral ligaments are immobilized in a shortened position (e.g., metacarpophalangeal joints).

   f. **Isometric exercises** within the cast are recommended. Allow the muscles to move within the limits of the cast.

2. **Fractures involving articular surfaces**

   a. **Reduce intraarticular fractures anatomically if possible.** If operative intervention is indicated, then a goal of internal fixation is to allow range of motion exercises or continuous passive motion within the first 2 or 3 days postoperatively.

   b. **If anatomic restitution cannot be achieved**, then early motion may allow mobile fragments to be molded into a better position. This motion should improve the potential of fibrocartilage resurfacing. Early movement is difficult to define, but some movement should be started within the first week.

3. **Between these two groups**, there is a considerable degree of overlap. If it is anticipated that a complicated and often incomplete open reduction and internal fixation is not secure enough to allow early movement of the joint, then it may be better to treat the fracture nonoperatively. The **objective** is the **best possible final range of movement and function.**

## REFERENCES

1. Bingold AC. On splitting plasters. *J Bone Joint Surg Br.* 1979;61:294-295.
2. Pope MH, Callahan G, Lavarette R. Setting temperatures of synthetic casts. *J Bone Joint Surg Am.* 1985;67:262-264.
3. Lavalette R, Pope MH, Dickstein H. Setting temperature of plaster casts. *J Bone Joint Surg Am.* 1982;64:907-911.

4. Boutis K, Babyn P, Gueree R, Willan A, Howard A. A splint was not inferior to a cast for distal radius fracture in children. *J Bone Joint Surg Am.* 2010;93:1507-1512.
5. Shore B, Hutchinson S, Harris M, et al. Epidemiology of cast saw injuries. *J Bone Joint Surg Am.* 2014;96:1-8.
6. Wytch R, Mitchell C, Ritchie IK, Wardlaw D, Ledingham W. New splinting materials. *Prosthet Orthot Int.* 1987;11:42-45.
7. Davids JR, Frick SL, Skewes E, Blackhurst DW. Skin surface pressure beneath an above-the-knee cast: plaster casts compared with fiberglass casts. *J Bone Joint Surg Am.* 1997;79:565-569.
8. Liu RW, Mehta P, Fortuna S, et al. Music playing in a cast room reduced heart rate in children. *J Ped Orthop.* 2007;27;831-833.
9. Wehbe MA. Plaster uses and misuses. *Clin Orthop Relat Res.* 1982;167:242-249.
10. Aita D, Bhave A, Herzenberg J, Paley D, Cannada L. The load applied to the foot in a patellar ligament-bearing cast. *J Bone Joint Surg Am.* 1998;80:1597-1602.
11. Shuler FD, Grisafi FN. Cast-saw burns; evaluation of skin, cast and blade temperatures generated during cast removal. *J Bone Joint Surg Am.* 2008;90A:2626-2630.

## SELECTED HISTORICAL READING

Charnley J. *The Closed Treatment of Common Fractures.* 3rd ed. Williams & Wilkins; 1972: 179-183.

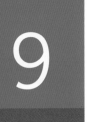

# 9 Orthopaedic Unit Care

Scott B. Marston and Jordan Barker

I. The orthopaedic unit must present a warm, friendly, and quiet atmosphere as an essential part of the treatment program. Most patients who enter the hospital are anxious and need reassurance from everyone on the unit. To have an effective team, it is necessary for everyone involved in the patient's care to understand the goals of the treatment program. To achieve this, careful and clear communication is required because it is recognized that the best run orthopaedic services are those that involve all of the personnel in the decision-making process. To maintain the best possible environment for patients and to ease the problems of communication, it is helpful to schedule and standardize activities and procedures. This principle is even more important with the current emphasis on shortened length of hospital stay.

II. **Rounds**

Rounds are important in that they constitute an evaluation for the benefit of the patient and an educational experience for all of the participants. Be certain that the best interests of the patient are not sacrificed for education. Knowing that any nonverbal cue or word uttered in the presence of the patient can stimulate a reaction in her, him, or their family is fundamental to the art of healing. Maintaining a professional appearance is also important and includes proper attire. Portrayal of professionalism building confidence in the care team. The focus of the interaction must center on the treatment of the patient and the disease process. Fascination, preoccupation, or engagement of the disease (or language to that effect) must be avoided. The patient must be regarded and respected, and all allusions to the disease or the treatment must be framed as a focus on the patient. The patient must be made to feel that he or she is receiving sympathetic attention as a living human being rather than being scrutinized like a specimen. This does not necessarily mean that scientific discussion is inappropriate at the bedside. However, in general, a highly technical debate or lengthy discussion should be conducted away from the bedside and out of the patient's hearing range or the patient should be offered an explanation of the context of the discussion in terms they can understand.

A. The **approach to the patient** must be direct and personal. Properly conducted, it can be an excellent teaching experience for those in attendance and help the patient understand his or her problems more completely. If the leader of the rounds addresses the patient with friendly words of inquiry or explanation and actively engages the patient in the discussion, the patient tolerates or welcomes these clinical discussions. When managed along these lines, rather than resenting visitations from large groups, most patients will relish the attention they are receiving and enjoy participating in the process.

B. Personal privacy is very important and is becoming more so. Before beginning rounds, if there are visitors present, a member of the team should ask the patient if he or she is comfortable having the visitors present during the interactions. If so, engaging the patients family and friends and making them aware of the patients diagnosis and activity restrictions can help with compliance. Drawing pictures and/or reviewing x-rays can help deepen their understanding.

C. **Present case histories at bedside only with the patient's permission.** Devote attention to examining the patient, giving advice, or obtaining further history. Refer to patients by name. References to age, sex, or race are out of place unless essential to the discussion and cannot be perceived by those in attendance.

D. **Sensitive humor** can be beneficial as long as the patient shares it. This is an art, carefully administered. Laughter can be cruel when the patient thinks that it is directed toward him or her.

E. **The head nurse should be an integral part** of rounds. The nurse prepares for rounds as well as participates in them. When the patient is examined, the nurse should be at the head of the bed to promote the comfort of the patient during the examination. The doctors and students have much to learn from the nurse in charge.

F. **Consultations** are an important part of patient care and are usually ordered by the attending physician with a statement as to the current care. One of the team members should directly contact the consultant to relay the purpose for the consult and any other pertinent information. Make every effort to assist the consultant. Frame the question, anticipate the need, and provide the appropriate data. The resident, physician assistant, or staff physician should inform the patient of the consultation and explain the purpose of the visit.

III. **Patient Evaluation and Documentation**

A. **Utilizing the electronic medical record (EMR).** Nearly all institutions have converted to an EMR. Spend time early on developing templates for routine tasks: consult notes, admit history and physical examinations (H&Ps), progress notes, brief op notes, and so on.

1. When using templates, use caution and remember that each patient is unique and your documentation should reflect this.
2. Avoid adding extraneous information; be thorough but concise.
3. Resist the temptation to cut and paste. Adding to the volume of the note may hinder communication by making it harder to find the relevant part of the record necessary to treat the patient. Your notes should be your notes.
4. Comply with Health Insurance Portability and Accountability Act (HIPPA) regulations. Only view medical records of patients for whom you are providing care. Physicians have lost their privileges for violating these rules.

B. **History and physical.** This vital document will be read and referenced by all future consulting physicians and teams; therefore, its accuracy and thoroughness is paramount.

1. **Chief complaint.** This is not a diagnosis, but the principle problem(s) from the patient's point of view.
2. **History of present illness.** Include relevant aspects of the injury mechanism, including dates and times.
3. **Patient profile**
   a. Medical and surgical history
   b. Medications
   c. Allergies. Include the type of reaction.
   d. Family history
   e. Social history. Include vocation, smoking/tobacco, alcohol, and drug use history.
   f. Hand dominance, as appropriate
4. **Review of systems**
5. **Physical examination**. It is of utmost importance to include a baseline, detailed neurovascular examination of the involved extremities.

6. **Laboratory results**
7. **Imaging findings.** Provide your own interpretation of X-rays.
8. **Assessment.** May be symptom-based or diagnosis-based, including differential diagnoses when uncertain, and a brief summary of your rationale.
9. **Plan**
   a. **Diagnostic** plan
   b. **Therapeutic** plan
   c. **Lesion-specific**, including splinting, protections, weight-bearing status
   d. **General orthopaedic**, including infection considerations, anticoagulation, rehabilitation, and discharge criteria
   e. **Patient education**
C. **Progress notes** should be written daily and as often as there is change in the patient's condition.
   1. **Subjective** data
   2. **Objective** data
   3. **Assessment**
   4. **Plan**
      a. **Diagnostic**
      b. **Therapeutic**
      c. **Patient education**
D. **Discharge summaries**
   1. **Dates of admission and discharge**
   2. **Master problem list** with the appropriate dates
   3. List of **operations and procedures**, including the dates
   4. **Description** of the inpatient problems
   5. **Physical examination**
   6. **Laboratory data**
   7. **Hospital course** for each problem, including laboratory data, treatment, and plans when appropriate
   8. **Discharge instructions**
      a. Diet, activity, wound care
      b. Discharge medications
      c. Follow-up
IV. **Inpatient Management**
   A. **Do not resuscitate (DNR)/do not intubate (DNI) status.** Discuss with the patient, power of attorney, and/or family regarding their wishes for resuscitation and intubation soon after admission.
   B. Clearly specify **weight-bearing** and **activity** orders so that nurses, physical/occupational therapists, consultants, and case workers may work harmoniously.
   C. **Pain control**
      1. **Acute pain** will result from injury as well as surgery and must be carefully controlled to optimize outcomes. Uncontrolled pain can result in prolonged hospital stays, readmission, a series of detrimental physiologic responses, including delirium in the elderly. Multimodal analgesia has been shown to be effective across multiple orthopaedic subspecialties, resulting in decreased acuity of postoperative care, decreased length of hospital stay, improved early range of motion, improved mobility, decreased persistent pain, increased patient satisfaction, fewer opioids consumed, and fewer opioid-related adverse effects. It has become the standard of care in pain management. Multimodal analgesia means utilizing two or more drugs with different mechanisms of action with the goal of gaining a synergistic effect from the combination as a whole, as well as limiting opioid use. Regimens may include local anesthetic infiltration, peripheral nerve blocks, neuraxial

blocks, acetaminophen, gabapentin, and nonsteroidal anti-inflammatory drugs, including cyclooxygenase-2-specific inhibitors.[1,2]

2. **Opioids** should always be used with caution. There has been a significant rise in the quantity of opioids prescribed in the United States over recent years, accompanied by an unfortunate rise in opioid-related deaths. Though powerful analgesics, the benefit of these drugs must be considered in light of their side effects. Side effects include hypotension, oversedation, respiratory depression, ileus, postoperative nausea and vomiting, confusion, constipation, and itching. Another less-understood and paradoxical side effect is opioid-induced hyperalgesia, which increases pain with narcotic use, and is associated with large doses. Certain patients are at particularly high risk of oversedation and respiratory depression and should be monitored carefully. They include those with sleep apnea, morbid obesity, snoring, age over 61, opioid naiveté, longer general anesthetic time, preexisting pulmonary or cardiac disease, thoracic or other surgical incisions that may impair breathing, smoking, and concomitant use of other sedating drugs (benzodiazepines, antihistamines, sedatives, or other central nervous system depressants).[1,2]

3. **Integrative medicine**, which includes acupuncture, acupressure, massage, healing touch, music therapy, aromatherapy, and reflexology, has been shown to improve pain scores and can serve as a useful adjunct to any pain control regimen.[3]

4. **Chronic pain.** Chronic pain can be described as ongoing or recurrent pain, lasting beyond the usual course of active illness or injury or 3-6 months. Patients with a history of chronic pain and/or chronic opioid use should be managed with extra care. A detailed history of prior medications should be obtained to avoid withdrawal and uncontrolled pain. Consider a consultation from the pain management service to assist in these circumstances.

D. **Hypnotics** (sleeping pills) should be used with caution, particularly in the elderly. Trazadone and melatonin are generally safe and tolerated well.

E. **Antiemetics.** The effects of anesthesia postoperatively, as well as narcotics, can result in nausea and emesis. In conjunction with the anesthesia team, order antiemetics postoperatively to limit this side effect.

F. **Nutrition/diet orders**

1. Diet orders must take into consideration the patient's existing medical problems, such as a history of aspiration, carbohydrate portions in diabetes, water and salt intake in hyponatremia, mineral levels in dialysis, vegetable selection during warfarin use, and so forth.

2. Malnutrition is a common finding among orthopaedic patients, particularly among the elderly, obese, and diabetic patients. Malnutrition is associated with increased complications and can be diagnosed by standardized scoring tools, anthropometric measurements, or serologic laboratory values, most commonly, albumin.[4]

3. Consider a nutrition consultation if there is concern for malnutrition.

G. **If preoperative preparation is necessary:**

1. Make sure the patient is **medically optimized** for surgery. This will include a thorough medical work up and discussion with the internal medicine service when appropriate.

2. **Surgical prep often includes a** 10-minute chlorhexidine (Hibiclens) or povidone-iodine (Betadine) scrub before surgery.[5-7] If the patient is ambulatory, the scrub is most easily accomplished by a shower with chlorhexidine or hexachlorophene soap at home the night before surgery. Shaving hair from the operative field should be done in the preoperative holding area or operating room with mechanical shavers. Small nicks or

lacerations often occur with conventional razors and can become colonized and increase the risk of a postoperative infection.[5]

3. **Laboratory data.** Patients undergoing a surgical procedure usually have a hemoglobin test within 30 days of surgery. In patients with a history of infection related to the planned surgery, the erythrocyte sedimentation rate (ESR) and C-reactive protein (CRP) should be obtained. If the age of the patient (generally older than 50 years) or the history indicates, a chest X-ray and electrocardiogram (ECG) are appropriate. Whenever blood transfusion is deemed likely, autologous blood donation can be considered, though the efficacy and cost-effectiveness remain controversial.[8-10] Because this is not possible for acute trauma cases, the use of intraoperative suction-collection-filtering-retransfusion (cell saver) may also be considered. Help your team anticipate these needs.

H. **Antibiotics** should be used prophylactically for most orthopaedic procedures.[11,12] Cephazolin, a broad-acting first-generation cephalosporin, is the preferred antibiotic and is to be administered within 60 minutes of skin incision and continued every 8 hours for 24 hours postoperatively[11,12]; however, a single dose may be just as efficacious. For longer cases, cephazolin should be redosed every 4 hours during the procedure.[11,12] For those allergic to penicillin or cephalosporins, clindamycin or vancomycin may be considered.

Recent evidence suggests 30% of postoperative hip surgical site infections may be due to gram-negative organisms compared to 10% in the knee. Therefore, many surgeons are adding Gentamicin or Aztreonam to their preoperative prophylactics regimen for hip patients.[13]

I. **Prevention of venous thromboembolism (VTE)** is a high priority in orthopaedic trauma and postoperative patients. In addition to early mobilization when able, mechanical and chemical prophylaxis should be considered early in the treatment course.

1. **Mechanical prophylaxis**, in the form of thromboembolic deterrent (TED) hose and pneumatic compression devices, has been shown to decrease the rates of deep vein thrombosis (DVT) and should be considered in patients when able. If patients are at high risk for bleeding because of hemophilia or liver disease, mechanical prophylaxis alone may be appropriate.[14] Care should be taken when using these devices in patients with frail skin or high risk for ulcer, such as diabetic neuropathy.

2. **Chemical prophylaxis** comes in many forms, with each drug class exhibiting unique risks and benefits. In general, the benefit of preventing blood clots needs to be weighed against the increased risk of postoperative hematoma formation and wound drainage, which may predispose to infection.[15]

   a. **Warfarin** is a vitamin K antagonist. If chosen for VTE prophylaxis, it must be monitored closely with the international normalized ratio. Despite the burden of frequent monitoring, warfarin has been shown to be an effective deterrent to VTE.

   b. **Acetylsalicylic acid (aspirin)** works as an irreversible COX-1,2 inhibitor, which disrupts platelet aggregation. Guidelines by the American College of Chest Physicians and the American Academy of Orthopaedic Surgeons have recommended aspirin as an effective agent for VTE prophylaxis.[15] Large retrospective studies have demonstrated no difference in 81 mg BID versus 325 mg BID in prevention of VTE in elective hip and knee arthroplasty.[15,17]

   c. **Unfractionated heparin** is an antithrombin III activator. The standard dosage is 5,000 IU subcutaneously every 8 hours. Benefits of heparin include a relatively short half-life, which makes it a convenient drug perioperatively. Monitoring for heparin-induced thrombocytopenia includes daily complete blood count (CBC) laboratory draws to assess platelet levels.

d. **Low-molecular-weight heparin,** often in the form of enoxaparin, is also an antithrombin III activator, but with less activity against thrombin compared with unfractionated heparin. Low-molecular-weight heparin is recommended as the agent of choice by the Orthopaedic Trauma Association and should be initiated within 24 hours unless there are contraindications. The usual starting dose is either 40 mg daily or 30 mg every 12 hours, but it is adjusted according to body mass index. Routine laboratory monitoring is not necessary.[17] If enoxaparin is to be continued after discharge, ask the nursing staff to educate the patient and their family regarding home administration techniques.

e. **Direct Xa inhibitors,** such as apixaban and rivaroxaban, have become more popular in recent years given their convenient dosing schedules, efficacy in prevention of VTE, and lack of need for laboratory monitoring. One concern, however, is the lack of availability of a reversal agent.[17]

**J. Urinary retention.** Indications for bladder catheterization include prolonged anesthesia, poor patient mobility, and inability to void. Prolonged anesthesia is often defined as a case longer than 3 hours. The decision for a catheter is a joint decision between the surgeon and the anesthesia team and is optimally discussed with the patient preoperatively. This decision is best made if there is clear communication between the surgeon and the anesthesia team about case length, comorbidities, expected blood loss, fluid parameters, trauma status, postoperative nursing needs, and so on. If the bladder has been overdistended, it may take several days to regain normal tone and function. If this occurs, consider a urology consult. If the patient requires catheterization, it should be done with a small catheter with a 5-mL balloon. Some argue that the catheter should be left in place until the patient is ambulatory or is off narcotics; others argue that the catheter should be removed as soon as the patient is alert enough to urinate to limit possible urinary tract infections.[19] As common as catheter usage is, literature-based guidance on catheter usage is deficient. In general removal of the catheter in the recovery room with in and out catheterization if necessary is the best choice.

**K. Bowel regimen.** Bowel problems are best addressed preemptively. A mix of bulking agents, stool softeners, lubricants, and laxatives may make the patient's course more comfortable if given before there is a problem. This is particularly true of bedbound patients on narcotics, which slow the alimentary tract. Docusate sodium (Colace), 100 mg BID, is usually satisfactory, but it may be necessary to supplement this with 30 to 60 mL of milk of magnesia at bedtime. Mineral oil is a useful stool softener/lubricant, but it should be administered with caution because it may interfere with vitamin absorption. Suppositories and enemas may be necessary if less invasive methods are ineffective.

**L. Skin.** Pressure sores are often prevented by thoughtful nursing care.[20, 21] Pressure problems are common over the sacrum and heels. Patients who are unable to change position frequently following surgery or trauma must be turned frequently by the staff. Dressings that cover these common areas must be applied anticipating the inability to move or protect. When exposed, skin checks for redness are critical, especially on newly injured patients, unconscious patients, patients with dementia, patients with spinal cord injury or spina bifida, splinted extremities, and extremities in traction. The problem is exacerbated in paraplegic and quadriplegic patients or in patients with concomitant head injury. If the orthopaedic condition does not allow frequent change in position, consider using special flotation mattresses or rotating beds.[21] Check the skin during rounds.

**M. Common *pre*operative orders** for an orthopaedic procedure
1. **Diet**—nothing by mouth before surgery, usually 8 hours before, or after midnight for a case the following day
2. **Activity**
3. **Vital signs**
4. **Preoperative scrub or shower** with chlorhexidine, povidone-iodine, or hexachlorophene
5. **Laboratory data and other testing.** Check with specialists and anesthesia team.
6. **Hematocrit/hemoglobin**
7. **Urinalysis**
8. **Chest X-ray** if patient is older than 50 years
9. **ECG** if patient is older than 50 years and no recent ECG results are available
10. **ESR** and **CRP** if there is a history of infection
11. **Blood typed and cross matched** if significant loss is anticipated. The use of an intraoperative "cell saver" should be anticipated and used when blood loss is anticipated to be more than 500 mL. Similarly, the use of a tourniquet can limit blood loss and should be planned
12. **Antibiotics** if indicated (hold preoperative antibiotics if intraoperative cultures are to be obtained)
13. **Analgesics**
14. **Hypnotic**

**N. Common *post*operative orders** for an orthopaedic procedure
1. **Diet, including supplementary shakes. Consider a nutrition consult if necessary.**
2. **Activity or position**
3. **Ice, elevation** if appropriate
4. **Weight-bearing status**
5. **Physical therapy** with surgery-specific restrictions/limitations
6. **Occupational therapy**
7. **Vital signs**—record intake and output if indicated
8. **Patient turning, coughing, incentive spirometry, and deep breathing encouraged** every 1 to 4 hours.
9. **Urinary catheter or straight catheter orders if no urine** is produced within 8 hours postoperatively.
10. **Pain medication**
11. **Hypnotic**
12. **Multivitamin**
13. **Postoperative labs.** CBC and basic metabolic panel (BMP) generally obtained postoperative days 1 and 2.
14. **Postoperative X-rays** if indicated
15. **Physician on-call notified** for blood pressure less than 90/60, pulse greater than 100, or temperature greater than 38.3°C.
16. **Anticoagulation therapy**
17. **Postoperative antibiotics**
18. **Bowel program**
19. **Social service consultation** if needed for disposition

**V. Orthopaedic Tips for Students**
**A. Involvement of medical, nursing, and physician assistant students on the orthopaedic team**
1. Discuss expectations and goals with your residents and attendings at the beginning of the rotation.
2. There should be a balance among exposure to the clinic, hospital rounds, and the operating room.

3. Get to know the office staff who will have schedules and related educational opportunities. Know to whom you should report or ask questions.
4. Consider giving a presentation to the orthopaedic team, if possible, centered around a particular patient you found interesting.
5. Try to gain exposure to the various subspecialties of orthopaedics.

**B. Advice on how to be useful and get the most out of your rotation**
1. Start early. If possible, round and review patients before the team.
2. Communicate with all. Ask questions of the nurses, staff, residents, and consultants.
3. Know the plan. The plan is dynamic and will evolve. Know the contingencies that would change the plan. Offer to help execute the next step in care.
   a. For surgery, check on the completion of the preparations. Check and confirm nothing by mouth (NPO) status, pending laboratory values, pending imaging, surgical consents, and consultant evaluations.
   b. For the postoperative period, ensure adequate pain medication and follow-up on postoperative images and laboratory values (e.g., hemoglobin, electrolytes). Question the need for urinary catheters and discontinue them as early as possible.
   c. For discharge and follow-up, help get them ready. When appropriate, communicate with the therapists, nurses, and social workers.
4. Contribute energy and be willing to help with tasks such as dressing changes, suture removal, and so forth.
5. Be careful about what information you give directly to the patient. Err on the side of caution. **Never** be the first one to give the patient bad news (unless specifically directed otherwise by the staff physician).
6. Read, study, and ask. Prioritize the study of anatomy and the physical examination.

**C. Principles specific to orthopaedics**
1. Handle bone with the care it needs. It may look hard and impenetrable, but it is living tissue. Protect it from inflammation, infection, avascularity, and abnormal stresses and motions.
2. Handle joints with the care they require. Restore alignment, anatomy, and soft tissue. Remember that the implications for bone injury, whether diaphyseal, metaphyseal, or periarticular, have specific implications for each of the joints of the limb.
3. Be precise in your assessment of pain. Most patients in orthopaedics present with pain as their chief complaint. Knowing your anatomy and refining your examination techniques will yield accurate diagnoses.
4. Remember the soft tissues. Fractures are soft-tissue injuries with a broken bone inside, and often the soft tissue is the rate-limiting step of the treatment.
5. Appreciate anatomy. Seek to restore it in both closed and open forms of treatment.
6. Anticipate future problems. The orthopaedist is often the only one to understand the long-term implications of musculoskeletal deformity and disease.
7. Consider the patient as a whole. Psychosocial disharmony may be at the heart of the patient's chief complaint.
8. Always go to the operating room with plan A, B, and C in mind.
9. Learn and execute excellent dressing techniques.
10. Recognize that children are different, their problems are different, and their needs are different. Things happen in children that do not happen in adults, and the injuries and their responses are age and site dependent.

a. The anatomy is different. The supracondylar area of the elbow goes through a remodeling phase between ages 4 and 8 in which the bone becomes very thin, hence the higher rate of fractures in this age group. There are other classic patterns (triplane fractures and Tillaux fractures of the ankle). There is no substitute for simply knowing the patterns that occur, watching for them, and treating their idiosyncrasies.

b. The physiology is different. The blood supply to certain areas (femoral head, epiphyseal fragments) passes through a period of vulnerability. Their ability to heal is different.

**D. Principles of the attending/team leader**

1. Be a clinician. Suppress and delay the inclination to define the problem solely with an X-ray. Take a history, know the patient, and **examine** the patient.

2. Remember the simple things such as ice, heat, rest, elevation, and reassurance.

3. Understand inflammation. Understand what it is and is not in orthopaedics. Know when it is primarily part of the pathology (rheumatoid arthritis, bursitis) and when it is part of the healing (fractures, sprains).

**E. Work well with others**

1. Be an effective part of the team. Know and respect the roles of the professionals around you. They will help to anticipate the needs of the patients, communicate, and administer cost-efficient care.

2. Do what is necessary to facilitate orderly transfer of care. This is done through direct communication with those assuming the care. It is not by hospital note or by the assumption of the role of others. Live or phone conversation is best.

**F. Students presenting at rounds.** It is one of the great exercises in the study of medicine to learn by presenting a case. The exercise gives the student presenters a focus to bring principles and practice together, which they will do innumerably during their careers. It gives the expert an opportunity to illustrate specifics and generalities. It gives everyone an opportunity to interact.

1. Be organized and know the case.

2. Know the radiographs and advanced imaging. Be sure to have reviewed them before the case because you can be sure that as soon as they are presented, a roomful of very smart, conscientious, experienced people will begin to critique them for orderliness, quality, relevance, subtle cues, and missed lesions.

3. Listen for the pearls to drop. The best conferences are a mix of academics and practical considerations playing off one another. There will be insights about diagnosis, technique, decision-making, and people.

4. Speak the language. There is a language of fractures. Varus, valgus, proximal, distal, fracture type and classification, and soft-tissue injury class are part of the presentation exercise. If you use an eponym (i.e., Colles, Barton's, Bennetts), expect to be asked the origin and meaning of the name. Almost all classification systems have inadequacies or shortcomings; be prepared to discuss these. Be prepared to show additional studies that help define the pathology if the plain films cannot. Remember that the best classification systems also include mechanism, pathophysiology, treatment, and prognosis.

5. Show courage. If you are in trouble, do not expect to be rescued too early. Orthopaedists enjoy watching a competent student struggle with forming a concept or discovering a truth. Do not bail or defer to the staff or teachers too early. Remember, you are probably one of hundreds of students that the members of the conference have seen in this circumstance, and they will want you to succeed, overcome, and grow. If someone asks you to present, it is a compliment of sorts. Rise up to it.

6. **Never** lie. If you are presenting a case that you have never seen, say so early. If there is missing data, say that too. If you do not know the answer, simply say, "I don't know, but I will find the answer and get back to you."

### G. Final thoughts

1. *Primum non nocere*. Know your limitations. One of the great hazards in medicine is the practitioner who rises to a level of incompetence and does not pull back from it. Periods of growth (including being a medical or PA student) carry risks of failure for both patient and doctor or PA.
2. Take good medical care of your patients. There is no substitute for seeing (actually seeing and examining) your patients.
3. Respect patients as humans. Communicate respectfully and honestly. Apologize when late and give a reasonable explanation when it is appropriate. Make eye contact. Shake hands often (where culturally appropriate), and give consolation, sympathy, empathy, and sensitivity to what they may be feeling emotionally and physically.
4. Have reverence for the history and process that put you in this remarkable circumstance. The principles you apply were discovered at great cost over centuries. When the exam room door closes, it will be you, the patient, and those principles.
5. Be supportive of your colleagues. You may feel that the patient has been poorly or inadequately served somehow, but it may only add to their suffering to give a colleague misgivings or guilt about how they should have done things differently, and this should rarely, if ever, be discussed in front of the patient. Conversely, if you appreciate or have confidence in a consultant or colleague, say so.
6. Remember to learn professionalism in addition to orthopaedics.

## REFERENCES

1. Jones J Jr, Southerland W, Catalani B. The importance of optimizing acute pain in the orthopedic trauma patient. *Orthop Clin North Am*. 2017;48(4):445-465.
2. Goodman SB. Multimodal analgesia for orthopaedic procedures. *Anesth Analg*. 2007;105(1):19-20.
3. Dusek JA, Finch M, Plotnikoff G, et al. The impact of integrative medicine on pain management in a tertiary care hospital. *J Patient Saf*. 2010;6:48-51.
4. Cross MB, Yi PH, Thomas CF, Garcia J, Della Valle CJ. Evaluation of malnutrition in orthopaedic surgery. *J Am Acad Orthop Surg*. 2014;22(3):193-199.
5. DeRogatis MJ, Mahon AM, Lee P, Issack PS. Perioperative considerations to reduce infection in primary hip and knee arthroplasty. *JBJS Rev*. 2018;6:1-9.
6. Darouiche RO, Wall MJ, Itani KM, et al. Chlorhexidine-alcohol versus povidone-iodine for surgical-site antisepsis. *N Engl J Med*. 2010;362:18-26.
7. Saltzman MD, Nuber GW, Gryzlo SM, et al. Efficacy of surgical preparation solutions in shoulder surgery. *J Bone Joint Surg Am*. 2009;91:1949-1953.
8. Kamath AF, Pagnano MW. Blood management for patients undergoing total joint arthroplasty. *JBJS Rev*. 2013;1:1-11.
9. Benli IT, Akalin S, Duman E, et al. The results of intraoperative autotransfusion in orthopaedic surgery. *Bull Hosp Jt Dis*. 1999;58:184-187.
10. Tan TL, Shohat N, Rondon AJ, et al. Prophylactic antibiotic prophylaxis in total joint arthroplasty: a single dose is as effective as multiple doses. *J Bone Joint Surg Am*. 2019;101:429-437.
11. Fletcher N, Sofianos D, Berkes MB, et al. Prevention of perioperative infection. *J Bone Joint Surg Am*. 2007;89:1605-1618.
12. Boxma H, Braekhuizen T, Patka P, et al. Randomized controlled trial of single-dose antibiotic prophylaxis in surgical treatment of closed fractures: the Dutch Trauma Trial. *Lancet*. 1996;347:1133-1137.
13. Bosco JA, Tejada PRR, Catanzano AJ, et al. Expanded gram-negative antimicrobial prophylaxis reduces surgical site infection in hip arthroplasty. *J Arthroplasty*. 2016;31(3):616-621.
14. Scolaro JA, Taylor RM, Wigner NA. Venous thromboembolism in orthopaedic trauma. *J Am Acad Orthop Surg*. 2015;23(1):1-6.

15. Parvizi J, Huang R, Restrepo C, et al. Low-dose aspirin is effective chemoprophylaxis against clinically important venous thromboembolism following total joint arthroplasty. *J Bone Joint Surg Am*. 2017;99(2):91-98.
16. Lieberman, JR, Heckmann, N. Venous thromboembolism prophylaxis in total hip arthroplasty and total knee arthroplasty patients: from guidelines to practice. *J Am Acad Orthop Surg*. 2017;25(12):789-798.
17. Flevas DA, Megaloikonomos PD, Dimopoulos L, et al. Thromboembolism prophylaxis in orthopaedics: an update. *EFORT Open Rev*. 2018;3(4):136-148.
18. Brown GA. Venous thromboembolism prophylaxis after major orthopaedic surgery: a pooled analysis of randomized controlled trials. *J Arthroplasty*. 2009;24(6 Suppl):77-83.
19. Carpiniello VL, Cendron AM, Altman HG, et al. Treatment of urinary complications after total joint replacement in elderly females. *Urology*. 1988;32:186-188.
20. Bonnaig N, Dailey S, Archdeacon M. Proper patient positioning and complication prevention in orthopaedic surgery. *J Bone Joint Surg Am*. 2014;96A:1135-1140.
21. Allman RM, Walker JM, Hart MK, et al. Air-fluidized beds or conventional therapy for pressure sores: a randomized trial. *Ann Intern Med*. 1987;107:641-648.

## SELECTED HISTORICAL READINGS

American Academy of Orthopaedic Surgeons. Information statement: recommendations for the use of intravenous antibiotic prophylaxis in primary total joint arthroplasty. AAOS; 2004.

Harris WH, Athanasoulis CA, Waltron AC, et al. Prophylaxis of deep-vein thrombosis after total hip replacement, dextran and external pneumatic compression compared with 1.2 or 1.3 grams of aspirin daily. *J Bone Joint Surg Am*. 1985;67:57-62.

Henny CP, Odoom JA, Ten Cate H, et al. Effects of extradural bupivacaine on the haemostatic system. *Br J Anaesth*. 1986;58:301-305.

Jensen JE, Jensen TG, Smith TK, et al. Nutrition in orthopaedic surgery. *J Bone Joint Surg Am*. 1982;64:1263-1272.

Kay SP, Moreland JR, Schmitter E. Nutritional status and wound healing in lower extremity amputations. *Clin Orthop Relat Res*. 1987;217:253-256.

McKenzie PJ, Wishart HY, Smith G. Long-term outcome after repair of fractured neck of femur: comparison of subarachnoid and general anaesthesia. *Br J Anaesth*. 1984;56:581-585.

Means JH. *The Amenities of Ward Rounds and Related Matters*. Massachusetts General Hospital Print Shop; 1942.

Michelson JD, Lotke PA, Steinberg ME. Urinary bladder management after total joint replacement surgery. *N Engl J Med*. 1988;319:321-326.

Schaeffer AJ. Catheter-associated bacteriuria. *Urol Clin North Am*. 1986;13:735-747.

Thorburn J, Louden JR, Vallance R. Spinal and general anaesthesia in total hip replacement: frequency of deep vein thrombosis. *Br J Anaesth*. 1980;52:1117-1121.

Weed LL. *Medical Records, Medical Education, and Patient Care*. 2nd ed. Year Book; 1970.

# 10 Traction

Marc F. Swiontkowski

## I. Objectives

Although traction is being used with decreasing frequency for fracture care outside of developing nations, a knowledge of these effective principles is necessary for special indications or situations in which equipment or expertise is not available or patient comorbidities do not permit operative intervention. Traction remains a useful temporizing method in the severely injured patient with femoral shaft or pelvic/acetabular fractures.[1]

**A.** Traction maintains the **length** of a limb as well as **alignment and stability** at the fracture site. Treating femoral fractures with fixed skeletal traction is an example.

**B.** Traction can **allow joint motion** while maintaining the alignment of the fracture. For example, the Pearson attachment on a Thomas splint allows knee movement during traction treatment of a femoral fracture; overbody or lateral skeletal traction allows elbow motion while maintaining the alignment of a humeral fracture.

**C.** Traction can **overcome muscle spasm** associated with bone or joint disease. An example is Bucks traction, which is sometimes recommended for patients with hip injuries.

**D.** **Edema is reduced** in an extremity by a traction unit that elevates the affected part above the heart.

## II. Essential Materials

The bed must have a firm mattress or a bed board. Elevate the head or the foot of the bed using either shock blocks or the bed's intrinsic elevation system. Attach an overhead frame, trapeze, and side rails to the bed so that the patient can shift position. Traction equipment includes bars, pulleys, ropes, weight hangers, skeletal traction apparatus, and, in some instances, plaster cast materials. Various figures in this chapter show the type and placement of equipment about the bed.

## III. Skin Traction

**A.** Skin traction may be used as a definitive method of treatment as well as a first aid or temporary measure. The **traction force** applied to the skin is transmitted to the bone through the superficial fascia, deep fascia, and intermuscular septa. Skin damage can result from too much traction force. The maximum weight recommended for skin traction is 10 lb or less, depending on the size and age of the patient. If this much weight is used, discontinue the skin traction after 1 week. If less weight is used and if the skin is inspected biweekly, skin traction may be safely used for 4 to 6 weeks. Pediatric patients need skin inspection on a more frequent basis.

**B.** **Application**

1. **Carefully prepare the skin** by removing the hair as well as washing and drying the area.

2. **Avoid placing adhesive straps over bony prominences.** If bony prominences are in the area of strap application, cover them well with cast padding before the adhesive straps are applied. Always use a spreader bar to avoid pressure from the traction rope on bony prominences.

3. Make the **adhesive straps** from adhesive tape, moleskin adhesive, or a commercial skin traction unit consisting of foam boots with Velcro straps.

Place the straps longitudinally on opposite sides of the extremity, with free skin left between the straps to prevent any tourniquet effect. Attach the free ends of these straps to the spreader bar. Hold the straps in place by encircling the extremity with an adhesive or elastic wrap. Then apply the traction rope to the spreader bar.

4. Support the leg in traction with pillows or folded bath blankets without contact under the heel to **prevent edema and irritation of the heel**.

## IV. Skeletal Traction[2]

**A. Definition.** Skeletal traction is applied through direct fixation to bone.

**B. Equipment**

1. **Kirschner wire** is a thin, smooth wire with a diameter of 0.0360 to 0.0625 in. The advantages of Kirschner wire are that it is easy to insert and that it minimizes the chance of soft-tissue damage or infection. The disadvantage is that it rotates within an improper bow and can cut through osteoporotic bone. These complications are minimized using the proper traction bow. Even though Kirschner wire is small in diameter and flexible, it can withstand a large traction force when the proper traction bow is used. This special bow (Kirschner bow) provides the wire with rigidity by applying a longitudinal tension force (Fig. 10-1). If properly placed and not improperly stressed, the wire does not break and causes less bone damage than the larger Steinmann pins.

2. **Steinmann pins** vary in diameter from 0.078 to 0.19 in and come in smooth and threaded forms. Because they are large enough to have inherent stability, the Steinmann pin bow (Bohler bow), which attaches to these pins, does not exert tension along the pin as does the Kirschner traction bow. The two types of pins should be readily recognized and used with the appropriate bow (Fig. 10-1).

3. **Factors to be considered**

   a. **Nonthreaded wire or pin** is smaller, more uniform, less easily broken, more easily inserted, and removed with less twisting than the threaded type. A disadvantage is that it can slide laterally through the skin and bone. Even with careful attention, it can move enough to disturb the traction or predispose to a pin tract infection.

   b. The **threaded wire or pin** has stress risers at each thread, breaks more easily, must be larger in diameter to gain the same strength, and takes a longer time to insert. In inserting a threaded pin, one is tempted to go rapidly with the hand or battery powered drill, which creates an undue amount of heat. On the other hand, because the threads prevent lateral slippage of the pin, this type is preferable to the nonthreaded variety for long-term (longer than 1 to 2 weeks) traction.

4. The wires and pins are available with two types of points. One is a **trocar**, a blunted point that tends to grind through the bone with relatively little cutting ability. The other is a **diamond-shaped point**, a modified type of drill that passes through bone more easily and with less heating. Wires and pins that are dull, sharpened off-center, or bent should not be used. These wander during insertion and create a hole that is too large.

5. Note that pins and wires are frequently used as **internal fixation** devices for fractures; such use is discussed in **Chapter 11** and the chapter on hand fractures, **Chapter 21**.

**C. Pin and wire insertion guidelines**

1. Pin or wire insertion is a surgical procedure, so **some form of consent** is needed, at least with a witness in attendance who signs a note in the medical record attesting that informed consent was obtained. A signed, witnessed surgical consent is preferred. The site of pin application should be signed with a surgical marking pen, and a time out should be held as if the procedure were being done in the operating room.

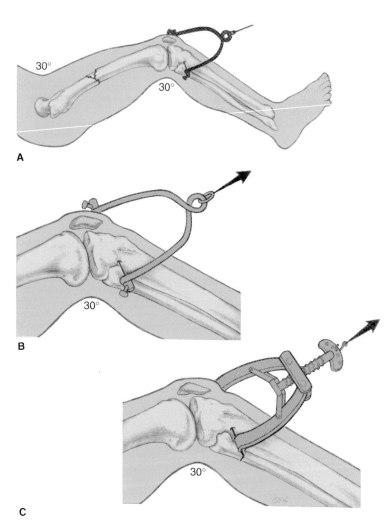

**Figure 10-1.** Traction bows. When using skeletal traction to treat femoral fractures, the knee is kept in slight flexion **(A)**. Proximal tibial traction is reserved for adults. To avoid physeal injury in children with resultant recurvation deformity, distal femoral traction proximal to the distal femoral physis is used. For larger Steinmann pins, a Bohler bow is used **(B)**. The tensioning capabilities of the Kirschner bow allow the use of smaller Kirschner wires **(C)**.

2. Establish the **status of neurovascular structures with a thorough clinical examination** before inserting the pins. Placement of the pins requires knowledge of the specific anatomy and the location of vital structures. **Rule:** Always start the pin on the side where the vital structures are located. This gives better control and better avoidance of these structures. For instance, start an olecranon pin on the medial side to avoid the ulnar nerve.

3. **Skin preparation.** The skin should be free of signs of infection. Follow aseptic procedures, using a topical germicidal antiseptic, drapes, mask, and gloves.
4. It is difficult to obtain enough **anesthesia** to block the periosteum completely. Anesthetize the skin and subcutaneous tissue with 1% lidocaine on the starting side of the bone. Go down to the periosteum with the needle tip and insert enough lidocaine around this area to produce some anesthesia. If there is pain as the pin is inserted and approaches the bone, inject more anesthetic. Drill the pin approximately halfway through the bone, get an idea where it will come out, and then anesthetize the opposite side. In a case in which the wire penetrates two bones, such as the tibia and fibula, it is impossible to anesthetize the area between the two bones. Tell the patient ahead of time that this may be painful for a few seconds but that as soon as the drilling stops, the pain will cease. If done in the emergency department, conscious sedation should be utilized.
5. **Skin incision.** When starting the procedure, pass the wire or pin through a stab wound made with a no. 11 blade. If only a puncture wound is made by the pin, **tight** skin adherence to the pin predisposes to an infection. If an infection with abscess does occur, drain it by extending the stab wound. Dress the pin site with sterile 4 × 4s on each side with Betadine solution applied. Change the dressings daily.
6. Pins and wires should be inserted using a **hand drill** rather than a power tool whenever possible. The time saved using power equipment is expended in preparation time. There is also a tendency to use too high a speed with power drills and generate too much heat, thereby promoting the development of bone necrosis around the pin insertion, resulting in a ring sequestrum. The smaller the pin and the slower the rotation of the hand drill, the faster the pin is inserted. Adequate support of the limb from adequate assistance must be available so that, as the pin is being inserted, the limb does not shift and cause the patient further pain.
7. Traction wires or pins are **best placed in the metaphyses**, not in dense cortical bone. Use caution to avoid epiphyseal plate damage, which can result in a growth disturbance. In skeletally immature patients, the pin should be inserted under fluoroscopic control to avoid the physis. In the area of the tibial tubercle, assume in female patients younger than 14 years and in male patients younger than 16 years that the epiphyseal plate is open. Because of the risk of physeal injury in the proximal tibia, choose the distal femur for skeletal traction in younger patients if possible. Ideally, pass the pin through only skin, subcutaneous tissue, and bone. Avoid muscles and tendons.
8. **Do not violate a fracture hematoma** by skeletal wires or pins for traction, or the equivalent of an open fracture will result.
9. **Do not penetrate joints** with traction wires or pins because pyarthrosis can occur. Do not enter the suprapatellar pouch with distal femoral wires or pins. Here again, inserting the pin under fluoroscopic control can avoid these complications.
10. **Points to remember** about wire or pin insertion:
    a. Chuck the wire or pin so that a length of just **2 to 4 in is exposed** to prevent wandering and bending.
    b. **Tighten chuck sufficiently** to prevent score marks that are sources of metal corrosion and fracture.
    c. Be certain that the wire **does not bend** as it is inserted.
    d. Use the proper traction bow (Fig. 10-1).

**D. Specific areas of insertion**
1. **Metacarpals.** Place the wire through the metaphyseal–diaphyseal junction of the index and middle metacarpals. To facilitate insertion, push the first dorsal interosseous muscle in a volar direction and palpate the

subcutaneous portion of the bone. Angle the wire to pass through the index and middle metacarpals and to come out the dorsum of the hand to preserve the natural arch.

2. **Distal radius and ulna.** Usually place the wire or pin through both the radius and the ulna. This site is rarely used.

3. **Olecranon.** Take care to avoid an open epiphysis. Do not place the pin too far distally because this causes elbow extension, and it is more comfortable to pull through a flexed elbow than an extended elbow. Use a moderate-sized wire or pin and insert it from the medial side to avoid the ulnar nerve. Use a very small traction bow.

4. **Distal femur.** Start on the medial side, anterior enough to avoid the neurovascular structures. This insertion is best accomplished by placing the pin 1 in inferior to the abductor tubercle. If the pin will be used for traction on a fracture table for delayed intramedullary nailing, make sure that it is placed far anterior, off the coronal midline to avoid incarceration by the intramedullary nail. Fluoroscopy should be used to help the surgeon avoid an open physis.

5. **Proximal tibia.** Place the wire or pin 1 in inferior and ½ in posterior to the tibial tubercle, starting on the lateral side to avoid the peroneal nerve. Take extreme care to avoid an open physis or apophysis; if the anterior portion of the proximal tibial epiphyseal plate is violated, genu recurvatum can occur.

6. **Distal tibia and fibula.** Start the pin 1 to 1½ fingerbreadths above the most prominent portion of the lateral malleolus to avoid the ankle mortise. Insert it parallel to the ankle joint and angulate it slightly anteriorly. The surgeon should feel the pin pass through the two fibular cortices and then the two tibial cortices. Pass the pin through both bones to avoid the tendons and neurovascular structures. If the pin is placed too far proximally, the foot rests on the bow, and a pressure sore may occur.

7. **Calcaneus.** Generally, select a large diamond-point pin. The preferred insertion site is 1 in inferior and posterior from the lateral malleolus or 1¾ in inferior and 1½ in posterior from the medial malleolus. Because of the position of the tibial nerve, the medial starting site is preferred. The position of the sural nerve on the lateral side of the heel must be avoided. If the pin is placed too far posteriorly, it causes a calcaneal (plantar flexed) position of the foot. If the pin is placed too far inferiorly, it may cut out of the bone. If the pin is placed too far superiorly, it can enter the subtalar joint and also spear the flexor tendons or tibial nerve and/or artery. Infections that are difficult to treat often occur when the calcaneus is used for long-term traction.

**V. Cervical Spine Traction[3]**

**A. Neck halter traction** is the simplest of the different types of cervical spine traction, but usually is not used in the treatment of acute cervical spine fractures or dislocations, being reserved for chronic conditions such as a cervical radiculopathy. Apply the traction to the mandible and occiput with a soft, commercially made halter.

1. When **continuous traction** is used with the patient in the supine position, the attached weight should not exceed 10 lb (5 lb is usually sufficient). With the patient sitting, approximately 8 lb may be added to the attached weight to account for the weight of the head. The total attached weight should not exceed 15 lb with the patient in the sitting position. The traction should not be strictly continuous, but used for 30 to 60 minutes followed by rest intervals to allow jaw motion and relieve pressure on the skin.

2. If **intermittent traction** for short periods is used three times daily, up to 30 lb may be used.

3. **Problems** associated with head halter traction are related to the weight used and the position of the neck. The optimum position is usually neutral or in slight flexion. Temporomandibular joint discomfort can ordinarily be relieved by changing the direction of traction force or decreasing the attached weight. Symptoms from local skin pressure may be relieved by the above methods or by appropriate padding.

B. **Skull tong traction** is a form of cervical spine traction and is applied by one of the many types of skull calipers (tongs) (Fig. 10-2). The most satisfactory caliper is screwed into the skull without the need for previous trephining and does not penetrate more than a preset depth. The Gardner-Wells tongs are recommended (Fig. 10-3).[4] With this type of apparatus, heavy traction can be applied to the skull for as long as required. It is especially useful for cervical spine fractures and dislocations. Perform the following procedures after the scalp is cleaned and draped; local shaving is sufficient, but is not absolutely mandatory.

1. The **Gardner-Wells skull traction tongs** are easy to insert. After preparing the skull, position the tongs below the temporal crest and tighten. A spring device within the tong points automatically sets the correct depth and tension. Then the indicator protrudes 1 mm from the knob of the tong, at which time the correct pressure (equivalent to 6 to 8 in/lb) is exerted. Retighten these pins in a sequential manner to the same value the next day, and then do not tighten them again unless loosening occurs.

2. Keep the head end of the frame slightly elevated so that the patient's body acts as countertraction.

3. Initiate cervical traction at 10 to 15 lb and incrementally increase only after checking the appropriate roentgenograms. Initiating traction at higher weights can occasionally result in marked distraction of ligamentous injuries. For definitive traction, Crutchfield's rule of 5 lb per level starting with 10 lb for the head allows for a maximum range of 30 to 40 lb for a C5-C6 injury.

C. **Fixed halo skull traction.** The halo device, originally introduced by Nickel and Perry,[5,6] can be used alone for traction or combined with a vest or cast.

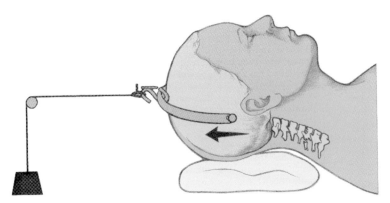

**Figure 10-2.** Tong traction. This treatment is used for most cervical fractures and dislocations. The points are positioned just above the ear pinnae. Padding can be used to generate more flexion or extension of the cervical spine as is indicated for reduction based on lateral cervical roentgenograms.

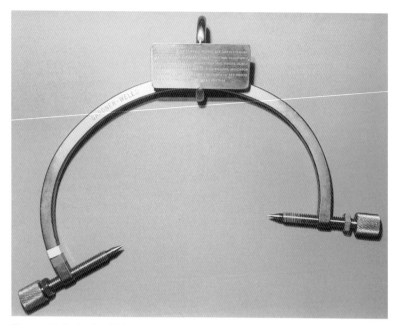

**Figure 10-3.** Gardner-Wells tongs.

1. **Materials**
   a. **Halo ring** (five standard sizes available). Carbon fiber rings are preferred because radiographs and magnetic resonance imaging (MRI) scans can be obtained without distortion
   b. **Five skull pins** (one spare included)
   c. **Two torque screwdrivers**
   d. **Four positioning pins**
   e. **A wooden board** (4 in × 15 in × ¼ in)
2. **Application** procedures are modified from those described by Young and Thomassen[7] and Botte et al.[5]
   a. **Shave and trim hair** around the pin sites (optional). The pin sites should be 1 cm above the lateral third of the eyebrow and the same distance above the tops of the ears in the parietal and occipital areas. Place the halo just inferior to the greatest circumference of the head (Fig. 10-4).
   b. Position the patient supine on a bed with the head extended beyond the edge. **Have the head supported** by an assistant's hands or by a 4-in-wide board placed under the head and neck.
   c. Place a **sterile towel** under the patient's head. This step is not necessary if an attendant is holding the head.
   d. Select a halo ring that allows for **1.5 cm clearance circumferentially**. If MRI studies are anticipated, an MRI-compatible ring and pins must be used (carbon fiber material).
   e. The halo ring, skull pins, and positioning pins should be autoclaved or gas sterilized.
   f. The assistant, wearing gloves, **positions** the halo ring around the head with the raised portion of the ring over the posterior part of the skull.

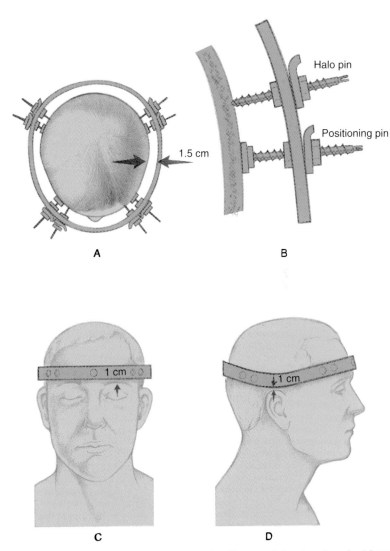

**Figure 10-4.** Principles of a halo ring application. The correct ring size allows for 1.5 cm of clearance **(A)**. Positioning pins are used to stabilize the ring while the skull pins are inserted **(B)**. The proper position of the ring is 1 cm above eyebrows and ear pinnae **(C, D)**.

Use positioning pins and plates to place the ring in the proper attitude and to equalize the clearance around the head.
g. Infiltrate the skin with local **anesthetic** at the four pin sites.
h. The **skull pins** should be at a 90° angle to the skull and turned to finger tightness. The skull pins are designed so that no scalp incisions or drill holes are needed. The shape of the point draws the skin under

it and does not cause bleeding. Try to avoid puckering of the skin at the pin site. If puckering does occur, remove the pins, flatten the skin, and repenetrate.

   i. Both operators use the **torque screwdrivers** simultaneously, turning opposing skull pins. Gain increments of 2 in/lb evenly up to the maximum desired by the physician. A suggested maximum is 4½ in/lb for children and 6 to 8 in/lb for adults.

   j. **Remove the positioning pins**.

   k. Incorporate the **support rods** of the halo apparatus into the plaster body jacket, as shown in Fig. 8-5, or use a sheepskin-lined molded plastic body jacket that is commercially available or custom made by an orthotist (Fig. 8-6).

   l. **Tangential roentgenographic views** or a computed tomography (CT) scan of the skull can be ordered to check the depth of the skull pins, but neither is routinely necessary.

  3. **Care of pin sites**

   a. **Clean** around the pins with peroxide solution using a cotton swab twice daily. Antibiotic or Betadine ointments are not recommended.

   b. **Check the torque** of the pins for the first few days. **Note:** If the patient complains of repeated looseness or if the proper torque cannot be gained, move the pin to another place on the ring by the aforementioned method. Do not remove a loose pin until the fifth replacement pin is inserted.

## VI. Upper Extremity Traction

  **A.** **Dunlop or modified Dunlop skin traction.** This type of traction is occasionally useful for the management of supracondylar humeral fractures.[8] Place the patient supine and suspend the arm in skin traction with the shoulder abducted and slightly flexed. In addition, slightly flex the elbow. Modification of this type of traction provides counteraction on the humerus, and this can be achieved with the arm over the edge of the bed and counterweight suspended from a felt cuff over the humerus, or with a felt cuff over the forearm pulling laterally with the elbow flexed (Fig. 10-5). Two disadvantages of Dunlop traction are that it cannot be applied over skin injuries and that elevation of the humeral fracture above the level of the heart is not possible with this method.

  **B.** **Overbody or lateral skeletal traction**

   1. In the management of extraarticular humeral shaft and metaphyseal fractures, it is occasionally desirable to maintain the shoulder in flexion without abduction but with the elbow at a right angle by placing the arm over the body. Maintain this position through olecranon skeletal traction, which allows some flexion and extension of the elbow if the traction pin is properly inserted. Because the hand and wrist usually tire in this position, support the wrist with a plaster splint. Skeletal traction through the olecranon may also be used in the lateral position (Fig. 10-6).

   2. A special, rarely used adaptation of upper extremity olecranon traction may be made by **placing the patient in a shoulder spica cast** that incorporates an olecranon pin into the plaster to apply fixed skeletal traction. This adaptation allows the patient to be ambulatory.

## VII. Lower Extremity Traction

  **A.** **Apply Buck extension skin traction** (Fig. 10-7) to the lower extremity to reduce muscle spasms about the knee or hip. However, do not use this form of traction for back conditions. Control rotation to some extent by placing the leg on a pillow with sandbags on the lateral side of the ankle. Although Buck traction is commonly recommended for hip fractures, its use should be limited in duration. For intracapsular fractures, keep the hip flexed to increase

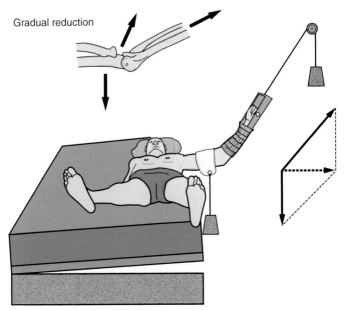

Gradual reduction

**Figure 10-5.** Modified Dunlop traction. A weight of 1 to 5 lb is usually required. Associated circulatory embarrassment might be aggravated by increasing elbow flexion.

hip capsule volume and thereby limit pain. The effectiveness of this type of traction in decreasing pain has not been demonstrated.[9,10]

B. **Hamilton-Russell traction** (Fig. 10-8) may be used for hip or femoral fractures, especially in children weighing 40 to 60 lb. Accomplish the traction with either skin traction or distal tibial skeletal traction plus a sling placed beneath the posterior distal thigh (avoid pressure in the popliteal fossa). A rope is attached to the sling and goes first to an overhead pulley, then to a pulley at the foot of the bed, next to a pulley on the foot plate attached to the spreader bar, then to a fourth pulley at the end of the bed, and finally to the attached weight. Analysis of the vector forces shows that the traction applied to the leg is increased considerably by moving the overhead pulley toward the foot of the bed. If this type of traction is used on a child, one usually attaches 3 lb to the traction apparatus. Produce a countertraction with the patient's body weight by elevating the foot of the bed.

C. **Split Russell traction** has the same indications and vector forces as Hamilton-Russell traction. The difference is that split Russell traction uses two separate ropes and weights, as shown in Fig. 10-9.

D. **Charnley traction unit** (boot) is useful for applying skeletal traction to a lower limb and is recommended for routine use (Fig. 10-10). This limits rotational forces on the limb controlling alignment, maintains the ankle in neutral position, and limits the stress on the traction bow. The unit is assembled by inserting a wire or pin through the proximal end of the tibia and then incorporating the wire or pin in a shortleg cast. The advantages are as follows:

1. The foot and ankle are maintained in a neutral **functional position**.
2. The limb is suspended in a cast, and there is no pressure on the calf muscles or peroneal nerve.
3. **Movement** of the skeletal pin or wire is **reduced** to a minimum.

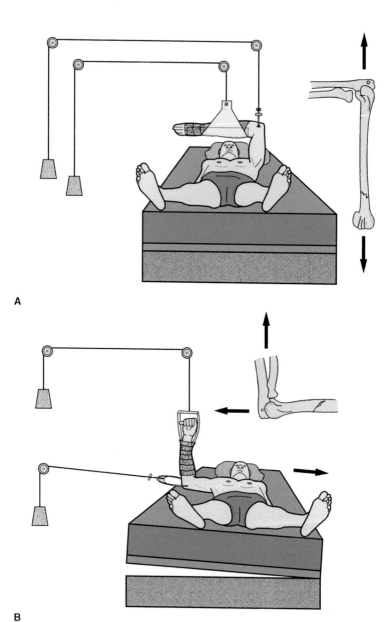

**Figure 10-6.** Olecranon pin traction. **A:** Overbody traction. Note that the elbow joint can move without disturbing the fracture. The hand and wrist rest in a plaster splint. **B:** Lateral traction.

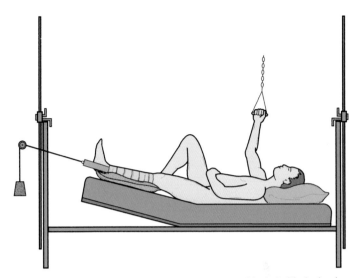

**Figure 10-7.** Buck extension skin traction. Note the elevation of the foot of the bed and support under the calf. Protect the fibular head and malleoli. A weight of 5 to 7 lb of traction is sufficient.

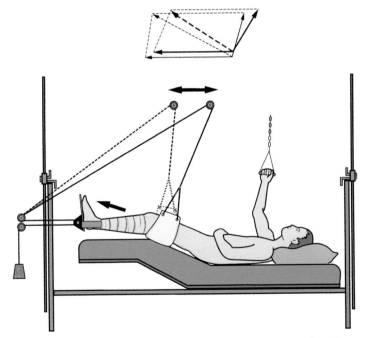

**Figure 10-8.** Hamilton-Russell traction. Note that the resultant force on the femur is a summation of vector analysis and depends on the position of the overhead pulley. Change the angulation of the distal fragment by moving the single overhead pulley.

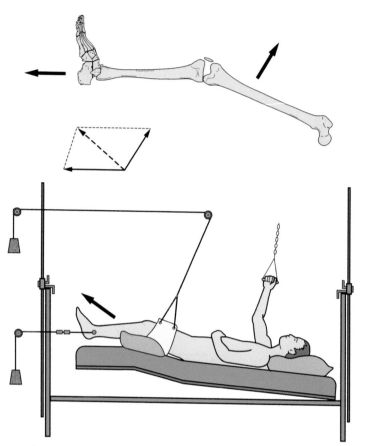

**Figure 10-9.** Split Russell traction is the same as Hamilton-Russell traction except that two separate ropes and weights are used instead of one.

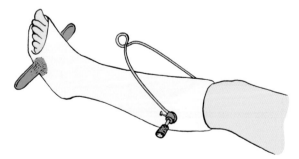

**Figure 10-10.** Charnley traction unit consisting of a skeletal wire or pin incorporated into a shortleg cast, which has a crossbar fixed to the sole. The unit is commonly employed for femoral fractures treated with skeletal traction.

**E. Balanced suspension skeletal traction** provides a direct pull on either the tibia or the femur through a wire pin. Rest the lower extremity on a stockinet or a cloth towel stretched over a Thomas splint. The splint, with or without a Pearson attachment, is balanced with counterweights to suspend the leg in a freely floating system. Attach separate suspension ropes to both sides of the proximal full-ring Thomas splint, run the ropes through overhead pulleys, and fasten weights to ropes at either end of the bed but not over the patient. Control rotation of the ring by individually adjusting the amount of attached weight. Suspend the distal end of the splint from a single rope to an overhead pulley, with the weight attached to the rope at one end of the bed. For safety reasons, place no weights over the patient. Control rotation of the extremity by a light counterweight attached to the side of the splint or by a crossbar attached to the plaster cast. The Charnley traction unit (boot) is ideally suited for both balanced suspension and fixed skeletal traction (which is discussed next) (Fig. 10-11). A **Pearson attachment** allows for flexion motion of the knee joint, which is an advantage, especially for those in traction for a long period or for those who have a comminuted tibial plateau fracture.

**F.** Use fixed skeletal traction in the initial treatment of femoral fractures in patients who will go on to intramedullary nailing or who need to be transported either in the hospital or to another facility. This limits shortening of the fracture which will facilitate later closed reduction and intramedullary fixation.

1. In the rare situation in which the fracture must be reduced before traction is applied, the apprehensive patient or the patient with a transverse fracture usually requires general or regional anesthesia.

2. Apply the Charnley traction unit to the lower leg if duration of traction is planned beyond a week or so.

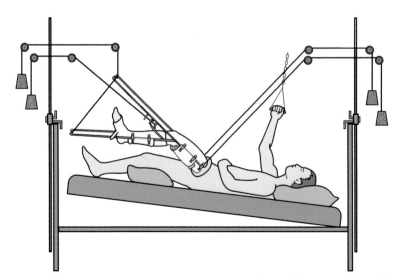

**Figure 10-11.** With balanced suspension traction, the various weights are adjusted until satisfactory alignment and suspension of the femoral fracture are achieved within the Thomas splint. Note the Charnley traction unit, firm mattress, bed board, and master pad. Wrap an elastic bandage about the thigh and splint to minimize the acute swelling.

3. Select a full- or half-ring Thomas splint that is 2 in greater than the proximal thigh.[2] This leeway is critical because a ring that is too tight causes distal edema and one that is too loose is ineffective. The ring must fit against the fibrofatty tissue in the perineum and the medial arch of the buttocks. The half ring is placed against the ischium and the strap tightened snugly against the anterior thigh.

4. While the leg is supported in traction, place the ring on the limb. Attach a single **master sling** of nonextensible cloth (a double-thickness cloth towel is ideal) measuring 6 to 9 in long to the splint beneath the fracture. Adjust tension to support the limb. If the sling is too tight, it causes excessive flexing of the proximal fragment; if it is too loose, it does not control the fracture. Attach this sling to the splint with several clamps.

5. Make a supporting or master pad that is 1 to 1½ in thick and 6 to 9 in long from an abdominal dressing or a folded towel. Insert a safety pin into the pad to assist localization of the pad on roentgenograms. Place this pad beneath the fracture and adjust it to maintain the normal anterior bow of the femur. A single sling is placed on the Thomas splint distally to support the shortleg cast.

6. **Check the reduction with follow-up radiographs.** End-on reduction for transverse fractures is ideal in adults; take care to avoid excessive distraction of the fracture if traction is the planned definitive treatment. If the patient will have delayed intramedullary nailing, maintain some (5 to 10 mm) distraction, which will aid in intraoperative reduction. In children, bayonet apposition is preferred. With the oblique fracture, it is important to feel bone-on-bone contact to be certain there is no soft-tissue interposition. If there is interposition, it can usually be dislodged by manipulation. Then assess length, alignment, and rotational positions and attach traction to the end of the splint. Extend two ropes from the Steinmann pin around the sides of the splint and attach them to the splint end. Tape two tongue blades together to form a Spanish windlass to adjust tension. After the first day or 2, when muscle spasm subsides, only slight traction is necessary to maintain the appropriate alignment. It might not be possible to gain full length initially because of tense swelling of the thigh. Attach a second pad or C-clamp to add cross-traction if needed for better alignment, particularly in the more transverse fracture patterns.

7. **Suspend the splint** to allow patient mobility in bed and to reduce edema. Fig. 10-12 depicts the completed setup.

8. **Follow-up care**, particularly in the first few weeks, is important. Wash the skin beneath the ring daily with alcohol, dry thoroughly, and powder with talc every 2 hours. The conscious patient may perform this care each hour and massage the skin to improve blood supply. If it is necessary to relieve skin pressure under the ring, apply traction directly from the end of the splint; slight distraction is preferred when intramedullary nailing is to be delayed for more than 24 hours. Be careful, however, not to cause distraction at the fracture site when using fixed skeletal traction as the definitive treatment because it will produce a nonunion. Start quadriceps exercises within the first few days and continue on an around-the-clock basis. All the elements outlined earlier are essential for effective utilization of fixed skeletal traction.

## VIII. Complications of Skeletal Traction

A. An **infection** of the pin tract is a common complication, but its incidence is reduced when the previously stated guidelines for pin and wire insertion are carefully followed. If an infection with a small sequestrum occurs, it is wise

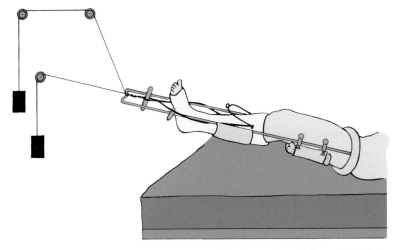

**Figure 10-12.** Fixed skeletal traction. Note the Charnley traction unit, the method of adjusting traction force through the windlass, the position of the master pad, and the traction on the end of the Thomas splint to relieve skin pressure on the proximal thigh. Place an elastic bandage around the thigh and splint to help control edema.

to remove the pin, curette the pin tract, and replace the pin in the operating room under adequate anesthesia. The infection usually subsides satisfactorily with antibiotic therapy.

**B. Distraction** of bone fragments at the fracture site is avoided by frequently measuring extremity length, using roentgenograms to check the position of fragments, and by keeping traction weights to a minimum. Distraction is best assessed by lateral roentgenograms because anteroposterior roentgenograms may not be perpendicular to the fracture and may underestimate the distraction. Distraction can predispose to a delayed union or nonunion of the fracture.

**C.** Use heavy traction with care and close observation to avoid **nerve palsy**. If paralysis does occur, adjust and possibly abandon the traction.

**D. Pin breakage** is unusual, but can occur if very heavy traction is used for long periods, especially in a restless patient. To protect the pin, incorporate it into plaster in the manner of the Charnley traction unit. Decrease the potential of metal corrosion and fracture using a wire or pin that is not scored.

## REFERENCES

1. Scannell BP, Waldrop NE, Sasser HC, Sing RF, Bosse MJ. Skeletal traction versus external fixation in the initial temporization of femoral shaft fractures in severely injured patients. *J Trauma.* 2010;68:633-640.
2. Obey MR, Berkes MB, McAndrew CM, Miller AN. Lower extremity skeletal traction following orthopaedic trauma: indications, techniques, evidence. *JBJS Rev.* 2019;7:1-10.
3. Wang JH, Daniels AH, Palumbo MA, Eberson CP. Cervical traction for treatment of spinal injury and deformity. *JBJS Rev.* 2014;2:1-10.
4. Gardner WJ. The principle of spring-loaded points for cervical traction. *J Neurosurg.* 1973;39:543-544.
5. Botte MJ, Byrne TP, Garfin SR. Application of the halo device for immobilization of the cervical spine utilizing an increased torque pressure. *J Bone Joint Surg Am.* 1987;69A:750-752.

6. Garfin SR, Botte MJ, Centeno RS, Nickel VL. Osteology of the skull as it effects halo pin placement. *Spine*. 1985;10:696-698.
7. Young R, Thomassen EH. Step-by-step procedure for applying a halo ring. *Orthop Rev*. 1974;3:62.
8. Finsen V, Borset M, Buvik GE, Hauke I. Preoperative traction in patients with hip fractures. *Injury*. 1992;23:242-244.
9. Jerre R, Doshé A, Karlsson F, et al. Preoperative skin traction was not useful for hip fractures. *J Bone Joint Surg Am*. 2001;83:303.
10. Henry BJ, Vrahas MS. The Thomas splint: questionable boast of an indispensable tool. *Am J Orthop*. 1996;25:602-604.

## SELECTED HISTORICAL READINGS

Charnley J. *The Closed Treatment of Common Fractures*. 3rd ed. Williams & Wilkins; 1972.
Nickel VL, Perry J, Garret A, et al. The halo. *J Bone Joint Surg Am*. 1968;50A:1400.

# 11 Operating Room Equipment and Techniques

Marc F. Swiontkowski

## I. Preparation for Surgery
### A. Scheduling surgery
1. **Prepare the patient** so that the risks, goals, and benefits of the selected procedure are understood. The patient or legal next of kin should know the nature of the patient's condition, the nature of the proposed treatment, the alternative treatments, the anesthetic risks, the anticipated probability for success, and the possible risks. Explain the postoperative dressings, casts or splints, exercise program, and other special requirements. When the patient has been so informed and has all questions answered, obtain a signed operative permit and mark the surgical sites with your initials.
2. **Review the technique** of the proposed operation. At the time surgery is scheduled, be confident that the patient's condition meets the appropriate indications for the proposed surgery. Know the anatomy and the surgical approaches involved in the selected surgical procedure. Carefully plan the procedure with the proper alternatives to reduce the length of time the wound is open. Be sure that all special equipment, implants, assistance, and time are available as expected. Complete any necessary digital templating of roentgenograms and preoperative planning drawings.[1]
### B. Before surgery
1. **Patient preparation.** Check to make sure the physical examination, chest roentgenogram, electrocardiogram, hemoglobin/hematocrit, and other indicated preoperative studies do not contraindicate surgery. Obtain a preoperative consultation from a specialist in internal medicine for all patients with unstable medical conditions. Many centers require preoperative primary care clearance for all patients. Order blood or type and screen, tetanus prophylaxis, and special medications as indicated. If an extremity operation is planned, be sure that the nails are properly trimmed and cleaned. Have the patient, family, and support system begin planning early for postdischarge or postoperation disposition needs, such as transportation home, wheelchairs, hospital beds, wheelchair access to the home, and commodes.
2. **Antibiotics**[2]
   a. **Preoperative antibiotics** should be administered for surgeries that are associated with a high risk of postoperative deep wound infection, for example, when any implant is inserted, when the operation results in a hematoma or dead space, when the anticipated operating time is greater than 2 hours, or when the surgeon is operating on bones, joints, nerves, or tendons.[3,4] Various studies have shown immediate preoperative and postoperative antibiotics to be beneficial with surgery involving musculoskeletal tissues.[2,4-6,19] See **Chapter 4** for utilization of antibiotics with open wounds. The duration of antibiotic therapy can be limited to 24 hours postoperatively without increasing the risk of infection.
   b. The **timing** of the antibiotic therapy is as important as **dosage**. Ideally, the antibiotic level should be highest when the tourniquet is inflated or the surgical hematoma (potential culture medium) is formed. Thus, the

antibiotics **must be given before surgery within 30 minutes of the incision**. Because the highest blood levels with intravenous (IV) administration are achieved immediately, the ideal time to give IV antibiotics is when the patient is in the preoperative area or operating room during the 10- to 15-minute period just before the tourniquet is inflated or before the surgical incision is made. The antibiotics are readministered at the recommended intervals throughout the operative procedure (generally every 3 to 4 hours). The surgeon must also be aware of the effect of blood loss on the antibiotic levels. If the blood loss equals one-half of the patient's volume, approximately one-half of the effective amount of the antibiotics has also been lost. The interval between the recommended doses for that patient, therefore, must be cut into half.

c. The authors recommend using one of the **first-generation cephalosporins**, which are bactericidal for staphylococcal and streptococcal bacterial specimens are usually found in wound infections following musculoskeletal surgery. The recommended antibiotics are listed in Table 11-1.

3. Patients who have been on long-term steroid therapy may need adjustments made in their **steroid dosage** when they undergo surgery or other major stress. The following is the simplest published regimen that the authors have found.[7] The hospital service should be consulted to confirm the dosage plan:

a. On the **day of surgery**, order hydrocortisone sodium succinate (Solu-Cortef), 100 mg IV, to be given with the premedication before surgery.

b. Use the **same dose** on the **first postoperative day**.

c. Use 50 mg of **hydrocortisone** on the **second postoperative day**.

d. Use 25 mg of **hydrocortisone** on the **third postoperative day** and then continue only with the patient's normal oral daily dose.

| TABLE 11-1 | Recommended Prophylactic Antibiotics for Orthopaedic Surgical Procedures (Open Trauma, Joint Replacement, Bone, Joint, Tendon, Ligament, and Nerve Surgery)[a] | | |
|---|---|---|---|
| **Bactericidal Antibiotics** | **Dosage for Adults** | **Notable Contraindications** | **Possible Complications** |
| Cefazolin[b] (Kefzol or Ancef) | 1–2 g q6–8h | History of an anaphylactic reaction to a penicillin drug requires careful usage; with renal insufficiency, the dose must be adjusted to the creatinine clearance | Cephalosporins occasionally cause a false-positive urine reaction with the Clinitest tablets (use test tape instead) and rarely cause blood dyscrasias, overt hemolytic anemia, or renal dysfunction; cephalothin frequently causes a positive Coombs test |
| Vancomycin[c] | 1 g initially, then 500 mg, q6h | With impaired renal function, dose must be adjusted to patient's creatinine clearance | Rapid IV administration can cause hypotension, which could be especially dangerous during induction of anesthesia, so administer at rate of no more than 10 mg/min |

[a]Antibiotics should be given immediately postoperatively and then one dose (IV) or up to 24 to 48 hours after surgery.
[b]Cefazolin can also be given intramuscularly (IM).
[c]For hospitals in which *Staphylococcus aureus* and *Staphylococcus epidermis* frequently cause wound infection or for patients allergic to cephalosporins.

4. **Surgery in patients with insulin-dependent diabetes mellitus.** It is imperative that patients develop a preoperative plan to adjust medications prior to surgery. Insulin doses may be reduced the night before and the morning of surgery at the discretion of the patients' diabetes management team. The duration of time diabetic patients are made NPO should be minimized to reduce unexpected fluctuation in blood sugar levels. Trauma associated with surgery can increase stress hormones in the body, such as cortisol and catecholamine levels, which can result in a hyperglycemic state. Patients who develop hyperglycemia while as inpatients have a higher chance of wound healing issues, infection, and prolonged recovery time. A common postoperative protocol is to use an insulin sliding scale on both type 1 and 2 diabetics until a normal diet is resumed. Oral glycemic control agents such as Metformin are usually restarted when the patient resumes a normal diet.[26]

   a. **In the morning before surgery**, the patient should omit breakfast and take about one-half of the normal insulin dose subcutaneously (SQ). Again, the hospital service should be consulted before final orders are placed.

   b. **After surgery**, use a **glucose measuring instrument every 4 to 6 hours** to monitor blood glucose levels. The following **sliding scale** is useful: If the glucose level is greater than 350 mg per dL, give 15 units regular insulin SQ. If the level exceeds 250 mg per dL, give 10 units regular insulin SQ.

   c. Return patients to their usual insulin dosage regimen as soon as they return to their normal activity level and to their usual American Diabetic Association diet.

5. **Surgery in patients with hemophilia.** Medical management of a patient with hemophilia who needs surgery requires precise assays of **factor levels** and **prior survival studies** of replacement factors to learn the effect of inhibitors and the biologic half-life in a particular patient. Aim to achieve 100% plasma levels just before anesthetics for surgery are administered. Maintain the level at 60% of normal for the first 4 days and more than 40% for the next 4 days. A level of 100% is also necessary for manipulation of a joint under anesthesia and for removal of pins. A 40% level is needed for suture removal. Levels of 20% are maintained for postoperative physical therapy for as long as 4 to 6 weeks after major joint surgery. Forty units of factor per kilogram of body weight administered just before anesthesia (unless survival studies done before surgery show that higher doses are needed) usually achieves close to 100% plasma factor levels. The hematology service should be contacted for assistance before placing the final orders.

## C. Day of surgery

1. Be sure the **anesthesia** technique proposed is adequate in terms of duration, muscle relaxation, and ability to position the patient properly.[8,9] Use of surgical checklists is strongly advised.[10] Supervise **positioning, preparing, and draping** so that the planned procedure could be accomplished without difficulty.[10] As the assistant prepares the patient, the surgeon can go to the instrument table with the scrub nurse and review major instruments required and implant from start to finish, outlining the planned procedure. The surgeon can also indicate what may be needed if any complications arise. The idea is to ensure that all equipment is immediately available, to review the procedure in the surgeon's mind, and to prepare the entire surgical team so that the team and surgeon can work together efficiently. See **Appendix E** for the position and draping of the patient. See **I.C.4.c** for a discussion of skin preparations.

2. **Pneumatic tourniquets**[11-13,23]

a. When a tourniquet is to be used, the necessary **apparatus** includes a cuff with a smooth, wrinkle-free surface that is a proper size. Select a tourniquet so that the width of the cuff covers approximately one-third of the patient's arm length. Check the tubing for leaks. The tourniquet machine should have a safety valve release/alarm because excessively high pressures can cause paralysis. The inflating device must allow rapid attainment of desired pressure.

b. Plan surgery to **minimize** the **operative time** and, as a consequence, the **tourniquet time**.[14] The conventional safe maximum inflation time of the tourniquet is 2 hours. The cuff may be applied about the arm or thigh but generally not about the forearm. There is no evidence that padding between the cuff and the skin is of any value, and such padding can cause skin wrinkles. Apply a plastic sheet with the adhesive edge placed on the skin distal to the tourniquet and cover the tourniquet with the plastic sheet as shown in Fig. 11-1, thereby preventing skin preparation solutions from getting underneath the cuff. Exsanguinate the limb with an Esmarch rubber bandage or with elevation of the limb above the patient's heart for 60 seconds before inflating the tourniquet. An Esmarch bandage should not be used in cases of tumors or infection. Flexing the knee or elbow before inflating the tourniquet makes positioning and closure easier and prevents the possible complication of a ruptured muscle, which can rarely occur by forced flexion of a tourniquet-fixed muscle. Rapidly inflate to the desired pressure. This is 175 to 250 mm Hg in the upper extremity, depending on the arm circumference and the patient's systolic blood pressure, and 250 to 350 mm Hg in the lower extremity, depending on thigh circumference.[11,15] Tissue pressure is always somewhat lower than tourniquet pressure, but at 30-cm circumference, it is close to 100%, declining to

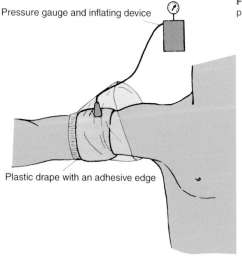

Pressure gauge and inflating device

Plastic drape with an adhesive edge

**Figure 11-1.** Application of a pneumatic tourniquet.

70% at 60 cm circumference.[11,15-17] The pressures should be decreased for infants and small children. Immediately after deflation, remove or loosen the cuff to prevent a venous congestion from proximal constriction of the extremity. If the tourniquet is deflated and reinflated during surgery, the time for reversal of the tourniquet-produced ischemia is proportional to the tourniquet time; that is, approximately 20 minutes is required for reversal after 2 hours of tourniquet time. In addition, tourniquet effects occur more rapidly after repeated use, and there is probably some summation of these effects. Double tourniquets are used for IV-required anesthesia (Bier blocks).[18] Individual variations such as age, vascular supply of the limb, condition of the tissues, and vascular diseases all influence the patient's tolerance to tourniquet usage. In general, avoid using tourniquets in trauma cases except where dissection around major nerves is required.

c. **Complications** of tourniquets include blisters and chemical burns (from "prep" solutions that leak under the tourniquet) of the skin, swelling, stiffness, and paralysis. Electromyographic changes have been demonstrated following the use of a tourniquet even within the approved time ranges.

3. The following is a **summary of Occupational Safety and Health Administration (OSHA) regulation No. 1920, "Bloodborne Pathogens,"** emphasizing staff and surgeon responsibilities.

a. **Wash hands immediately after removing gloves.**

b. **Wash** (with soap and water) **any exposed skin** (or flush mucous membranes) **immediately** (or as soon as feasible) **after contact with blood or potentially infectious materials.**

c. **Do not bend, cut, recap, or remove needles or other sharps.** If recapping is the only feasible method, it must be done using a mechanical device or the one-handed method.

d. **Do not eat, drink, smoke, apply cosmetics or lip balm, or handle contact lenses** in work areas where there is a reasonable likelihood of occupational exposure.

e. **Perform all procedures involving blood or potentially infectious material as to minimize spraying and splattering.**

f. If **outside contamination of transport containers** is possible (or there is a potential for puncture), place potentially infectious material in a second container to **prevent leakage during handling.**

g. **Use personal protective equipment** such as gloves, face shields, masks, gowns, shoe covers, and so on in situations in which there is risk of exposure to blood or potentially infectious material.

h. **Following an exposure, complete an incident report identifying the route of exposure and source individual.** A tube of the patient's blood should be drawn, labeled "spin," and held until the patient's consent can be obtained. The employee health nurse is to be contacted for testing as indicated.

i. **Hepatitis B virus immunization is recommended for all employees** and is usually available by contacting the employee health nurse. The authors believe that every surgeon is responsible for knowing his or her own human immunodeficiency virus, hepatitis B, and hepatitis C serologic status.

4. **Prevention of surgical wound infections**[19]

a. Operating room rituals are designed to **decrease infection**. Despite the best designs, wound contamination and subsequent wound infection continue. It is generally conceded that most wounds become contaminated; however, usually only those with devitalized tissue, large dead space with accumulating hematoma, or foreign bodies become frankly infected. A study of the possible sources of coagulase-positive staphylococci that contaminated surgical wounds during 50 operations revealed that bacteria of bacteriophage types that were present only in the air were found in 68% of the wounds; 50% of wounds contained bacteria of bacteriophage types that were found in the patient's nose, throat, or skin; 14% had bacteriophage types found in the noses and throats of members of the scrubbed surgical team; and 6% of the wounds had bacteriophage types found on the hands of the scrubbed surgical team. Maximum contamination occurs early in the operative procedure when there is a considerable amount of air circulation caused by individuals moving about the room.[3] After the air quiets, the rate of contamination is less, but an increased exposure time allows increased contamination. It is important to keep traffic in the operating room to an absolute minimum, to walk slowly, and to avoid fanning the air with quick opening of the doors, drapes, and towels.

b. Studies show considerable variation in the **filtration efficiency of different masks**. Cloth masks are only about 50% efficient in filtering bacterial organisms and are rarely used. Numerous disposable masks have a bacterial filtration efficiency greater than 94% according to the manufacturers. Fiberglass-free masks are probably safer. Prolonged use (averaging 4½ hours of operation time) and the use of moist masks do not impair the ability to filter, except in the case of cloth masks. As the surgical masks work on a filtration principle, double masking can actually increase air contamination with bacteria because double masking makes transportation of air through the mask pores more difficult and forces more unfiltered air to escape along the sides of the mask.[18]

c. Although airborne contamination is by far the most important source of contamination, **skin contamination** does occur. Even with the use of 1% or 2% tincture of iodine, the deeper areas of the epidermis are not bacteria free. With a 1% concentration, no cases of skin irritation have occurred. If a higher concentration is used, however, the excess iodine should be removed with alcohol after 30 seconds. One 5-minute scrub with povidone-iodine is as effective as a 10-minute scrub in reducing bacterial counts on the skin and keeping them down for as long as 8 hours. A 7.5% povidone-iodine (Betadine) skin disinfectant yields 0.75% available iodine. More recent work shows that **chlorhexidine gluconate** (Hibiclens) may be the scrub detergent of choice for both the surgeon and the patient.[20-22] A comparative study among hexachlorophene (pHisoHex), povidone-iodine, and chlorhexidine showed the latter to be probably the most effective. There was a 99.9% reduction in resident bacterial flora after a single 6-minute chlorhexidine scrub. The reduction of flora on surgically gloved hands was maintained over the 6-hour test period. In addition, the pharmacology of chlorhexidine is reportedly more effective against gram-positive and gram-negative organisms, including *Pseudomonas aeruginosa*.

   *Recent research has shown that currently used skin prep solutions may not eliminate P. acnes contamination around the shoulder, especially in males.*[31]

d. **Extremity draping.** Adhesive plastic drapes do not totally eliminate the patient's skin as a possible source of infection. Drape the extremities as described in **Appendix E**.

e. **Intraoperative procedures** to prevent postoperative wound infection include the elimination of any large collection of blood. A hematoma is an excellent potential culture medium. Wound suction is used whenever one anticipates continued bleeding into the wound; however, their use in fracture, joint replacement, and spine surgery has not been proven to decrease the incidence of wound infection. Surgical wounds are carefully irrigated to remove any potential contaminated residue before closing. In vitro experiments using bacitracin 50,000 units plus polymyxin B sulfate (Aerosporin) 50 mg in a liter of saline or lactated Ringer's solution have shown that 100% of *Staphylococcus aureus*, *Escherichia coli*, the *Klebsiella* organisms, and *P. aeruginosa* bacteria were killed by a 1-minute exposure to the antibiotic solution.[23] *Staphylococcus epidermidis* organisms were also killed. Only the *Proteus* organisms showed significant resistance to this antibiotic irrigation (only 3% to 22% were killed). *Proteus* organisms are uncommon as a cause of immediate postoperative infections in musculoskeletal surgery, however, when the wounds are not previously contaminated or infected. Data indicate that irrigation of surgical wounds with a solution containing bacitracin and polymyxin B sulfate or bacitracin and neomycin could potentially lower the incidence of postoperative infections.[24] A large number of patients are sensitive to neomycin, so its use is generally discouraged. Polymyxin B is sometimes difficult to obtain from the manufacturer. In this situation, some surgeons use a dilute Betadine solution as a topical antibiotic irrigant; however, this solution is toxic to tissue. Data confirming that antibiotic irrigants are superior to sterile saline in preventing surgical wound infection are generally lacking in orthopaedic surgery. Splash basins are a source of bacterial contamination and should not be used.

f. **The incidence of infection increases in wounds open for longer than 2 hours.** Whether this is a result of the increased exposure to the air, failure of masks, skin contaminants, or more trauma in the wound is not certain. Even with lengthy surgical cases, with good surgical technique, the rate of deep wound infection on "clean" orthopaedic cases should not exceed 1%.

g. **Laminar air flow systems** appear to be an effective means of reducing postoperative infection rates as long as the flow of air is kept laminar or streamlined across the operative area (e.g., during hip surgeries). These systems are not effective if the air becomes turbulent across the operative area because, for example, of the position of people in the operating room (e.g., during knee replacement surgery).[25]

h. **Hooded surgical exhaust systems** are effective but can be cumbersome.[18]

i. **Whenever a subsequent surgical wound infection** occurs in a clean, uneventful surgical case (particularly two to three cases within a month or two), consider a **nasal culture** from all those present at the time of the procedures.

5. **Malignant hyperthermia**

a. **Pathophysiology.** The target organ in malignant hyperthermia is skeletal muscle. Certain triggering events, such as the administration of volatile anesthetics or succinylcholine, precipitate release of calcium from the calcium-storing membrane (sarcoplasmic reticulum) of the muscle cell. The abnormal transport of calcium results in recurrent sarcomeric contractions and consequent muscle rigidity. The metabolic rate is accelerated, causing heat and increased carbon dioxide production with accelerated oxygen consumption. Core body temperature increases.

b. **History.** This potentially fatal syndrome is an autosomal dominant metabolic disease. In 40% of reported cases, an orthopaedist is the first to encounter this disorder. The incidence in the United States is approximately 1:1,000. The syndrome is associated more frequently with patients having congenital and musculoskeletal abnormalities: kyphosis, scoliosis, hernia, recurrent joint dislocations, club foot, ptosis, or strabismus. Malignant hyperthermia can occur at any age but is most likely to occur in a young individual. After exposure to an anesthetic (or other stress), body temperature may rapidly increase.

c. **Examination.** A rapid elevation in body temperature is noted early; however, it may become present late or not at all. Cardiac arrhythmias are usually concurrent, can progress to ventricular tachycardia, and may end in ventricular fibrillation with subsequent death. The soda lime canister may turn blue and become palpably hot. Tetanic muscle contractions occur in approximately 60% of cases. Like so many conditions in orthopaedics, early recognition is crucial. Temperature and electrocardiographic monitoring during surgery is mandatory. A rapid temperature elevation (even from an initial subnormal temperature), tachycardia, hypertonia of skeletal muscle, unexplained hyperventilation, overheated soda lime canister, dark blood, sweating, and blotchy cyanosis are all indicative of possible malignant hyperthermia.

d. **Treatment**

i. **Prevention**

(a) Obtain a **careful past history and family history**, inquiring especially about fatal or near-fatal experiences following emotional, physical, traumatic, or surgical stress or about a relative who died of an obscure cause in the perioperative period.

(b) Dantrolene (approximately 12 mg per kg body weight) used IV is one of the mainstays of treatment and probably works by reducing calcium outflow from the sarcoplasmic reticulum into the myoplasm.

(c) **Avoid** the use of **volatile anesthetics (Fluothane)** and **succinylcholine (Anectine)** in high-risk patients.

ii. **Management** of an evolving malignant hyperthermia syndrome

(a) Immediately **discontinue all anesthetic agents and muscle relaxants** and terminate the surgical procedure as quickly as possible.

(b) **Hyperventilate with oxygen.**

(c) **Use IV sodium bicarbonate**, 4 mL per kg body weight, and repeat as necessary until blood gases approach normal.

(d) Administer **mannitol**, 1 g per kg body weight, and furosemide (Lasix), 1 mg per kg body weight, which help maintain urine output to clear myoglobin and excessive sodium.

(e) Treat hyperkalemia with approximately 50 mg of **IV** glucose with 50 units of **insulin**.

(f) Control arrhythmias.

(g) **Cool the patient** with immersion in ice water and expose to an electric fan to facilitate evaporation. Refrigerated saline or Ringer's lactate administered IV is helpful. Maintain cooling procedures until the body temperature is less than 38°C.

(h) **Physiologic monitoring** by electrocardiography and measurement of the central venous pressure, blood gases every 10 minutes, volume and quality of renal output, serum electrolytes, glucose, serum glutamic oxaloacetic transaminase, creatine phosphokinase, and blood urea nitrogen is important.

(i) Good **prognostic signs** are lightening of the coma (often heralded by restlessness), return of reflexes, return to normal temperature, reduced heart rate, improved renal output, and return of consciousness.

e. **Complications**
  i. **Weakness and easy fatigability** persist for several months.
  ii. **Death** owing to ventricular fibrillation can occur within 1 or 2 hours from the onset of the condition. If death occurs later, it is usually a result of pulmonary edema, coagulopathy, or massive electrolyte and acid–base imbalance. If the patient dies after several days in a coma, the cause is usually renal failure or brain damage.

## II. Orthopaedic Operating Room Instruments and Their Usage

A. **Introduction.** Much of the remaining discussion is modified from a psychomotor skills course originally organized for the University of Washington Department of Orthopaedic Surgery residents by F. G. Lippert III, MD, in the 1980s.

B. **Techniques for checking the function of grasping-type surgical instruments.**[26] The breakdown of high-quality instruments is often the direct result of their misuse. Forceps, hemostats, needle holders, and clamps are frequently misused in orthopaedic surgery. They can be misapplied to various pins, nails, screws, and plates when pliers are not readily available. They are also misused to clamp large sponges, tubing, and needles.

  1. It is annoying to a surgeon and hazardous to the patient when **forceps or a hemostat** springs open. This mishap is caused by forceps malalignment, worn ratchet teeth, or lack of tension at the shanks.
     a. Start the equipment check by visually checking **jaw alignment** by closing the jaws of the forceps lightly. If the jaws overlap, they are out of alignment. Then, determine whether the teeth are meshing properly on forceps with serrated jaws. In addition, try to wiggle the instrument with the forceps open and holding one shank in each hand. If the box has considerable play or is very loose, the jaws are usually malaligned and the forceps need repair.
     b. To check the **ratchet teeth** on instruments, clamp the forceps to the first tooth only. A resounding snap should be produced. Then hold the instrument by the box lock and tap the ratchet teeth portion of the instrument lightly against a solid object. If the instrument springs open, it is faulty and needs repair.
     c. Test the **tension between the shanks** by closing the jaws of the forceps lightly until they barely touch. At this point, there should be clearance of 1/16 in or 1/8 in between the ratchet teeth on each shank.
  2. To test the function of the **needle holder**, first clamp the needle in the jaws of the holder, then lock the instrument on the second ratchet tooth. If the needle can be turned easily by hand, set aside the instrument for repair. When the instrument is new, it holds a needle securely on the first ratchet tooth for a considerable time. Needle holders such as a Crile, Wood, Derf, or Halsey, used in plastic surgery, should hold at least a 6-0 suture. Needle holders such as Castroviejo or Kalt should hold a 7-0 suture.

C. **Surgical exposure instruments.** There are various methods for testing the efficiency of **surgical scissors**. The Mayo and Metzenbaum dissecting scissors should cut four layers of gauze with the tips of their blades. Smaller scissors (less than 4 in long) should be able to cut two layers of gauze at the tips. All scissors should have a fine, smooth feel and require only minimum pressure by the blades to cut properly. The scissors action should not be too loose or too tight. Check the tips of the scissors for burrs or for excessive sharpness. Closed tips of the scissors should not be separated or loose. The precise setting of the blade is very important. Sharpening surgical scissors is a skilled procedure, usually requiring an exceptional craftsman to properly grind and set the blades.

1. **Periosteal elevators**
   a. Periosteal elevators are instruments designed to **strip (or elevate) periosteum from bone**. As the instrument is pushed along the surface of the bone, the soft tissue is lifted from the underlying bone. Periosteal elevators are thus instruments for blunt dissection and are designed to follow bony surfaces without gouging into the bone or wandering off into the soft tissues. They are also useful in blunt separation of other tissue planes such as in the exposure of the hip joint capsule. The use of periosteal elevators is most satisfactory in areas where tissue planes are not too firmly adherent. At bony attachments of a ligament or capsule, collagen fibers plunge deeply into the bone so that the elevator does not slide within a tissue interspace; sharp dissection with a scalpel is more appropriate here. In fracture fixation, periosteal stripping, which can adversely affect blood supply and bone healing, should be minimized wherever possible.
   b. Elevators are made in **different sizes and shapes**. They may be narrow or wide. Sharp corners allow insertion of the instrument into a tissue plane or beneath the periosteum. On the other hand, most blade corners are rounded to avoid producing damage when pressure is applied to the central portion of the blade.
   c. The **technique** of making a periosteal incision with a scalpel before the elevator is used helps form well-defined edges. When periosteum is being elevated from bone, the first rule of safety is to always keep the blade against bone. If the instrument is allowed to slip off into the soft tissues, vessels and nerves can be damaged. It is important to use two hands whenever possible to have a stable grasp on the instrument and to maintain fine control. A gentle rocking motion while advancing the blade produces more even results (Fig. 11-2). Although periosteal elevators need not be honed to the same sharp edge required for bone-cutting osteotomes, they do require some tissue-penetrating ability to be most effective. Nevertheless, they should not be so sharp as to incise soft tissue instead of stripping it.

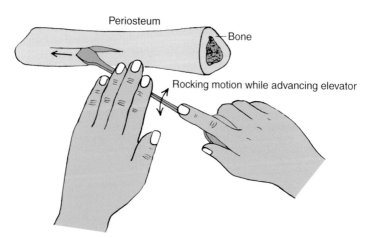

**Figure 11-2.** Proper use of a sharp-edged periosteal elevator. (From Spolek G. Unpublished data, 1974 with permission.)

d. **Important guidelines for tool selection and usage**
  i. Select the **correct size**. Generally, use a small elevator for small bones and a large elevator for large bones.
  ii. Select the **correct shape**. Usually, a sharp elevator is used to elevate periosteum and a rounded elevator to dissect soft tissue.
  iii. The **periosteum is incised with a scalpel**.
  iv. The **corner of the elevator** is used to reflect a periosteal edge.
  v. The **periosteum is elevated evenly** without tearing.
  vi. The elevator is **kept on the bone**.
  vii. The **bone is not engaged** by the elevator.
  viii. A **rocking motion** is used while advancing the elevator.
  ix. **Two hands** are used, one for power and one for stability and dissecting.
  x. **Overpenetration** into the soft tissues by the elevator **should be avoided**.
  xi. A **gentle technique** must be used.

D. **Bone-cutting instruments: osteotomes, gouges, and mallets**
  1. The **major difference** between an osteotome and a chisel is that an osteotome bevels on both sides to a point, whereas the chisel has a bevel on only one side (Fig. 11-3). The term **osteotome** is made up of **osteo**, which means "bone," and **tome**, which means "to cut"; the purpose of the tool is to cut bone. The cut should be produced under excellent control; otherwise, the bone can be split. Osteotomes come in different shapes and sizes. There are different types of handles that make for differences in holding and striking surface capabilities.
  2. **Selection of instruments**
    a. **Chisels** are used to remove bone from around screws and plates instead of osteotomes because they can be easily sharpened when the edges are nicked from being hit against the metal. It is better to keep a set of chisels specifically for removing metal implants.
    b. **Osteotomes** are used to cut bone and to shave off osteoperiosteal grafts. In fusion procedures, they are used to remove the cartilage and subchondral bone as well as to perform "fish scaling" of the surface of bone for bone graft union.

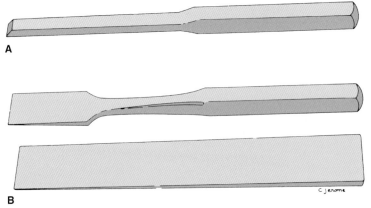

A

B

C Jerome

**Figure 11-3.** Differences between an osteotome and a chisel. **A:** A chisel. **B:** Two types of osteotome.

    c. **Gouges** are used to provide strips of cancellous bone graft from the iliac crest. They are also used to clean out the cartilage and subchondral bone from concave joint surfaces.

    d. **Mallets** are used to produce power to drive the aforementioned tools through bone and cartilage.

3. **Proper technique**

    a. The dominant hand is used to grasp the mallet, which strikes the back of the instrument and drives it through bone. **While hitting the osteotome through bone of increasing density,** notice that the sound becomes high pitched and the osteotome moves a shorter distance with each blow. In addition, there is a tightening or holding quality about the osteotome so that it moves less freely. This tightness is an indication that bone is coming under more tension and that a split of the bone is about to occur. Decrease the tension by working the osteotome back and forth through the bone. Occasionally, it is necessary to remove the osteotome to take a different direction or a slightly different angle. It is frequently important to prescore the bone so that the cutting goes directly toward it instead of splitting the bone in an unwanted area.

    b. **Precautions** include preventing the osteotome from sliding off the bone or from cutting through the bone rapidly and then plunging into soft tissue. The nondominant hand merely supports and directs the osteotome against bone until it gets started but does not apply any major pressure on the tool. Starting the cut is best accomplished by placing the osteotome at right angles to the bone, then angling the tool only after the initial score and cut have begun. These precautions protect both the patient and the hands of the assistant.

4. Specific **maintenance** is necessary in the handling and sharpening of the tools. The sharpening of an osteotome or a gouge is a difficult and critical procedure that must be undertaken with great caution. If the tool is overheated during sharpening, the temper is lost. The loss can be recognized by the bluish-gray color of the metal in contrast to the silvery color usually associated with stainless steel. In addition, care must be taken in cleaning and handling the tools while they are on a surgical table so that the ends do not become damaged by other instruments. Keep them in a rack during the sterilization process, not in a basin with other tools.

E. **Bone saws and files.** In general, the operator must control the amplitude, direction, and length of force applied to the saw. The use of saline irrigation to disperse heat is always recommended.

    1. The proper use of **Gigli saw** includes making a scribe mark at the start of the technique if possible. The surgeon must be careful not to drop or tangle the saw cable, to keep the cable at approximately 90°, and to use the middle two-thirds of the saw while applying a constant, steady tension. Excess body movement should be avoided to produce a straight bone cut. The use of saline coolant is recommended.

    2. A **bone file** or rasp is usually used to round the edge of a bone cut. Both hands should be used to control the direction of the tool and only a forward force should be applied.

F. **General bone screw biomechanics**

    1. **Holes** are generally drilled in bone not only for the purpose of inserting screws to hold orthopaedic implants but also for reduction clamps. Careful, even compulsive, attention to detail in selecting equipment and in drilling holes properly is vital to the performance of an implanted fixation device. The interlocking threads of screw and bone overlap by less than 0.02 in. Any failure of equipment or technique that decreases this margin drastically reduces the holding power of the screw. Given the severe loading environment

in which most orthopaedic implants operate, the holding power of a screw is an important matter. Force concentrations that occur when a screw fails to hold properly can result in a rapid failure of the implant.

2. **Drill bits**[1]

a. **Common defects in equipment.** As hole drilling is frequently taken for granted (the major attention being paid to the implant itself), drill bits come to the operating room in various stages of disrepair.

    i. A **dull point** is one of the most serious and least noticed defects. When the point is sharp, virtually all heat generated in drilling is carried away in the bone chips that are formed. Even slight dullness drastically increases friction between the point and the bone. This friction causes excessive heating and can affect the strength of the bone around the hole as well as cause inefficient cutting, which results in an oversized hole.

    ii. The flutes should be examined for **nicks and gouges** that score the walls of the hole, causing excessive heating and oversized holes; if identified, the drill bit should be discarded.

    iii. A drill with a **scored shank** does not sit straight in the chuck and causes the same trouble as a drill sharpened off-center.

    iv. Drill bits of the **wrong size** are sometimes selected. A difference of just one-hundredth of an inch is enough to diminish the holding power of a screw severely, even though insertion of the screw appears normal.

    v. A **bent drill bit** causes the same difficulty as a drill bit sharpened off-center. One cannot tell whether a drill bit is bent by simply looking at it; it must be rotated in the fingers. Even small **bends** create holes that are irregular, and the drill bit is very susceptible to breakage.

b. **Technique**

    i. Prevent the drill point from **wandering off-center**.

        (a) To keep the point from **wandering on penetration** and to protect surrounding soft tissues, use an appropriate-sized **drill guide**. Start the hole perpendicular to the surface. When bone penetration begins, shift to the desired direction. Always use saline to cool the drill bit.

        (b) Thin surgical drill bits are flexible, and if the drill is inadvertently held **slightly off perpendicular** when starting the hole, the point may bend the opposite way, making the point wander.

        (c) If the drill bit is **not positioned properly in the chuck** or if debris is present in the chuck or on the shank, the drill bit may wander off-center. Another error involves insertion of the drill bit too deeply into the chuck, which causes damage to the flutes when the drill is tightened. Check the drill for these problems before proceeding.

    ii. **Tighten the chuck down.** If the chuck is loose, it can rotate relative to the drill and score the shank.

    iii. **Too little force** (not too much force) is a common defect in technique. Push hard enough to cause a constant progression of the drill bit; otherwise, too much energy is being dissipated as friction rather than as cutting, causing excessive heating.

    iv. **Avoid overpenetration.** Slow the drill motor when the drill bit tip begins penetrating (noted by a change in resistance) and finish with care. With care, the surgeon will note that the pitch of the sound made by the drill drops just before penetration of the cortex. The tip should not penetrate more than one-eighth of an inch through the opposite cortex.

v. When the drill bit breaks through the opposite cortex, **keep it rotating in the same direction as you back it out**. The chips are thus carried out with the drill bit instead of being left in the hole.

vi. Drill motors should be **lubricated frequently**. Special surgical lubricants are available. Do not use mineral oil or ordinary oil because they are not permeable by steam and can harbor bacteria and spores even after autoclaving.

vii. Battery packs for power equipment should be kept charged with backups available.

c. **Adhere to the following points when using drills:**

i. **Choose the correct drill bit.** Reject dull, scored, bent, oversized, and incorrectly pointed drill bits. In general, use new drill bits for each case.

ii. **Insert the drill bit correctly in the chuck** with the drill bit centered and the chuck tightened on the shank only. Use quick release systems whenever possible to avoid potential problems.

iii. **Tighten the chuck sufficiently.**

iv. **Start the drill hole perpendicular to the surface**; then change to the desired direction.

v. **Maintain adequate pressure** on the drill to promote cutting and lessen heat production.

vi. **Maintain the proper direction** of the hole and penetrate the far cortical wall carefully, with the drill bit minimally penetrating.

vii. **Keep the drill rotating while backing it out** in order to clear the hole of bone chips.

3. **Screws**[1]

a. **Cortical bone screws** are fully threaded and come in various sizes for different sized bones. Non–self-tapping screws require a tap to cut the threads into the bone before insertion (Fig. 11-4).

b. **Cancellous bone screws** have a thinner core diameter plus wider and deeper threads to better grip the "spongy" bone. They are fully or partially threaded. Tapping is required only through the cortical surface.

c. **Lag screw fixation** can be achieved either with a partially threaded cancellous screw or by drilling a "gliding hole" (of the same size as the outer thread diameter) for the near cortex, allowing a cortical screw to produce lag compression.

d. Large, medium, and small (7.3 to 3.5 mm) **cannulated cancellous bone screws** are designed to pass over a guidewire. With this type of system, the surgeon can place a guidewire exactly where desired so that the cannulated drill, tap, and screw pass over this wire for precise placement. Care must be taken to not drill beyond the tip of the guidewire during predrilling as the wire will come out with the drill bit.

e. **Length of screw.** Drilling the proper hole is only the first step in firmly fixing the screw into the bone. The second part is selecting a screw that is of adequate length.[27]

i. To use a **depth gauge** properly, do not insert the gauge any farther than necessary. Be sure to have hooked the far end of the hole and not an intermediate point. Consider allowing additional length (usually 2 mm) over the scale reading on the depth gauge when choosing the screw length.

ii. A **self-tapping screw** has a tapered point whose holding power is further reduced by the flutes cut for tapping purposes. The *distal 2 mm of the self-tapping screw has no holding power at all, and the next 2 mm has very little. Screw lengths are measured from the proximal edge of the chamfered head to the distal point of the screw* (Fig. 11-4). If a screw is installed in a plate, additional length

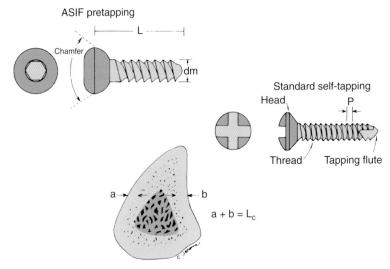

**Figure 11-4.** Comparison between Association for the Study of Internal Fixation (ASIF) and standard cortical bone screws.

must be allowed. Given the fact that bone screws hold principally in cortical bone, a screw that is short by 4 mm may lose 50% of its holding power.

  iii. When a screw is inserted on a *subcutaneous border of bone*, the hole should be *countersunk* before the depth is measured and the screw inserted.

  iv. **Tighten the screw snugly and no more,** so as not to strip the threads of the bone when inserting the screw. Retighten cortical screws three times to allow for the obligate loss of strain between screw and bone resulting from loss of fluid in the bone and stress relaxation.

**G. General principles of plating** are described in the following paragraphs and generally follow the concepts and techniques advocated by the Association for the Study of Internal Fixation (AO/ASIF) group, which supplies the most widely used fracture fixation implants in use. The plates are listed by their general biomechanical functions.[13]

  1. Protection or **neutralization plates** are used in combination with lag or other screws and protect the screw fixation in diaphyseal fractures. Without the plates, the screw fixation by itself does not withstand much loading and does not allow for early range of motion. The lag screws provide for most of the interfragmental compression and the plate protects the screws from torsion, bending, and shearing forces (Fig. 11-5).

  2. The dynamic compression plate (DCP) brings compression to the fracture site by its design. Recently, low-contact dynamic compression plates (LCD-CPs) and point contact plates have been developed that allow greater freedom in screw insertion through the plate and also limit the pressure necrosis effect of the plate on the cortical bone surface[1] (Figs. 11-6 to 11-8).

  3. By their nature, many epiphyseal and metaphyseal fractures are subject to compression and shearing forces. Lag screws are used to reconstruct the normal anatomy, but they cannot overcome the forces of shear and bending because of the thin cortical shells in these areas, especially in

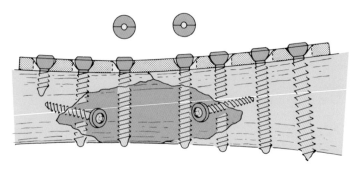

**Figure 11-5.** Application of a conventional or neutralization internal fixation plate. The neutral drill guide is used. Neutralization plate allows for more loading of the fracture than simple lag screw fixation.

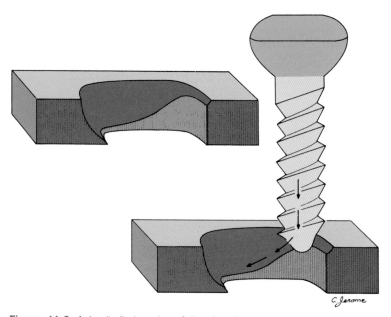

**Figure 11-6.** A longitudinal section of the dynamic compression plate (DCP) screw hole. Insertion of the Association for the Study of Internal Fixation (AO/ASIF) screw causes self-compression of the fracture site by the plate by sliding down an inclined cylinder to a horizontal one. (From Mueller ME, Allgöwer M, Schneider R, Willenegger H. *Manual of Internal Fixation*. 2nd ed. Berlin, Germany: Springer-Verlag; 1979:71 with permission.)

comminuted fractures. The fixation is supplemented with supporting or buttress plates to prevent subsequent fracture displacement from shear or bending stresses. Specially designed buttress plates include the T plate, the T **buttress plate**, the L buttress plate, the lateral tibial head plate, the spoon plate, the cloverleaf plate, and the condylar buttress plate. Additional plates for special locations (e.g., proximal and distal tibia, calcaneous) have recently been marketed.

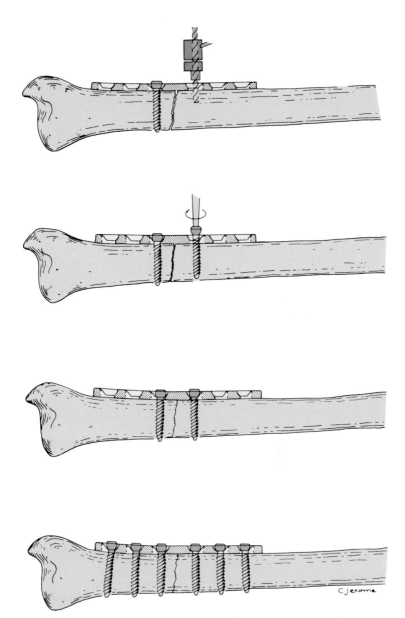

**Figure 11-7.** Application of self-compression plate. The load drill guide is used for placement of the second drill as shown in the top illustration. The other holes are drilled with the neutral drill guide. (From Mueller ME, Allgöwer M, Schneider R, Willenegger H. *Manual of Internal Fixation*. 2nd ed. Berlin, Germany: Springer-Verlag; 1979:67, 75 with permission.)

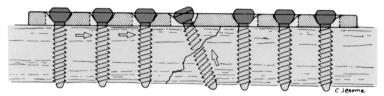

**Figure 11-8.** Dynamic compression plate with lag screw. The compression through the plate is applied first; then the lag screw is added to prevent a shear force on the lag screw.

4. Over the past decade, locking plates have been developed to add rigidity in metaphyseal fracture areas where angulatory stresses are highest. The sides of the screw heads are threaded and rigidly engage the threaded holes in the plate. Specially shaped plates have been developed for metaphyseal applications all over the skeleton by every implant manufacturer. The same technology has been developed for diaphyseal plate applications to help with clinical situations of extreme osteoporosis where the screw/plate/bone interface is at risk because of poor bone purchase with the screw threads.

5. To restore the load-bearing capacity of an eccentrically loaded fractured bone and minimize the forces borne by the fixation device, it is necessary to absorb the tensile forces (the result of a bending movement) and convert them into compressive forces. This requires **tension band fixation**, which exerts a force equal in magnitude but opposite in direction to the bending force (assuming the bone is able to withstand compression).[1] Therefore, comminuted fractures should be treated with other fixation devices or protected longer from bending moments.

   a. Ideally, **tension band plating** techniques are used on the femur, humerus, radius, and ulna.[1]

   b. **Tension band wire internal fixation**

      i. The **purpose** of tension band wire internal fixation is to secure the fragments of fractures in such a way that the application of normal forces (muscle forces, loads generated by walking) produces a compression of the fragments at the fracture site instead of pulling the fragments apart. The advantage of this technique is that the fixation is secure enough to allow early (if not immediate) use of the limb. Indications for tension band wiring are generally in the treatment of avulsion fractures at the insertion of muscles, tendons, or ligaments. If one has to deal with a rotational component or when accurate reduction of the fragments is vital, introduce two parallel Kirschner wires before the insertion of the tension band. The tension band then is passed around the wire ends.

      ii. The tension band **principle** works only when there are applied natural forces that tend to bend the bone at the fracture site. The olecranon, patella, and tip of the fibula are examples of such sites. Fig. 11-9 describes the principles of tension band wire internal fixation for the treatment of a transverse fracture of the olecranon.

      iii. As shown in Fig. 11-9, **a single-screw fixation without a tension wire loop is not adequate** because the screw bends with triceps activity and only half the fracture site is placed in compression.

      iv. It is evident that the wire is pulled in tension by the bending effect of the muscle force. Therefore, whatever force is exerted across the

**Figure 11-9.** The principles of tension band wire internal fixation as applied to a transverse fracture of the olecranon. Forces on an intact olecranon cause a bending moment. **A:** Same forces on a transverse fracture of the olecranon cause the fracture to open. **B:** Screw fixation provides only partial compression of fracture. **C:** Fixation of the cortex under tension creates equal compressive forces across the fracture site.

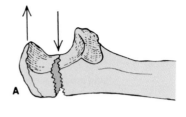

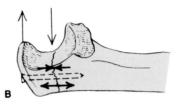

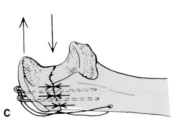

bony interface must be **compressive and equal** in magnitude to the force carried by the wire.

    v. Note that the tension band wiring **does not provide the desired rigidity for loading from all directions**. It is intended to resist only the strong tension forces applied through the action of specific muscles or through loading.

    vi. The **application** of tension band wire fixation is discussed in the treatment of olecranon fractures in **Chapter 19, III.B** and of patellar fractures in **Chapter 25, III.A.3**.

6. **Numerous other plates and screws** serve the aforementioned functions with various shapes and sizes to adapt to the local anatomy. They include straight and offset condylar blade plates, reconstruction plates (more easily contoured in all three planes, which make them optimum for use in the pelvis and distal humerus), dynamic hip screws, dynamic condylar screws, and specialized locking plates where the screw head is threaded into the plate. These are especially useful in osteoporotic bone.

7. **Contouring internal fixation plates.** Internal fixation plates may be contoured to fit the bone before application. Such contouring increases the bone–plate interface area so that the loads normally carried by the bone can be transferred to the plate by friction rather than pure shearing on the bone screws. To contour a plate template, press the aluminum template of the proper length against the bone, then bend the plate to match. Plate

benders may be handheld singular, handheld pliers, and table-mounted bending presses. Locking plates in general should not be contoured, as the hole configuration will be distorted.

a. The **bending press** gets the most use because most contouring is two-dimensional. The anvil is adjustable so that the handle can be used in the position with the best control (near the end of its travel). The **hand press** is used mainly for small plates, for plates with a semitubular cross section, and reconstruction picks. There are three different anvils (straight, convex, and concave) to prevent squashing of the semitubular plates. The **bending irons** are for applying twists and are most conveniently used when the jaws are opened upward to prevent the plate from falling out and when the handles are on the same side of the plate. Theoretically, uniform twist occurs between the irons, so start with them at the ends of the desired twist length. Once the twist is started, move the irons closer together to get localized contours. DCPs are weakest through the holes, where most of the twist occurs, so try to position the irons to prevent excessive bends at any one hole. Use the press first because the plate does not fit the anvil if the bending irons are used to twist beforehand. LCDCPs have more uniform characteristics and do not bend at the holes. Fig. 11-10 illustrates the three types of instruments.

b. **Important guidelines in usage**

   i. Bend the plate to form a **smooth, continuous contour**. Because the press causes a single, rather abrupt bend directly beneath the plunger, a long continuous curve is best formed by several small bends rather than a few sharp bends.

   ii. **Avoid bends through screw holes** because they alter the shape of the countersunk surface of the hole so that the screw does not seat properly. If a bend must be made through a screw hole, go easy on the press handle because the plate is weaker at a hole and less force is required to bend it.

   iii. If the required contour contains a series of **shallow and sharp bends**, do the shallow ones (greatest radius of curvature) first and progressively work toward the sharper bends, as shown in Fig. 11-11. This procedure tends to produce smooth contours and allows easier template matching. Contouring to fit a bump or knoll on the bone surface requires three bends: two convex and one concave.

   iv. **Do not overbend but ease into a contour** (see Fig. 11-11). Overbending requires straightening, which, besides being time-consuming work, hardens the plate in that area and thus reduces the strength of the plate.

   v. When contouring the plate, do not match the template exactly, but rather alter (underbend or overbend) the shape so that there is a **1- to 2-mm clearance between the plate and the bone at the site of a transverse fracture**. This technique causes compression of the cortex opposite the plate when the screws are tightened.

   vi. **Minimize scratching or marking of the plate surface.** If the surface is scratched, a potential corrosion site is created. Therefore, use the proper bending irons with smooth jaws rather than vise grips.

H. **Cerclage** is a technique of encircling a fractured bone with Parham-Martin band, stainless steel or titanium wire, Dall-Miles cable, or other nonabsorbable material to hold the fracture in reduction in conjunction with stronger, more permanent fixation. Cerclage is not recommended as a primary method of internal fixation of fractures. There are many techniques for applying cerclage wire.

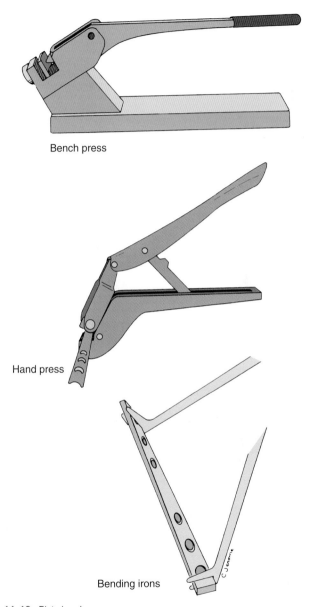

Bench press

Hand press

Bending irons

**Figure 11-10.** Plate benders.

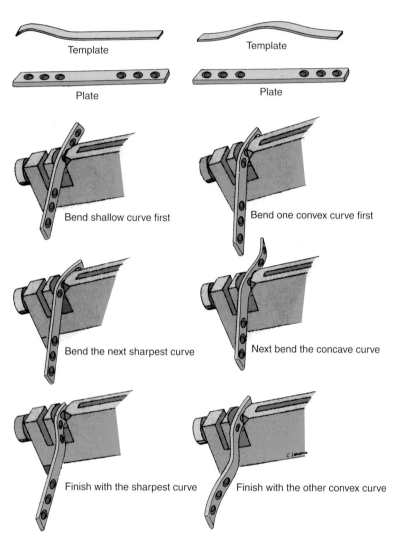

**Figure 11-11.** Steps in plate contouring.

1. **General rules of wire cerclage**
   a. **Avoid putting kinks in the wire.** Kinking is easy, particularly if the wire is coiled. Kinks result in stress concentrations that drastically reduce the fatigue strength of the wire.
   b. **Be sure that the loop around the bone is perpendicular to the long axis of the bone.** Otherwise, the loop may appear tight, but any slight movement causes it to shift and loosen.
   c. Use the cerclage wire only to hold the fracture site in reduction, not to apply compression. The wire is not strong enough to apply useful compression. Tighten the wire only until it is snug; be careful not to overtighten while making the knot.

d. Use the **proper-sized wire**; 18G is common and has sufficient strength. The area of the wire is a measure of its load-carrying capacity, which depends on the square of the diameter. Thus, the load-carrying capacity decreases considerably with even moderate decreases in radius.

2. **Wire tighteners**

a. The **Bowen wire tightener is an excellent tightener** (Fig. 11-12). Both wires are passed into the nose of the appliance and out the side. The outer wheel is turned to secure the wire against the inside cylinder. By turning the inside wheel, the inside cylinder is pulled up the handle of the device, effectively tightening the wire to the desired tension. The whole instrument is rotated to twist the wire, and the wires are then easily cut just distal to the last twist.

b. The **Kirschner wire traction bows** (see Fig. 11-1) have a mechanical advantage that varies with the jaw opening. The lowest mechanical advantage is in the fully closed position; this increases gradually with increasing jaw width. The average mechanical advantage for both the large and the small bows is 30:1. The last one-fourth inch of jaw opening coincides with a sudden increase in mechanical advantage of greater than 400:1, but this last one-fourth inch is rarely used.

c. **Comparison of knot strength.** The types of knots described here were tied in 20G steel wire and pulled apart in a tension test machine:

   i. Type of knot/maximum force before failure
     (a) ASIF loop/15.8 lb
     (b) Twist (one turn)/23.2 lb
     (c) Twist (three turns)/24.2 lb
     (d) Square knot/59.0 lb

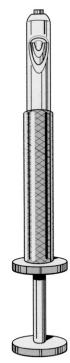

**Figure 11-12.** The Bowen wire tightener.

ii. These results do afford some conclusions. An ASIF loop is the weakest and is heavily dependent on careful knot formation for its strength. The twist is 47% stronger, but additional turns beyond the first 360° turn do not significantly increase the strength of the knot. The reason for using several twists is to provide some residual resistance after untwisting begins, although whether this resistance actually occurs has not been determined. The square knot is the strongest of all. Failure occurs by wire fracture just below the knot.

## I. Principles of intramedullary nailing

1. An intramedullary nail allows for internal splinting with a fixation device in the medullary canal. The **possibility of gliding along the dynamically locked nail promotes compression forces at the fracture site, and the stability from the long working length of the nail provides stiffness.**

2. This necessary reaming of the canal and resulting disruption of the endosteal blood supply in a severely open fracture that already has disruption of the periosteal blood supply may increase the chance for a nonunion or infection. In these situations, the use of a smaller **unreamed nail** seems to provide satisfactory results. Because these smaller unreamed nails have less mechanical stability, they generally require interlocking (placing one or two screws across the cortex and nail superiorly and inferiorly).[1] The incidence of implant failure by fatigue fracture is much greater than the larger diameter implants inserted with reaming.

3. In addition to the aforementioned indications, the treatment of complex fractures requires an **interlocking nail** to prevent excessive shortening and rotation. It is recommended to always statically lock the nail to avoid malrotation and shortening, which can occur related to unrecognized minimally displaced cracks.

## J. External skeletal fixation

1. The **use of external fixation**, particularly in the treatment of comminuted or open fractures, **has regained popularity**. Lambotte (1902) is generally given credit for the first use of external pin fixation. Anderson (1934), Stader (1937), and Hoffman (1938) all popularized a technique of external skeletal fixation. Vidal and Adrey, using the Hoffman approach, further refined the technique. Most recently, Ilizarov developed and popularized the ring fixator with small wire transfixion for use in limb lengthening, bone transport, and fracture fixation. More recent frame designs incorporate thin wire and half pin options with corresponding computer programs to plan correction of deformity where they are used in reconstruction applications.

2. Multiple external fixators are currently on the market. Regardless of which technique is used, certain **basic principles** must be followed:

   a. The insertion of the pins and the attachment of the external skeletal fixation is a major procedure performed in the operating room **following all normal operating room procedures**.

   b. The skin and fascia must be incised so that there is **no shear stress on these structures** that could result in necrosis.

   c. The **pins** must be **inserted slowly** with a hand chuck after predrilling with a saline-cooled drill bit to avoid heat necrosis of bone.

   d. There must be a **minimum of two pins above and two pins below the fracture**. Three pins add a small amount of stability in some systems. Maximal fracture stability is achieved using half pins separately within each bone segment, with wide separation, and by placing the connecting bar as close to the skin as possible. Additional stability is attained by stacking a second bar (this must be done by planning ahead because parallel pins are required in some systems) or using a second row of pins and connecting bar.

e. **Terminally threaded half pins** are used to prevent loosening and sliding of the unit in the bone.

f. Avoid motion of skin and fascia against the pins.

g. Use **strict aseptic techniques** when dressing the pin sites.

h. **Avoid distraction.** Make adjustments to ensure coaptation or impaction of the fracture fragments during the course of healing.

i. Studies have clearly shown that **external fixation devices can be used to treat fractures to union**. It was previously thought that the devices should be removed as soon as fractures are stabilized and be replaced by casts or cast-braces, if necessary, to allow weight bearing across the fracture to stimulate healing.

j. External fixation is a complex procedure that **requires skill and attention to detail**.

3. Possible **indications** for external skeletal fixation include the comminuted Colles fracture and comminuted or open fractures of the tibia, particularly in the proximal and distal ends where intramedullary nailing is less feasible and the risk of infection from the more extensive soft-tissue stripping required for plating is significant. A common indication is with open ankle fractures or ankle fractures that are irreducible and have significant skin damage. The external fixator allows for fracture stabilization until skin healing is adequate enough for open reduction and internal fixation. The apparatus should be used with caution for fractures in the humerus, femur, and pelvis because of the higher incidence of pin tract infection and pin loosening. Patient acceptance is also higher with other devices. The thin wire fixator technique developed by Ilizarov has made application in the metaphyseal region more secure, but because of the use of these "through" pins, the anatomic knowledge required in inserting them is greater. The Ilizarov frames are useful for fracture management, bone transport, and limb lengthening.

K. **Obtaining bone graft material** is a common procedure in orthopaedics. On most occasions, the iliac crest is used for the graft, although various bone grafts are available. After closure of the wound, installation of 0.5% bupivacaine without epinephrine reduces the postoperative pain. The following is the recommended surgical technique:

1. **For removal of a small amount of bone**, tension the skin over the iliac bone and cut to the ilium between the external oblique and the gluteal fascia without entering muscle. A small periosteal flap is excised with sharp dissection from the superior aspect of the crest. A window is then cut through the cortical bone between the inner and the outer tables. The periosteum is not stripped from the bone so pain is less.

2. **For removal of sizable grafts**, the surgeon must decide whether to use the anterior or posterior part of the iliac crest. Often, the choice is dictated by the position of the patient during operation. Anticipating the possible need for iliac bone grafting for proper positioning, prepping, and draping is required for the smooth flow of the operation. Whenever possible, the patient should be positioned so that the area of the posterior superior iliac spine can be used.

a. **Removal of bone from the anterior part of the iliac crest.** The skin incision must be long enough to allow a comfortable exposure of the anterior 4 to 5 in of the iliac crest. Sharp dissection is used to expose the crest. A periosteal elevator is used to expose the inner or outer surface of the ilium. The bone may then be removed by an osteotome or gouge. Care should be taken not to involve both tables of the ilium to minimize hematoma formation and postoperative pain and deformity. One should also be careful to avoid the anterior superior spine for reasons of cosmesis as well as to prevent injury to the lateral femoral cutaneous nerve. Absorbable gelatin sponges (Gelfoam) may be used to help control bleeding. The wound may be closed over suction drainage, but drains are not routinely used.

b. **Removal of bone from the posterior iliac crest.** An oblique incision is made over the iliac crest approximately 1 to 2 in lateral to the midline. The incision is not extended far enough over the crest to involve the superior cluneal nerves. The periosteum from the outer table is lifted with the periosteal elevator, and the detached muscles are protected with warm, moist lap sponges. Cancellous strips are then removed, and care should be taken not to enter the sacroiliac joint. Excessive bleeding is helped by absorbable gelatin sponges. The wound may be closed over suction drainage on rare occasion with excessive bleeding.

c. **Removal of bicortical grafts.** These are wafers of bone taken from the iliac crest with the bone removed as a single block with both cortices. Generally, bicortical grafts are used in vertebral body fusions and in situations in which a structural graft is required. The same surgical techniques described in the preceding sections (**II.J.2.a** and **b**) are used, except that the incision and the donor site is between the anterior (or posterior) superior iliac spine and the most cephalad portion of the iliac crest. Bicortical graft donor sites are nearly always symptomatic for a significant postoperative period and often are deforming cosmetically.

**L. Basic skin suture techniques**

1. **General principles**

   a. Do not close the wound **if it may possibly be contaminated** (as in many open fractures). Delayed closure 3 to 5 days later is always preferable in doubtful cases.

   b. If skin edges are battered and ragged, debride them so that healthy tissues are brought together.

   c. Good **closure of subcutaneous tissues** is the key to good skin closure.

   d. **Approximate**, do not strangulate.

   e. **Cutting needles with monofilament suture or thin wire** are used for skin. Skin staples are also used frequently. Cotton and silk sutures are not recommended for skin closure because of the increased inflammatory response to these materials and because of the wick effect that can draw organisms into the wound.

   f. Before making a long incision, **mark it out with a surgical marking pen and make a crosshatch every 2 cm**. Then, when closing, make sure the crosshatches match up. Never make skin marks with a knife or needle because scarring results.

   g. **Steri-Strips** are useful adjuncts for skin closure, but they should never be applied when the skin is under significant tension. They also can impede drainage because they provide a fairly watertight closure.

   h. Consider placing a film of Polysporin ointment or a Betadine nonadherent dressing over the closed incision before applying outer dressings.

   i. Use **pickups**, rather than pincers, **as skin hooks**.

2. **Types of skin suture.** All types of skin closure rely on good subcutaneous suturing to provide strength and to relieve some of the tension from the skin edges.

   a. The needle path with a **box** or simple suture is perpendicular to the dermis. The depth of each half of the suture is equal. When tying the knot, have the edges just touch, as shown in Fig. 11-13. Never tie the knot so tightly that the skin bunches up.

   b. Start the **everting** suture as for a large box-type closure, then reverse the direction, thus making a minibox suture of just the dermis. Match the depth in the opposite side, as shown in Fig. 11-14. Tie the knot so that the slightest skin pucker results.

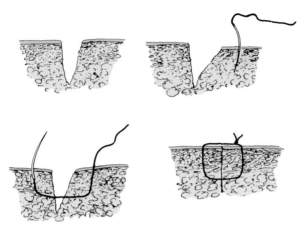

**Figure 11-13.** Technique for a box suture.

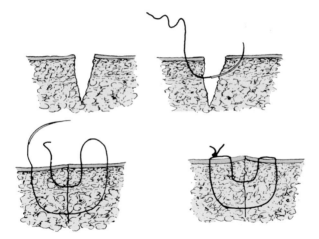

**Figure 11-14.** Technique for an everting suture.

c. An **intradermal** (or subcuticular) suture is entirely in the dermis and does not hold together with appreciable skin tension. Begin the closure several centimeters from the end of the wound and pass the needle from the starting point to the dermis at the apex of the wound. Obtain a secure amount of dermis on one side and then the other. Match the exit point on one side of the dermis with the entrance point on the other side, that is, directly opposite and of equal depth, as shown in Fig. 11-15. Occasionally, pull the ends of the suture back and forth so that it slides well. End the suture as it was begun. The ends of the suture may be knotted or taped to the skin to prevent them from pulling out. The suture line is then splinted with Steri-Strips.

d. The **"near-far/far-near"** suture may be used when the skin must be closed under some tension. Begin with a deep box-type suture that is

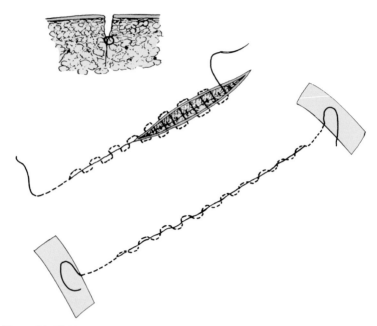

**Figure 11-15.** Technique for an intradermal (subcuticular) suture.

near the wound edge on one side and far from it on the other. Complete the technique with a box-type suture with the near and far sides reversed. Tie the suture so the skin edges are approximated (Fig. 11-16). It has been said that this technique should not be used with suture diameter greater than 3-0 as this suture will break before excessive tension is delivered to the wound edges.

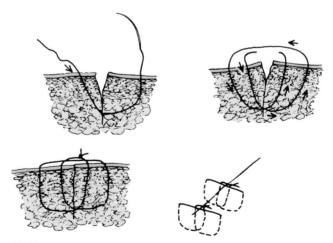

**Figure 11-16.** Technique for a "near-far/far-near" suture.

The **Donati skin suture** technique, which was popularized by the AO/ASIF group, is another modified mattress suture technique. It is useful when closing skin under tension. The suture courses deeply across the wound and then goes through the subdermal area without exiting the skin on the second side. Begin with a deep box-type suture on the first side of the wound. Pass back into the original side and exit between the wound and the original entrance site (Fig. 11-17).

3. **Adhesives for Superficial Wound Closure**

Adhesives for superficial wound closure are an increasingly popular option for total knee and hip replacement patients. Tissue adhesives provide a skin closure with high tensile strength that is cosmetically pleasing and easy to maintain. Skin adhesives also provide increased skin profusion by avoiding overtensioning of the skin at the time of closure. Adhesives are most successful when used in combination with a meticulous multilayered wound closure. Prior to the use of an adhesive closure, the patient should be medically optimized and have no known allergies/sensitivities to adhesives such as surgical glues and acrylates (eyelash extensions or fake nails). Prior to administering a topical adhesive, a layered wound closure is necessary starting with the fascial layer, followed by the elimination of any subcutaneous dead space, then a complete subcutaneous closure, and finally a subcuticular closure, if necessary. During skin closure, the skin edges should be well aligned to avoid gapping, overlaying, or dog earing of the skin. Minimizing drainage from the wound at the time of topical adhesive application is essential to allow the adhesive to appropriately adhere to the skin. It is important to allow appropriate adhesive drying time prior to breaking sterile technique or removing the surgical drape as the adhesive does not become occlusive from bacteria or other environmental elements until the drying process is complete. Once dry, tissue adhesives such as DERMABOND (2-octyl-cyanoacrylate; Ethicon Inc.) provide a mechanical barrier to microbial penetration.[28] Tissue adhesives must be completely dry before placing a dressing on top; otherwise the final dressing will become "glued" to the skin. Waiting for the adhesives to completely dry prevents disruption of the occlusive bond and the incisional healing process when the dressing is removed. Tissue adhesives have been

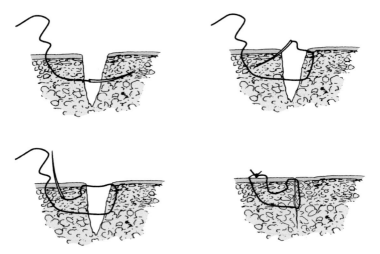

**Figure 11-17.** Technique for a Donati suture.

associated with less wound drainage requiring fewer dressing changes postoperatively than other closure techniques.[29,30] However, there are no current data that suggest tissue adhesives reduce superficial wound infections postoperatively compared to other closure methods.[27]

# REFERENCES

1. Müller ME, Allgöwer M, Schneider R, et al. *Manual of Internal Fixation*. 3rd ed. Springer-Verlag; 1990.
2. Castles JJ. Clinical pharmacology of glucocorticoids. In: McCarty DJ, ed. *Arthritis and Allied Conditions*. 9th ed. Lea & Febiger; 1979:399.
3. McKenzie PJ, Loach AB. Local anaesthesia for orthopaedic surgery. *Br J Anaesth*. 1986;58:779-789.
4. Raj PR, Cacodney A, Cannella J. Useful nerve blocks for pain relief and surgery. In: Browner B, ed. *Skeletal Trauma*. WB Saunders; 1992.
5. Martin JT. Complications associated with patient positioning. *Anesth Analg*. 1988;67(suppl 4S):1.
6. Reid HS, Camp RA, Jacob WH. Tourniquet hemostasis. A clinical study. *Clin Orthop Relat Res*. 1983;177:230-234.
7. Sapega AA, Heppenstall RB, Chance B, et al. Optimizing tourniquet application and release times in extremity surgery. A biochemical and ultrastructural study. *J Bone Joint Surg Am*. 1985;67:303-314.
8. Shaw JA, Murray DG. The relationship between tourniquet pressure and underlying soft-tissue pressure in the thigh. *J Bone Joint Surg Am*. 1982;64:1148-1152.
9. Moore MR, Garfin SR, Hargens AR. Wide tourniquets eliminate blood flow at low inflation pressures. *J Hand Surg Am*. 1987;12:1006-1011.
10. McLaren AC, Rorabeck CH. The pressure distribution under tourniquets. *J Bone Joint Surg Am*. 1985;67:433-438.
11. Neimkin RJ, Smith RJ. Double tourniquet with linked mercury manometers for hand surgery. *J Hand Surg Am*. 1983;8:938-941.
12. Nelson JP, Glassburn AR Jr, Talbott RD, et al. The effect of previous surgery, operating room environment, and preventive antibiotics on postoperative infection following total hip arthroplasty. *Clin Orthop Relat Res*. 1980;147:167-169.
13. Peterson AF, Rosenberg A, Alatary SD. Comparative evaluations of surgical scrub preparations. *Surg Gynecol Obstet*. 1978;146:63-65.
14. Scherr DD, Dodd TA, Buckingham WW Jr. Prophylactic use of topical antibiotic irrigation in uninfected surgical wounds. A microbiological evaluation. *J Bone Joint Surg Am*. 1972;54:634-640.
15. Lidwell OM. Clean air at operation and subsequent sepsis in the joint. *Clin Orthop Relat Res*. 1986;211:91-102.
16. Van Roekel HE, Thurston AJ. Tourniquet pressure: the effect of limb circumference and systolic pressure. *J Hand Surg Br*. 1985;10:142-144.
17. Pencer G. What you should know about surgical instruments. *Surg Team*. 1974;3:39.
18. Salaasa T, Swiontkowski M. Surgical attire and the operating room; role in infection process. *J Bone Joint Surg Am*. 2014;96:1485-1492.
19. Ponce B, Raines B, Reed R, et al. Surgical site infection after arthroplasty: comparative effectiveness of prophylactic antibiotics. *J Bone Joint Surg Am*. 2014;96:970-977.
20. Neu HC. Cephalosporin antibiotics as applied in surgery of bones and joints. *Clin Orthop Relat Res*. 1984;190:50-64.
21. Rosenberg AD, Wambold D, Kraemer L, et al. Ensuring appropriate timing of antimicrobial prophylaxis. *J Bone Joint Surg Am*. 2008;90:226-232.
22. Fletcher N, Sofianos D, Berkes MB, et al. Prevention of perioperative infection. *J Bone Joint Surg Am*. 2007;89:1605-1618.
23. Noordin S, McEwen JA, Kragh JF Jr, et al. Current concepts review. Surgical tourniquets in orthopaedics. *J Bone Joint Surg Am*. 2010;92:1318-1322.
24. Saltzman MD, Nuber GW, Gryzlo SM, et al. Efficacy of surgical preparation solutions in shoulder surgery. *J Bone Joint Surg Am*. 2009;91:1949-1953.
25. Ostrander RV, Botte MJ, Brage ME. Efficacy of surgical preparation solutions in foot and ankle surgery. *J Bone Joint Surg Am*. 2005;87:980-985.
26. Duggan EW, Carlson K, Umpierrez GE. Perioperative hyperglycemia management: an update. *Anesthesiology*. 2017;126(3):547-560.

27. Kim K. A meta-analysis and systematic review evaluating skin closure after total knee arthroplasty—what is the best method? *J Arthroplasty*. 2017;32(9):2920-2927.
28. Krishnan R, MacNeil SD, Malvankar-Mehta MS. Comparing sutures versus staples for skin closure after orthopaedic surgery: systematic review and meta-analysis. *BMJ Open*. 2016;6(1):e009257. doi:10.1136/bmjopen-2015-009257
29. Yuenyongviwat V. A randomised controlled trial comparing skin closure in total knee arthroplasty in the same knee: nylon sutures versus skin staples. *Bone Joint Res*. 2016;5:185-190. doi:10.1302/2046-3758.55.2000629
30. Gromov K, Troelsen A, Raaschou S, et al. Tissue adhesive for wound closure reduces immediate postoperative wound dressing changes after primary TKA. A randomized controlled study in simultaneous bilateral TKA. *Clin Orthop Relat Res*. 2019;477(9):2032-2038.
31. Hsu JE, Bumgarner M, Matsen F. Propionibacterium in shoulder arthroplasty: what we think we know today. *J Bone Joint Surg Am*. 2016;98(7):597-606.

## SELECTED HISTORICAL READINGS

Arnold WD, Hilgartner MW. Hemophilic arthropathy. *J Bone Joint Surg Am*. 1977;59:287-305.

Bagby GW. Compression bone-plating: historical considerations. *J Bone Joint Surg Am*. 1977;59:625-631.

Bechtol CO, Ferguson AB, Laign PG. *Metals and Engineering in Bone and Joint Surgery*. Williams & Wilkins; 1959.

Bowers WH, Wilson FC, Green WB. Antibiotic prophylaxis in experimental bone infections. *J Bone Joint Surg Am*. 1973;55:795-807.

Boyd RJ, Burke JF, Colton T. A double-blind clinical trial of prophylactic antibiotics in hip fractures. *J Bone Joint Surg Am*. 1973;55:1251-1258.

Brod JJ. The concepts and terms of mechanics. *Clin Orthop Relat Res*. 1980;146:9-17.

Dineen P. Microbial filtration by surgical masks. *Surg Gynecol Obstet*. 1971;133:812-814.

Ha'eri GB, Wiley AM. The efficacy of standard surgical face masks: an investigation using "tracer particles." *Clin Orthop Relat Res*. 1980;148:160-162.

Ha'eri GB, Wiley AM. Wound contamination through drapes and gowns: a study using tracer particles. *Clin Orthop Relat Res*. 1981;154:181-184.

Hamilton HW, Booth AD, Lone FJ, et al. Penetration of gown material by organisms from the surgical team. *Clin Orthop Relat Res*. 1979;141:237-246.

Hargens AR, McClure AG, Skyhar MJ, et al. Local compression patterns beneath pneumatic tourniquets applied to arms and thighs of human cadavera. *J Orthop Res*. 1987;5:247-252.

Heppenstall RB, Scott R, Sapega A, et al. A comparative study of the tolerance of skeletal muscle in ischemia. Tourniquet application compared with acute compartment syndrome. *J Bone Joint Surg Am*. 1986;68:820-828.

Hoffmann R. Rotules á os pour la reduction dirigé, non sanglante, des fractures (ostéotaxis). *Helv Med Acta*. 1938;5:844-856.

Jacobs JK, Burrus R, Heyssel RM, et al. Evaluation of draping techniques in prevention of surgical-wound contamination. *JAMA*. 1963;184:293-294.

Jardon OM, Wingard DW, Barak AJ, et al. Malignant hyperthermia. A potentially fatal syndrome in orthopaedic patients. *J Bone Joint Surg Am*. 1979;61:1064-1070.

Katz JF, Siffert RS. Tissue antibiotic levels with tourniquet use in orthopaedic surgery. *Clin Orthop Relat Res*. 1982;165:261-264.

Matthews LS, Hirsch C. Temperatures measured in human cortical bone when drilling. *J Bone Joint Surg Am*. 1972;54:297-308.

Noordin S, McEwen J, Kragh J Jr, et al. Surgical tourniquets in orthopaedics. *J Bone Joint Surg Am*. 2009;2958-2967.

Post M, Telfer MC. Surgery in hemophilic patients. *J Bone Joint Surg Am*. 1975;57:1136-1145.

Whiteside LA, Lesker PA. The effects of extraperiosteal and subperiosteal dissection. II. On fracture healing. *J Bone Joint Surg Am*. 1978;60:26-30.

Williams DN, Gustilo RB. The use of preventive antibiotics in orthopaedic surgery. *Clin Orthop Relat Res*. 1984;190:83-88.

# 12 Acute Management of Spine Trauma

Robert A. Morgan

## I. Introduction

Spine trauma needs to be understood in the context of the overall care of the patient. It is often present in the polytraumatized patient, complicating their hospital care as well as resulting in worsened outcomes at all stages.

**A. Initial evaluation and management.** Optimal outcome following acute spinal injury depends on early recognition of injury and appropriate management to prevent further injury. Adherence to principles of advanced trauma life support (ATLS) makes it mandatory that all patients with a mechanism of injury compatible with spinal injury should be assumed to have a spinal cord injury until proven otherwise. Any history of loss of consciousness or presenting complaints of numbness, tingling, or weakness should alert the practitioner to the presence of a possible spinal cord injury. Additionally, complaints of pain along a radicular dermatome or any bilateral pain or weakness should be clues to the possibility of a spinal cord injury. Brachial plexus injury or other peripheral nerve injuries should be considered diagnoses of exclusion in the setting of trauma. A detailed physical examination that includes cranial nerve function is required, as well as swallowing and phonation where possible. Manual motor testing of the upper and lower extremities, sensory testing of the upper and lower extremities, and reflex testing including the documentation of presence or absence of pathologic reflexes such as Hoffmann and Babinski need to be conducted. Although a great deal of information may be established from a gait examination, it is rarely useful in the acute trauma setting. In the neurologic examination, a detailed rectal examination is critical in defining the patient's neurologic status to include the presence or absence of rectal tone as well as perianal sensation. Finally, a detailed physical examination requires inspection and palpation of the entire spinal column looking for open wounds or ecchymosis, as well as palpations of any step-offs or deformities. A careful physical examination can identify ligamentous disruption in the spine, particularly in patients who may not be able to undergo magnetic resonance imaging (MRI) for more detailed imaging.

**B. Imaging studies**

1. **Radiographs**

   a. Standard radiographic evaluation of the cervical spine includes the lateral, open mouth odontoid, and anterior–posterior (AP) plain radiographs. Lateral view detects up to 85% of significant cervical spine injuries provided that the occipitocervical and cervicothoracic junctions are visualized. Missed fractures at the cervicothoracic junction may occur despite apparently normal lateral radiograph.[1] Orthogonal oblique views do not increase the sensitivity of plain film evaluation and add radiation exposure and cost to the examination. AP and lateral radiographs of the thoracic and lumbar segments are indicated as screening films in the presence of pain or abnormal physical examination findings in these regions and in cognitively impaired patients who cannot cooperate in physical examination, including obtunded patients. Noncontiguous spinal trauma is common, with reported incidence rates of up to 19%,[2] and the presence of an injury anywhere in the spine should prompt radiographic evaluation of the entire spine.

b. Important points to consider in interpreting plain radiographs include the following:

i. Any alteration in the alignment of the vertebral bodies. Straightening of the cervical spine can result from muscle spasms or from positioning the patient's head in slight flexion.

ii. Any step-off in the line of the posterior intervertebral facet joints.

iii. Any increase in the width of the retropharyngeal space in front of the vertebral bodies (normal is 4 to 6 mm at C3 and 15 to 20 mm at C6). This rule does not apply in a crying child.

iv. Any fracture lines in a vertebral body or in the posterior elements.

v. Any increase of distance between two spinous processes.

vi. Any displacement of the spinous process on the cephalad side, which is toward the side of any unilateral dislocation on the AP film.

vii. Any indication that the body of one vertebra has moved forward in relation to another on the lateral roentgenogram because such movement usually indicates a dislocation or fracture–dislocation of one or both joint facets at that level. If the amount of displacement is more than half the width of the vertebral body, the dislocation is bilateral and the spine is extremely unstable.

2. **Computed tomography (CT) scanning** can provide rapid and detailed assessment of the spine. This should include high-resolution imaging (2- to 3-mm collimation and 1.5-mm pitch) from the occiput to T1 with sagittal and coronal reconstructions. Several studies have demonstrated high levels of sensitivity (90%) and specificity (100%) of screening CT scanning in polytrauma patients.[3-5] CT scanning represents an evolving standard of care in the evaluation of cervical spine and cervicothoracic junction injuries for cervical injuries[6,7]; CT scanning represents the standard of care in all patients when

a. Poorly visualized areas are encountered on plain films.

b. Visualization of T1 is not improved with gentle downward traction on the arms, swimmer's views, or oblique views.

c. Fractures or dislocations are identified elsewhere in the spine.

d. In patients who are intubated, as plain films miss up to 17% of injuries to the upper cervical spine in the presence of an endotracheal tube.

3. **MRI** is less sensitive, less specific, and less cost-effective than the plain film series or screening CT for the identification and evaluation of cervical fracture.[8] However, MRI is extremely sensitive and specific for the evaluation of the paravertebral soft tissues, including the spinal cord, intervertebral discs, and ligamentous structures.[9] With the increasing use of MRI, the incidence of identifying noncontiguous fractures has increased to 41% versus the standard reported 10% to 15%. Patients with abnormal neurologic findings, particularly incomplete injuries, should undergo MRI scanning of the relevant spinal segment(s) to visualize the spinal cord and nerve roots.

4. **Dynamic fluoroscopy.** Passive flexion and extension stressing of the cervical spine, performed by an experienced physician under fluoroscopy, has a reported sensitivity of 92.3% and specificity of 98.8% for detecting significant ligamentous injuries and instability of the cervical spine.[10] Although some centers support the use of this technique in clearing the spine of unconscious patients, the risk of neurologic deterioration may outweigh its benefits, especially given the widespread availability of CT and MRI.[10]

C. **Clearance of spine in trauma patients.** Although protection of the spine is mandatory at all stages of managing the traumatized patient, clearance of the spine should take place only after potential life-threatening injuries have been stabilized.

1. In the cognitively intact patient who is not under the effect of drugs or alcohol and who is cooperative, clinical clearance of the spine may be possible. Although case reports of bony and ligamentous spinal injuries in such patients do exist, unstable spinal injuries and neurologic deterioration in these patients have not been reported. Accordingly, routine radiographic evaluation in such cases is not indicated. However, the physical examination findings of neck or back pain, neurologic abnormalities, bruising, spinal deformity, pain with active range of motion, or significant distracting nonspinal injuries should prompt further investigation.[11]

2. Obtunded or uncooperative patients as well as alert patients with physical examination findings consistent with spinal injury should be maintained on spinal precautions until thorough clinical and radiographic evaluation of the spine has been completed, which should occur in an expedited fashion. A prospective study of consecutive blunt trauma patients admitted to a single institution demonstrated 99.75% sensitivity for CT scanning in its ability to clear clinically significant cervical spine injuries. Although the recommendation is that CT be used as a sole modality to radiographically clear the cervical spine in obtunded trauma patients, there is separate clinical evidence to suggest that the spondylotic cervical spine may present a specific clinical category where CT scanning is unreliable in determining stability and will miss clinically significant injuries. In an obtunded or unreliable patient, CT scan has a negative predictive value of up to 90.9% for ligamentous injury and a negative predictive value of 100% for instability in the nonspondylotic patient.[7]

3. In a prospective cohort study comparing the Canadian C-spine rule (CCR) versus the Nexus low-risk criteria in patients with trauma, the sensitivity and specificity of CCR were 99.4% and 40.4%, respectively. The CCR mandates that any patient with a high-risk factor, including age greater than 65, in trauma or dangerous mechanism, or complaints of paresthesias in extremities should proceed to imaging studies. Any patient without a high-risk factor who instead has a low-risk factor allowing for the safe assessment of range of motion, including simple rear-end motor vehicle collision, or sitting position in the Emergency Department, or ambulatory at any time, or delayed onset of neck pain, or absence of midline cervical spine tenderness may proceed to range-of-motion examination, including the ability to rotate the neck actively 45° to the left and to the right. This would indicate a patient whose cervical spine is considered "cleared".

D. **Fracture stability.** As described by White and Panjabi,[12] stability refers to the spine's ability to maintain patterns of displacement and movement under normal physiologic loads without incapacitating pain, progressive deformity, or increasing neurologic deficit. The isolated but unstable spine fracture at the spinal cord level results in complicated management throughout the patient's hospital and posthospital course. Stable fractures are important to recognize in that they are often a marker for other injuries, particularly intrathoracic or intraabdominal injury.

1. **Acute spinal instability** most directly impacts the spine's ability to protect neural elements, including spinal nerves and the spinal cord from further injury, and may be clinically manifested as neurologic deficit or severe intractable pain.

2. **Glacial instability** represents the spine's tendency to deform over time and is manifested by clinical deformity as well as progressive debilitating pain.
   a. Osteoporosis is an underlying medical condition that may result in glacial instability in an otherwise apparently stable fracture pattern.
3. **Radiographic and anatomic features.** Determination of instability varies with the injured spinal segments, with the occipitocervical junction having different characteristics radiographically and anatomically, indicating instability when compared with the subaxial cervical spine, the cervicothoracic junction, the thoracic spine, the thoracolumbar junction, the lumbar spine, and the lumbosacral spine. Each region has unique characteristics and will be discussed as a separate section. Additionally, the spinal cord represents a distinct entity within the spine with unique injury characteristics and will be discussed as a separate section of the spine.

## II. Fractures, Dislocations, and Fracture–Dislocations

A. **Craniocervical junction.** The craniocervical junction, or occipitocervical junction, represents a unique combination of osteologic and ligamentous structures allowing a tremendous range of motion in flexion and extension at the occipital condyles and C1, a tremendous range of rotation at the junction of C1 and C2, and a transition zone between the unconstrained motion at the occipital to C2 levels and the more constrained subaxial cervical spine occurring osteologically through C2.

1. **Craniocervical junction injury patterns**
   a. **Craniocervical dislocation.** Craniocervical dislocations or occipitocervical dislocations represent a loss of ligamentous integrity between the occiput, C1, and C2. This is best identified by the Harris lines,[13,14] with a measurement of greater than 14 mm indicating a craniocervical dislocation.[1] The key feature in understanding these injuries is that the ligamentous constraints linking the occiput to C2 are destroyed in this injury pattern, resulting in global instability. The exact displacement of the skull relative to the dens may be quite fluid and variable depending on the time imaging is obtained. Prior work classifying the dislocation pattern based on the location of the occiput relative to C2 is not useful for determining either prognosis of injury or treatment modalities as any of the displacement patterns represents global instability. The basion to the tip of the dens interval is less than 12 mm in 95% of the patients; greater than 12 mm is considered abnormal. The basion–axial interval is the basion to the posterior dens and is between 4 and 12 mm in 98% of the patients. Greater than 12 mm indicates anterior subluxation, and less than 4 mm indicates posterior subluxation.
      i. **Clinical features.** Wallenberg syndrome is defined by lower cranial nerve deficits (Fig. 12-1). Horner syndrome, cerebellar ataxia, Bell (fifth cranial nerve) cruciate paralysis, and contralateral loss of pain and temperature are they physical signs.[15,16]
      ii. **Additional imaging studies.** CT angiogram to evaluate the vertebral artery given the relative tethering of the vertebral artery around the craniocervical junction is indicated. An MRI including the brain stem and cervical spine is necessary to evaluate for any concurrent cord or brain stem injury as well as for the presence of traumatic dural tear.
      iii. **Acute management.** Sandbag placement around the head with consideration of halo vest placement, as well as airway control to include early elective intubation. Often these injuries are so severe

---

[1]The interested reader is referred to the OTA PowerPoint presentation on Upper Cervical Spine Injuries for diagrammatic representations and further detail.

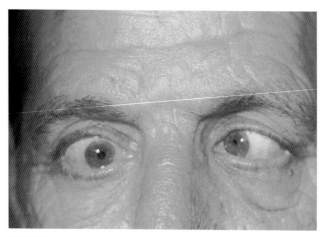

**Figure 12-1.** Right cranial nerve VI palsy. (From Tasman W, Jaeger E. *The Wills Eye Hospital Atlas of Clinical Ophthalmology.* 2nd ed. Lippincott Williams & Wilkins; 2001, with permission.)

that the patient presents with intubation from the field, but if this has not occurred, retropharyngeal swelling can predictably become so severe as to require emergent intubation, which would be associated with a high mortality rate.

iv. **Operative intervention.** In a patient who is otherwise medically stable, the standard of care should be considered, including an occiput to C2 posterior instrumented spinal fusion. Upright radiographs should be obtained before discharge.

v. **Morbidity and mortality.** Craniocervical dislocations in general have historically been associated with a greater than 50% mortality rate, although the promulgation of ATLS techniques and broader penetration of advanced emergency medical services have contributed to an increased survival of patients with these injuries. Additionally, this injury pattern can represent a spectrum, as described by Bellabarba et al.,[15] with a craniocervical sprain representing a less severe form of this injury.

2. **Occipital condyle fractures**
   a. **Type I** represents an impaction fracture with bilateral impaction fractures representing an axially unstable fracture pattern.
   b. **Type II** is an extension of basilar skull fracture and is typically a stable injury.
   c. **Type III** represents an alar ligament avulsion and is potentially highly unstable.[17,18] A 50% missed injury rate is associated with craniocervical dislocations, with one-third of these having neurologic worsening while in the hospital.[15,19]

3. **C1 ring injuries**
   a. **Atlas fractures.** Fractures of the atlas include relatively trivial fractures such as posterior ring fractures associated with hyperextension injuries, unstable injury patterns such as the burst fracture or "Jefferson" fracture (Figs. 12-2 and 12-3), as well as lateral mass fracture separation.
      i. **Imaging.** The key imaging study for assessing C1 ring injuries is the open mouth odontoid view that may be approximated with the coronal plane reconstruction of a thin-cut CT scan. This is used to assess

**Figure 12-2.** Jefferson fracture.

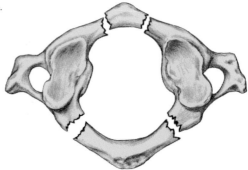

the integrity of the transverse atlantal ligament, which is a key stabilizer of this level. Separation of the lateral masses of greater than 6.9 mm indicates the rupture of the transverse atlantal ligament and an unstable fracture pattern. Additionally, the vertebral artery is at risk for injury, and a CT angiogram is an important study to obtain to evaluate any acute injury. Late instability at this level, if left untreated, puts the patient at risk for a thrombotic cerebrovascular accident.

   ii. **Treatment.** Acute management of these injuries consists of reduction, typically in a halo vest, and operative stabilization of unstable injuries. Nondisplaced fractures may be treated in a cervical collar or a halo and necessitates close clinical follow-up. Although fracture union may be achieved with nonoperative means, there can be resultant atlantoaxial instability that puts the patient at risk for late neurologic deterioration. A fracture separation of the lateral mass frequently results in progressive torticollis if left untreated. Upright radiographs should be obtained before discharge.

4. **Fractures of the axis (C2)**
   a. **Odontoid.** The most common fracture of the second cervical vertebra is a fracture of the odontoid. This column of bone is necessary for rotation at the craniocervical junction. The appropriate mechanics of C1 and C2 are primarily ligamentous restraints, including the transverse

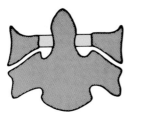
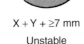

X + Y + ≥7 mm

Stable          Unstable

**Figure 12-3.** Jefferson fractures. When a comminuted fracture of C1 shows bilateral overhang of the lateral masses that total 7 mm or more, rupture of the transverse ligament has probably occurred, rendering the spine unstable. (From White AA III, Panjabi MM. *Clinical Biomechanics of the Spine.* JB Lippincott; 1978:203, with permission.)

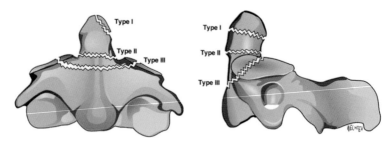

**Figure 12-4.** Odontoid fractures shown in anteroposterior and lateral views. Type I is an oblique fracture through the upper part of the odontoid caused by alar ligament avulsion. Type II is through the base of the odontoid. Type III is through the upper portion of the vertebral body. Illustration by John Wechter.

atlantal ligament and the apical ligaments, as well as an expanse of the posterior longitudinal ligament, which, when combined, makes the cruciate ligaments across the dorsal portion of the dens. Additionally, the tectorial membrane, a continuing expanse of the posterior longitudinal ligament, provides stability between the occiput and C2.

i. **Fracture classification** (Fig. 12-4).

(a) **Type I** odontoid fracture involves the attachment of the apical ligament and represents a potentially unstable craniocervical junction injury. Most commonly, this is actually a nonfused ossicle and an incidental finding. In the acute trauma setting, an occult craniocervical junction injury must be ruled out.

(b) **Type II** odontoid fracture typically involves the midportion of the odontoid and may be subdivided into Type IIA, IIB, and IIC,[20] with ramifications for operative intervention.[2] The hallmark of the Type II odontoid fracture is that it is at high risk for nonunion. The significance of this nonunion needs to be considered in management planning. Low-energy odontoid fractures, typically encountered in the elderly with minor trauma, may be quite tolerant of a nonunion that is otherwise stable in flexion and extension and does not cause debilitating pain. A stable pseudarthrosis is the common result of nonoperative management of these fractures in this patient population. Given the relatively high risk of perioperative mortality and morbidity in elderly patients with an odontoid fracture, a stable pseudarthrosis may be considered a good treatment outcome. Unstable fractures that result in debilitating pain, progressive deformity, neurologic deficit, or risk for progressive neurologic deficit are best treated operatively regardless of patient's age or comorbidities. These injury patterns are often associated with upper cervical cord injuries, as well as the potential for vertebral artery injury, indicating the utilization of MRI, magnetic resonance angiography (MRA), and/or CT angiography. Upright radiographs should be obtained before discharge.

b. Traumatic spondylolisthesis (Fig. 12-5) of the axis (Hangman fracture). Mechanically, this represents a separation of the posterior ring from the vertebral body of C2, typically occurring through the pars that represents a transition zone at C2 from the craniocervical junction to the subaxial cervical spine.

[2]Interested readers are referred to OTA PowerPoint presentation on upper cervical spine injuries for further description and details.

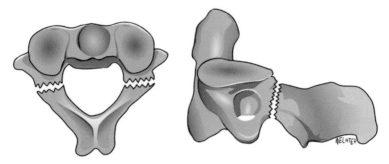

**Figure 12-5.** Effendi Type I fracture. Illustration by John Wechter.

    i. **Type I** fractures through the pars are uncommonly associated with spinal cord injury, and typically may be treated in a closed fashion with a cervical collar or halo thoracic brace.

    ii. **Type II** fractures that involve a portion of the body of C2 are more commonly associated with spinal cord injury because of the translation of the partially intact ring across the spinal canal. This injury may also be treated in a closed fashion. It should be noted that the status of the C2-3 disc is critical in determining appropriate treatment modality as Type IIA fracture tends to displace in traction because of the torn posterior longitudinal ligament and posterior disc.

    iii. **Type III** injury will be grossly unstable in traction.

**B. Subaxial cervical spine.** The subaxial cervical spine begins at the C2-3 articulations and extends down to the cervicothoracic junction, which is essentially the rostral aspect of C7.

    1. **Classification.** The mechanics of fractures in the subaxial cervical spine are similar throughout the region and have been classified by numerous authors with the goal of a system that is both descriptive and prognostic, with the additional characteristic of assisting operative decision-making. Currently, a "perfect" classification system does not exist. The current primary role of classification systems of subaxial cervical spine injuries is that of pedagogical usage. In this regard, the classic Allen–Ferguson description of injuries (Fig. 12-6) combining mechanical loading and displacement is helpful for understanding the injury patterns, as well as for communicating the types of injuries. The columnar theory of Holdsworth continues to have merit and is used in all other classification systems as a basis for describing the injury patterns. This includes an anterior column consisting of the entire vertebral body and disc and a posterior column consisting of the posterior ligamentous complex including the posterior elements. Additional systems have been developed to aid in operative decision-making and include the Subaxial Injury Classification (SLIC) as well as the AO subaxial cervical spine injury classification systems.[21,22] These systems emphasize the importance of the posterior ligamentous complex as a stabilizer.

    2. **Types of injury.** The individual injury patterns include distraction flexion, compression flexion, vertical compression, compression-extension, distraction extension, and lateral bending injuries.

        a. Distraction flexion (Fig. 12-7) injuries are among the most common injuries in the subaxial cervical spine seen in high-energy trauma. These

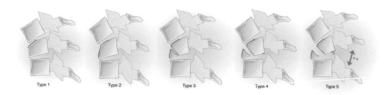

**Figure 12-6.** Allen and Ferguson classification of closed, indirect, fractures, and dislocations of the cervical spine. **A:** Type 1—blunting of anterior–superior vertebral margin. **B:** Type 2—anterior–inferior beaking and loss of anterior vertebral height. **C:** Type 3—fracture of the beak. **D:** Type 4—posterior–inferior vertebral body displacement ≤3 mm into canal. **E:** Type 5—posterior displacement ≥3 mm, with displacement of facets and spinous processes. *Indicates failure of PLL (Posterior Longitudinal Ligament). **Indicates failure of the entire posterior ligament complex.

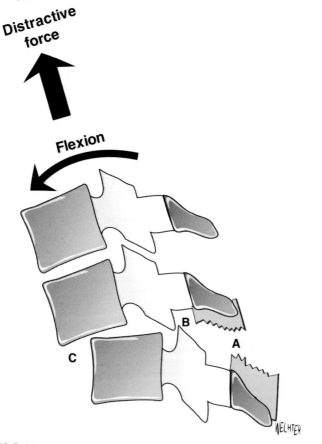

**Figure 12-7.** Distractive-flexion (DF) injury: Posterior ligamentous disruption **(A)** followed by facet subluxation. The facets will progressively sublux and dislocate unilaterally and then bilaterally **(B)**, which leads to the vertebral body displacing anteriorly **(C)**. Illustration by John Wechter.

injuries result from the restrained thorax and unrestrained head in a sudden deceleration, such as when hitting a wall in a motor vehicle. The constellation of injuries in a graded scale in the Allen–Ferguson system represents sequential failure of restraining mechanisms. The injury typically begins dorsally and progresses ventrally as increasing disruption and instability are encountered.

i. **Imaging.** The hallmark of this injury pattern is disruption of the facet joints and widening of the interspinous process distance, with or without subluxation of the vertebral bodies. This is evident on both CT scanning and plain radiographs, but subtle widening of the facet joints and interspinous process distance may be the only indicator of an extremely unstable injury that has spontaneously reduced in the supine position. MRI characteristics include disruption of the supraspinous and interspinous ligament complex with folding or rolling of the ligaments evident, along with disruption of the ligamentum flavum, with folding or rolling of the ligament. Facet joint effusions will also be present, when varying amount of vertebral body increased signal. Less commonly, soft-tissue injury is evident ventral to the cervical spine (Fig. 12-8). Subluxation of

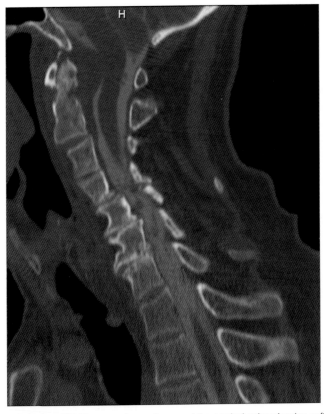

**Figure 12-8.** Computed tomography myelogram of the cervical spine showing soft-tissue mass effect encroaching upon and compressing the spinal cord.

the vertebral bodies is commonly seen when the facet joints begin to uncouple and dislocate. A 25% subluxation of the rostral vertebral body on the caudal vertebral body often represents a unilateral facet fracture or dislocation and is a combined translation and rotation, often resulting in unilateral nerve root injury. Bilateral facet dislocations, or fracture–dislocations, often result in 50% subluxation of the rostral vertebral body on the caudal vertebral body and are most commonly associated with spinal cord injury.

ii. **Treatment.** Management of these injuries in the acute setting is directed toward minimizing further injury to the neural elements, particularly the spinal cord, as well as protecting the patient from the adverse effects related to their spinal cord injury, which will be discussed in the section on spinal cord injury. Closed reduction of facet joint dislocations is often performed under general anesthesia with cervical traction and intraoperative fluoroscopy. Once the facet joints have been reduced, MRI is often performed before definitive surgical stabilization.

iii. Cervical orthoses are indicated for patient transport, and any unstable injury is best managed operatively. Upright **radiographs** should be obtained before discharge.

b. **Compression flexion** (Fig. 12-9) injuries often result in a similar injury pattern to the distraction flexion injuries. However, the posterior

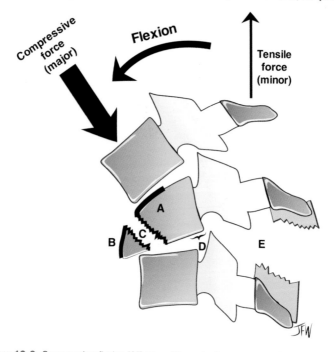

**Figure 12-9.** Compression-flexion (CF) injury: The major force, compression, causes anterior blunting of the vertebral body initially **(A)**, beaking **(B)**, followed by oblique fracture **(C)**, and ultimately posterior translation of the vertebral body **(D)**. In late stages, posterior distractive forces (minor) cause posterior ligamentous failure, manifested radiographically by distraction of the facets and transverse processes **(E)**. Illustration by John Wechter.

ligamentous complex will be variably affected. Severe compression flexion injuries, also known as "teardrop" or "quadrangular" fractures, are highly unstable and represent a failure of the ventral cervical spine as well as the posterior ligamentous complex. Spinal cord injury is commonly associated with this injury pattern, which may be seen typically after a water diving accident. Initial management of these injuries consists of reduction, like the distraction flexion injuries. For injuries not involving the posterior ligamentous complex, nonoperative management of the neurologically intact patient with an orthosis including cervical collars or halo vests may be appropriate, particularly in isolated injuries. In patients with progressive neurologic deficits and an intact posterior ligamentous complex, a ventrally based operative procedure such as a corpectomy would be considered a traditional method of treatment. Injury patterns including disruption of posterior ligamentous complex require an anterior- and posterior-based approach, although isolated posterior approaches using a screw-based construct may be useful in some circumstances. Stand-alone posterior wiring without ventral reconstruction results in loss of stabilization and progressive kyphosis. Upright radiographs should be obtained before discharge.

  c. **Distraction extension** (Fig. 12-10) injuries are typically represented by compression fractures of the posterior elements, including spinous process and lamina, with avulsion fractures ventrally around the disc space. These are typically seen in elderly patients after relatively low-energy falls; hence, osteophyte fractures are commonly identified in this

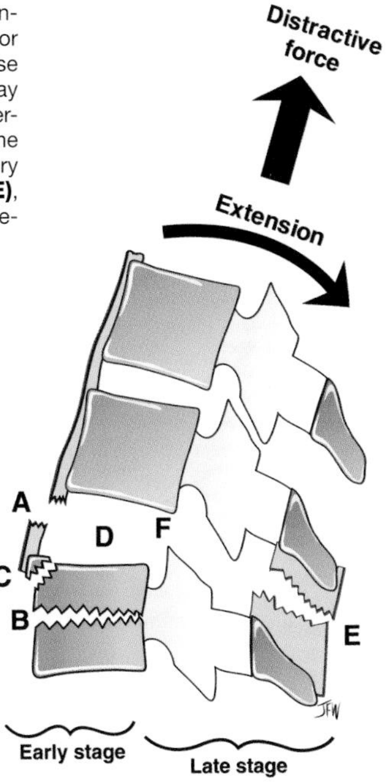

**Figure 12-10.** Distractive–extension (DE) injury: Initially, anterior tension injures the anterior ligamentous complex **(A)** or causes a transverse fracture of the vertebral body **(B)**. There may also be an avulsion fracture of the anterior vertebral margin **(C)**. Radiographic widening of the disc space is often seen **(D)**. Progressive injury involves the posterior ligamentous complex **(E)**, with resultant posterior translation of the vertebral body **(F)**. Illustration by John Wechter.

patient population. These are typically stable injuries but higher-energy fractures may result in frank mechanical instability. This injury pattern is commonly associated with a central cord syndrome, which will be discussed later. Management of these fractures in the acute setting relates to the identification of the fracture that is best characterized on a thin-cut CT scan with sagittal reconstructions, as well as supplemental MRI obtained for any evidence of neurologic deficit or for potential preoperative planning. Operative management of these injuries typically consists of an anterior cervical discectomy and fusion at the injured level. However, the severely spondylotic spine may be better treated with a laminoplasty or laminectomy and instrumented arthrodesis posteriorly if multiple levels need to be addressed. Upright radiographs should be obtained before discharge.

d. **Compression-extension** (Fig. 12-11) injuries present with failure of the posterior elements before the ventral elements, but in the more severe injury patterns presents with complete dislocation of the cervical spine. Lateral flexion injuries typically present as fractures into the foramen transversarium, with higher stage injuries presenting with the potential for lateral mass separations, which may also represent a subtype of extension injury. Lateral mass separations are unstable and

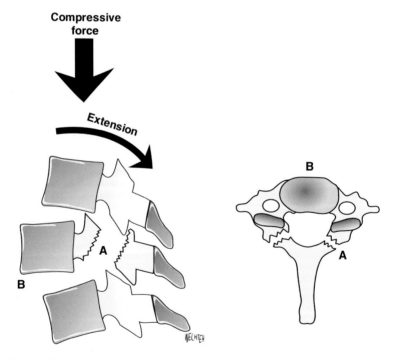

**Figure 12-11.** Compressive–extension (CE) injury: Fracture of the vertebral arch (lamina/pedicle/articular process) occurs first **(A)**, allowing movement of the vertebral body **(B)**, *unilateral* arch disruption allows rotatory subluxation while *bilateral* disruption permits anterior translation of vertebral body. Illustration by John Wechter.

require operative intervention. Fractures into the foramen transversarium are markers for injury of the vertebral artery and require further evaluation including CT angiography.[23] Upright radiographs should be obtained before discharge.

   e. **Vertical compression** (Fig. 12-12) injuries without a flexion or extension component will typically result in either a traumatic disc herniation or a burst fracture. Similar to burst fractures in the thoracolumbar spine, these may be stable or unstable and may be initially managed nonoperatively unless there is neurologic deficit. If the posterior ligamentous complex is intact, these injuries may be managed with a ventral corpectomy only. Upright radiographs should be obtained before discharge.

**C. Cervicothoracic junction.** Cervicothoracic junctional injuries, encompassing the region from C6 to approximately T4, may be classified in the same **manner** as subaxial cervical spine injuries.

   1. **Initial management** is the same, with an attempt at closed reduction being indicated for any neurologically impaired patient. This reduction would typically be undertaken with Gardner–Wells tongs or a halo ring (Fig. 12-13). Closed reduction maneuvers will be difficult to assess at the cervicothoracic junction. Additionally, the traction weight required may often exceed 70 lb.

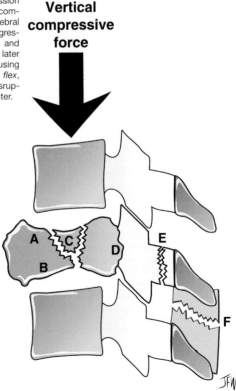

**Figure 12-12.** Vertical compression (VC) injury: The primary vertical compressive force initially causes vertebral cupping **(A, B)**, followed by progressive vertebral comminution **(C)** and retropulsion into the canal **(D)**. In later stages, the neck may *extend*, causing a posterior arch fracture **(E)** or *flex*, causing posterior ligamentous disruption **(F)**. Illustration by John Wechter.

**Vertical compressive force**

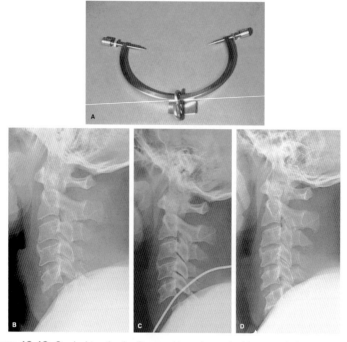

**Figure 12-13.** Cervical traction is often used to reduce spinal fractures before surgical stabilization. **A:** Gardner–Wells tongs are fixated into the skull and weights are applied to these tongs to provide traction. **B, C, D:** A 35-year-old man who was involved in a motor vehicle accident and suffered a spinal cord injury as a result of subluxation with C5-6 bilateral jumped facets. **B:** The initial lateral radiograph shows greater than 50% subluxation of C6 on C7 and bilateral jumped facets at this level. **C:** The patient was placed in 35 lb of cervical traction and the C5-6 interspace widened. **D:** At 50 lb of cervical traction, the facets and the subluxation were reduced. (From Eric D, Schwartz, Adam E, et al. *Spinal Trauma: Imaging, Diagnosis, and Management.* Lippincott Williams & Wilkins; 2007, with permission.)

2. **Imaging** of these injuries is difficult with plain radiography, with plain radiographs being unable to adequately image C7–T1 and the upper thoracic spine extending down to T5 in most patients. A CT scan of the cervical spine with reconstructed images should be considered the standard for imaging of the cervicothoracic junction, and any CT scan of the cervical spine should extend down to T4 to be considered an adequate image.

3. **Orthotic management** is similar to the subaxial cervical spine but requires a junctional thoracic extension to adequately immobilize this region. A halo vest applies improved stabilization of this region, particularly relative to its ability to stabilize the subaxial cervical spine.

4. **Operative management** of fractures in this region will be more commonly approached posteriorly because of the stresses applied at this junction and the need for increased mechanical stability. C6-7 and C7–T1 may be appropriate for anterior approaches, particularly at the C6-7 level. Upright radiographs should be obtained before discharge.

**D. Thoracic spine injuries.** The hallmark of thoracic spine injuries is the associated risk of cardiac or pulmonary injury, and any significant thoracic spine injury must be expected to have an associated pulmonary contusion, particularly when associated with multiple rib fractures. Additionally, any spinal cord injury present in the thoracic spine has a dismal prognosis for recovery. The use of steroids in an attempt to lessen this tends to aggravate the patient's pulmonary condition and results in worsened outcomes, and hence should be avoided.

1. **Initial evaluation** of these injuries includes standard chest X-ray as part of ATLS protocols. A thoracic radiograph may be useful as part of a screening protocol; however, detailed evaluation of the fractures requires a thin-cut CT scan with coronal and sagittal plane reconstructions.

2. **Classification** of thoracic fractures is often a reflection of an extension of the thoracolumbar fracture classification system devised by Denis and is a three-column system consisting of an anterior column, a middle column, and a posterior column. As this is not entirely applicable to the thoracic spine, a fourth column of the thoracic spine, the rib articulation with the sternum, is also described. The posterior ligamentous complex, as in the subaxial cervical spine and cervicothoracic junction, remains the key determinant of mechanical stability at this level.

3. **Operative approaches** remain primarily posterior throughout the **thoracic** spine, particularly with the utilization of extracavitary approaches to the ventral thoracic spine, which are particularly useful in the setting of pathologic fractures related to malignancy. Standing radiographs should be obtained before discharge.

E. **Thoracolumbar fractures.** The thoracolumbar junction is marked by a transition from the stable and relatively immobile thoracic spine to the more mobile lumbar spine. This transition zone is bounded rostrally by the so-called floating ribs at T11 and T12, with the more stable segment being T10 entering into the mechanically true thoracic spine. Caudally, this region is bounded by the rostral extent of L4 at which point we transition into the lumbosacral junction.

1. **Classification** schema applicable to the thoracolumbar spine are inappropriately applied to other regions of the spine. Useful classification schemes in the thoracolumbar spine include the AO classification system as well as the Denis classification system.

a. **AO classification system**

i. **AO Type A** fractures represent axial loading fractures and are typified by compression-type injuries. It should be noted that a "stable" burst fracture represents a spectrum of Type A injuries and that the involvement of the middle column does not significantly affect prognosis. Unstable burst fractures are defined by a greater than 30° relative kyphosis, loss of vertebral body height of greater than 50%, or biplanar deformity on AP X-ray. These are markers for ligamentous complex integrity or loss of ligamentous integrity and are also represented by MRI with evidence of disruption of the posterior ligamentous complex. Stable burst fractures are characterized by a less than 20° to 30° kyphosis, less than 50% lumbar canal compromise, or less than 30% thoracic canal compromise. Relative indications for surgery include a single-level lumbar vertebral body height loss of greater than 50%, single-level thoracic vertebral body height loss of greater than 30%, combined multilevel height loss of greater than 50%, or relative segmental or combined kyphosis of greater than 30°.

ii. **AO Type B** fractures represent flexion or extension injuries with the integrity of the posterior ligamentous complex again being the key factor in determining whether an injury is "stable" or "unstable."

Additional injuries that are important to identify include the hyperextension injuries that are common in patients with ankylosis conditions of the spine. An additional category of injury includes the Chance fracture (Fig. 12-14), which is most commonly seen in pediatric lap belt injuries.

iii. **AO Type C** injuries represent the complex fracture–dislocations and shear injuries, as described by Denis and Holdsworth.[24]

2. **Initial treatment** of thoracolumbar fractures is similar to that described for thoracic fractures, with an initial period of bed rest with log rolling for evaluation of stability and associated injuries, as well as a determination to be made about definitive management. Although definitive management may consist of a prolonged period of bed rest, it is typically only used in extraordinary circumstances where a patient would not otherwise tolerate an intervention. Both fracture healing and neurologic recovery are seen with nonoperative management.[25] Although bracing may be used as an adjunct to nonoperative management, it is not helpful in preventing progressive deformity and should generally only be considered for ambulatory patients. Complications of bracing include deformity and pressure

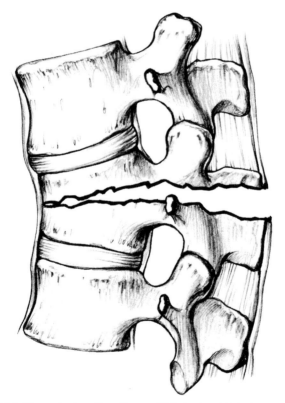

**Figure 12-14.** Chance fracture. (From Hansen ST, Swiontkowski MF. *Orthopaedic Trauma Protocols*. Raven; 1993:221, with permission.)

sores that may be particularly troublesome in the critically ill patient or spinal cord injured patient.

3. **Operative management** includes kyphoplasty for osteoporotic fractures, percutaneous stabilization, as well as formal open procedures with anterior procedures typically performed for injuries associated with spinal cord injury, although posterior-only-based solutions are useful for the management of the spinal cord injured patient as well. Standing radiographs should be obtained before discharge.

**F. Low lumbar and lumbosacral junction injuries**

1. Most commonly, these injuries include transverse process and isolated spinous process fractures that are otherwise considered stable but should be noted as a marker for underlying solid organ or viscous injury. These injuries may be treated with elastic bracing as an adjunct to pain management. Traumatic spondylolisthesis is often encountered in these levels, particularly at L4 and L5, and is most commonly treated nonoperatively with elastic bracing immobilization. Progressive deformity or neurologic deficits are indications for operative intervention. Burst fractures as described for the thoracolumbar region have typically been treated in a nonoperative fashion at these levels. However, late deformity is a particular problem across the lumbosacral junction. As this problem is more and more identified, operative intervention is more commonly undertaken because of the difficulty with nonoperative stabilization across the lumbosacral junction, with braces only being effective down to the rostral extent of L4 and no bracing being effective for preventing deformity progression. Additionally, in the polytraumatized patient, prolonged sitting or supine position results in permanent loss of lumbar lordosis, which leads to a developmental flat back deformity. Because of the typically poor hold in the sacral pedicle screws, iliac fixation is often required for adequate mechanical stabilization across the lumbosacral junction. Standing radiographs should be obtained before discharge.

**G. Sacral fractures**

1. Multiple classification systems exist for the description of sacral fractures and typically involve the transition between the axial skeleton and the appendicular skeleton. Isler and Ganz[26] described the effect of fractures related to the lumbosacral articulations. Roy-Camille et al.[27] identified the axial fractures of the sacral body and their effects. Denis[28] described three zones of injury (Fig. 12-15), with Type I being the sacral ala, Type II being the foraminal zone, and Type III encompassing the central canal. Type III fractures may be subdivided into H-type, U-type, lambda-type, and T-type patterns. Less commonly described but occasionally encountered fractures include the vertical fracture through the S1 body. Fractures of the sacrum may result in neurologic injury in up to 25% of fractures.[29] The L5 root may be injured in Zone 1 injuries as it traverses the anterior–superior border of the S1 vertebral body and sacral ala. Additionally, injury to the anal and urethral sphincters with lower sacral roots may be missed if a detailed neurologic examination is not performed. In the series by Denis et al., 57% of patients with a Zone 3 injury had a neurologic deficit, 28% neurologic injury rate in Zone 2 fractures, and only 6% injury in Zone 1 fractures.

2. Treatment of sacral fractures largely depends on neurologic injury, deformity, and stability of the lumbosacral junction or pelvic ring. Most sacral fractures are associated with pelvic ring injuries and treated to reconstruct the pelvis ring, as discussed in a separate section. Angular kyphosis across the sacrum or comminution of the sacrum associated with sacroiliac (SI) joint dislocation may be well treated with triangular osteosynthesis as

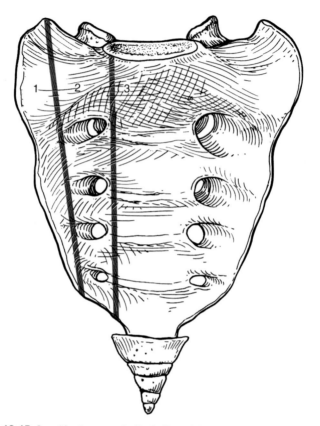

**Figure 12-15.** Sacral fracture zones by Denis. (From John WF, Sam WW, et al. *The Adult and Pediatric Spine.* Lippincott Williams & Wilkins; 2004, with permission.)

described by Schildhauer et al.[30,31] Percutaneous screws for U-type sacral fractures may be associated with progressive angular displacement, and more stable fixation methods such as triangular osteosynthesis should be considered for these injuries. Neurologic injury as an indication for operative intervention should be approached cautiously as 80% of initial nerve injuries improve regardless of treatment modality,[28] and nerve injuries related to transection of the nerve are reported in up to 35% of these injuries, which would not be affected by operative intervention.

**III. Spinal Cord Injury**

The incidence is 10,000 to 12,000 cases per year, with 85% being males 16 to 30 years of age. Fifty percent of all spinal cord injuries are complete. Fifty to sixty percent of spinal cord injuries are cervical, and the immediate mortality for complete cervical spinal cord injury is 50%.[32] (National spine injury.) Expected neurologic recovery, 70% to 85% of patients with complete tetraplegia will gain at least one additional level, and if a patient has a motor grade 2/5 at a given level 1 week out from injury, 100% of patients gain functional strength at the next level down.[33] In incomplete tetraplegia, 90% gain at least one upper extremity motor level,[33] with the majority of improvement seen in the first 6 to 9 months.[34] Ambulation after spinal cord injury can be expected in 46% of the patients with incomplete tetraplegia at 1 year and 76% of incomplete paraplegics at 1 year.[35]

**A. American Spinal Injury Association (ASIA) classification** (Fig. 12-16).

1. **Complete spinal cord injuries.** Injuries at a level of the spinal cord below which there is no sensory or motor function. This is classified as an ASIA A injury. This term is only applicable after spinal shock has resolved.

2. **Incomplete injuries.** These represent injuries to the spinal cord in which there is some motor or sensory function below the level of injury. This preservation of function may be quite subtle, with sacral sparing being the only indicator that the spinal cord is not completely disrupted. This is further classified into ASIA B, C, D, or E.

   a. **ASIA B** injuries represent loss of motor function below the level of the injury with some sensory function present.

   b. **ASIA C** injuries represent some motor function preservation below a muscle grade 3/5.

   c. **ASIA D** injuries represent useful motor function preservation greater than or equal to grade 3/5.

   d. **ASIA E** injuries represent normal motor function.

   e. Incomplete injuries are also described by spinal cord syndromes that include the following:

      i. **Anterior cord syndrome** represents loss of the ventral motor function of the spinal cord with preservation of dorsal sensory function.

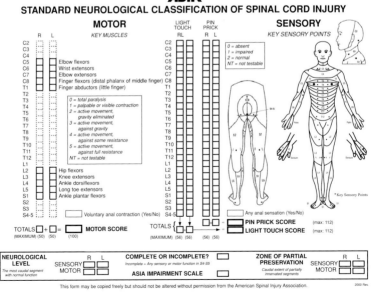

**Figure 12-16.** Standard neurologic classification form for spinal cord injury. (From American Spinal Injury Association. *International Standards for Neurological Classification of Spinal Cord Injury,* Revised 2002. American Spinal Injury Association, with permission.)

ii. **Brown–Sequard syndrome** causes loss of ipsilateral motor and dorsal column function along with contralateral pain and temperature sensation.

iii. **Posterior cord syndrome**, which is uncommonly encountered in trauma, represents a loss of proprioception and other sensory function, with preservation of motor function.

iv. **Central cord syndrome**, commonly seen in hyperextension injuries particularly in the elderly, represents a greater loss of function (including sensory and motor) in the upper extremities than in the lower extremities, although significant impairment in the lower extremities can also be noted in dense central cord syndromes. This has the best prognosis for recovery of any of the incomplete spinal cord syndromes.

B. **Other neurologic syndromes** in trauma to be aware of include the following:

1. **Wallenberg syndrome** (see the section on occipitocervical dislocation)

2. **Conus medullaris syndrome**, an injury occurring at the base of the spinal cord typically at the region between T12 and L1, resulting in relatively normal sensory and motor function except for the sacral roots with loss of bowel and bladder control as well as sensation in the sacral nerve roots. This must be differentiated from a cauda equina syndrome as the cauda equina syndrome has a much better prognosis.

3. **Cauda equina syndrome** typically presents as a bilateral lower extremity loss of sensory and motor function that may or may not include bowel and bladder function.

4. **Transient quadriplegia** (a spinal cord concussion) represents a transient loss in the ability of the spinal cord to transmit neurologic signals but without permanent injury to the spinal cord. Transient quadriplegia typically spontaneously resolves over 48 hours. This is most commonly seen in athletes with some element of congenital stenosis. Multiple episodes of transient quadriplegia are a contraindication to return to play. This must be differentiated from spinal cord injury without radiographic abnormality (SCIWORA).

5. **SCIWORA** is a condition found in pediatric patients because of the differential elasticity of the vertebral column when compared with the spinal cord. These patients present with a spinal cord injury demonstrable on MRI but not on plain radiographs or typically CT scan. This represents a true spinal cord injury and should be differentiated from transient quadriplegia.

C. **Initial management** of the spinal cord injured patient

1. After a detailed neurologic examination with attention to protecting the cervical spine during evaluation with neutral inline stabilization, the patient must be protected from further injury. This is best accomplished in a hospital setting by keeping the patient in a semirigid cervical orthosis (examples include Miami J or Aspen collar) and keeping the patient on flat bed rest for the duration of the further diagnostic work-up. The patient should not be kept on a backboard or sliding board as pressure necrosis can begin quite rapidly, particularly in the spinal cord injured patient with impaired sensation and motor function. The spine board does not provide any improved stabilization over simple bed rest in the hospital setting, and it is a critical patient care step to remove the patient from the spine board as quickly as possible once the patient has been removed from the ambulance. Once the patient has been removed from the spine board, any transfers or rolling must be performed with a team approach to lifting and moving the patient to include maneuvers such as the log roll or six-person lift. This allows the person to be safely transported for further diagnostic

work-up. The primary goal of diagnostic imaging at this point is to evaluate the spine for stability as well as to evaluate the extent of the spinal cord injury. Any patient with a neurologic deficit must have an MRI as part of the diagnostic work-up unless it is otherwise contraindicated.

**D. Definitive management** of spinal cord injury

1. Definitive management of spinal cord injury involves two areas of concern: anatomic and physiologic.

   a. **Anatomic concerns.** The primary anatomic concern is residual spinal cord compression. In dislocated segments, the residual compression may be relieved rapidly by emergent reduction, as discussed earlier. If a reduction has been performed and residual compression persists, or if there is no dislocated segment and residual compression is present, operative intervention is indicated to decompress the spinal cord. The timing of this intervention is a complex discussion beyond the scope of this manual. A secondary consideration after decompression of the neural element is stabilization of unstable segments. The primary goal of stabilization of unstable segments is to create an optimal mechanical environment for the spinal cord to spontaneously heal, particularly in incomplete injuries. Additionally, this prevents progressive deformity or severe intractable pain. Mechanical stabilization is particularly important after decompressive procedures as adequate decompression of the spinal cord in the trauma setting often increases instability in the affected segment. Although exact methods of stabilization are a complex discussion and beyond the scope of this manual, they were briefly discussed earlier.

   b. **Physiologic concerns.** In the acute setting, primary attention must be given to maintaining adequate perfusion of the spinal cord to ensure adequate delivery of oxygen and removal of waste products to optimize spinal cord recovery. Several studies have suggested maintaining a mean arterial pressure of greater than 85 for 5 to 7 days optimizes spinal cord recovery. At a minimum, hypotension must be avoided to prevent a spinal cord infarction or extension of the injury. This may require pharmacologic pressors and is always best accomplished in the intensive care unit (ICU) setting. Currently, the only indicated pharmacologic intervention in the spinal cord injured patient is pressor support, particularly in the patient with neurogenic shock.

2. **Steroids**

   a. Currently, there is no level 1 evidence for the utilization of steroids or any pharmacologic agent for the amelioration of spinal cord injury.[36]

   b. **Shock syndromes associated with spinal cord injury**

      i. **Spinal shock** represents a transient condition that may be described as a "concussion" of the spinal cord or temporary disruption in the ability of the spinal cord to transmit signals. This will be variably associated with permanent injury but will initially manifest itself as a complete injury. This typically resolves by 48 hours but may persist up to 6 weeks. Spinal shock may be associated with, but must be differentiated from, neurogenic shock.

      ii. **Neurogenic shock** is a physiologic condition manifesting itself secondary to disruption of sympathetic pathways controlling blood pressure and heart rate. This will be clinically evident as a relative bradycardia in the setting of hypotension. Initial treatment is volume resuscitation, particularly in the trauma patient who may have combined hypovolemic and neurogenic shock. Pharmacologic management is indicated and helpful in the management of this syndrome and typically involves both alpha and beta agonists.

## IV. Particular Considerations in Spine Trauma

### A. Blunt vertebral artery injury

1. Incidence rate is 33% in a cervical spine fracture–dislocation.[37] Vertebral artery injury incidence, rate of stroke in untreated samples, is up as high as 14% and decreases to near 0% with the institution of antiplatelet therapy.[37]

### B. Gunshot wounds to the spine

1. Gunshot wounds to the spine associated with a perforated viscous are initially treated with antibiotics and evaluated for stability. The stability assessment in gunshot wounds is not the same as that for blunt trauma and can be controversial. A minimum of 2 days of broad-spectrum antibiotics is indicated, with 2 weeks of intravenous (IV) antibiotics for viscous penetrations being ideal. Bullet removal does not appreciably alter outcome and may be associated with an unacceptably high risk of cerebrospinal fluid leak.[38–40]

### C. The stiff spine

1. A spine may become ankylosed through various conditions, including ankylosing spondylitis, diffuse idiopathic skeletal hyperostosis, posttraumatic and postoperative, as well as any number of congenital anomalies. Any patient complaining of pain after trauma in the region of an arthrodesed spine warrants advanced imaging studies to rule out any associated fracture. Fractures associated with the ankylosed spine are presumed to be unstable and in patients with ankylosing spondylitis are highly unstable and associated with a high risk of neurologic deterioration if treated in a nonoperative fashion or if identified in a delayed fashion. (Chapman) Typically, imaging studies include an MRI. However, patients unable to obtain an MRI secondary to pacemakers or other implants or medical stability may be assessed with a bone scan to equal effect. There is limited role for nonoperative management of these types of fractures. However, in selected patients with diffuse idiopathic skeletal hyperostosis, nonoperative management may be successful.

### D. The osteoporotic spine

1. Patients with osteoporosis are at risk for glacial deformity and recurrent insufficiency fractures. These may commonly be missed on plain radiographs and CT, and either a bone scan or MRI is warranted to evaluate for these injuries. There continues to be a role for kyphoplasty in the treatment of the osteoporotic fracture for pain control, structural support, and augmentation of implants in operative interventions.[41] Up to 50% of patients who sustain a fragility fracture of the lumbar spine sustain another vertebral fracture in the same year. Patients should be aware that prior vertebral fracture is the best predictor of subsequent fractures, and treatment for osteoporosis can help prevent this fracture cascade.[42]

## SELECTED HISTORICAL READINGS

Anderson LD, D'Alonzo RT. Fracture of the odontoid process of the axis. *J Bone Joint Surg Am*. 1974;56:1663-1674.

Bohler L. Fracture and dislocation of the spine. In: Bohler L, Bohler J, eds. *The Treatment of Fractures*. 5th ed. Grune & Stratton; 1956.

Bohlman HH. Acute fractures and dislocations of the cervical spine. An analysis of three hundred hospitalized patients and review of the literature. *J Bone Joint Surg Am*. 1979;61:1119-1142.

Braakman R, Vinken PJ. Unilateral facet interlocking in the lower cervical spine. *J Bone Joint Surg Br*. 1967;49:249-257.

Chance GQ. Note on a type of flexion fracture of the spine. *Br J Radiol*. 1948;21:452.

Clawson DK. Low back pain. *Northwest Med*. 1970;69:686-689.

Dawson EG, Smith L. Atlanto-axial subluxation in children due to vertebral anomalies. *J Bone Joint Surg Am.* 1979;61:582-587.

Denis F. The three column spine and its significance in the classification of acute thoracolumbar spinal injuries. *Spine (Phila Pa 1976).* 1983;8(8):817-831.

Dickson JH, Harrington PR, Erwin WD. Results of reduction and stabilization of the severely fractured thoracic and lumbar spine. *J Bone Joint Surg Am.* 1978;60:799-805.

Fielding JW, Cochran GB, Lawsing JF III, et al. Tears of the transverse ligament of the atlas. A clinical and biomechanical study. *J Bone Joint Surg Am.* 1974;56:1683-1691.

Fielding JW, Hensinger RN, Hawkins RJ. Os odontoideum. *J Bone Joint Surg Am.* 1980;62:376-383.

Griswold DM, Albright JA, Schiffman E, et al. Atlanto-axial fusion for instability. *J Bone Joint Surg Am.* 1978;60:285-292.

Holdsworth F. Fractures, dislocations, and fracture-dislocations of the spine. *J Bone Joint Surg Am.* 1970;52:1534-1551.

Hohl M. Soft-tissue injuries of the neck in automobile accidents. Factors influencing prognosis. *J Bone Joint Surg Am.* 1974;56:1675-1682.

Johnson RM, Hart DL, Simmons EF, et al. Cervical orthoses. A study comparing their effectiveness in restricting cervical motion in normal subjects. *J Bone Joint Surg Am.* 1977;59:322-339.

Rand RW, Crandall PH. Central spinal cord syndrome in hyperextension injuries of the cervical spine. *J Bone Joint Surg Am.* 1962;44:1415-1422.

Schatzker J, Rorabeck CH, Waddell JP. Fractures of the dens (odontoid process). An analysis of thirty-seven cases. *J Bone Joint Surg Br.* 1971;53:392-405.

Schneider RC, Livingston KE, Cave AJ, et al. "Hangman's fracture" of the cervical spine. *J Neurosurg.* 1965;22: 141-154.

Spence KF Jr, Decker S, Sell KW. Bursting atlantal fracture associated with rupture of the transverse ligament. *J Bone Joint Surg Am.* 1970;52:543-549.

Stauffer ES. Current concepts review: internal fixation of fractures of the thoracolumbar spine. *J Bone Joint Surg Am.* 1984;76:1136.

## REFERENCES

1. Tan E, Schweitzer ME, Vaccaro L, et al. Is computed tomography of nonvisualized C7-T1 cost-effective? *J Spinal Disord.* 1999;12(6):472-476.

2. Miller CP, Brubacher JW, Biswas D, et al. The incidence of noncontiguous spinal fractures and other traumatic injuries associated with cervical spine fractures: a ten year experience at an academic medical center. *Spine (Phila Pa 1976).* 2011;36(19):1532-1540.

3. Humphry S, Clarke A, Hufton M, et al. Erect radiographs to assess clinical stability in patients with blunt cervical trauma. *JBJS* 94;1-4,2012.

4. Nuñez DB Jr, Zuluaga A, Fuentes-Bernardo DA, et al. Cervical spine trauma: how much more do we learn by routinely using helical CT? *Radiographics.* 1996;16(6):1307-1318.

5. Nuñez DB Jr. Helical CT for the evaluation of cervical vertebral injuries. *Semin Musculoskelet Radiol.* 1998;2(1):19-26.

6. Blackmore CC, Ramsey SD, Mann FA, et al. Cervical spine screening with CT in trauma patients: a cost-effectiveness analysis. *Radiology.* 1999;212(1):117-125.

7. Hogan GJ, Mirvis SE, Shanmuganathan K, et al. Exclusion of unstable cervical spine injury in obtunded patients with blunt trauma: is MR imaging needed when multi-detector row CT findings are normal? *Radiology.* 2005;237(1):106-113.

8. Vaccaro AR, Kreidl KO, Pan W, et al. Usefulness of MRI in isolated upper cervical spine fractures in adults. *J Spinal Disord.* 1998;11(4):289-293.

9. Vaccaro AR, Falatyn SP, Flanders AE, et al. Magnetic resonance evaluation of the intervertebral disc, spinal ligaments, and spinal cord before and after closed traction reduction of cervical spine dislocations. *Spine (Phila Pa 1976).* 1999;24(12):1210-1217.

10. Davis JW, Kaups KL, Cunningham MA, et al. Routine evaluation of the cervical spine in head-injured patients with dynamic fluoroscopy: a reappraisal. *J Trauma.* 2001;50(6): 1044-1047.

11. Stiell IG, Clement CM, McKnight RD, et al. The Canadian C-spine rule versus the NEXUS low-risk criteria in patients with trauma. *N Engl J Med.* 2003;349(26):2510-2518.

12. White AA III, Panjabi MM. *Clinical Biomechanics of the Spine.* JB Lippincott; 1978.

13. Harris JH Jr, Carson GC, Wagner LK. Radiologic diagnosis of traumatic occipitovertebral dissociation: 1. Normal occipitovertebral relationships on lateral radiographs of supine subjects. *AJR Am J Roentgenol.* 1994;162(4):881-886.

14. Harris JH Jr, Carson GC, Wagner LK, et al. Radiologic diagnosis of traumatic occipitoverte-bral dissociation: 2. Comparison of three methods of detecting occipitovertebral relationships on lateral radiographs of supine subjects. *AJR Am J Roentgenol*. 1994;162(4):887-892.

15. Bellabarba C, Mirza SK, West GA, et al. Diagnosis and treatment of craniocervical dislo-cation in a series of 17 consecutive survivors during an 8-year period. *J Neurosurg Spine*. 2006;4(6):429-440.

16. Sweet J, Ammerman J, Deshmukh V, et al. Cruciate paralysis secondary to traumatic atlan-tooccipital dislocation. *J Neurosurg Spine*. 2010;12(1):19-21.

17. Anderson PA, Montesano PX. Morphology and treatment of occipital condyle fractures. *Spine (Phila Pa 1976)*. 1988;13(7):731-736.

18. Tuli S, Tator CH, Fehlings MG, et al. Occipital condyle fractures. *Neurosurgery*. 1997;41(2):368-376.

19. Matava MJ, Whitesides TE Jr, Davis PC. Traumatic atlanto-occipital dislocation with survival. Serial computerized tomography as an aid to diagnosis and reduction: a report of three cases. *Spine (Phila Pa 1976)*. 1993;18(13):1897-1903.

20. Grauer JN, Shafi B, Hilibrand AS, et al. Proposal of a modified, treatment-oriented classifi-cation of odontoid fractures. *Spine J*. 2005;5(2):123-129. doi: 10.1016/j.spinee.2004.09.014

21. Aarabi B, Walters BC, Dhall SS, et al. Subaxial cervical spine injury classification systems. *Neurosurgery*. 2013;72(suppl 3):170-186. doi: 10.1227/NEU.0b013e31828341c5.

22. Vaccaro AR, Koerner JD, Radcliff KE, et al. AOSpine subaxial cervical spine injury classifica-tion system. *Eur Spine J*. 2016;25(7):2173-2184. doi: 10.1007/s00586-015-3831-3

23. Rizzolo SJ, Cotler JM. Unstable cervical spine injuries: specific treatment approaches. *J Am Acad Orthop Surg*. 1993;1(1):57-63.

24. Magerl F, Aebi M, Gertzbein SD, et al. A comprehensive classification of thoracic and lumbar injuries. *Eur Spine J*. 1994;3(4):184-201.

25. Rechtine GR II, Cahill D, Chrin AM. Treatment of thoracolumbar trauma: comparison of com-plications of operative versus nonoperative treatment. *J Spinal Disord*. 1999;12(5):406-409.

26. Isler B, Ganz R. Classification of pelvic ring injuries. *Injury*. 1996;27(suppl 1):3-12.

27. Roy-Camille R, Saillant G, Gagna G, et al. Transverse fracture of the upper sacrum. Suicidal jumper's fracture. *Spine (Phila Pa 1976)*. 1985;10(9):838-845.

28. Kempen DH, Delawi D, Altena MC, et al. Neurologic outcomes after traumatic transverse sacral fractures. *JBJS Reviews*. 2018;6:1-11.

29. Mehta S, Auerbach JD, Born CT, et al. Sacral fractures. *J Am Acad Orthop Surg*. 2006;14(12):656-665.

30. Schildhauer TA, Ledoux WR, Chapman JR, et al. Triangular osteosynthesis and iliosacral screw fixation for unstable sacral fractures: a cadaveric and biomechanical evaluation under cyclic loads. *J Orthop Trauma*. 2003;17(1):22-31.

31. Schildhauer TA, Josten C, Muhr G. Triangular osteosynthesis of vertically unstable sacrum frac-tures: a new concept allowing early weight-bearing. *J Orthop Trauma*. 1998;12(5):307-314.

32. National Spinal Cord Injury Statistical Center. *Annual Report*. University of Alabama; 2003.

33. Zlotolow DA, Bethany L, Pahys JM. Team approach: treatment and rehabilitation of patients with spinal cord injury resulting in tetraplegia. *JBJS Reviews*. 2019;7:1-11.

34. Waters RL, Adkins R, Yakura J, et al. Donal Munro lecture: functional and neurologic recov-ery following acute SCI. *J Spinal Cord Med*. 1998;21(3):195-199.

35. Waters RL, Adkins R, Yakura J, et al. Prediction of ambulatory performance based on motor scores derived from standards of the American Spinal Injury Association. *Arch Phys Med Rehabil*. 1994;75(7):756-760.

36. Consortium for Spinal Cord Medicine. Early acute management in adults with spinal cord injury: a clinical practice guideline for health-care professionals. *J Spinal Cord Med*. 2008;31(4):403-479.

37. Miller P, Fabian TC, Croce MA, et al. Prospective screening for blunt cerebrovascular injuries: analysis of diagnostic modalities and outcomes. *Ann Surg*. 2002;236(3):386-393.

38. Romanick PC, Smith TK, Kopaniky DR, et al. Infection about the spine associated with low-velocity-missile injury to the abdomen. *J Bone Joint Surg Am*. 1985;67(8):1195-1201.

39. Glolaj JP, Eismont FJ. Gunshot wounds to the spine. *JBJS Rev*. 2015;3:1-9.

40. Duz B, Cansever T, Secer HI, et al. Evaluation of spinal missile injuries with respect to bullet trajectory, surgical indications and timing of surgical intervention: a new guideline. *Spine (Phila Pa 1976)*. 2008;33(20):E746-E753.

41. Becker S, Chavanne A, Spitaler R, et al. Assessment of different screw augmentation tech-niques and screw designs in osteoporotic spines. *Eur Spine J*. 2008;17(11):1462-1469.

42. Cloutier D. Osteoporosis: a comprehensive review. *JBJS J Orthop Phys Assist*. 2015;3(3):18-31.

# 13 Disorders and Diseases of the Spine

David Polly

## I. Low Back Pain

Low back pain is ubiquitous in the population, with 50% to 90% of persons having back pain at some point in their lives, and with an annual incidence of 15% to 40%. It is the most common cause of activity limitation in persons younger than 40 years. Fortunately, most patients with back pain will improve with time and will not require extensive studies beyond a good history and physical examination. However, it is important for the clinician to identify patients for which a more urgent or advanced evaluation is needed.

**A. History-taking in the patient with low back pain.** A thorough history is important in determining the etiology of back pain. Important elements of the history are listed in Table 13-1. These elements derived from the history can collectively indicate a specific diagnosis.

Although the common causes are benign and self-limiting, it is extremely important to be aware of "red flags" and rule out the dangerous causes that require urgent and advanced evaluation (Table 13-2). These red flags include progressive neurologic deficits, night pain, pain at rest, fever, and loss of bowel or bladder control. The common patient with back pain is between the ages of 20 and 50 years and has no signs or symptoms of systemic illness. Be on the alert for back pain in the young and the old. A history of night sweats, fever, weight loss, and fatigue may be indicative of a malignancy or an infection. It is also important to elicit any past low back injuries and family history of back problems and to determine forms of treatment that the patient has received and their effects on the pain, as these may provide diagnostic clues.

| TABLE 13-1 | Pertinent Elements of History in a Patient with Low Back Pain |
| --- | --- |
| Duration and onset of pain | |
| Location | |
| Character | |
| Aggravating factors/activities | |
| Alleviating factors/activities | |
| Radiation | |
| Associated numbness, weakness, or bowel or bladder disturbance | |
| Temporality | |
| Constitutional symptoms | |
| Prior back injury and surgery | |
| Treatment received and response to treatment | |
| Review of systems | |

| TABLE 13-2 | "Red Flags" in Patients Presenting with Back Pain |
|---|---|
| Concern for malignancy | |
| Age > 50 | |
| Previous history of cancer | |
| Unexplained weight loss | |
| Pain unrelieved by bed rest | |
| Pain lasting > 1 mo | |
| Failure to improve within 1 mo | |
| Acute trauma | |
| Concern for infection | |
| Erythrocyte sedimentation rate > 20 mm | |
| Intravenous drug abuse | |
| Urinary tract infection | |
| Skin infection | |
| Fever | |
| Concern for compression fracture | |
| Corticosteroid use | |
| Concern for neurologic problem | |
| Sciatica | |
| New bowel or bladder incontinence | |

B. **Physical examination.** The physical examination complements a good history in the process of arriving at a differential diagnosis. The examination begins with observing the patient's gait as well as the body position chosen by the patient (patients with acute sciatica may choose to avoid sitting in a slouched position, as this places extra pressure on the impinged nerve root). The back should be exposed, and one should look for any redness or warmth and hairy patches or skin defects. The presence of muscle atrophy or asymmetry should also be noted. Next, the range of motion of the spine is tested. Pain that is aggravated by flexion generally indicates a disc problem, whereas pain that is aggravated by extension points to stenosis, facet arthritis, or spondylolysis. Palpation should then be performed. Spinous process tenderness may indicate an acute osteoporotic fracture, whereas tenderness in the area of the posterior superior iliac spine indicates pain from the sacroiliac (SI) joint. A palpable step-off between the spinous processes indicates a spondylolisthesis. A complete motor and sensory examination including deep tendon reflex testing is essential. Dermatomal sensory deficits and muscle weakness may show a pattern, indicating impingement of a specific nerve. A straight-leg raise is generally performed with the patient in the supine position, but can be done first with the patient in the seated position when the patient's physical symptoms seem disingenuous. In patients where there is a concern for cauda equina syndrome (CES), a rectal examination and perianal sensation pinprick testing should be performed. Finally, an examination of the hip joint should be routinely performed, as there is significant overlap in clinical picture between hip and spine disorders. To evaluate the SI joint, there are several key tests. The Fortin finger test is where the patient points directly to the posterior–superior iliac spine. The five physical examination tests are flexion abduction external rotation (FABER), thigh thrust, pelvic gapping, pelvic compression, and Gaenslen's test. It is useful to identify the posterior hip joint to the patient (this is number 1) and then the posterior–superior iliac spine (PSIS—this is number 2). When performing the tests, asking the patient if it hurts at #1 or #2 helps to clearly define a positive or negative test result. If three or more are positive, there is an 85% positive predictive value that the SI joint is symptomatic.[1]

**C. Causes of low back pain.** Low back pain is a symptom, not a disease, and the pathologic basis of the pain frequently lies outside the spine.

1. **Vascular back pain.** Abdominal aortic aneurysms or peripheral vascular disease may give rise to backache or symptoms resembling sciatica.
2. **Neurogenic back pain.** Tension, irritation, and compression of lumbar nerves and roots may cause pain down one or both legs. Lesions anywhere along the central nervous system, particularly of the spine, may present with back and leg pain.
3. **Viscerogenic back pain.** Low back pain may be derived from disorders of the organs in the lesser abdominal sac, the pelvis, or the retroperitoneal structures, such as the pancreas and kidneys. Renal stones can present as severe back pain.
4. **Psychogenic back pain.** Clouding and confusion of the clinical picture by emotional overtones may be seen. A pure psychogenic component is rare.
5. **Spondylogenic back pain.** Common conditions causing spondylogenic back pain are outlined in Table 13-3.
   a. **Disc degeneration** is by far the most common cause of back pain. Disc degeneration may occur anywhere along the spine and produce neck pain, thoracic spine pain, or lumbar or low back pain. Disc degeneration may be associated with nerve root irritation, which would then result in radicular leg pain.
      i. **Anatomy.** The spine provides stability and a central axis for the limbs that are attached. The spine has to move, transmit weight,

| TABLE 13-3 | Common Conditions Causing Spondylogenic Back Pain |
|---|---|
| 1. Disc degeneration | |
| 2. Spondylolisthesis | |
| 3. Trauma | |
| Myofascial sprains/strains | |
| Fractures | |
| 4. Infection (bacterial tuberculosis) | |
| 5. Tumor (benign, malignant, metastatic) | |
| 6. Rheumatologic | |
| Ankylosing spondylitis/spondyloarthropathy | |
| Fibrositis/fibromyalgia | |
| 7. Metabolic | |
| Osteoporosis | |
| Osteomalacia | |
| Paget's disease | |

and protect the spinal cord. When viewed from the side, the thoracic spine is concave forward (kyphosis), and the cervical and lumbar regions are concave backward (lordosis).

ii. **Vertebral components**

(a) Each segment of the vertebral column transmits weight through the vertebral body anteriorly and the facet joints posteriorly. Between adjacent bodies are the intervertebral discs, which are firmly attached to the vertebrae. The disc consists of an outer annulus fibrosus, which is made up of concentric layers of fibrous tissue, and a central avascular nucleus pulposus, which consists of a hydrophilic gel made of protein, polysaccharide, collagen fibrils, sparsely chondroid cells, and water (88%). The spinal cord and cauda equina are found within the spinal canal. At each intervertebral level, nerve roots leave the canal through the intervertebral foramina.

(b) A functional spinal unit or motion segment consists of two adjacent vertebrae and the intervertebral disc. It forms a three-joint complex with the disc in front and two facet joints posteriorly. The facet joints, like other joints in the body, have capsules, ligaments, muscles, nerves, and vessels. Changes in one joint affect the other two. Narrowing of the disc space, therefore, may result in malalignment of the facet joints and, with time, may lead to wear-and-tear degenerative arthritic changes in those joints.

iii. Normal aging is associated with a gradual dehydration of the disc. The nucleus pulposus becomes desiccated, and the annulus fibrosus develops fissures parallel to the vertebral end plates running mainly posteriorly. Small herniations of nuclear material may squeeze through the annular fissures and may also penetrate the vertebral end plates to produce Schmorl's nodes. If the nuclear material impinges against a nerve, it may produce nerve root irritation. The flattening and collapse of the disc results in osteophytes along the vertebral bodies. Malalignment and displacement of the facet joints is an inevitable consequence of disc space collapse, leading to osteophytes that may narrow the lateral or subarticular recess of the spinal canal or the intervertebral foramina. This narrowing of the spinal canal or the intervertebral neural foramina is called *spinal stenosis*.

iv. Pain from disc degeneration without nerve root irritation. There are three patterns of low back pain associated with disc degeneration: **acute incapacitating backache**, which may occur a few times in a person's life and not be a regular problem; **recurrent aggravating backache**, which is the most common type and is associated with regular periods of recurrence and remission of back pain; and **chronic persisting backache**, which is most difficult to treat.

(a) The back pain associated with disc degeneration is mechanical in nature. It is aggravated or brought on by activity and relieved by rest in the acute phase. Rest as a treatment strategy should be limited to 1 to 2 days. There may be a referred component of back pain into the legs, but this is usually down the back of the legs and rarely goes beyond the knee. The low back pain may be due to periods of hard work, prolonged standing or walking, or prolonged sitting in one position. The peak incidence of back pain in the general population is in the 40s and 50s. This is the time when the discs have collapsed and there is relative instability at the motion segment. The natural history, however, is for the spine to eventually stabilize with increased fibrosis around the facet joints and the discs. As the patient gets older, the physical demands become less and the spine becomes stiffer. The incidence of mechanical back pain, therefore, declines beyond the 60s.

(b) Patients who give a history of fever, weight loss, malaise, night and rest pain, morning stiffness, and colicky pain should be carefully evaluated for the possibilities of infection, tumor, spondyloarthropathy, or viscerogenic back pain.

v. **Disc degeneration with root irritation**

(a) Nerve root irritation and compression may be due to an **acute disc herniation** or may be associated with **spinal stenosis**. Acute disc herniation results in **sciatica**, which typically presents with severe, incapacitating pain that radiates from the back down the leg. There may be associated paresthesias, numbness, motor weakness, or reflex changes. The pain may be constant and is frequently aggravated by coughing, sneezing, and straining. Intradiscal pressure is increased in a bending and sitting position, especially if lifting is performed, therefore increasing the amount of pain. The pain may be lessened by lying down.

(b) The **most frequent sites of disc herniation** are within the spinal canal, resulting in impingement of the traversing nerve root. Less commonly, a disc herniation may be located laterally in the foramen, resulting in impingement of the exiting nerve root. The leg pain or sciatica is accompanied by signs of nerve root tension, which can be diagnosed by a positive straight-leg raising test, bowstring sign, or Lasègue test.

(c) In **spinal stenosis**, the leg pain or radicular pain is brought on by prolonged walking or standing (neurogenic claudication). The pain may be associated with paresthesias and is relieved by sitting or stooping. There are few physical findings or neurologic deficits unless the condition has been present for a long time and is advanced. Neurogenic claudication associated with spinal stenosis should be distinguished from vascular claudication caused by peripheral vascular disease.

vi. **Neurology of the lower extremities.** The nerve roots leaving the spine at each segmental level may be affected by acute disc herniations, bony foraminal stenosis, or stenosis associated with both soft-tissue and bony compression. The nerve root may be affected within the central spinal canal either in the subarticular recess or in the intervertebral foramen. Both the traversing and the exiting nerve roots may be affected. For example, the L5 root traverses below the L4–L5 disc level and exits laterally under the pedicle of L5. The S1 nerve root traverses below the L5–S1 disc level and exits laterally under the pedicle of S1. The location of the disc herniation will determine which nerve root is affected. Posterior lateral disc herniations generally affect the nerve root at the traversing level. The less-common lateral recess and foraminal disc herniations affect the exiting nerve root at the affected level. For instance, an L4–L5 posterior lateral disc herniation would affect the L5 nerve root. A foraminal herniation at that L4–L5 level would affect the L4 nerve root. It is important to correlate the patient's symptoms and physical findings with the abnormalities seen on radiographs, magnetic resonance imaging (MRI) scans, and computed tomography (CT) studies. It is important, therefore, to have knowledge of the nerve roots and their distal innervation. The main nerve roots are listed in Table 13-4.

b. **Sacroiliac joint pain.** 15% to 30% of low back pain is actually from the SI joint. **Physical** examination can reliably identify this.

i. **Imaging studies**

(a) **Radiographs** may appear normal or demonstrate disc space narrowing, osteophyte formation, or instability on lateral flexion and

| TABLE 13-4 | Neurology of the Lower Extremity | | |
|---|---|---|---|
| Root | Muscles | Sensation | Reflex |
| L2 | Hip flexion | Anterior thigh (proximal) | None |
| L3 | Knee extension (quadriceps) | Anterior thigh (distal) | Patellar |
| L4 | Anterior tibialis | Medial leg | Patellar |
| L5 | Extensor hallucis longus | Lateral leg and dorsum of foot | None |
| S1 | Gastrocsoleus peroneus longus and brevis | Lateral foot | Achilles |

extension views. They are usually not helpful in acute low pain, because it has been demonstrated that there is no clear-cut correlation between low back pain and the presence of disc space narrowing on plain radiographs.[2] In general, radiographs should not be obtained until the pain has persisted 6 weeks because most pain episodes are self-limited. However, in patients with red flags such as rest pain, night pain, or a history of significant trauma, anteroposterior and lateral X-rays should be obtained.

(b) **Myelograms** are invasive and are less commonly used. They may be used in combination with CT scans in patients who have complex problems or **who** have had multiple surgeries and instrumentation. Myelograms should be ordered either by or with direct consultation of the treating surgeon.

(c) **CT scans** are generally helpful when MRI scans cannot be obtained. They provide excellent definition of the osseous anatomy. Pars fractures are **clearly** identified with CT scans.

(d) **MRI scans** of the lumbar spine are noninvasive, provide detailed **anatomic** imaging, and show compromise of neural structures.

(e) **Bone scans** of the spine and pelvis are useful if tumor and infection are suspected, although these abnormalities can also be picked up easily on an MRI scan. A single-photon emission computed tomography (SPECT) scan will distinguish between a symptomatic and an asymptomatic spondylolysis.

(f) **Indications for imaging acutely in low back pain.** Acute imaging is indicated only if there is a history of trauma, concern for infection or tumor, presence of a neurologic deficit, suspicion for osteoporosis, and acute fracture.

c. **Spondylolisthesis.** Spondylolisthesis is the forward slippage of one vertebra on another. Spondylolysis is the presence of a bony defect of the pars interarticularis, which may result in spondylolisthesis. The incidence of spondylolysis/spondylolisthesis in the asymptomatic population is 3% to 5%. Spondylolysis and spondylolisthesis are common causes of back pain in children and adolescents. It is unclear how common this entity results in back pain in adult patients. Factors that indicate a higher probability of slip progression in children and adolescents include female gender, skeletal immaturity (pregrowth spurt), and greater than 50% slip. These patients must be followed much more closely, particularly if they are gymnasts or perform other activities that place extra stress on their posterior–lateral elements.

  i. **Classification**
    (a) **Dysplastic**
    (b) **Isthmic**

    (c) **Traumatic**
    (d) **Pathologic**
    (e) **Degenerative**

  ii. **Dysplastic spondylolisthesis** is caused by congenital abnormality of the lumbosacral articulation, including deficiency and malorientation of the facets. **Isthmic spondylolisthesis** results from a defect in the pars interarticularis, allowing forward slippage of the vertebrae. It may be related to an acute fracture, a fatigue fracture, or an elongation or attenuation of an intact pars interarticularis. **Traumatic spondylolisthesis** is caused by an acute fracture of the pedicle, lamina, or facet. **Pathologic spondylolisthesis** results from an attenuation of the pedicle caused by the weakness of bone (e.g., osteogenesis imperfecta). The most common type is **degenerative spondylolisthesis**, which results from degeneration of the disc and facet joints, resulting in instability.

  iii. The **Meyerding grading system** is used to indicate the percentage of displacement of the superior vertebral body on the inferior vertebral body as follows: grade I, 0% to 25%; grade II, 25% to 50%; grade III, 50% to 75%; grade IV, 75% to 100%; and grade V, greater than 100% spondyloptosis.

  iv. **Etiology.** The initial onset of a spondylosis lesion occurs at approximately 8 years of age. History of minor trauma may exist. The onset of symptoms coincides closely with either the adolescent growth spurt or the repetitive athletic activity. It is thought to originate in a stress or fatigue fracture. The shear stresses are greater on the pars interarticularis when the spine is extended. Such stresses are seen with certain activities (e.g., back walkovers in gymnastics, carrying heavy backpacks, heavy lifting).

  v. **Clinical findings in isthmic spondylolisthesis.** Patients who are symptomatic present with an insidious onset of low back pain during the adolescent growth spurt that may also radiate to the buttocks of posterior thighs. The pain is noted to be exacerbated by extension of the lumbar spine. Inspection of the back for scoliosis should be performed. A few patients do have nerve root or radicular pain in the lower extremities. Hamstring tightness or spasm is commonly found in symptomatic patients. A palpable step-off may be felt at the level of the slip.

  vi. Anteroposterior and lateral radiographs are helpful in making the diagnosis to demonstrate the slip. An undisplaced spondylolysis is best seen on the oblique views of the lumbar spine. The "Scottie dog" sign describes the appearance of the facet joints and pars interarticularis on the oblique radiographs. A break in the "Scottie dog" neck represents the pars fracture in spondylolysis. For the young patient with back pain felt to be due to spondylolysis/spondylolisthesis, it is important to institute activity modification and close follow-up. If symptoms persist, then consultation is advised. Bracing may be considered if there is persistent pain that is not resolved by activity modification. There is no urgency about surgical treatment of spondylolisthesis unless serial radiographs have demonstrated progression of the slip or if there is a significant neurologic impairment.

**D. Treatment**

  1. **Treatment of acute nonradicular back pain.** The key elements of initial treatment include analgesia and patient education. Use of nonsteroidal antiinflammatory drugs (NSAIDs) as the first-line treatment for back pain

has demonstrated benefit.[3,4] The addition of short duration treatment (several days) with muscle spasm medication appears beneficial.[5,6] The use of muscle relaxants in conjunction with NSAIDs appears to have a beneficial effect.[7] Patients with more severe pain may require opioid medication, but this should be used judiciously and tapered as the pain subsides.

In the past, activity modification and bed rest had been advocated for acute low back pain management. However, studies have shown that bed rest provides no benefit over maintaining activities as tolerated and may in fact have detrimental effects.[8,9]

There is no definitive evidence supporting the effectiveness of physical therapy in acute low back pain treatment, although aerobic exercise has a positive correlation with spine health.[10] Manual therapy (such as chiropractic, osteopathic, or physical therapy applied manual techniques) appears to shorten the duration and intensity of symptoms.[11] There is no role for surgery in the treatment of acute, low back pain. The use of guidelines appears to have some benefit, but has had variable use to date.[12]

2. **Treatment of acute sciatica.** Initial treatment is directed at making the symptoms tolerable for the patient until the natural history of improvement occurs. This involves the **use** of NSAIDs and muscle relaxants as necessary. The use of short-term oral steroids can also be effective for severe sciatica. Opioid medication can be given in severe cases, but no longer than 7 days. The exception to this nonoperative approach is in patients with CES, where surgical decompression is required within 24 to 48 hours of onset to maximize the probability of neurologic recovery.[13,14] Progressive neurologic deterioration without CES is also a relative indication for expedited surgery. There is recent evidence that transforaminal epidural steroid injections (ESIs) may avoid surgery in a number of patients.[15]

If unacceptable pain persists at 4 to 6 weeks, then surgical treatment is of benefit. A recent randomized trial comparing operative and nonoperative treatment for acute disc herniation showed superior outcomes with surgical management.[16]

3. **Treatment of lumbar spinal stenosis.** Neurogenic claudication is a chronic disease that develops slowly, but is usually progressive.[17] Given its insidious course, it is always reasonable to consider nonoperative options first. In addition, most patients are older and may have comorbidities that make them poor surgical candidates. Nonoperative measures include NSAIDs and physical therapy. ESIs may be given three to four times in a 6-month period. The data to support the efficacy of nonoperative treatment are limited.

In patients with severe pain and functional loss, surgical intervention may be considered. The benefit of lumbar decompression over nonoperative treatment in patients with at least 12 weeks of persistent symptoms has been shown in recent randomized trials.[18,19]

In patients with both lumbar stenosis and degenerative spondylolisthesis, there are good data indicating the benefit of decompression and fusion.[20–22] There is much debate about the benefit of spinal instrumentation in combination with fusion. Spinal instrumentation increases the fusion rate. Successful fusion provides better clinical results than do pseudarthrosis.[20]

4. **Treatment of chronic low back pain.** There are differences in natural history, treatment, and prognosis between acute and chronic low back pain. The treatment of chronic back pain is a challenging and controversial subject.[23] The difficulty lies in diagnosing the specific pain generator. There are many confounding variables, such as workers compensation,

smoking, litigation, diabetes, and psychological issues.[24-27] The pain generator could be disc degeneration, facet degeneration, chemically mediated nerve irritation, or other as yet undefined mechanisms.[28] Because these patients are such a variable cohort, conflicting data arise from studies with highly variable entry criteria.

There is great variability in recommended nonoperative treatment with highly variable results. There is consensus that **education** is a vital component of treatment.[29-32] Patients should be taught proper posture, correct spine biomechanics in everyday activities, and the dos and don'ts of back care. The use of **exercise programs** focusing on core strengthening and flexibility exercises has demonstrated benefit in these patients.[33,34] Medications that are used for chronic back pain include **NSAIDs, muscle relaxants, and antidepressants**.[4,6,35] Fluoroscopic-guided lumbar injections are frequently used in patients with lumbar disc herniation or lumbar stenosis before surgery is considered. Foraminal injections are an effective treatment option for relieving radicular symptoms associated foraminal stenosis. Lumbar facet arthritis is often treated with lumbar facet joint injections and radiofrequency ablation of the nerves that innervate the facet joint.

Judicious use of opioid medication may be considered in patients with severe debilitating pain, with the awareness of the potential for dependence.

There is also variability in surgical treatment recommendations ranging from uninstrumented posterior fusion, instrumented posterior fusion, various interbody fusion techniques, and minimally invasive techniques using these same strategies to the newest technologies for motion preservation, such as artificial disc replacement or posterior ligamentous tethering devices. A prospective randomized trial looking at chronic low back pain treatment demonstrated the effectiveness of surgery compared with nonoperative treatment,[36] indicating that surgery is an option in patients with persistent disabling pain who have exhausted nonoperative measures.

For patients who have SI pain, nonoperative treatment is the first-line therapy. There is limited quality of evidence for nonsurgical management effectiveness; however, it is lower cost and lower risk. If nonoperative treatment fails, then minimally invasive surgical treatment is reasonable (Polly[37] INSITE 2-year results, Dengler[38] iMIA 2-year results).

## II. Deformities of the Spine

There are three basic types of spinal deformity: **scoliosis, kyphosis**, and **lordosis**.

### A. Scoliosis

1. Scoliosis is a side-to-side curvature when the spine is viewed in the coronal plane. This deformity may be flexible and reactive, or fixed and structural. In the former, there is no structural change, and the deformity is correctable. There are three causes of a flexible scoliosis: **postural, compensatory** (to another curve, pelvic tilt, or short leg), and **sciatic**. In structural scoliosis, there is a three-dimensional deformity. The vertebrae are deformed and are rotated toward each other. The resulting rotation of all the attachments and appendages of the vertebrae, such as ribs and processes, results in asymmetry of the body, waistline, and paravertebral prominences, as well as shoulder elevation.

2. The broad **categories of structural scoliosis** are as follows:
   a. Idiopathic (infantile, juvenile, and adolescent)
   b. Osteopathic (congenital)
   c. Neuropathic (cerebral palsy, poliomyelitis)
   d. Myopathic (muscular dystrophies)
   e. Connective tissue (Marfan syndrome, Ehlers-Danlos syndrome)
   f. Neurofibromatosis

3. Scoliosis is also seen in other disease processes, such as spinal cord injuries, infections, metabolic disorders, and tumors.
4. **Curve types**
   a. A **structural curve** is a segment of the spine with lateral curvature lacking normal flexibility.
   b. A **primary curve** is the first or earliest of several curves to appear. A compensatory curve is a curve above or below a major curve. It may progress to become a fixed or secondary curve.
5. **Adolescent idiopathic scoliosis.** This is the most common type and has no known cause. It presents around puberty and may progress until skeletal maturity has been reached. There may be one, two, or three curves occurring most frequently in the thoracic and lumbar spine.
   a. **Risk factors for progression of adolescent idiopathic scoliosis.** Progression is related to the size of the curve, area of the spine involved, and physiologic age of a patient. Large thoracic curves progress to a greater degree than single lumbar or thoracolumbar curves. The younger the skeletal age, the more likely the curve progression. Progression is less likely to progress in boys than in girls.
6. **Clinical findings.** Presentation of a painless deformity occurs between the ages of 10 and 15 years. If severe and persistent pain is present, the possibility of a tumor (most commonly osteoid osteoma), sciatic scoliosis, or spondylolysis should be considered. The rotational deformity is more noticeable on forward flexion, creating a paravertebral prominence. Other clinical features include shoulder elevation, neckline prominence on side asymmetric waistline, or prominent hip. The term *spinal imbalance* refers to the head or the trunk being off-center with respect to the pelvis. Clinically, this can best be measured by dropping a plumb line from the base of the skull. Any deviation of the line from the gluteal cleft measures the amount of spinal imbalance to the left or right. A complete history and physical examination is performed to exclude other causes of scoliosis.
   a. The **history** of a patient with spinal deformity should include age when the deformity was first noted, the perinatal history, age at menarche, and the family history of scoliosis. In children and adolescents, scoliosis is generally not painful. If persistent pain is present, appropriate diagnostic tests should be performed to exclude bony or spinal tumor, herniated discs, or other abnormalities. The patient is examined undraped, except for undershorts, and asymmetries in the shoulder, scapular, waistline, and pelvic region are identified. The balance of the thoracic area over the pelvis is assessed. The C7 plumb line test is used to evaluate the balance of the head over the pelvis and the range of motion of the spine in flexion and extension. Side bending is also observed. The patient should also be inspected from the side for the evaluation of kyphosis or lordosis. The forward bend test is useful to identify areas of asymmetry in the paravertebral areas. Prominence of the scapula or rib on one side is called a "rib hump." A complete neurologic examination should be performed. Pubertal stages in girls and boys are assessed. Leg length from the anterior–superior iliac spine to the medial malleoli is measured. The lower extremities are evaluated for deformities or contractures.
7. **Radiographic evaluation** includes full-length views of the entire spine in a standing position. The angle of curvature is measured. The size of the curve is measured by the **Cobb method**. The upper and lower end vertebrae are identified. These are the vertebrae that are maximally tilted into the curve. A line is drawn along the superior end plate of the upper end vertebra, and a second line is drawn parallel the inferior end plate of

the lower end vertebra. Perpendicular lines are drawn from these lines. The intersection of the two perpendicular lines is the Cobb angle. Radiographs are also used to evaluate the degree of skeletal maturity. The **Risser classification** measures skeletal maturity based on the degree of iliac apophysis ossification from anterolateral to posteromedial.

8. **Treatment.** The natural history of these curves varies. Some curves remain the same, others progress, and yet others progress relentlessly. The goal of treatment is to prevent curve progression. Serial radiographs are obtained every 4 months until skeletal maturity. Risk of curve progression is highest in younger patients with larger curves.

   a. **Bracing** is indicated in the growing patient with curves of 20° to 40°. Bracing the body and torso indirectly exerts forces on the spine (e.g., pressure pads on ribs attached to convex vertebrae) and may prevent further curve progression, but does not straighten the curvature.

   b. **Surgery** is indicated for curves greater than 40° in the skeletally immature patient who has failed conservative treatment. Anterior or posterior instrumentation is performed to correct the curvature and stabilize the spine. Bone grafting is added to achieve spinal fusion.

   c. **Kyphosis**

      i. The gentle posterior curvature of the normal thoracic spine when viewed from the side (sagittal plane) is kyphosis. The normal range is 20° to 40°. Excessive posterior curvature beyond normal is also referred to as *kyphosis*.

      ii. **Adolescent round back** (postural kyphosis) is a flexible deformity evenly distributed throughout the thoracic spine and without any structural changes. It may be due to lax ligaments or poor muscle tone and is associated with other postural defects, such as flat feet. Treatment is the same as for Scheuermann kyphosis.

      iii. **Structural kyphosis** refers to stiff curves with vertebral wedging. It is seen in Scheuermann disease and osteoporosis (round back of old age). This type of kyphosis has underlying structural change and usually has a local sharp posterior angulation, also termed *kyphus*, which may also be seen in fracture or infection.

      iv. **Classification**
         (a) **Postural kyphosis**
         (b) Scheuermann disease
         (c) Myelomeningocele
         (d) Traumatic kyphosis
         (e) Postsurgical kyphosis
         (f) Postradiation kyphosis
         (g) Metabolic disorders
         (h) Skeletal dysplasia
         (i) Tumors

      v. **Scheuermann disease (adolescent kyphosis).** This is a growth disorder of uncertain etiology involving the vertebral growth plates.

   d. **Clinical findings**

      i. There are two types based on location. The **classic form** of Scheuermann disease occurs in the thoracic spine. Criteria for diagnosis include wedging of at least 5° of three adjacent vertebrae and end-plate irregularity. This type is twice as common in girls as in boys. The painless deformity is usually first noticed by parents. Pain may occur, but is a rare symptom. Onset is usually around 10 years of age. A distinct hump at the apex of the kyphosis is frequently noted. The deformity is accentuated on forward flexion, and its rigidity prevents correction on extension.

    ii. The **lumbar form** of Scheuermann disease occurs more commonly in adolescent boys. They present with chronic mechanical lumbar pain, which may improve with maturation.

    iii. The Cobb method of measuring kyphosis is used to measure the degree of angulation, and a value greater than 45° to 50° in the thoracic spine is significant.

9. **Treatment.** A progressive kyphosis of the thoracic spine in a skeletally immature patient is treated with a **Milwaukee brace** until maturity. Surgery is reserved for cases with curves greater than 75° that have pain or are unresponsive to bracing. Lumbar Scheuermann disease is not responsive to bracing. It is treated by exercises and antiinflammatories if painful.

## REFERENCES

1. Petersen T, Laslett M, Juhl C. Clinical classification in low back pain: best-evidence diagnostic rules based on systematic reviews. *BMC Musculoskelet Disord.* 2017;18(1):188.
2. Boden SD. The use of radiographic imaging studies in the evaluation of patients who have degenerative disorders of the lumbar spine. *J Bone Joint Surg Am.* 1996;78:114-124.
3. van Tulder MW, Scholten RJ, Koes BW, et al. Nonsteroidal anti-inflammatory drugs for low back pain: a systematic review within the framework of the Cochrane Collaboration Back Review Group. *Spine (Phila Pa 1976).* 2000;25:2501-2513.
4. Koes BW, Scholten RJ, Mens JM, et al. Efficacy of non-steroidal anti-inflammatory drugs for low back pain: a systematic review of randomised clinical trials. *Ann Rheum Dis.* 1997;56:214-223.
5. Browning R, Jackson JL, O'Malley PG. Cyclobenzaprine and back pain: a meta-analysis. *Arch Intern Med.* 2001;161:1613-1620.
6. Deyo RA. Drug therapy for back pain. Which drugs help which patients? *Spine (Phila Pa 1976).* 1996;21:2840-2849; discussion 2849-2850.
7. Cherkin DC, Wheeler KJ, Barlow W, et al. Medication use for low back pain in primary care. *Spine (Phila Pa 1976).* 1998;23:607-614.
8. Malmivaara A, Häkkinen U, Aro T, et al. The treatment of acute low back pain—bed rest, exercises, or ordinary activity? *N Engl J Med.* 1995;332:351-355.
9. Hagen KB, Hilde G, Jamtvedt G, et al. The Cochrane review of bed rest for acute low back pain and sciatica. *Spine (Phila Pa 1976).* 2000;25:2932-2939.
10. van Tulder M, Malmivaara A, Esmail R, et al. Exercise therapy for low back pain: a systematic review within the framework of the Cochrane collaboration back review group. *Spine (Phila Pa 1976).* 2000;25:2784-2796.
11. Cherkin DC, Deyo RA, Battié M, et al. A comparison of physical therapy, chiropractic manipulation, and provision of an educational booklet for the treatment of patients with low back pain. *N Engl J Med.* 1998;339:1021-1029.
12. McGuirk B, King W, Govind J, et al. Safety, efficacy, and cost effectiveness of evidence-based guidelines for the management of acute low back pain in primary care. *Spine (Phila Pa 1976).* 2001;26:2615-2622.
13. Ahn UM, Ahn NU, Buchowski JM, et al. Cauda equina syndrome secondary to lumbar disc herniation: a meta-analysis of surgical outcomes. *Spine (Phila Pa 1976).* 2000;25:1515-1522.
14. Kohles SS, Kohles DA, Karp AP, et al. Time-dependent surgical outcomes following cauda equina syndrome diagnosis: comments on a meta-analysis. *Spine (Phila Pa 1976).* 2004;29:1281-1287.
15. Riew KD, Yin Y, Gilula L, et al. The effect of nerve-root injections on the need for operative treatment of lumbar radicular pain. A prospective, randomized, controlled, double-blind study. *J Bone Joint Surg Am.* 2000;82:1589-1593.
16. Weinstein JN, Lurie JD, Tosteson TD, et al. Surgical versus nonoperative treatment for lumbar disc herniation: four-year results for the Spine Patient Outcomes Research Trial (SPORT). *Spine (Phila Pa 1976).* 2008;33:2789-2800.
17. Spivak JM. Degenerative lumbar spinal stenosis. *J Bone Joint Surg Am.* 1998;80:1053-1066.
18. Weinstein JN, Tosteson TD, Lurie JD, et al. Surgical versus nonsurgical therapy for lumbar spinal stenosis. *N Engl J Med.* 2008;358:794-810.
19. Weinstein JN, Tosteson TD, Lurie JD, et al. Surgical versus nonoperative treatment for lumbar spinal stenosis four-year results of the Spine Patient Outcomes Research Trial. *Spine (Phila Pa 1976).* 2010;35:1329-1338.

20. Kornblum MB, Fischgrund JS, Herkowitz HN, et al. Degenerative lumbar spondylolisthesis with spinal stenosis: a prospective long-term study comparing fusion and pseudarthrosis. *Spine (Phila Pa 1976).* 2004;29:726-733; discussion 733-734.

21. Knaub MA, Won DS, McGuire R, et al. Lumbar spinal stenosis: indications for arthrodesis and spinal instrumentation. *Instr Course Lect.* 2005;54:313-319.

22. Berven S, Deeptee J, O'Neill C, et al. Team approach: degenerative spinal deformity. *JBJS Rev.* 2017;5:1-9.

23. Hanley EN Jr, David SM. Lumbar arthrodesis for the treatment of back pain. *J Bone Joint Surg Am.* 1999;81:716-730.

24. Guest GH, Drummond PD. Effect of compensation on emotional state and disability in chronic back pain. *Pain.* 1992;48:125-130.

25. Koleck M, Mazaux JM, Rascle N, et al. Psycho-social factors and coping strategies as predictors of chronic evolution and quality of life in patients with low back pain: a prospective study. *Eur J Pain.* 2006;10:1-11.

26. Blake C, Garrett M. Impact of litigation on quality of life outcomes in patients with chronic low back pain. *Ir J Med Sci.* 1997;166:124-126.

27. Goldberg MS, Scott SC, Mayo NE. A review of the association between cigarette smoking and the development of nonspecific back pain and related outcomes. *Spine (Phila Pa 1976).* 2000;25:995-1014.

28. Luoma K, Riihimäki H, Luukkonen R, et al. Low back pain in relation to lumbar disc degeneration. *Spine (Phila Pa 1976).* 2000;25:487-492.

29. Albaladejo C, Kovacs FM, Royuela A, et al. The efficacy of a short education program and a short physiotherapy program for treating low back pain in primary care: a cluster randomized trial. *Spine (Phila Pa 1976).* 2010;35:483-496.

30. George SZ, Teyhen DS, Wu SS, et al. Psychosocial education improves low back pain beliefs: results from a cluster randomized clinical trial (NCT00373009) in a primary prevention setting. *Eur Spine J.* 2009;18:1050-1058.

31. Andrade SC, Araújo AG, Vilar MJ. Back school for patients with non-specific chronic low-back pain: benefits from the association of an exercise program with patient's education. *Acta Reumatol Port.* 2008;33:443-450.

32. Tavafian SS, Jamshidi A, Mohammad K, et al. Low back pain education and short term quality of life: a randomized trial. *BMC Musculoskelet Disord.* 2007;8:21.

33. Casazza BA, Young JL, Herring SA. The role of exercise in the prevention and management of acute low back pain. *Occup Med.* 1998;13:47-60.

34. Anshel MH, Russell KG. Effect of aerobic and strength training on pain tolerance, pain appraisal and mood of unfit males as a function of pain location. *J Sports Sci.* 1994;12:535-547.

35. Alcoff J, Jones E, Rust P, et al. Controlled trial of imipramine for chronic low back pain. *J Fam Pract.* 1982;14:841-846.

36. Fritzell P, Hägg O, Wessberg P, et al. 2001 Volvo Award Winner in Clinical Studies: lumbar fusion versus nonsurgical treatment for chronic low back pain: a multicenter randomized controlled trial from the Swedish Lumbar Spine Study Group. *Spine (Phila Pa 1976).* 2001;26:2521-2532; discussion 2532-2534.

37. Polly DW, Swofford J, Whang PG, et al. Two-year outcomes from a randomized controlled trial of minimally invasive sacroiliac treatment vs. non-surgical management for sacroiliac joint dysfunction. *Int J Spine Surg.* 2016;10:28.

38. Dengler J, Kools D, Pflugmacher R, et al. Randomized trial of sacroiliac joint arthrodesis compared with conservative management for chronic low back pain attributed to the sacroiliac joint. *J Bone Joint Surg Am.* 2019;101(5):400-411.

# 14

# Fractures of the Clavicle

Peter A. Cole and Temi Ogunleye

## I. General Information

A. **Anatomy, epidemiology, and mechanism.** The clavicle is the main stabilizer between the axial and appendicular skeleton. It is wider and tubular proximally as seen in an axial X-ray projection, but flattens toward its distal end in the anteroposterior (AP) plane. Any force absorbed by the upper extremity transmits to the thorax through the clavicle. Its S-shaped curve accommodates the axial and rotational forces that act upon it, as well as those of elevation and flexion–extension through the sternoclavicular joint proximally and acromioclavicular joint distally. This fact, in addition to its superficial location, explains why it is vulnerable to injury. It has been estimated to be one of the most commonly fractured bones, at 3.8% of all fractures.[1]

Whereas older, classic articles[2,3] on clavicle fractures indicated that nonunion after fracture occurred less than 1% of the time, many contemporary series have revealed a higher rate. A systematic review of 2,144 clavicle fractures by Zlowodzki et al.[4] detailed a 15.1% nonunion rate in displaced clavicle fractures. Risk factors for nonunion include advancing age, female gender, completely displaced clavicle fractures with no bony contact, distal clavicle fractures, and comminuted fractures.[5] These variables do not provide absolute indications for surgery, but should be taken into consideration for treatment decision-making.

Most often, clavicle fractures result from a blow to the shoulder, such as during a fall to the turf, although they may also result from a direct hit to the collarbone. These fractures are commonly seen in all ages, but especially now in the osteoporotic elderly as lifestyles have become more active. The incidence of clavicular fractures in men aged 65 and 80 is 49.4 and 61.2 per 100,000 population/year, respectively, and in woman aged 65 and 80, 61.2 and 106.6 per 100,000 population/year, respectively.[6]

B. **Classification.** Allman[7] classified these fractures according to whether they were proximal, middle, or distal one-third injuries and noted that the middle one-third fracture was by far the most common. More recently, the Arbeitsgemeinschaft für Osteosynthesefragen (AO)/Orthopaedic Trauma Association (OTA) has updated their fracture classification, which includes several new subsets of clavicular fractures.[8] Eighty percent of clavicular fractures occur in the mid-diaphysis, whereas 15% are in the distal one-third and 5% in the proximal one-third.

C. Distal one-third clavicle fractures should be characterized further as to whether they are intraarticular or extraarticular and whether the clavicular shaft is displaced superiorly, which would imply disruption of the coracoclavicular ligaments.[2,9]

## II. Diagnosis

A. **History and physical examination.** The patient presents with pain and deformity localized to the clavicle, often accompanied by ecchymosis and tenting of the skin. The deformity common to the middle third fracture is caused by the proximal diaphyseal fragment being pulled by the sternocleidomastoid muscle. The deformity is accentuated by the weight of gravity on the upper extremity pulling downward on the distal fragment. Examination will frequently reveal bony crepitus and should include inspection of the skin for punctures or lacerations consistent with an open fracture. As the clavicle is directly anterior to the brachial plexus and the subclavian vessels, examination should also include neurovascular assessment, particularly in injuries associated with high-energy mechanisms.

**B. Radiographs.** A standard AP view of the clavicle usually confirms the diagnosis of a fracture. Adding 15° of tilt to the X-ray gantry (caudad for posteroanterior [PA]; cephalad for AP) aids fracture visualization by limiting overlying structures in the X-ray field. Radiographic protocols must be defined to better describe displacement, and a well-accepted protocol has not been widely adopted; however, a single AP view is not adequate for assessment.

At our institution, the senior author instituted a protocol for more accurate assessment of fracture displacement. A bilateral panoramic view of both shoulders to measure clavicular shortening is performed (Fig. 14-1) in addition to a supine and upright AP view of the shoulder to assess dynamic displacement (Fig. 14-2). Upright films often reveal many times greater displacement and angulation; thus, this X-ray is the more relevant position for measurement when the patient can tolerate. Fracture location, degree of comminution, and displacement (both vertical translation and medialization) should be assessed. These factors are used to determine how the patient will be managed. Often, in the setting of polytrauma, a chest X-ray provides the initial radiographic diagnosis. Surrounding structures such as the scapula and ribs should be inspected for injury as well.

Repeat X-rays of the shoulder are warranted on a weekly basis for the first 3 weeks if nonoperative treatment is chosen because clavicle fractures have a propensity to displace and shorten in the early peri-injury period.[10]

**III. Treatment**

**A. Nonoperative.** Extraarticular fractures displaced less than 1 cm should be treated with a simple sling for comfort. A figure 8 strapping splint has been used historically but has largely been abandoned as there is no evidence suggesting either technique is superior in terms of radiographic and functional outcomes.[11] In 2015, a randomized controlled trial that included both adults and pediatric clavicle fractures found that use of the broad-arm simple sling offers similar functional outcomes and union rate when compared to the

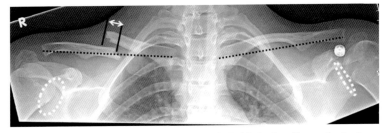

**Figure 14-1.** Panoramic clavicle view of a midshaft clavicle fracture. Two methods of measuring shortening are illustrated. Measuring the difference in clavicle length has been shown to have a high interreader reliability; however, it is imperative that the X-ray technician ensures proper patient position when taking the X-ray. In this particular view, the lengths of the injured and uninjured clavicle are almost equivalent, while there is clearly enough fragment medialization to consider operative management. Comparing glenoid fossa symmetry is helpful in assessing the presence of rotation in the patient or shoulder.

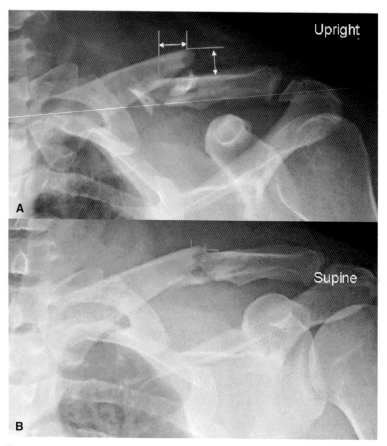

**Figure 14-2. A:** Anteroposterior (AP) clavicle view with patient upright at the time of X-ray. There is marked medialization and vertical displacement of the clavicle fracture. **B:** AP clavicle view was obtained the same day with the patient supine. The fracture is minimally displaced in this position. Obtaining both upright and supine views is helpful to appreciate fracture stability as well as the amount of displacement.

figure 8 sling. However, the key difference is that the simple sling provides better pain relief, and therefore the study advocates its use in midshaft fractures of the clavicle.[12] Intraarticular distal clavicle fractures most often warrant nonoperative treatment if the coracoclavicular ligaments are intact and there remains some cortical apposition between fragments. In the case of intraarticular clavicle fractures, the patient should be warned of the possibility of arthritic symptoms. This outcome can be treated on a delayed basis with distal clavicle resection. In children, a couple of weeks of relative immobilization is all it takes before callus begins to provide the splinting necessary for healing of the bone ends. Despite displacement, preadolescents should be treated nonoperatively in all cases on account of their remodeling potential. In adults, 3 to 4 weeks of such immobilization will provide the same relief. Patients can then begin to advance their motion and shoulder use as allowed by symptoms.

**B. Operative.** There are several indications for operative management of clavicle fractures.

1. The clearest indication is the case of an open fracture, which requires irrigation, debridement, and stabilization. The most common form of internal fixation is with plate and screws.

2. Fractures lateral to the coracoid may be associated with torn coracoclavicular ligaments, in which case the shaft of the clavicle tends to displace superiorly. This injury variant is associated with a higher rate of nonunion. Conservative management should be discussed with the patient and placed in the context of the patient's activity level, hand dominance, age, and comorbidities. If this lateral fracture variant is displaced more than 1 cm, strong consideration should be given to openly reduce and fix the fracture. Numerous fixation techniques exist; however, the optimal technique is highly dependent on the size of the lateral fragment, intraarticular extension, and presence of associated ligament injury. There are several choices of technique and implants for treating distal clavicle fractures. Two such implants include the Hook Plate (Synthes USA, Paoli, PA), and the Endo Button (Arthrex, Naples, FL), but simple tension band wiring techniques can also be successfully used.

   A multicenter randomized controlled trial showed a lower nonunion rate after plate fixation of fully displaced midshaft clavicle fractures compared with nonoperative treatment in a sling, but this study found that there was no difference in functional outcomes or general symptoms and limitations.[13] Distal clavicle locking plates from several manufacturers that are precontoured and have the capacity for locking screws to capture the small or comminuted distal fragments are widely available.

3. Another relative indication for surgery is medialization more than 2 cm, as determined by the amount of overriding of the clavicle shaft fragments (Figs. 14-1 and 14-3). McKee et al.[14] documented poorer performance on endurance testing and DASH scores in patients with more than 2 cm of shortening. In addition, McKee et al. have shown that corrective osteotomy for symptomatic malunions can improve function and strength.[15]

4. If the neck of the scapula (glenoid) is fractured along with the clavicle, this is also a relative indication for surgery. In such a circumstance, a displaced clavicle fracture should be fixed to stabilize the "floating shoulder." This injury complex implies that the glenohumeral joint has no support and is one type of a double disruption of the superior shoulder suspensory

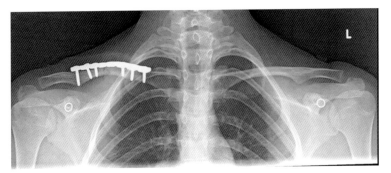

**Figure 14-3.** Postoperative X-rays of fracture illustrated in **Fig. 14-1**. A 2.7 limited-contact dynamic compression (LCDC) plate with six locking screws was used. At least six cortices of fixation should be obtained on either side of the fracture for adequate stability.

complex.[16] Other authors have suggested the alternative of scapula fixation in that setting instead, and yet others have advocated fixation of both injuries.[17-21] The senior author's preference is to treat minimally displaced double lesions nonoperatively and to treat both the clavicle and scapula when displaced, with open reduction and internal fixation, which allows for immediate postoperative mobility.

**C. Follow-up.** Patients should be followed weekly for the first 3 weeks after injury to monitor healing and ensure further displacement has not occurred. Patients need reassurance that discomfort, crepitus, and deformity are expected during this phase of healing. The patient should be instructed to avoid forward flexion and horizontal adduction maneuvers during this healing phase to avoid displacement. After this juncture, passive and gentle active range of motion should be encouraged, as well as light lifting, guided by the patient's symptoms. Most often, excellent function is restored by 3 months postinjury, at which time all restrictions can be lifted assuming healing has been demonstrated radiographically. Radiographic healing can certainly take many more weeks in the elderly.

**D. Complications.** Complications do occur following operative and nonoperative intervention. Rates of nonunion and symptomatic malunion following nonoperative treatment may be higher than previously thought. A meta-analysis of recent studies showed that the rate of nonunion of displaced midshaft clavicular fractures was 15.1% after nonoperative care compared with 2.2% after plate fixation.[4] In 2017, a clavicle trial was performed on 332 patients with displaced midshaft clavicular fractures that concluded that the cumulative nonunion rate was 15%, which is consistent with the nonunion rate described in previous literature.[22] Intrinsic risk factors for nonunion include advancing age and female gender. Extrinsic factors include lack of cortical apposition and presence of comminution. In addition, patients should be counseled from the beginning that they should anticipate a lump in the region of the fracture if treated nonoperatively. Operative complications are predominately related to implant irritation requiring hardware removal; however, infection, nonunion, and implant failure have all been reported. In addition, there is a remote potential for catastrophic complications, such as pneumothorax or neurovascular injury. A study performed by McKnight et al. investigated postoperative complication rates after surgical management of nonunions compared with complication rates after open reduction internal fixation (ORIF) of acute fractures. The authors demonstrated a more than twofold increase in short-term complications and more than threefold increase of wound complication in the nonunion cohort.[23]

## Regions Hospital and the University of Minnesota Recommendations

### Clavicle Fractures

**Diagnosis:** Supine and upright 15° cephalad oblique view and a panoramic AP view of both shoulders to measure shortening

**Nonoperative treatment:** Sling for comfort: 2–4 weeks, institute range-of-motion exercises at 2 weeks and advance motion, strengthening, and function as allowed by symptoms. Begin removal of all restrictions after 3 months, depending on age and radiographic evidence for healing

**Indications for surgery:** Open fractures, vascular injuries, nonunions, or initial displacement of greater than 2 cm. Relative indications are displaced distal fractures, comminuted fractures, and simple fractures with no bony contact

**Recommended technique:** Anteroinferior plate of the clavicle after open reduction in slender patients, patients with simple transverse or short oblique patterns, or patients who use packs or straps over their shoulder. Superior plating is used in larger patients, comminuted fractures, and for nonunions owing to the biomechanical advantage on the tension side of this bone. Although many precontoured and locking plates can be used, 3.5 limited-contact dynamic compression (LCDC) plates for larger patients and 2.7 dynamic compression plates for small patients and adolescents are sufficient as well.

## REFERENCES

1. Court-Brown CM, Aitken SA, Forward D, et al. The epidemiology of fractures. In: Bucholz RW, ed. *Fractures in Adults.* 7th ed. Lippincott Williams & Wilkins; 2009.
2. Neer CS II. Nonunion of the clavicle. *J Am Med Assoc.* 1960;172:1006-1011.
3. Rowe CR. An atlas of anatomy and treatment of mid-clavicular fractures. *Clin Orthop Relat Res.* 1968;58:29-42.
4. Zlowodzki M, Zelle BA, Cole PA, Jeray K, McKee MD. Treatment of acute midshaft clavicle fractures: systematic review of 2144 fractures: on behalf of the Evidence-Based Orthopaedic Trauma Working Group. *J Orthop Trauma.* 2005;19(7):504-507.
5. Robinson CM, Court-Brown CM, McQueen MM, Wakefield AE. Estimating the risk of nonunion following nonoperative treatment of a clavicular fracture. *J Bone Joint Surg Am.* 2004;86-A(7):1359-1365.
6. Court-Brown CM, McQueen MM. Global forum: fractures in the elderly. *J Bone Joint Surg.* 2016;98(9):e36(1-7).
7. Allman FL Jr. Fractures and ligamentous injuries of the clavicle and its articulation. *J Bone Joint Surg Am.* 1967;49(4):774-784.
8. Meinberg E, Agel J, Roberts C, Karam M, Kellam J. Fracture and dislocation classification compendium—2018. *J Orthop Trauma.* 2018;32:S1-S10.
9. Robinson CM. Fractures of the clavicle in the adult. Epidemiology and classification. *J Bone Joint Surg Br.* 1998;80(3):476-484.
10. Plocher EK, Anavian J, Vang S, Cole PA. Progressive displacement of clavicular fractures in the early postinjury period. *J Trauma.* 2011;70(5):1263-1267.
11. Andersen K, Jensen PO, Lauritzen J. Treatment of clavicular fractures. Figure-of-eight bandage versus a simple sling. *Acta Orthop Scand.* 1987;58(1):71-74.
12. Ersen A, Atalar AC, Birisik F, Saglam Y, Demirhan M. Comparison of simple arm sling and figure of eight clavicular bandage for midshaft clavicular fractures: a randomised controlled study. *Bone Joint J.* 2015;97-B(11):1562-1565.
13. Woltz S, Stegeman S, Krijnen P, et al. Plate fixation compared with nonoperative treatment for displaced midshaft clavicular fractures: a multicenter randomized controlled trial. *J Bone Joint Surg Am.* 2017;99:106-112.
14. McKee MD, Pedersen EM, Jones C, et al. Deficits following nonoperative treatment of displaced midshaft clavicular fractures. *J Bone Joint Surg Am.* 2006;88(1):35-40.
15. McKee MD, Wild LM, Schemitsch EH. Midshaft malunions of the clavicle. Surgical technique. *J Bone Joint Surg Am.* 2004;86-A(suppl 1):37-43.
16. Goss TP. Double disruptions of the superior shoulder suspensory complex. *J Orthop Trauma.* 1993;7(2):99-106.
17. Cole PA, Gauger EM, Schroder LK. Management of scapula fractures. *J Am Acad Orthop Surg.* 2012;20:130-141.
18. Ramos L, Mencía R, Alonso A, Ferrández L. Conservative treatment of ipsilateral fractures of the scapula and clavicle. *J Trauma.* 1997;42(2):239-242.
19. Edwards SG, Whittle AP, Wood GW II. Nonoperative treatment of ipsilateral fractures of the scapula and clavicle. *J Bone Joint Surg Am.* 2000;82(6):774-780.
20. Leung KS, Lam TP. Open reduction and internal fixation of ipsilateral fractures of the scapular neck and clavicle. *J Bone Joint Surg Am.* 1993;75(7):1015-1018.

21. Herscovici D Jr. Open reduction and internal fixation of ipsilateral fractures of the scapular neck and clavicle. *J Bone Joint Surg Am.* 1994;76(7):1112-1113.
22. Ahrens P, Garlick N, Barber J, Tims EM; Clavicle Trial Collaborative Group. The clavicle trial: a multicenter randomized controlled trial comparing operative with nonoperative treatment of displaced midshaft clavicle fractures. *J Bone Joint Surg Am.* 2017;99:1345-1354.
23. McKnight B, Heckmann N, Hill JR, et al. Surgical management of midshaft clavicle nonunions is associated with a higher rate of short-term complications compared with acute fractures. *J Shoulder Elbow Surg.* 2016;25(9):1412-1417.

## SELECTED HISTORICAL READINGS

Neer CS II. Fractures of the distal third of the clavicle. *Clin Orthop Relat Res.* 1968;58:43-50.

# 15

# Sternoclavicular and Acromioclavicular Joint Injuries

Peter A. Cole and Temi Ogunleye

## I. Sternoclavicular Injuries

### A. General information

1. **Anatomy and mechanism.** The sternoclavicular (SC) joint is a diarthrodial joint between the medial clavicle and the clavicular notch of the sternum. Although there is little intrinsic osseous stability, the SC ligaments are reinforced by the costoclavicular ligaments, intraarticular disc ligament, interclavicular ligament, and joint capsule. Because of strong ligamentous support, injuries to the SC joint are rare, representing only 3% of shoulder girdle injuries.[1] In a quantitative anatomic description of the SC joint and its surrounding muscles, Lee et al. described the sternothyroid and sternohyoid inserting immediately posterior and inferior to the SC joint. They provide a definable layer between the posterior aspect of the SC joint and mediastinal structures.[2]

The SC joint is the only true articulation between the axial and appendicular skeleton and allows for motion in all planes. The majority of scapulothoracic motion occurs through the SC joint, which is capable of approximately 50° of upward elevation, 30° of combined anterior–posterior (AP) motion, and 30° of rotation around its long axis[3] (Fig. 15-1).

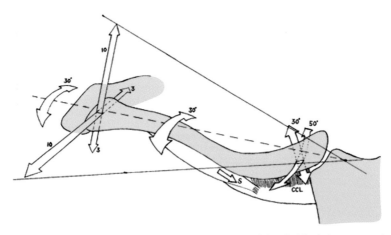

**Figure 15-1.** Diagram showing the relative displacement of the clavicle during movement of the shoulder. The lateral clavicle may translate in the cephalocaudal and anteroposterior planes. The medial clavicle must be able to translate in these planes and also rotate by as much as between 40° and 50° during overhead movement. CCL, costoclavicular ligament; S, subclavius. (From Sewell MD, Al-Hadithy N, Leu AL, et al. Instability of the sternoclavicular joint: current concepts in classification, treatment and outcomes. *Bone Joint J.* 2013;95:721-731, needs permission.)

The clavicle is the first long bone to ossify (fifth week in utero); however, the medial epiphysis is the last long bone ossification center to appear (18 to 20 years) and the last epiphysis to close (23 to 25 years).[4]

An SC injury usually represents a high-energy event; therefore, other injuries should be expected. Owing to the posterior proximity of critical structures such as the great vessels, phrenic and vagus nerves, trachea, and esophagus, associated injuries should be diagnosed promptly; vascular injury to the vessels preferably with a computed tomography (CT) angiogram.

The mechanism of injury can be from either a direct or an indirect force applied to the shoulder. A direct blow to the anteromedial clavicle can result in a posterior dislocation. In an indirect mechanism, a medial force vector compresses the shoulder and loads the SC joint. If the medial force drives the scapula posteriorly (retracted) along the thorax, the SC joint dislocates anteriorly, and if driven anteriorly (protracted), the SC joint dislocates posteriorly.

2. **Classification.** SC joint injuries can be classified by several ways, including the degree of instability, timing, direction, and cause.[1] The SC joint may sustain a simple sprain that is stable but painful, joint instability and subluxation, or frank dislocation, depending on the degree of ligament disruption.[5] More importantly, SC dislocations are described according to the direction of dislocation, **anterior or posterior** dislocation. Anterior dislocations are more common and less often associated with other injuries.

An important point to distinguish is the possibility of a medial clavicular physeal fracture that can displace anteriorly or posteriorly as well, thus mimicking a dislocation. This should be suspected in patients with SC joint injuries who are under 25 years of age. Most of these injuries heal and remodel without surgical intervention.[1]

As an aside, there is an atraumatic type of dislocation due to ligamentous laxity, which can manifest in arthritis, but emphasis in this chapter remains on the traumatic variety.

**B. Diagnosis**

1. **History and physical examination.** After inquiring regarding the mechanism of injury, the patient should be asked about the presence of shortness of breath and difficulty breathing or swallowing, particularly upon recognition of a posterior dislocation. Hoarseness, persistent cough, and stridor should be documented. Patients may have distended neck veins secondary to local venous congestion. Pain is well localized and associated with swelling and ecchymosis. There is usually a palpable and mobile prominence just anterior and lateral to the sternal notch in the case of an anterior dislocation, or perhaps a puckering of the skin with a sense of fluctuance due to a posterior dislocation. A persistent anterior prominence following anterior dislocation is not of any functional significance.[6] Chest auscultation and a thorough neurovascular examination to the ipsilateral extremity are important to document early. Some clinical findings include decreased active abduction and flexion in the scapular plane along with discomfort with cross body arm movements.[6]

2. **Radiographs.** AP radiographs of the chest or clavicle are often of limited usefulness when assessing for SC joint injuries. A **serendipity** X-ray view of the shoulder is a 40° cephalic tilt view centered on the manubrium.[4] In this view, an anterior dislocation will be manifested with a superior appearing clavicular head.

Once suspected, a CT examination with 2-mm interval cuts should also be obtained to visualize the location and extent of dislocation and evaluate the retrosternal region for soft-tissue and physeal injuries. If a vascular injury is suspected, the CT angiogram can be used to visualize the great vessels to assess for signs of vascular injury.

A magnetic resonance imaging (MRI) can be considered to further evaluate the anatomy of the SC joint and location of critical soft-tissue structures. An MRI may be helpful in distinguishing between a dislocation and physeal injury in children and young adults.

## C. Treatment

1. **Nonoperative.** Most SC injuries are anterior dislocations, and these may be treated nonoperatively with the expectation of potential cosmetic asymmetry usually associated with good functional results and resolution of pain.[7] An allograft reconstruction with an open reduction can be considered for avoidance of the substantial bump that is associated with expectant management. Closed reduction can be attempted; however, the joint usually will not remain reduced, and no brace has been demonstrated to be efficacious to maintain reduction. This expectant result also holds true for the growth plate injuries in patients under 22 years of age that are displaced anteriorly.

2. **Operative.** It is mostly agreed upon that surgical intervention for anterior SC joint dislocations is not clearly indicated and that the risks may outweigh the benefits of an open reconstruction of the joint.[5] Surgical reconstruction for anterior dislocations may be considered for dislocations associated with persistent symptoms, including instability, that negatively impact activities of daily living. Bak and Fogh performed a study in which 32 patients with chronic anterior unstable SC joint underwent reconstruction with a tendon autograft. The reconstruction resulted in prolonged improvement in shoulder function.[6]

A posterior dislocation should undergo a manipulative reduction to unlock the retrosternal clavicular head even if open reduction is necessary. The rationale for the need for closed reduction relates to the concern that impingement on critical structures may yield late sequelae from erosion, obstruction, or irritation.[8]

A pointed bone tenaculum may be useful to grasp the head of the clavicle and pull it back to its proper relation to the manubrium. A roll between the shoulder blades while the patient is supine, in combination with lateral traction of the abducted arm, is a helpful adjunctive maneuver. A closed reduction maneuver is usually unsuccessful and, even if reduced, may not stay reduced. Owing to possible violation of critical structures in the mediastinum, anesthesia should always be on hand to manage the airway, and a thoracic surgeon on standby during the procedure, because even though the likelihood of risk is minimal, the result of an associated injury could be catastrophic.

Many authors have described techniques for stabilization of the unstable SC joint using various tendon reconstructions, medial clavicle osteotomy or resection, and/or Kirschner wire fixation with mixed results.[9] A recent systematic review of literature assessing clinical outcomes of surgical management of SC joint dislocations concluded that ligament reconstruction using a tendon graft has the lowest rates of recurrent instability and complications, whereas open reduction and internal fixation techniques were associated with a higher rate of second operation (80%) for implant removal.[10] If fixation of a medial clavicle physeal or other medial clavicle fracture variant is desired with implants, attempts to provide even temporary fixation to the sternum is illogical because of the major mobility of the SC joint discussed earlier. Many authors warn against the use of any transfixing wires across the SC joint because of reports of wire migration. In the patient with an open physis, reduction of the dislocated distal fragment can be reinforced with heavy braided suture through drill holes in the distal fragment, capturing capsule and SC ligaments for repair.

3. **Follow-up.** A sling with an abduction pillow may be used for 1 month to support the extremity during the acute phase of pain during a period of relative immobility. Motion and function should be allowed to advance as discomfort allows. The **patient** may need reassurance for months during a period of gradually resolving symptoms. There is certainly a subset of patients who fail nonoperative management and develop chronic pain, instability, crepitance, and unacceptable discomfort.

4. **Complications.** Retrosternal dislocations are frequently missed because of the lack of physical examination findings in the context of a multiply injured patient.[11] Missed or late diagnosis of associated injuries of the mediastinum and brachial plexus may occur. With nonoperatively treated anterior dislocations, the patient should anticipate a significant prominence, which is a concern for some patients. Failure of fixation, hardware migration, and redislocation have also been reported after operative stabilization and are likely due to the high forces acting on this primary articulation between the upper extremity and the axial skeleton.[12] Lastly, arthritic symptoms of the SC joint are not uncommon, and many authors have described resection of the clavicular head to address refractory pain.[13]

## II. Acromioclavicular Injuries
### A. General information
1. **Anatomy and mechanism.** The acromioclavicular (AC) joint is a synovial, diarthrodial joint that contains a small, round meniscus composed of fibrocartilage much like the knee. The static linkage of the lateral clavicle to the upper extremity is via the coracoclavicular (CC) and AC ligaments as well as the joint capsule. The AC joint capsule is strongest at its superior and posterior margin.[14] In addition, the AC ligament provides stability in the AP plane.[15] The scapula is suspended from the clavicle via the CC ligaments, which run from the base of the coracoid from the undersurface of the clavicle (Fig. 15-2). The CC ligament is formed by the trapezoid and conoid ligaments, which provide stability in the superior–inferior (vertical) plane.[15]

The AC dislocation is commonly referred to as a shoulder separation. Owing to its vulnerable position on the lateral aspect of the shoulder, an AC dislocation is a common injury that occurs as the joint absorbs the direct forces generated with a blow to the shoulder. The most common mechanism is a fall directly onto the shoulder with the arm adducted.

2. **Classification** (Fig. 15-3). Tossy et al.[16] and Allman[17] originally developed classification systems for AC joint dislocations based on the degree of ligament injury and radiographic displacement and graded these as Types I to III. Rockwood modified this classification by adding three more types (IV, V, and VI), based on the directions of displacement.[18,19] The joint may sustain a simple strain with no displacement referred to as a **Type I**. The **Type II** injury is described as being displaced superiorly less than the diameter of the clavicle and is thought to be associated with complete tearing of the AC ligaments but relative sparing of the CC ligaments. The **Type III** dislocation represents complete disruption of the CC and AC ligaments with superior displacement. In 2014, the Upper Extremity Committee of International Society of Arthroscopy, Knee Surgery and Orthopaedic Sports Medicine (ISAKOS) implemented a new subclassification of the Rockwood Type III AC joint dislocations, including a Type IIIA variant, which is defined as a stable AC joint, and the Type IIIB variant, which is described as an unstable AC joint, with an overriding clavicle

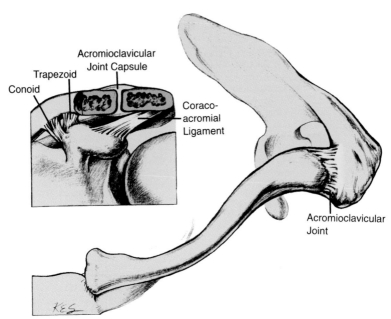

**Figure 15-2.** This illustration highlights the anatomy of the acromioclavicular joint. The joint capsule as well as the conoid and trapezoid portions of the coracoclavicular ligament are all static stabilizers of the acromioclavicular joint. (From Hansen ST, Swiontkowski MF. *Orthopaedic Trauma Protocols*. Raven Press; 1993:80, with permission.)

on AP radiographs with cross body adduction views.[20] A **Type IV** AC dislocation is complete and displaced posteriorly; whereas a **Type V** is an extreme variation of Type III, where the clavicle buttonholes through the trapezius into the subcutaneous tissue and thus is associated with much more stripping of the trapezius and deltoid. A Type III dislocation can be differentiated from a Type V based on the inability to reduce the AC joint in a Type V dislocation. The **Type VI** dislocation is an inferior dislocation under the coracoid process.

**B. Diagnosis**

1. **History and physical examination.** The history usually details a fall on the shoulder, and it is associated with well-localized pain. The AC joint is typically swollen and point tender. Another positive physical examination finding for AC joint abnormalities includes the cross body adduction test having a sensitivity of 77%. This test is performed with the arm flexed forward to 90° and adducted across the body adding a loading force with traction by the examiners hand.[21] If a visual or palpable step-off exists, or the distal clavicle feels reducible, there is at least a Type II injury.

2. **Radiographs.** Typically, an AP X-ray of the shoulder reveals the injury, although imaging of the joint can be enhanced with a 10° cephalic tilt centered on the shoulder, known as the Zanca view. Although the absolute distance from the superior coracoid to the inferior clavicle (CC distance) has a normal range of 1.1 to 1.3 cm, it can vary radiographically.[22] Visualization of both the AC joints on the same large X-ray cassette helps

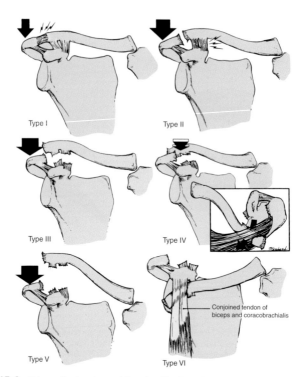

**Figure 15-3.** Schematic drawings of the classification of ligamentous injuries that can occur to the acromioclavicular ligament. Type I: A mild force applied to the point of the shoulder does not disrupt either the acromioclavicular or the coracoclavicular ligaments. Type II: A moderate-to-heavy force applied to the point of the shoulder will disrupt the acromioclavicular ligaments, but the coracoclavicular ligaments remain intact. Type III: When a severe force is applied to the point of the shoulder, both the acromioclavicular and coracoclavicular ligaments are disrupted. Type IV: In this major injury, not only are the acromioclavicular and coracoclavicular ligaments disrupted but also the distal end of the clavicle is displaced posteriorly into or through the trapezius muscle. Type V: A violent force has been applied to the point of the shoulder, not only rupturing the acromioclavicular and coracoclavicular ligaments but also disrupting the deltoid and trapezius muscle attachments and creating an irreducible separation between the clavicle and the acromion. Type VI: Another major injury is an inferior dislocation of the distal end of the clavicle to the subcoracoid position. The acromioclavicular and coracoclavicular ligaments are disrupted. (From Rockwood CA, Williams GR, Young DC. Injuries to the acromioclavicular joint. In: Rockwood CR, Green DP, Bucholz RW, et al., eds. *Fractures in Adults*. 4th ed. Lippincott–Raven; 1996:1354, with permission.)

to understand relative displacement. A bilateral Zanca view to view both the AC joints in a single view is recommended to evaluate relative displacement.[15] An increase in CC distance of 5 mm or greater than 25% usually indicates a complete tear of the CC ligaments.[23] Weighted stress radiographs are not necessary and needlessly painful.

**C. Treatment**

1. **Nonoperative.** Type I and II AC injuries should be treated nonoperatively with the expectation of good functional results and usually with complete resolution of pain.[24] Ice should be provided in the acute setting to relieve

swelling, as well as a sling to support the arm. A closed reduction of a Type II injury will not remain reduced, and no brace has been proven to be efficacious in this regard.

As for Type III dislocations, clinical studies comparing operative versus nonoperative treatment seem to indicate that there is no benefit from surgical treatment,[24-30] although some experts believe that the overhead throwing athlete and manual laborer should undergo reconstruction.[18] Currently, there is controversy in regard to optimal treatment of this variant of AC joint dislocation. A randomized controlled trial performed by the Canadian Orthopaedic Trauma Society on operative versus nonoperative treatment of Type III injuries concluded that both patient- and surgeon-based outcomes scores were superior in the nonoperative group at 6 weeks and 3 months after injury. In addition, patients in this cohort were able to return to work earlier than those who underwent surgical repair.[26] A later study performed by the same organization suggested that the nonoperative group had better Disability of the Arm, Shoulder, and Hand (DASH) score and Constant Shoulder Score at 6 weeks, 3 months, and 6 months.[27]

2. **Operative.** Many surgical procedures have been described to repair an AC dislocation with the goal of obtaining and maintaining AC joint reduction. The strategy is either to provide primary fixation of the AC joint or to augment the CC ligaments to maintain a reduced joint. Some surgeons advocate a combination of these two strategies to maintain the reduction against the great forces acting to displace the clavicle. Although each strategy can be employed in the acute or delayed setting, if a ligament reconstruction is done late, it is usually combined with a distal clavicle resection.

Some surgical techniques to restore AC joint stability include reconstruction of CC ligament with autograft or allograft tendon and articular fixation with Kirschner wires, hook plate, or suture buttons.[28] The most widely known procedure is the Weaver–Dunn,[31] and many surgeons augment some variation of this repair with fixation across the clavicle, into the coracoid, or around the base of the coracoid and clavicle like a sling. The Weaver–Dunn itself involves transferring the AC ligament through the end of a resected distal clavicle; however, this procedure has tended to fall out of favor because of the potential role of the AC ligament in glenohumeral joint stability as it may help to prevent superior escape of the humerus in the setting of rotator cuff incompetence.

The hook plate concept is a popular option for acute AC joint dislocations.[18,32] The plate is fixed to the cephalad border of the distal clavicle, and a terminal plate extension is placed under the acromion so the clavicle is reduced and restrained from springing cephalad. This can be employed either alone or in conjunction with CC ligament augmentation. The plate is routinely removed at 3 months, requiring a second operation. Primary hook plate fixation is a simple, consistent, and reproducible technique that reliably restored AC joint alignment with a high rate of patient satisfaction.[26] An attempt to repair the AC joint as well as the CC ligaments should augment the use of this implant.

Another fixation concept is the "Tightrope Technique" (Arthrex, Naples, FL), which is being used by some surgeons as a minimally invasive option for fixation.[33,34] This provides fixation between the coracoid process and the clavicle and can be performed arthroscopically or through a mini-open approach. A 2017 systemic review and meta-analysis performed by Arirachakaran et al. reports that suture button fixation has higher shoulder function scores and lower postoperative pain compared to hook plate fixation; however, there are higher complication rates.[28] The jury is out as to which technique is best, if even better than nonoperative treatment for Type III injuries.

3. **Follow-up.** As is the case with the SC dislocation, a sling may be used for a few weeks to support the extremity during the acute phase of pain, whether treated with or without surgery. Motion is advanced as discomfort allows. Shorter or longer periods with relative rest are required according to which injury is present. Often, the Type I and II injuries cause pain for a longer period than the Type III injuries because of partial communication of the joint surfaces and tethering of partially torn ligamentous structures. The patient may need reassurance for months during a period of gradually resolving symptoms. Patients should understand that any implants placed across the AC joint should be removed at approximately 3 months post-op to prevent erosion of the acromion.

4. **Complications.** Occasionally, symptomatic posttraumatic osteolysis or arthritis of the AC joint develops. An arthroscopic or open resection of the distal clavicle can be done with results that have generally been favorable.[35] However, this should be reserved for those patients without evidence of CC ligament insufficiency or AC joint instability, as resection may further destabilize the distal clavicle.

Patients who undergo nonoperative management are at risk of poor cosmetic outcomes of their shoulder.[36] Most of the complications related to surgery relate to failure of fixation, causing chronic symptomatic instability. Hardware failure such as cutout of CC fixation on either the clavicular or coracoid side of a CC ligament reconstruction is well described, as well as acromial osteolysis or periimplant acromion fractures from hook plates that are left in too long underscore the technically demanding nature of the reconstruction.

## Regions Hospital Treatment Recommendations

### Acromioclavicular Injuries

**Diagnosis:** AP shoulder radiograph, 10° cephalad oblique radiograph, clinical examination.

**Treatment:** Grades I, II, and some III, sling for comfort for 7 to 10 days, then range of motion exercises.

**Indications for surgery:** Grades IV to VI, and some grade III. Young patients, athletes, and manual laborers should be considered for surgical treatment, as well as patients who do not accept the unsightly cosmetic deformity as an acceptable outcome.

**Recommended technique:** Hook plate application and CC ligament repair and augmentation; plate removal at 3 months.

## REFERENCES

1. Yeh GL, Williams GR Jr. Conservative management of sternoclavicular injuries. *Orthop Clin North Am.* 2000;31:189-203.
2. Lee JT, Campbell KJ, Michalski MP, et al. Surgical anatomy of the sternoclavicular joint: a qualitative and quantitative anatomical study. *J Bone Joint Surg Am.* 2014;96(19):e166.

3. Sewell MD, Al-Hadithy N, Leu AL, et al. Instability of the sternoclavicular joint: current concepts in classification, treatment and outcomes. *Bone Joint J.* 2013;95:721-731.
4. Wirth MA, Rockwood CA Jr. Disorders of the sternoclavicular joint. In: Rockwood CA Jr, Matsen FA III, Wirth MA, et al., eds. *The Shoulder.* Vol 1. 4th ed. WB Saunders; 2009:527-560.
5. Groh GI, Wirth MA. Management of traumatic sternoclavicular joint injuries. *J Am Acad Orthop Surg.* 2011;19:1-7.
6. Bak K, Fogh K. Reconstruction of the chronic anterior unstable sternoclavicular joint using a tendon autograft: medium-term to long-term follow-up results. *J Shoulder Elbow Surg.* 2014;23(2):245-250.
7. de Jong KP, Sukul DM. Anterior sternoclavicular dislocation: a long-term follow-up study. *J Orthop Trauma.* 1990;4:420-423.
8. Groh GI, Wirth MA, Rockwood CA Jr. Treatment of traumatic posterior sternoclavicular dislocations. *J Shoulder Elbow Surg.* 2011;20:107-113.
9. Spencer EE Jr, Kuhn JE. Biomechanical analysis of reconstructions for sternoclavicular joint instability. *J Bone Joint Surg Am.* 2004;86:98-105.
10. Kendal JK, Thomas K, Lo IK, et al. Clinical outcomes and complications following surgical management of traumatic posterior sternoclavicular joint dislocations: a systemic review. *J Bone Joint Surg.* 2018;6(11):e2.
11. Thomas DP, Davies A, Hoddinott HC. Posterior sternoclavicular dislocations—a diagnosis easily missed. *Ann R Coll Surg Engl.* 1999;81:201-204.
12. Flatow EL. The biomechanics of the acromioclavicular, sternoclavicular, and scapulothoracic joints. *Instr Course Lect.* 1993;42:237-245.
13. Rockwood CA Jr, Groh GI, Wirth MA, et al. Resection arthroplasty of the sternoclavicular joint. *J Bone Joint Surg Am.* 1997;79:387-393.
14. Fukuda K, Craig EV, An KN, et al. Biomechanical study of the ligamentous system of the acromioclavicular joint. *J Bone Joint Surg Am.* 1986;68:434-440.
15. Li X, Ma R, Bedi A, Dines DM, Altchek DW, Dines JS. Management of acromioclavicular joint injuries. *J Bone Joint Surg Am.* 2014;96(1):73-84.
16. Tossy JD, Mead NC, Sigmond HM. Acromioclavicular separations: useful and practical classification for treatment. *Clin Orthop Relat Res.* 1963;28:111-119.
17. Allman FL Jr. Fractures and ligamentous injuries of the clavicle and its articulation. *J Bone Joint Surg Am.* 1967;49:774-784.
18. Collins DN. Disorders of the acromioclavicular joint. In: Rockwood CA Jr, Matsen FA III, Wirth MA, et al., eds. *The Shoulder.* Vol 1. 4th ed. WB Saunders; 2009:453-526.
19. Rockwood CA Jr. Injuries to the acromioclavicular joint. In: Rockwood CA Jr, Green DP, eds. *Fractures in Adults.* Vol 1. 2nd ed. JB Lippincott; 1984:860-910.
20. Beitzel K, Mazzocca AD, Bak K, et al. ISAKOS upper extremity committee consensus statement on the need for diversification of the Rockwood classification for acromioclavicular joint injuries. *Arthroscopy.* 2014;30:271-278.
21. Chronopoulos E, Kim TK, Park HB, et al. Diagnostic value of physical tests for isolated chronic acromioclavicular lesions. *Am J Sports Med.* 2004;32(3):655-661.
22. Bearden JM, Hughston JC, Whatley GS. Acromioclavicular dislocation: method of treatment. *J Sports Med.* 1973;1:5-17.
23. Williams GR, Nguyen VD, Rockwood CA Jr. Classification and radiographic analysis of acromioclavicular dislocations. *Appl Radiol.* 1989;18:29-34.
24. Taft TN, Wilson FC, Oglesby JW. Dislocation of the acromioclavicular joint: an end-result study. *J Bone Joint Surg Am.* 1987;69:1045-1051.
25. Bannister GC, Wallace WA, Stableforth PG, et al. The management of acute acromioclavicular dislocation. A randomised prospective controlled trial. *J Bone Joint Surg Br.* 1989;71:848-850.
26. Canadian Orthopaedic Trauma Society. Multicenter randomized clinical trial of nonoperative versus operative treatment of acute acromio-clavicular joint dislocation. *J Orthop Trauma.* 2015;29:479-487.
27. Mah JM; Canadian Orthopaedic Trauma Society. General health status after nonoperative versus operative treatment for acute, complete acromioclavicular joint dislocation: results of a multicenter randomized clinical trial. *J Orthop Trauma.* 2017;31(9):485-490.
28. Arirachakaran A, Boonard M, Piyapittayanun P, et al. Post-operative outcomes and complications of suspensory loop fixation device versus hook plate in acute unstable acromioclavicular joint dislocation: a systematic review and meta-analysis. *J Orthop Traumatol.* 2017;18:293-304.
29. Galpin RD, Hawkins RJ, Grainger RW. A comparative analysis of operative versus nonoperative treatment of grade III acromioclavicular separations. *Clin Orthop Relat Res.* 1985;193:150-155.

30. Smith MJ, Stewart MJ. Acute acromioclavicular separations. A 20-year study. *Am J Sports Med.* 1979;7:62-71.
31. Weaver JK, Dunn HK. Treatment of acromioclavicular injuries, especially complete acromioclavicular separation. *J Bone Joint Surg Am.* 1972;54:1187-1194.
32. Sim E, Schwarz N, Höcker K, et al. Repair of complete acromioclavicular separations using the acromioclavicular-hook plate. *Clin Orthop Relat Res.* 1995;314:134-142.
33. DeBerardino TM, Pensak MJ, Ferreira J, et al. Arthroscopic stabilization of acromioclavicular joint dislocation using the AC graftrope system. *J Shoulder Elbow Surg.* 2010;19:47-52.
34. Scheibel M, Dröschel S, Gerhardt C, et al. Arthroscopically assisted stabilization of acute high-grade acromioclavicular joint separations. *Am J Sports Med.* 2011;39:1507-1516.
35. Martin SD, Baumgarten TE, Andrews JR. Arthroscopic resection of the distal aspect of the clavicle with concomitant subacromial decompression. *J Bone Joint Surg Am.* 2001;83:328-335.
36. Chang N, Furey A, Kurdin A. Operative versus nonoperative management of acute high-grade acromioclavicular dislocations: a systematic review and meta-analysis. *J Orthop Trauma.* 2018;32(1):1-9.

## SELECTED HISTORICAL READING

Urist MR. Complete dislocation of the acromioclavicular joint; the nature of the traumatic lesion and effective methods of treatment with an analysis of 41 cases. *J Bone Joint Surg Am.* 1946;28:813-837.

# 16 Acute Shoulder Injuries

Jonathan P. Braman and Alicia K. Harrison

## I. General Principles

A. **Anatomy.** The shoulder is the most mobile joint in the body, and this significant range of motion allows for the positioning of the hand in space. The larger humeral head articulates with a relatively small glenoid; therefore, there is little constraint for the glenohumeral joint from the bony anatomy. This construct allows for the shoulder's extreme range of motion. Static and dynamic stabilizers provide additional constraint. The labrum acts to increase the depth of the glenoid concavity and provide additional stability. The glenohumeral ligaments (superior, middle, and inferior) stabilize the joint in various shoulder positions. The supraspinatus, infraspinatus, subscapularis, and teres minor, which make up the rotator cuff, act as important dynamic shoulder stabilizers and play a very important role in the mobility of the glenohumeral joint. The parascapular muscles are equally essential to normal shoulder function because these muscles function to position the scapula and glenoid appropriately in space. If the scapula is not stabilized by these muscles, the glenoid cannot act as a stable base with which the humeral head may articulate. It is the complexity of this joint that provides great mobility, although such extreme mobility may at times place the shoulder at increased risk for injury.

B. **Differential diagnosis.** The most common acute shoulder injuries include glenohumeral dislocation, rotator cuff injury, and fractures. It is, however, essential to consider other possible etiologies in a patient presenting with acute shoulder pain, including cervical disc disease (C5 nerve root), brachial neuritis, pleural irritation, tumors, and cardiac disease.

## II. Shoulder Dislocations

A. **Classification.** Shoulder instability is classified by the position of the humeral head with respect to the glenoid (anterior, inferior, posterior, or multidirectional). Shoulder dislocations typically include cases documented radiographically or those involving a formal manipulative reduction. Dislocations are further characterized by timing or chronicity (acute, recurrent, chronic) and by etiology (traumatic or atraumatic). Anterior dislocations are by far the most common. Patient age at the time of the first dislocation is a significant predictor of both accompanying injury and the patient's risk of recurrent dislocation. The risk of recurrent dislocation has been shown to be inversely proportional to age; the classic article found that one-third of patients aged 20 years or younger at the time of the initial dislocation went on to require surgery for recurrent dislocation.[1]

B. **Anterior dislocations**
   1. **Mechanism of injury.** Anterior dislocations may occur in various mechanisms. Traumatic anterior dislocations classically result when the arm is forced into an abducted, externally rotated position at the extreme range of motion. In patients with multidirectional instability (MDI), ligamentous laxity, or multiple recurrent instability (especially including bone loss), an anterior dislocation may occur with little trauma in a broad range of shoulder positions.

2. **Examination.** A thorough examination of the shoulder is essential in the patient sustaining an acute shoulder injury. The appearance of the shoulder in the setting of an anterior dislocation is squared off with prominence of the posterolateral acromion and a hollow appearance of the posterior shoulder. The patient typically holds the arm in an adducted position, and attempts at range of motion of the shoulder are extremely painful and mechanically limited. A thorough neurovascular examination of the upper extremity is essential before any reduction attempts are made because axillary nerve injuries are commonly seen in glenohumeral dislocations and must be documented before manipulation of the shoulder. One prospective study found that as many as 54% of patients with glenohumeral dislocations had an axillary nerve injury, and neurologic complications were more common in patients aged 50 years or older.[2]

3. **Imaging.** All patients with a suspected dislocation of the shoulder should have a complete series of shoulder X-rays. This should include an anteroposterior (AP), true AP in the plane of the scapula (Grashey view), a transscapular ("Y") view, and an axillary view. The combination of these orthogonal views will not only clearly demonstrate the direction of the dislocation but also allow for the recognition of any associated fractures.

4. **Initial treatment**
   a. **Reduction without general anesthesia.** Prompt reduction of the dislocation is important not only to relieve the patient's pain but also to minimize the risk of associated neurologic injuries, because this risk increases in shoulders that remain dislocated over 12 hours.[3] To achieve a gentle and pain-free reduction, muscle relaxation and pain relief are required. The patient may be provided intravenous (IV) pain medication and sedation, although an intraarticular lidocaine block is equally effective as well.[4] For this block, 10 to 20 mL of 1% plain lidocaine is injected into the glenohumeral joint. Multiple methods of reduction can then be effective when applied correctly.
      i. **Prone reduction (Stimson technique).** The patient is placed prone on the examination table or stretcher with the involved arm and shoulder hanging over the edge of the table. A 10-lb weight is suspended from the patient's wrist or may be held in the patient's hand. If good analgesia and relaxation are present, the shoulder may reduce in this position without further manipulation.
      ii. **Reduction by traction.** The patient is positioned supine, and additional IV sedation is administered. An assistant provides countertraction, whereas the physician grasps the forearm of the involved shoulder and gently pulls in a line of 30° of abduction and 20° to 30° of forward flexion. Countertraction may be effectively applied by placing a folded sheet around the thorax and applying linear traction in the opposite direction of the reduction force. Sustained traction for 5 minutes may be necessary. Vigorous and forceful attempts at reduction should be avoided. Firm, constant pressure is often effective in reducing the joint as long as the patient is adequately sedated.
   b. **Reduction under anesthesia.** If the aforementioned methods fail or if a proximal humerus fracture (other than a tuberosity fracture) is present, a reduction under general anesthetic with complete muscle relaxation is indicated. The shoulder typically reduces easily with little risk of further damage to the glenohumeral joint or its surrounding structures. The posterior humeral head may be impaled on the anterior glenoid if an anterior dislocation is difficult to reduce. Accentuating the deformity by first adducting and external rotating the humerus can

"unlock" the humeral head and allow for traction and internal rotation to reduce the shoulder. Forceful external rotation on an impaled humeral head can result in a fracture of the humeral surface.

5. **Postreduction treatment.** The length of immobilization has not been shown to have any effect on the incidence of redislocation.[5] The shoulder should only be immobilized for 1 to 2 weeks as needed for pain control after a dislocation or subluxation episode. A range of motion and rotator cuff strengthening program is initiated early, avoiding the extremes of external rotation and abduction. Patients are allowed to return to sports and other activities when the shoulder has normal range of motion and strength without pain. There is a trend toward early magnetic resonance imaging (MRI) arthrogram in first-time dislocations in teenagers and young adults who engage in athletic activities. The recurrent dislocation rate is upward of 70% in this age group, and subsequent dislocations can result in continued bone loss of the glenoid. Given this high rate of recurrence, MRI arthrogram and early stabilization after a first-time dislocation is a reasonable treatment option.

6. **Recurrent dislocations or subluxations.** The same standards for examination and imaging should be applied in cases of recurrent instability. It remains important to rule out any accompanying injury, particularly to the bony constraints of the glenoid and humerus. Occasionally, if the event is witnessed and the evaluation suggests a recurrent dislocation without fracture, then an attempt for reduction can be made before radiographic imaging. For patients with recurrent instability, these events can have significant effects on the quality of life. For these patients, surgical intervention is indicated and may be critical to establish shoulder stability.

7. **Accompanying injuries**
   a. **Bankart lesions.** In 1923, Bankart described a lesion (now referred to as the *Bankart lesion*) seen in concert with shoulder dislocations in which the anterior capsule and labrum are avulsed from the glenoid.[6] In some cases, the capsule and labrum remain attached to a bony fragment, which fractures off the glenoid (bony Bankart). One classic study found a Bankart lesion in 97% of patients younger than 24 years who were treated surgically for their first-time dislocation.[7] This same study identified a 90% recurrence rate for instability in this same patient population treated nonoperatively. These findings led the authors to suggest a strong association between the Bankart lesion and recurrent instability.
   b. **Hill-Sachs lesion.** When the humeral head dislocates anterior to the glenoid fossa, a compression fracture may occur on the posterolateral humeral head (Hill-Sachs lesion) from impaction of the head on the anterior edge of the glenoid. When this fracture leads to significant bone loss of this portion of the humeral head, the shoulder is at increased risk of recurrent dislocation as the region of bone impaction engages the glenoid.
   c. **Rotator cuff tears.** Rotator cuff tears are occasionally found in association with glenohumeral dislocation, typically in patients older than 40 years,[8] with the incidence of rotator cuff tear after acute dislocation in patients older than 40 years reported to be in the range of 35% to 86%. For patients older than 40 years in whom range of motion and strength do not improve within 2 to 4 weeks after the injury, MRI or ultrasound is indicated to assess for rotator cuff tear.
   d. **Neurologic injury.** Neurologic injuries are frequently seen in association with shoulder dislocations. The axillary nerve and musculocutaneous nerve are most commonly injured, although complete brachial

plexopathies have been described. Most injuries represent a neuropraxia, and a return to preinjury motion and strength is typical in these cases. However, multiple studies have documented permanent nerve injuries in association with shoulder dislocation.[2,9]

8. **Surgical management.** There are different approaches to surgical management of anterior shoulder instability. As mentioned previously, recent literature would suggest that surgical management may be indicated for repair of Bankart lesions in younger patients (less than 24) after a first-time traumatic dislocation.[7] More debate exists regarding operative versus nonoperative management in older individuals. Certainly for patients with recurring instability episodes, surgical management is a very reasonable treatment. Shoulder stabilization may be performed either open or arthroscopically. Depending on patient risk factors, equivalent results may be seen for open and arthroscopic management.[10-12] Recurrent instability has been found to be more common in younger patients and contact athletes, with more recent studies suggesting recurrent instability is more common with arthroscopic versus open repair.[13,14]

**C. Posterior dislocations**

1. **Mechanism of injury.** Posterior instability results from a fall on an adducted and forward flexed arm, although it may also occur in sporting events in which a posteriorly directed force is applied to the outstretched elevated arm. A compression fracture of the anterolateral aspect of the humeral head may also occur (reverse Hill-Sachs lesion). As with anterior shoulder instability, in younger individuals, an avulsion of the posterior labrum with a small fragment of the posterior glenoid rim (reverse Bankart lesion) may occur. Seizures or electrocution are more frequently reported as a mechanism for posterior instability.

2. **Examination.** Many posterior dislocations are misdiagnosed or missed acutely, especially when a humeral neck fracture allows the arm to "derotate" through the fracture site. It is particularly important to recognize the examination and radiographic hallmarks of a posterior dislocation. Patients with a posterior shoulder dislocation classically hold the arm in extreme internal rotation with severe pain with attempted external rotation. The coracoid is also very prominent anteriorly in these patients. Posterior dislocations that go undetected in the emergency department (ED) can have disastrous consequences, including avascular necrosis of the humeral head.

3. **Roentgenograms.** The AP view is often incorrectly interpreted as normal, but one should recognize the classic marked internally rotated position of the proximal humerus, which is often described as a "light-bulb" sign. The true AP will often also reveal the classic finding of overlap of the humeral head on the glenoid (Fig. 16-1). A transscapular "Y" view and an axillary view will clearly demonstrate the posterior position of the humeral head (Fig. 16-2).

4. **Treatment.** Adequate muscle relaxation via IV sedation is essential. Reduction is most easily achieved by translating the humerus posteriorly, followed by lateral translation of the proximal humerus with gentle, controlled manipulation of the humerus anteriorly to the reduced position. Postreduction treatment is similar to that for anterior dislocation (see **B.5**), except that internal rotation and adduction extremes are avoided. If the shoulder dislocates immediately after being reduced, the arm should be placed in external rotation and abduction to maintain stability. Some posterior dislocations (particularly those resulting from seizures) may have large reverse Hill-Sachs lesions that cause further instability episodes.

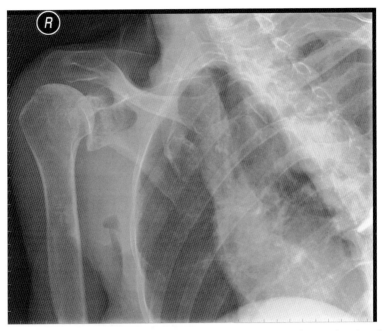

**Figure 16-1.** True anteroposterior of the shoulder revealing the classic finding of overlap of the humeral head on the glenoid (or "double density") found with posterior dislocations of the glenohumeral joint.

5. **Recurrent dislocations.** Recurrent posterior instability is most commonly seen in collision athletes and, rarely, includes recurrent locked dislocations. In this setting, arthroscopic posterior labral repair is the treatment of choice. When recurrent locked dislocations occur, they are often secondary to large reverse Hill-Sachs lesions and/or posterior bony Bankart lesions. Nonoperative management is rarely effective in stabilizing these shoulders, and surgical management to reconstruct the bone loss or repair a large labral repair may be necessary. In some cases, particularly with large bone defects, or in the revision setting, glenoid osteoplasty or bone block capsulorrhaphy may be necessary. For patients with atraumatic recurrent posterior instability, treatment should involve physical therapy and activity or lifestyle restrictions, with consideration given to surgical management if nonoperative treatment is ineffective.

**D. Multidirectional instability**

1. **Mechanism of injury.** MDI is diagnosed when there is clinical evidence that the shoulder is unstable and symptomatic in two or more directions. The initial instability event is atraumatic, and the patient may actually be able to voluntarily dislocate the shoulder.

2. **Examination.** The typical patient is often young, with MDI seen regularly in adolescent athletes. Seventy-five percent of patients with MDI are ligamentously lax,[15] and a sulcus sign is often seen. These patients will, on examination, have evidence of instability in both the anterior and posterior directions.

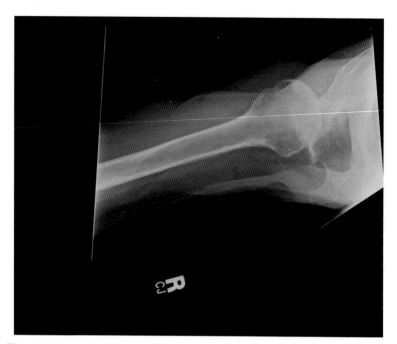

**Figure 16-2.** An axillary view clearly demonstrating the posterior position of the humeral head.

3. **Imaging.** Often, radiographs are normal, given the atraumatic nature of these instability events. The presence of a Hill-Sachs, reverse Hill-Sachs, or Bankart lesions is rare.

4. **Treatment.** Nonoperative treatment is strongly advised and has been found to be effective for 88% of patients with MDI.[16] Surgical treatment may be considered for patients in whom extensive nonoperative treatment is ineffective and quality of life is significantly limited by shoulder instability. If surgical intervention is to be pursued, it must address the multi-directional nature and the ligamentous laxity frequently at the source of the problem.

E. **Inferior dislocations.** Inferior dislocations (also called *luxatio erectae*) are rare. The patient's arm is locked in an overhead position (Fig. 16-3A, B). Reduction is obtained by IV sedation and relaxation. The arm is then reduced with lateral distraction, while it is brought out of an abducted position.

III. **Acute Rotator Cuff Tears**

A. **Mechanism of injury.** Acute tears of the rotator cuff are rare, but typically occur in young patients with significant trauma or patients older than 40 years in the setting of a shoulder dislocation (see **7.c**). Age-related degenerative rotator cuff tears are much more common (see Chapter 17).

B. **Examination** (see Chapter 17).

C. **Imaging.** It is important to evaluate the patient for a greater tuberosity fracture because avulsion of a fragment of the tuberosity may be pulled off with the rotator cuff. This is best addressed with a complete series of shoulder X-rays (see **B.3**). Young individuals who are suspected of having a rotator cuff

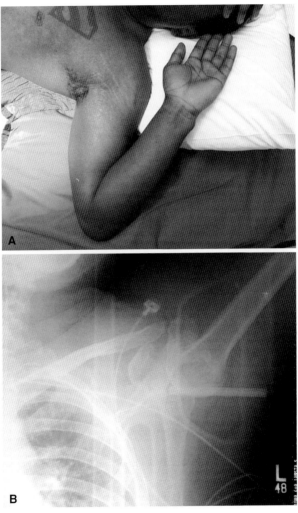

**Figure 16-3. A, B:** Inferior dislocation (luxatio erecta). The patient's arm is locked in an overhead position.

tear on history or examination should undergo an MRI scan or an ultrasound evaluation to assess the status of their rotator cuff.

- **D. Treatment.** In young or active patients with a true acute rotator cuff tear, early operative repair is indicated. Early repair is also indicated in those cases associated with a displaced avulsion fracture of the greater tuberosity.[17]

IV. **Ruptures of the Long Head of the Biceps Brachii**
- **A. Mechanism of injury.** Injuries of the long head of the biceps (LHB) tendon may occur with forceful elbow flexion or forearm supination. Many cases are associated with ongoing rotator cuff problems and age-related tendon degeneration. Steroid use for body conditioning is another etiology.

**B. Examination.** A visible asymmetry of the injured versus noninjured upper arm is evident when the patient flexes the biceps muscle. This deformity is referred to as a "Popeye" sign. In the acute setting, swelling may obscure this deformity. Over time, ecchymosis often arises, although it may take time to become visible on the skin. It is often dependent and can go all the way to the wrist.

**C. Treatment.** Ruptures of the LHB tendon are treated nonoperatively. The indications for repair are cosmetic because rupture or tenotomy of the LHB tendon results in little functional loss, except in patients who have avocational or vocational need for maximal supination strength or endurance.

## REFERENCES

1. Hovelius L, Augustini BG, Fredin H, et al. Primary anterior dislocation of the shoulder in young patients. A ten-year prospective study. *J Bone Joint Surg Am*. 1996;78(11):1677-1684.
2. Toolanen G, Hildingsson C, Hedlund T, et al. Early complications after anterior dislocation of the shoulder in patients over 40 years. An ultrasonographic and electromyographic study. *Acta Orthop Scand*. 1993;64(5):549-552.
3. Perlmutter GS, Apruzzese W. Axillary nerve injuries in contact sports: recommendations for treatment and rehabilitation. *Sports Med*. 1998;26(5):351-361.
4. Miller SL, Cleeman E, Auerbach J, et al. Comparison of intra-articular lidocaine and intravenous sedation for reduction of shoulder dislocations: a randomized, prospective study. *J Bone Joint Surg Am*. 2002;84-A(12):2135-2139.
5. Hovelius L. Anterior dislocation of the shoulder in teen-agers and young adults. Five-year prognosis. *J Bone Joint Surg Am*. 1987;69(3):393-399.
6. Bankart AS. Recurrent or habitual dislocation of the shoulder-joint. *Br Med J*. 1923;2(3285): 1132-1133.
7. Taylor DC, Arciero RA. Pathologic changes associated with shoulder dislocations. Arthroscopic and physical examination findings in first-time, traumatic anterior dislocations. *Am J Sports Med*. 1997;25(3):306-311.
8. Stayner LR, Cummings J, Andersen J, et al. Shoulder dislocations in patients older than 40 years of age. *Orthop Clin North Am*. 2000;31(2):231-239.
9. Alnot JY, Liverneaux P, Silberman O. Lesions to the axillary nerve. *Rev Chir Orthop Reparatrice Appar Mot*. 1996;82(7):579-589.
10. Fabbriciani C, Milano G, Demontis A, et al. Arthroscopic versus open treatment of Bankart lesion of the shoulder: a prospective randomized study. *Arthroscopy*. 2004;20(5):456-462.
11. Voos JE, Livermore RW, Feeley BT, et al. Prospective evaluation of arthroscopic Bankart repairs for anterior instability. *Am J Sports Med*. 2010;38(2):302-307.
12. Bottoni CR, Smith EL, Berkowitz MJ, et al. Arthroscopic versus open shoulder stabilization for recurrent anterior instability: a prospective randomized clinical trial. *Am J Sports Med*. 2006;34(11):1730-1737.
13. Kasik CS, Rosen MR, Saper MG, et al. High rate of return to sport in adolescent athletes following anterior shoulder stabilisation: a systematic review. *J ISAKOS*. 2019;4(1):33-40.
14. Hohmann E, Tetsworth K, Glatt V. Open versus arthroscopic surgical treatment for anterior shoulder dislocation: a comparative systematic review and meta-analysis over the past 20 years. *J Shoulder Elbow Surg*. 2017;26(10):1873-1880.
15. Neer CS II, Foster CR. Inferior capsular shift for involuntary inferior and multidirectional instability of the shoulder. A preliminary report. *J Bone Joint Surg Am*. 1980;62(6):897-908.
16. Burkhead WZ Jr, Rockwood CA Jr. Treatment of instability of the shoulder with an exercise program. *J Bone Joint Surg Am*. 1992;74(6):890-896.
17. Bassett RW, Cofield RH. Acute tears of the rotator cuff. The timing of surgical repair. *Clin Orthop Relat Res*. 1983;175:18-24.

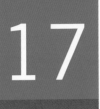

# Nonacute Shoulder Disorders

Jonathan P. Braman and Alicia K. Harrison

## I. Rotator Cuff Disorders

A. **Anatomy.** Four muscle-tendon units make up the rotator cuff: the subscapularis, supraspinatus, infraspinatus, and teres minor. The supraspinatus and infraspinatus are innervated by the suprascapular nerve, the subscapularis by the upper and lower subscapular nerves, and the teres minor by the axillary nerve. Rotator cuff disease is a spectrum of disorders ranging from what many refer to as "impingement" to rotator cuff tendinopathy to massive full-thickness tears. The role of impingement in rotator cuff disease remains a point of debate within the Orthopaedic Surgery field. Some propose that narrowing of the subacromial space leads to rotator cuff injury,[1] whereas others believe there is no causal relationship between the two.[2] The subacromial space involves the area from the undersurface of the acromion and the acromioclavicular (AC) joint superiorly to the coracoacromial ligament and coracoid anteriorly to the humeral head inferiorly. The subacromial bursa exists within the subacromial space above the rotator cuff.

B. **Mechanism of injury.** Proponents of impingement as a cause of rotator cuff disease suggest that a narrow subacromial space leads to compression of the rotator cuff against the overlying acromion and to eventual tearing of the rotator cuff. Undersurface spurring of the AC joint, instability of the glenohumeral joint, or changes in the shape of the acromion are suggested as the most common reasons for rotator cuff compromise. The resultant subacromial space narrowing and the patient's symptoms from this narrowing are referred to as **impingement syndrome**. The earliest stage of rotator cuff disease involves bursitis and tendinosis, which in some patients may progress to full-thickness cuff pathology. Others discard the concept of impingement and instead identify intrinsic components such as age-related degeneration or diminished blood supply to the tendon as the primary etiology for rotator cuff disease. Most likely, it is a combination of many of these factors that leads to the development of rotator cuff disease.

C. **History.** The typical patient with cuff disease is over age 40 and reports anterolateral shoulder or arm pain that is worse with the arm away from body or overhead activities. Many patients also find that pain is worse when lying recumbent at night.

D. **Examination.** As with most musculoskeletal examinations, one begins with visual inspection. Inspection of the shoulder girdle may identify visible atrophy of the supraspinatus or infraspinatus fossa, which suggests advanced cuff disease. Either a chronic massive rotator cuff tear or suprascapular nerve compression can cause atrophy of the muscle bellies that may be visible on inspection. Active and passive shoulder motion must be assessed in addition to rotator cuff strength. Supraspinatus weakness may be present with rotator cuff tears, and significant external rotation and forward flexion weakness often indicates that a large rotator cuff tear is present. Evocative maneuvers such as Neer and Hawkins tests are often referred to as impingement tests and may give some indication of rotator cuff disease.

E. **Imaging.** A complete series of shoulder radiographs should be obtained. Cystic changes within the greater or lesser tuberosity may be suggestive of chronic rotator cuff disease. Radiographs may illustrate superior humeral migration relative to the glenoid or rounding off of the greater tuberosity, which are changes seen with more advanced or chronic cuff tears. If rotator cuff disease is suspected with symptoms persisting despite nonoperative treatment or if a sizable full-thickness rotator cuff tear is suspected, a magnetic resonance imaging (MRI) is an appropriate next step in patient evaluation. For patients in whom an MRI is contraindicated, a computed tomography (CT) arthrogram or ultrasound is the best way to image the rotator cuff. In the hands of an experienced ultrasonographer, ultrasonography can also provide visualization of rotator cuff pathology and even assess the level of atrophy of the rotator cuff musculature.

F. **Diagnosis.** As previously mentioned, rotator cuff disease represents a wide spectrum of pathology from bursitis and tendinopathy to full-thickness rotator cuff tears. Diagnosis of a particular patient's rotator cuff injury is made based on history, symptoms, response to nonoperative treatment, and finally additional imaging in the form of MRI, CT arthrogram, or ultrasound.

G. **Treatment**
   1. **Bursitis/tendinopathy/impingement**
      a. **Nonoperative treatment**
         i. **Physical therapy.** The mainstay of treatment for patients without rotator cuff tears is physical therapy (PT). PT is typically the first line of treatment for patients with bursitis or rotator cuff tendinopathy and most nonacute shoulder pathology. The focus of treatment for these nonacute disorders includes regaining the patient's normal range of motion first through a stretching program. This may include the addition of modalities to diminish pain. Once range of motion is normalized, patients can be taught home exercises to improve strength and shoulder biomechanics. A focus on scapular stabilization is an essential component of rehabilitation for patients with chronic shoulder problems as this optimizes mechanics through the shoulder's range of motion. A trial of several months of dedicated PT is reasonable before considering surgery in the setting of many nonacute shoulder disorders.
         ii. **Injections.** Limited use of injections may be effective in the treatment of nonacute shoulder disorders. For example, a subacromial injection with a corticosteroid and an analgesic can be beneficial in this population. Of note, a prospective randomized clinical trial has not shown that inclusion of steroid in the injection solution improves outcome.[3] Resolution of a patient's pain or improvement in rotator cuff strength after the injection provides important information about the potential etiology of the patient's symptoms. In addition, injections are often most helpful for patients with nonacute shoulder pathology who are otherwise unable to perform PT on account of pain.
      b. **Operative treatment** is a reasonable option for patients who fail a reasonable (approximately 6 month) course of nonoperative treatment. Surgical management may include a bursectomy, recession of the coracoacromial ligament, and/or an anterior acromioplasty. These procedures may be completed through either open or arthroscopic techniques. Rotator cuff repair is extremely effective at providing improvements in pain and function and has been shown to be cost-effective as well.[4] Arthroscopic techniques have the benefit of allowing a thorough

examination of the glenohumeral joint for any concomitant pathology and improved cosmesis and may provide quicker pain relief and return to activity postoperatively.

2. **Rotator cuff tears**

   a. **Nonoperative management.** Although rotator cuff tears do not heal without surgery, a number of patients may not require surgical repair. Nonsurgical management is typically indicated for more sedentary patients or those whose activities do not demand normal shoulder strength. These patients may have improvement in their pain and function with PT alone. PT was effective in treating atraumatic rotator cuff tears in approximately 75% of patients in a large study.[5] It is also important to note that some rotator cuff tears are not reparable based on the size of the tear, retraction of the tendon, or advanced atrophy of their rotator cuff muscles.[6]

   b. **Operative management.** For many patients, rotator cuff repair offers the best chance at long-term improvement in shoulder pain and function.[7] This can be achieved both open and arthroscopically.[8] Some studies suggest that arthroscopic repair allows for a delayed initiation of a rehabilitation program by several weeks and months and potentially increased rates of tendon healing.[9]

3. **Calcific tendinitis.** This disorder involves consolidation of calcium within the substance of a rotator cuff tendon. This condition can be extremely painful, particularly when or if the calcium diffuses out of the tendon as it causes an acute inflammatory bursitis. This disorder is treated symptomatically and a subacromial injection with corticosteroid and lidocaine may diminish acute symptoms and allow the patient to participate in PT. "Needling" the deposit (which in some cases is palpable) with an 18G needle and providing a subacromial injection may help to diminish the size of the deposit.[10] This technique may also be done under ultrasound guidance. If needling or subacromial injections are ineffective in controlling the patient's symptoms, the calcific deposit can be excised arthroscopically.

4. **Long head of biceps (LHB) tendinitis** often accompanies rotator cuff disease and frequently responds to bicipital groove injections or PT. If nonoperative treatment does not provide lasting relief, surgical treatment in the form of a tenotomy or tenodesis of the LHB may be indicated.

5. **Superior labrum anterior to posterior (SLAP) tears.** SLAP tears are common, particularly in older populations. Initial treatment should include an appropriate trial of nonoperative management.[11] When nonoperative management is ineffective in controlling symptoms, surgical intervention may be considered. For the young patient, a SLAP repair may represent a reasonable option. However, there is concern surrounding the outcomes of SLAP repairs, particularly in overhead athletes.[11-13] For many patients, this lesion may also be successfully treated with a biceps tenotomy or tenodesis, particularly if the SLAP tear is addressed concomitantly with a rotator cuff repair.[14]

## II. Glenohumeral Disorders

There are many causes for loss of glenohumeral range of motion. The most common are glenohumeral arthritis or shoulder stiffness. Both of these disorders are characterized by a loss of active and passive range of motion. This differs from other disorders such as rotator cuff disease in which passive range of motion is typically more normal, even when active range of motion is limited by pain or weakness.

## A. Glenohumeral arthritis

1. **Etiology.** Loss of the normal articular cartilage may be due to degeneration (osteoarthritis), rheumatoid disease, or secondary to previous trauma. Osteoarthritis is by far the most common etiology. A history of glenohumeral dislocation, particularly recurrent instability, also significantly increases one's risk of glenohumeral arthropathy.[15]

2. **History.** Patients with glenohumeral arthritis very often report significant pain at night, either owing to increased pain while lying flat or due to difficulty lying on the shoulder. Most patients also present with significant stiffness, and losses of internal/external rotation can be particularly dramatic.

3. **Examination.** These patients most often exhibit a loss of active and passive range of motion although strength is frequently normal. The change in the articular surface geometry, coupled with capsular contracture, causes a mechanical block to motion in these patients. Some patients exhibit crepitus, particularly in the midrange of motion. It is extremely important to make note of any neurovascular deficits as these are unlikely due to the shoulder arthritis and should be further evaluated for an additional etiology. The age group and demographic group that have shoulder arthritis and many other shoulder problems can also have cervical spine disease, which can cause similar symptoms.

4. **Imaging.** Radiographic examination must include a complete shoulder X-ray series (anteroposterior [AP], Grashey, Y view, and axillary view). Narrowing of the glenohumeral joint space is best seen on the Grashey and axillary views and gives an indication of the severity of arthritis. Severe posterior glenoid erosion is best appreciated on the axillary view but may also be seen on the Y view. Preferential posterior glenoid wear, or "biconcavity" and a "ring osteophyte," typically forms around the humeral head in the setting of osteoarthritis, whereas periarticular erosions and central glenoid wear are more common in rheumatoid arthritis. An MRI scan is indicated to assess rotator cuff integrity and glenoid version preoperatively. In cases of severe glenoid bone loss, a CT scan with or without three-dimensional (3D) reconstruction may be helpful for surgical planning.

5. **Treatment**

   a. **Nonoperative treatment.** Nonoperative treatment is indicated for early or moderate osteoarthritis. Nonsteroidal anti-inflammatory medications are effective in many cases, especially when coupled with activity modification. Viscosupplementation has not been approved by the Food and Drug Administration (FDA) for use in the shoulder, although it may represent an option for those patients with moderate arthritis or those patients wishing to defer surgical treatment.[16] Infrequent corticosteroid injections are a reasonable treatment for patients with moderate-to-severe arthritis for whom surgical treatment is not an option, although repeat corticosteroid injections should not generally be used as a long-term treatment unless surgical remediation is impossible. PT directed at gentle range of motion may be beneficial in the early stages of arthritis, although these exercises generally exacerbate pain in patients with advanced disease.

   b. **Operative treatment.** In early stages of arthritis, an arthroscopic capsular release may provide some relief of symptoms. For the very young patient (<50 years) with arthritis, a humeral resurfacing with or without allograft resurfacing of the glenoid is a reasonable option. A hemiarthroplasty is typically indicated primarily for patients who wish to continue heavy manual labor (repetitive lifting >50 lb, impact activities). For almost all other patients, a total shoulder arthroplasty is the best surgical option for glenohumeral arthritis. Total shoulder replacement results in greater range of motion and pain relief compared with hemiarthroplasty.[17,18]

**B. Shoulder stiffness** (adhesive capsulitis/frozen shoulder)

1. **Etiology.** Shoulder stiffness can be either primary or secondary. Primary etiologies include idiopathic shoulder stiffness from capsular fibrosis. This disorder is more common in patients with endocrine disorders such as thyroid abnormalities or diabetes mellitus, although the exact pathologic mechanism is not well understood. Secondary stiffness can result after a period of disuse following shoulder injury or after surgery.

2. **History.** These patients typically report aching pain in the shoulder that may be constant, but is also frequently exacerbated by activities, especially those at the extremes of motion. Some patients report a very acute onset of pain that may then be followed by the loss of shoulder motion.

3. **Examination.** Both active and passive range of motion are diminished, and internal/external rotation as well as forward elevation may be diminished. Rotator cuff strength is frequently normal, but it can be very difficult to determine true rotator cuff function secondary to the patient's limited and frequently painful range of motion.

4. **Imaging.** Imaging should be normal in this setting but a complete four-view shoulder series is necessary to rule out other disorders that may cause pain and stiffness (such as arthritis or calcific tendinitis). If an MRI is obtained to rule out other pathology, decreased axillary pouch volume or thickening of the capsule may be seen.

5. **Treatment**

   a. **Nonoperative.** PT accompanied by a dedicated home-based stretching program is effective for 90% of the patients.[19] It is essential to educate the patients that symptoms can take a very long time to resolve, even up to 18 months. A glenohumeral corticosteroid injection can be effective for patients particularly in the earliest stage or for patients in whom pain prevents their full participation in PT.

   b. **Operative treatment.** Surgery involves capsular releases to improve range of motion and can be done either closed or arthroscopically. A subacromial bursectomy typically accompanies a capsular release in this setting. Operative intervention is typically not employed until the patient fails 12 months of a dedicated stretching program.

**III. AC Joint Disorders**

**A. Arthritis**

1. **Etiology.** AC joint osteoarthritis is a very common finding, particularly in individuals older than 50 years. Most are asymptomatic. Although osteoarthritis is most common, posttraumatic AC arthritis is seen after distal clavicle fractures and AC separations. AC joint pain is also seen in young patients who participate in regular weight lifting, although the radiographic changes in these patients are more subtle.

2. **History.** Patients typically point directly to the superior aspect of the AC joint when localizing their pain. Activities reproducing cross-body adduction or internal rotation behind the back may also aggravate the patient's symptoms. Some patients report pain with weight on the superior part of the AC joint (straps from purses or bags, or brassieres).

3. **Examination.** Patients have tenderness on palpation at the site of the AC joint. Cross-body adduction, internal rotation up the back, and extreme forward elevation are often painful. The active compression test is also often positive.[20]

4. **Imaging.** The typical complete four-view shoulder X-ray series is recommended. The AC joint is typically seen best in profile on the AP view. Osteophyte formation and joint space narrowing may be seen in osteoarthritis, whereas lytic changes in the distal clavicle are often seen in younger patients (distal clavicle osteolysis). These lytic changes are often best seen radiographically with a Zanca view.

5. **Treatment.** Management of AC arthritis is based primarily on symptom management and typically involves oral analgesics and, if necessary, a corticosteroid injection into the AC joint. If nonoperative treatment does not provide long-term relief of symptoms, a distal clavicle resection is indicated and may be done either arthroscopically or open.[21]

## IV. Scapulothoracic Disorders
### A. Scapulothoracic bursitis (snapping scapula)

1. **Etiology.** The scapula glides along the posterior chest wall, thereby acting to increase the range through which the arm or hand can be positioned. The bursa between the scapula and the thorax assists in allowing this gliding motion. Rarely, inflammation of this bursa or variable scapular anatomy causes scapulothoracic motion to become painful.

2. **History.** These patients may localize their pain to the posterior medial border of the scapula and describe crepitus with scapulothoracic motion.

3. **Examination.** Typically, the patient will demonstrate crepitus about the medial border of the scapula that may be palpable or even audible to the examiner.

4. **Imaging studies** are rarely diagnostic, but should include a shoulder series and complete imaging of the scapula to rule out any other pathology, including bone or soft-tissue tumors such as osteochondroma and elastofibroma dorsi.

5. **Treatment.** Management of this disorder involves dedicated PT to include parascapular strengthening and improved glenohumeral and scapulothoracic mechanics. For patients who are very symptomatic, a corticosteroid injection into the scapulothoracic bursa can be effective. Very rarely, if nonoperative methods do not provide long-term relief, an arthroscopic or open bursectomy and excision of the superior medial border of the scapula may be considered.[22]

### B. Winging of the scapula

1. **Etiology.** Scapular winging may result from dysfunction of the muscles that control the position of the scapula against the chest wall, involving the serratus anterior (innervated by the long thoracic nerve) or the trapezius (innervated by the spinal accessory nerve). Most often, this form of scapular winging involves some form of injury to the nerves innervating these muscles. Facioscapulohumeral muscular dystrophy is a rare cause of scapular winging. It is a form of muscular dystrophy that results in weakness of the facial and upper trunk muscles. Patients characteristically cannot whistle, and it can and may lead to unilateral or bilateral winging. Because of the autosomal dominant inheritance, it is frequently seen in families, albeit with variable penetrance. Scapular dyskinesia is a common finding in patients with glenohumeral dysfunction, but does not represent true scapular winging.

2. **History.** Patients typically report shoulder dysfunction in the form of weakness and a loss of active shoulder motion. Many patients also report the acute onset of shoulder pain at the same time. Some patients have a history of surgery or trauma in the region of the nerve affected, but most patients do not have a cause for their dysfunction. In these patients, the etiology may be a form of neuritis.

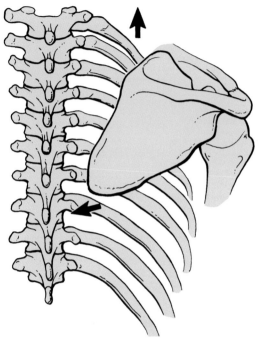

**Figure 17-1.** Position of the scapula with primary scapular winging because of serratus anterior palsy. The scapula pulls away from the back and does not protract on arm elevation. (From Kuhn JE, Hawkins RJ. Evaluation and treatment of scapular disorders. In: Warner JJP, Iannotti JP, Gerber C, eds. *Complex and Revision Problems in Shoulder Surgery*. Philadelphia, PA: Lippincott-Raven; 1997:357-375.)

3. **Examination.** Involvement of the long thoracic nerve or serratus anterior produces medial scapular winging, whereby the scapula is translated medially and superiorly (Fig. 17-1). This can be best visualized by having the patient raise the affected arm to the horizontal and push against the wall or the examiner's hand. Involvement of the spinal accessory nerve, trapezius, and rhomboids produces lateral scapular winging, in which the scapula elevates off the thorax and translates laterally. This is most commonly iatrogenic and can result from a biopsy or other surgical procedure that injures cranial nerve XI. In this form of injury, the shoulder may be found to have a more drooping posture and the patient may have a significant loss of shoulder abduction.

4. **Treatment** involves dedicated PT focused on parascapular strengthening and maintaining glenohumeral motion. Scapular winging because of neuromuscular dysfunction frequently takes 12 months or more to recover. If no recovery is seen after 12 to 24 months, surgical management may be considered. Operative treatment is complex, however, involving either tendon transfers or a scapulothoracic fusion.[23]

## REFERENCES

1. Bigliani LU, Ticker JB, Flatow EL, et al. The relationship of acromial architecture to rotator cuff disease. *Clin Sports Med.* 1991;10(4):823-838.
2. Goldberg BA, Lippitt SB, Matsen FA III. Improvement in comfort and function after cuff repair without acromioplasty. *Clin Orthop Relat Res.* 2001;(390):142-150.
3. Alvarez CM, Litchfield R, Jackowski D, et al. A prospective, double-blind, randomized clinical trial comparing subacromial injection of betamethasone and xylocaine to xylocaine alone in chronic rotator cuff tendinosis. *Am J Sports Med.* 2005;33(2):255-262.
4. Vitale MA, Vitale MG, Zivin JG, et al. Rotator cuff repair: an analysis of utility scores and cost-effectiveness. *J Shoulder Elbow Surg.* 2007;16(2):181-187.
5. Kuhn JE, Dunn WR, Sanders R, et al. Effectiveness of physical therapy in treating atraumatic full-thickness rotator cuff tears: a multicenter prospective cohort study. *J Shoulder Elbow Surg.* 2013;22(10):1371-1379.
6. Gladstone JN, Bishop JY, Lo IK, et al. Fatty infiltration and atrophy of the rotator cuff do not improve after rotator cuff repair and correlate with poor functional outcome. *Am J Sports Med.* 2007;35(5):719-728.
7. Millett PJ, Horan MP, Maland KE, et al. Long-term survivorship and outcomes after surgical repair of full-thickness rotator cuff tears. *J Shoulder Elbow Surg.* 2011;20:591-597.
8. Morse K, Davis AD, Afra R, et al. Arthroscopic versus mini-open rotator cuff repair: a comprehensive review and meta-analysis. *Am J Sports Med.* 2008;36(9):1824-1828.
9. Parsons BO, Gruson KI, Chen DD, et al. Does slower rehabilitation after arthroscopic rotator cuff repair lead to long-term stiffness? *J Shoulder Elbow Surg.* 2010;19(7):1034-1039.
10. Yoo JC, Koh KH, Park WH, et al. The outcome of ultrasound-guided needle decompression and steroid injection in calcific tendinitis. *J Shoulder Elbow Surg.* 2010;19(4):596-600.
11. Edwards SL, Lee JA, Bell JE, et al. Nonoperative treatment of superior labrum anterior posterior tears: improvements in pain, function, and quality of life. *Am J Sports Med.* 2010;38(7):1456-1461.
12. Neri BR, ElAttrache NS, Owsley KC, et al. Outcome of type II superior labral anterior posterior repairs in elite overhead athletes: effect of concomitant partial-thickness rotator cuff tears. *Am J Sports Med.* 2011;39(1):114-120.
13. Gorantla K, Gill C, Wright RW. The outcome of type II SLAP repair: a systematic review. *Arthroscopy.* 2010;26(4):537-545.
14. Franceschi F, Longo UG, Ruzzini L, et al. No advantages in repairing a type II superior labrum anterior and posterior (SLAP) lesion when associated with rotator cuff repair in patients over age 50: a randomized controlled trial. *Am J Sports Med.* 2008;36(2):247-253.
15. Hovelius L, Saeboe M. Neer Award 2008: arthropathy after primary anterior shoulder dislocation–223 shoulders prospectively followed up for twenty-five years. *J Shoulder Elbow Surg.* 2009;18(3):339-347.
16. Noël E, Hardy P, Hagena FW, et al. Efficacy and safety of Hylan G-F 20 in shoulder osteoarthritis with an intact rotator cuff. Open-label prospective multicenter study. *Joint Bone Spine.* 2009;76(6):670-673.
17. Izquierdo R, Voloshin I, Edwards S, et al. American Academy of Orthopaedic Surgeons Clinical Practice Guideline on: the treatment of glenohumeral joint osteoarthritis. *J Bone Joint Surg Am.* 2011;93(2):203-205.
18. Bryant D, Litchfield R, Sandow M, et al. A comparison of pain, strength, range of motion, and functional outcomes after hemiarthroplasty and total shoulder arthroplasty in patients with osteoarthritis of the shoulder. A systematic review and meta-analysis. *J Bone Joint Surg Am.* 2005;87(9):1947-1956.
19. Levine WN, Kashyap CP, Bak SF, et al. Nonoperative management of idiopathic adhesive capsulitis. *J Shoulder Elbow Surg.* 2007;16(5):569-573.
20. O'Brien SJ, Pagnani MJ, Fealy S, et al. The active compression test: a new and effective test for diagnosing labral tears and acromioclavicular joint abnormality. *Am J Sports Med.* 1998;26(5):610-613.
21. Flatow EL, Duralde XA, Nicholson GP, et al. Arthroscopic resection of the distal clavicle with a superior approach. *J Shoulder Elbow Surg.* 1995;4(1, pt 1):41-50.
22. Lehtinen JT, Macy JC, Cassinelli E, et al. The painful scapulothoracic articulation: surgical management. *Clin Orthop Relat Res.* 2004;(423):99-105.
23. Wiater JM, Flatow EL. Long thoracic nerve injury. *Clin Orthop Relat Res.* 1999;(368):17-27.

# 18

# Fractures of the Humerus

Ariel A. Williams

## I. Fractures of the Proximal Humerus

A. **Mechanism.** Proximal humerus fractures are seen in all age groups, but are more common in the elderly. In young adults, they are a result of high-energy trauma. In older patients, they often result from low-energy falls.[1]

B. **Physical examination.** Bruising and swelling of the shoulder and pain and crepitus with passive motion of the glenohumeral joint suggest a proximal humerus fracture. A careful neurologic examination is essential, as proximal humerus fractures and fracture–dislocations can be accompanied by axillary nerve and brachial plexus injuries.

C. **Radiographs.** Evaluation should include anteroposterior, true anteroposterior, and axillary lateral shoulder radiographs, as well as anteroposterior and lateral films of the humerus. Pain may limit motion, making obtaining an axillary lateral radiograph difficult. Assisting the patient by slowly and gently elevating the arm while they lie in a supine position can achieve sufficient elevation for axillary radiographs. Alternatively, a Velpeau view, obtained with the patient's arm resting at their side and their forearm across their chest, can also demonstrate fracture alignment.

D. **Treatment.** Neer divides proximal humerus fractures into six groups, as shown in Fig. 18-1, on the basis of the number of fracture fragments and the degree of displacement.[2] In order to be considered a displaced fragment, the fragment must be displaced more than 1 cm or angulated more than 45°. (Thus, a nondisplaced fracture is a Neer one-part fracture, no matter the number of fracture lines.) Although studies have shown a lack of interrater reliability in interpreting radiographs to accurately classify proximal humerus fractures,[3] the Neer classification remains the most often utilized.

1. **Fractures with minimal displacement (Neer one-part fractures).** Approximately 85% of all fractures of the proximal humerus fall into this category. These fractures are typically managed nonoperatively with a sling and early motion. Stability is usually afforded by some impaction at the fracture site and the preservation of soft-tissue attachments. Elbow, wrist, and hand range-of-motion exercises should begin immediately. Shoulder circumduction exercises (aka pendulum exercises) are initiated as soon as they can be tolerated, generally within 5 to 7 days. The patient is instructed to bend 90° at the waist, allowing the arm to either hang or swing in a gentle circle and avoid active contraction of the shoulder muscles.[2] Assisted forward elevation and assisted external rotation exercises in the supine position can generally be started approximately 10 to 14 days after injury. Some form of protection may be needed for 6 to 8 weeks; then more vigorous physical therapy may be prescribed, including wall climbing, overhead rope-and-pulley, passive range of motion, and rotator cuff strengthening exercises.[4]

2. **Neer two-part fractures.** Many displaced two-part fractures benefit from surgery. Surgical neck fractures generally occur with the arm in abduction. The rotator cuff is usually intact. The fracture site is often angulated more

Displaced fractures

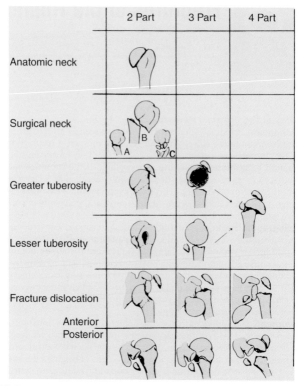

**Figure 18-1.** Neer's anatomic concept for standardizing the terminology of fractures of the proximal humerus. (From Neer CS II. Displaced proximal humeral fractures. Part I. Classification and evaluation. *J Bone Joint Surg Am*. 1970;52:1077-1089, with permission.)

than 45° or malrotated. Neurovascular injury can occur in this type of fracture because the shaft may be displaced into the axilla. This is more common in elderly patients with atherosclerotic (less compliant) arteries. If surgery is undertaken, the fracture may be reduced with abduction and flexion of the distal fragment and fixation accomplished with percutane- ously placed pins.[5] Alternatively, open reduction internal fixation can be performed with a locking plate and screws, obtaining more rigid fixation than percutaneous pins and allowing earlier initiation of range of motion postoperatively. Two-part fractures involving the anatomic neck are less common. Because of the blood supply to the humeral head, these frac- tures may lead to osteonecrosis. Greater and lesser tuberosity fractures are of special note because they compromise the rotator cuff insertions. Surgical fixation of tuberosity fractures can be accomplished with screws, nonabsorbable sutures, or tension band **wiring**. If the fracture fragment is very small, it can be excised and the rotator cuff repaired directly down to bone with suture anchors.

3. Neer (see Selected Historical Readings) states that open reduction is indicated for any displaced **three-part fracture** and that prosthetic replacement is preferable treatment for any displaced **four-part fracture**. This is due to the high rate of posttraumatic humeral head osteonecrosis in four-part fractures. We believe that, at best, these are difficult fractures to treat and that operative treatment should be undertaken only by surgeons with special expertise in managing shoulder trauma. Recently, there has been a shift in management of unstable displaced fractures, especially those in older patients with poor bone quality to reverse shoulder arthroplasty.[4]

4. **A fracture–dislocation of the shoulder**, whether anterior or posterior, may be reduced by a closed method under general anesthesia. If closed reduction fails, open reduction with internal fixation or prosthetic replacement (in older patients) is indicated.

**E. Complications**

1. The most common complication is **loss of some glenohumeral motion**, especially internal rotation and abduction. This often occurs as a result of malposition of the greater tuberosity. The best way to rehabilitate the glenohumeral joint is to start motion early and achieve primary fracture union. Careful attention to starting an early physical therapy program can markedly improve the end result. Home programs where exercises are performed by a motivated patient two to three times per day with weekly physical therapy monitoring seem to produce the best results. Open treatment may be indicated to achieve adequate stability of displaced fractures to allow early motion.

2. **Delayed union or nonunion** is not uncommon with displaced fractures, especially surgical neck fractures. When it occurs, some loss of joint motion generally results, regardless of subsequent treatment. If the patient experiences pain and loss of motion in association with the nonunion, the treatment is either replacement arthroplasty or internal fixation with bone grafting.

3. **Associated nerve and vascular damage** is not rare with displaced fractures and should be identified early so that prompt, effective treatment can be instituted. Involvement of the axillary, median, radial, and ulnar nerves is reported with nearly equal frequency.

4. **Osteonecrosis.** Avascular necrosis (AVN) of the humeral head is more likely to occur after three- or four-part fractures or fracture–dislocations, but can follow even innocuous appearing fractures. AVN is well tolerated in the upper extremity as it is frequently asymptomatic and patients have fairly good function.

5. If symptomatic, osteonecrosis is often managed with shoulder arthroplasty in older patients.

**II. Proximal Humeral Epiphyseal Separation**

A. **Anatomy.** The proximal humeral remains open until 14 to 18 years of age and accounts for about 80% of the length of the humerus. In younger children, significant angulation at the fracture site is well tolerated because of the remodeling potential of the growing proximal humerus.

B. **Radiographs.** Anteroposterior and axillary lateral radiographs typically illustrate the fracture. The most common pattern is a Salter–Harris type 2 injury, but numerous variations have been reported (see **Chapter 2 for description of the Salter–Harris classification**). Salter–Harris type 1 injuries are seen in neonates and in very young children.

C. **Treatment.** This fracture can often be reduced by closed methods with appropriate anesthesia. Reduction requires aligning the distal fragment to the proximal one, usually by abduction and external rotation of the distal fragment.

As long as the rotation of the two fragments relative to one another is correct, up to 70° of angulation can remodel to produce normal shoulder function up to 7 years of age. Up to 11 years in a girl and 12 years in a boy, 50% apposition is acceptable, but varus malalignment should not exceed 45° and rotary deformity must be minimal.[6,7] Treatment is then carried out in a sling with circumduction exercises. A hanging long arm cast is a useful way to use gravity to align fracture fragments in these fractures.

D. Open reduction is rarely indicated, but closed manipulation and percutaneous pin fixation should be considered if closed reduction fails to achieve an acceptable degree of correction and stability. The mature adolescent should be treated as an adult.

### III. Diaphyseal Humerus Fractures

A. **Mechanism.** Diaphyseal humerus fractures can be the result of high-energy trauma in young patients or much lower energy mechanisms in the elderly. The incidence of this fracture is bimodal, occurring at the highest rates in young adults and individuals of age 60 and older.[8,9] Although the fracture may occur in any part of the diaphyseal bone, the middle third is the most commonly involved.

B. **Physical examination** should be thorough to rule out any nerve or vascular damage. The time of onset of any nerve involvement must be accurately documented. The radial nerve travels through the spiral groove directly on the humeral shaft and is injured in approximately 11% of diaphyseal humerus fractures.[9] If the radial nerve is intact, the patient will be able to extend the wrist against gravity and extend the fingers as well as the thumb. If the radial nerve is not functioning, the patient will still be able to use the hand intrinsics to extend the fingers at the proximal interphalangeal joints. Do not be fooled.

There are three separate mechanisms by which the radial nerve may be injured.

1. **Damage at the time of injury** usually produces a neurapraxia, less commonly an axonotmesis or traction injury, and rarely a neurotmesis. Neurotmesis is most commonly associated with open fractures.[10]

2. **During the process of manipulation and immobilization,** neurapraxia can occur, and if the pressure is not relieved, it can become an axonotmesis. This is usually a result of the nerve being trapped between the fracture fragments.

3. **During the process of internal fixation,** neurapraxia or axonotmesis can develop from manipulation of the nerve.

C. **Treatment.** Initial fracture treatment includes immobilizing the arm against the chest with plaster coaptation splints, as shown in Fig. 18-2. The patient should begin hand and wrist range-of-motion exercises immediately to prevent stiffness. Two to 3 weeks after injury, the splint can be removed and the patient placed into a snug-fitting commercial or custom fracture brace.[11,12] Shoulder and elbow motion is then initiated. Bayonet apposition is acceptable as long as angular alignment is good. Distraction should be avoided and is generally a harbinger of nonunion.

Open reduction and internal fixation is indicated for open fractures, fractures with associated vascular injuries, Holstein–Lewis fractures (an oblique distal third fracture with radial nerve injury where the nerve can be trapped in the fracture), bilateral fractures, in the setting of massive obesity (where closed reduction and effective orthotic treatment is not possible), and for patients with polytrauma.[13] Plates and screws, reamed intramedullary (IM) nails, and flexible IM nails seem to be equally efficacious. IM nails can be placed without opening the fracture site, but they do result in a 20% to 30% incidence of postoperative shoulder pain and stiffness.[14] For this reason, plate fixation is the preferred method of operative stabilization in most settings.

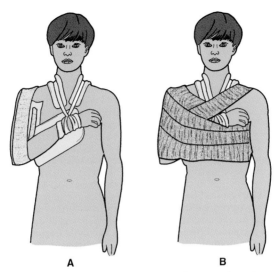

**A**                                    **B**

**Figure 18-2.** Treatment of the humeral shaft fractures. **A:** The first step is to apply coaptation splints to the arm and then to apply a commercial collar and cuff or one made of muslin. Stockinette should not be used because it stretches. The neck and wrist are padded beneath the collar and cuff with felt. **B:** After adequate padding in the axilla and beneath the forearm, the arm and forearm can be immobilized against the thorax with a swathe.

    **D. Treatment of an associated radial nerve injury.**
    **E.** Nerve involvement at the time of injury should be managed with observation, passive range-of-motion exercises of the wrist and fingers, and use of a radial nerve splint for the wrist and fingers. The prognosis for recovery is excellent, with 80% or more patients regaining full function, although recovery may take 1 year or longer. Based on a meta-analysis, Shao et al.[9] provided a treatment algorithm for humeral shaft fractures with radial nerve injuries that recommends observation as the initial treatment in most cases. If radial nerve function is present after the injury, but lost after closed reduction, the nerve should be explored in the operating room. Late nerve involvement is also an indication for exploration and neurolysis.
    **F. Complications.** Delayed unions and nonunions do occur and are best treated with compression plating and a cancellous bone graft. If nonunion occurs after IM nailing, plate fixation with bone grafting results in healing in approximately 90% of cases; repeat IM nailing is generally not advisable.
**IV. Supracondylar Humerus Fractures—Pediatric**
    **A. Mechanism.** Pediatric supracondylar humerus fractures most commonly result from a fall on an outstretched arm. The fracture propagates through the thin bone of the distal humerus between the olecranon fossa and the coronoid fossa.
    **B. Physical examination.** The elbow is typically markedly swollen and tender. Associated vascular and nerve injury is common, and the examiner must carefully document function of the radial, median, ulnar, posterior interosseous, and anterior interosseous nerves, as well as the quality of the radial pulse and capillary refill of the hand. Vascular damage, nerve damage, or marked displacement constitutes a surgical emergency. In addition, the examiner should

carefully examine the wrist and shoulder for tenderness or deformity and palpate the forearm compartments for signs of compartment syndrome.

C. **Radiographs.** Anteroposterior and lateral radiographs of the elbow and forearm should be obtained. The numerous growth plates at the elbow and their changing appearance during growth make interpreting pediatric elbow radiographs challenging. In some cases, radiographs of the opposite elbow can be helpful in making a diagnosis. In rare instances, a magnetic resonance imaging (MRI) may be necessary to determine the presence and character of an injury. However, MRI should be used sparingly in young children because of the need for sedation and/or general anesthesia so as to obtain an adequate examination.

D. **Treatment.** The Gartland Classification divides supracondylar humerus fractures into three types. Type I fractures are nondisplaced. The fracture line may not be visible on radiographs, the only sign of an underlying injury a lucency along the posterior distal humerus on the lateral view. This is the "posterior fat pad sign" caused by a hemarthrosis elevating the fat pad around the elbow. Type II fractures are displaced but the posterior cortex remains intact, acting as a hinge for extension of the distal fragment. In type III fractures, there is no cortical continuity between the proximal and distal fragments. This can lead to quite significant displacement. Type I fractures are treated nonoperatively in a cast for 3 to 4 weeks. The appropriate management for type II fractures is controversial. Some type II fractures can be treated nonoperatively, but there is no consensus on how these fractures are best identified.[15] If nonoperative treatment is elected, although it may be tempting to reduce the fracture by hyperflexing the elbow, the elbow should not be flexed more than 90° because of the ensuing risk of compartment syndrome. More displaced type II supracondylar fractures are typically treated with closed reduction and percutaneous pinning. This can be performed on an outpatient basis within a few days of injury.[16] All type III fractures require reduction and pinning. Because of the seriousness of the potential complications of compartment syndrome and neurovascular compromise with a type III supracondylar fracture, nearly all children with these injuries are admitted to the hospital to facilitate prompt surgical intervention and close monitoring of neurovascular status. As soon as the condition of the patient allows, a definitive reduction under general anesthesia is attempted. The technique of reduction is illustrated in Figs. 18-3 and 18-4. Pin configuration is controversial. Traditionally, crossed K-wires (one from the medial side and one from the lateral side) have been the predominant configuration. This requires small incisions to place the medial pin to be sure the ulnar nerve is not injured.[17] However, the use of several lateral pins has been shown to be equally efficacious at maintaining reduction while avoiding ulnar nerve injuries from the medial pin.[17] If the patient is seen late and the swelling is massive, an alternative is the use of Dunlop traction until the swelling resolves (see Fig. 10-5).

*In the younger child, there is some latitude in anteroposterior angulation or displacement.* The direction of the initial displacement provides a clue for the proper forearm position after reduction. If the initial displacement is medial, placing the forearm into pronation tightens the medial hinge, closes any lateral gap in the fracture line, and helps prevent subsequent cubitus varus. If the initial displacement is lateral, placing the forearm in supination tightens the lateral soft-tissue hinge, closes the medial aspect of the fracture line, and helps prevent cubitus deformity.

The use of **Baumann angle** to guide treatment was described in the German literature in 1929. To use this technique, bilateral radiographs of the distal humerus are necessary. A line is drawn down the center of the diaphysis of the humerus, and another is drawn across the epiphyseal plate

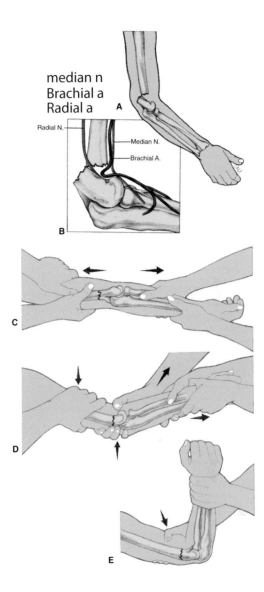

median n
Brachial a
Radial a   A

Radial N.

Median N.

Brachial A.

B

C

D

E

**Figure 18-3.** Reduction technique for supracondylar humeral fractures that occur with the elbow in flexion. **A:** Distal fragment is displaced posteriorly. **B:** The brachial artery may become entrapped at the fracture site. **C:** Restore length by applying traction against countertraction. **D:** With pressure directed anteriorly on the distal fragment, provide reduction. **E:** The reduction is generally stable with the elbow in flexion with the forearm pronated.

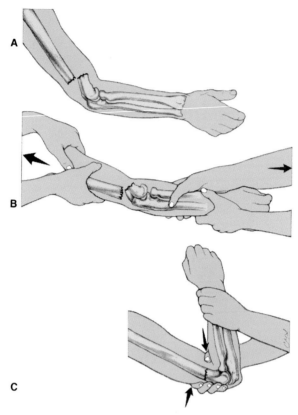

**Figure 18-4.** Reduction technique for supracondylar fractures that occur with the elbow in extension. **A:** The distal fragment is displaced anteriorly relative to the proximal fragment. **B:** Restore length by applying traction against countertraction. **C:** With pressure directed posteriorly on the distal fragment, the fracture is reduced. The elbow is then extended to enhance stability of the reduction in most circumstances.

of the capitellum. If the angle is 5° different from the unaffected side, the reduction is not complete and a significant abnormality in the carrying angle, such as cubitus varus, may result. The reduction is generally off in rotation. On the lateral radiograph, the anterior humeral line must pass through the capitellum to ensure that there is no malreduction with rotation or extension.

Open reduction may be necessary if repeated attempts at closed reduction fail. An anterior or lateral incision may be used to expose the fracture. The anterior incision may provide the easiest direct exposure because of the generally extensive damage to the brachial muscle by the fracture displacement. Splint the elbow in 20° to 30° of flexion after pinning the fracture to allow for swelling. The patient must be observed with frequent neurovascular checks for at least 24 hours for signs and symptoms of compartment syndrome. The pins are removed after 3 to 4 weeks, and intermittent active motion is started out of cast or splint. The splint is discarded. Stiffness may result from overzealous attempts of family, friends, and therapists to aid the child in regaining motion quickly. The child should be allowed to use the elbow, and the family should be reassured that he or she will gain extension of the joint with time and growth.

**Distal humeral epiphyseal slips** in younger children are rare, but when they occur, they should be treated as supracondylar fractures. This particular fracture pattern can be associated with nonaccidental trauma, and the provider should be alert to this possibility.

E. **Complications**
   1. Cubitus varus and valgus (varus is far more common)
   2. Loss of elbow motion
   3. Tardy ulnar nerve palsy

V. **Supracondylar and Intercondylar Fractures—Adults**
   A. **Mechanism of injury.** Distal humerus fractures often result from low-energy falls in elderly patients or high-energy trauma in young adults.
   B. **Physical examination.** The elbow is swollen, and the patient is unable to move the elbow actively in most cases. A careful neurologic examination should be documented. Ulnar nerve dysfunction is especially common with high-energy distal humerus fractures.
   C. **Radiographs.** Anteroposterior and lateral elbow and humerus radiographs should be obtained. A traction anteroposterior radiograph can help characterize comminuted fractures. Fractures vary from simple transverse supracondylar fractures to severely comminuted intraarticular fractures. Computed tomographic (CT) imaging of the elbow may be helpful for operative planning in cases with significant comminution.
   D. **Treatment.** Elbow stiffness develops rapidly in adults; therefore, early elbow and hand motion is the key to a good functional result. At the initial presentation, the fractured extremity should be placed in a well-padded posterior splint. Open reduction and internal fixation is the treatment of choice for most fractures.[18] Most fractures are visualized through an olecranon osteotomy, paratricipital or triceps splitting approach. The configuration of plates depends on the fracture pattern and surgeon preference, but fixation must be secure enough to allow early motion. Highly comminuted fractures should be referred to experienced fracture surgeons to prevent the situation of open reduction and unstable fixation.

   Patients undergoing internal fixation should be started on active range-of-motion exercises within 3 to 5 days of the procedure. Tenderness usually disappears in 4 to 6 weeks; the splint is then discarded, and further active elbow movement is encouraged. In the most comminuted fractures in elderly individuals, total elbow replacement is an alternative option to open reduction internal fixation.

   E. **Complications**
      1. **Heterotopic ossification** can lead to elbow stiffness and limited motion. Risk factors for heterotopic ossification include concomitant head injury, delay in operative intervention, and repeated surgeries. At this time, there is no evidence that routine heterotopic ossification prophylaxis in the form of indomethacin or radiation is indicated.[19]
      2. **Loss of motion** is common after these fractures, especially if the fracture is comminuted and extends into the joint.
      3. **Ulnar nerve dysfunction** can occur at the time of injury or because of manipulation of the nerve or swelling intraoperatively. Some surgeons routinely transpose the ulnar nerve at the time of operative fixation, but studies report conflicting evidence about the benefits of routine transposition.[19]

## VI. Lateral Condyle Fractures—Pediatric

A. **Mechanism.** The lateral condyle fracture may result from a fall on an out-stretched hand. Alternatively, the fracture may occur as a result of the common extensor origin avulsing the bone fragment. These fractures typically occur in young children, with the peak incidence occurring at age 6.

B. **Radiographs.** Routine anteroposterior and lateral elbow radiographs are obtained, but oblique films and films of the uninjured elbow are often needed to define the injury accurately. Occasionally, an MRI may be necessary to further delineate the injury.

C. **Treatment.** Nondisplaced fractures can be managed in a long arm splint or cast for 4 weeks. Close follow-up is necessary, with repeat films 3 to 5 days after the initial injury. If the fracture is displaced, the treatment of choice has traditionally been open reduction and fixation with Kirschner wires or a screw. However, closed reduction and percutaneous pinning in experienced hands may produce equivalent results.[20]

D. **Complications**
1. **Failure to achieve accurate reduction of the fracture** results in cubitus valgus, late arthritic changes, nonunion, and/or a tardy ulnar nerve palsy.
2. When the epiphysis is open, **overgrowth of the lateral condyle** occasionally occurs, with a resulting cubitus varus.
3. **Osteonecrosis of the lateral condyle** can occur after open reduction, especially if the soft tissues containing the vascular supply are stripped off of the posterior aspect of the condyle.

## VII. Medial Epicondyle Fractures

A. **Mechanism of injury.** The center of ossification of the medial epicondyle of the humerus appears at 5 to 7 years of age. Medial epicondyle fractures most commonly result from an elbow dislocation with avulsion of the fragment. The medial ligament of the elbow maintains its inferior attachment and pulls the medial epicondyle from the humerus. This fracture is most common in children ages 9 to 14, but it can also occur in adults.

B. **Physical examination.** The patient often presents with medial elbow pain and swelling, and some patients have associated ulnar nerve dysfunction.

C. **Radiographs.** Anteroposterior and lateral elbow radiographs are used to identify the position of the medial epicondyle. Radiographs of the normal elbow for comparison can be helpful to identify the amount of apophyseal displacement. If the elbow was dislocated and spontaneously reduces, the medial epicondyle fragment can become entrapped in the joint.

D. **Treatment.** Reduce any elbow dislocation by linear traction with sedation and assess the position of the fragment radiographically. If the fracture is less than 2 mm displaced, the injury can be managed with immobilization for 7 to 10 days, followed by early active motion. If the joint is not congruent, an entrapped bony fragment is likely.

Indications for surgery include bony fragments in the joint, valgus instability, or a fracture displaced more than 5 mm. Young overhead athletes with more mildly displaced fractures and those with high-energy injuries may also benefit from surgery.[21] The medial epicondyle fracture can be reduced and held by screw fixation. Pins can be used for smaller fragments (Fig. 18-5). If open reduction is undertaken, the ulnar nerve must be protected but need **not** be transposed anteriorly.

**Complications** are largely those of an elbow dislocation. Nonunion of the medial epicondyle fragment is common with nonoperative management but usually asymptomatic. A displaced medial epicondyle may result in valgus instability of the elbow.

E. If the medial epicondyle remains displaced, ulnar nerve problems are not uncommon.

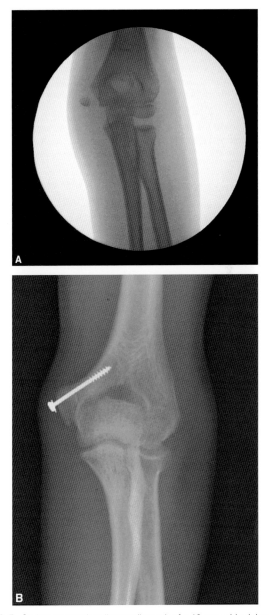

**Figure 18-5. A:** Anteroposterior elbow radiograph of a 16-year-old adolescent boy who injured his elbow while playing football demonstrates a displaced medial epicondyle fracture. **B:** Anatomic alignment following open reduction internal fixation with a small fragment screw and washer.

## HCMC Treatment Recommendations

### Proximal Humerus Fractures

**Diagnosis:** Anteroposterior shoulder radiograph with axillary view and transscapular lateral (shoulder trauma series) view. Consider computed tomography scan with reconstructions if a displaced three- or four-part fracture is noted on plain radiographs and the patient is a surgical candidate.

**Treatment:** Be sure that the humeral head is located. If the fracture is impacted or minimally displaced, apply sling for comfort and begin assisted range-of-motion exercises from 7 to 14 days.

**Indications for surgery:** Marked (>1 cm) displacement of tuberosity fragments, varus angulation of head, dislocated humeral head, head-splitting fracture, or open fractures.

**Technical options:** On the basis of age of the patient, type of fracture, and bone quality:

- Greater tuberosity fractures: open reduction and screw or tension band fixation
- Two-part surgical neck fractures: closed reduction and percutaneous pinning in pediatric fractures, plate or intramedullary nail fixation in adults
- Three-part fractures: closed reduction and pinning versus open reduction and internal fixation
- Four-part fractures, head-splitting fractures: prosthetic replacement is advisable for elderly patients with markedly comminuted fractures or those associated with humeral head dislocation

## HCMC Treatment Recommendations

### Humeral Shaft Fractures

**Diagnosis:** Anteroposterior and lateral humeral radiographs, physical examination. Be sure to check radial nerve function.

**Treatment:** Closed reduction and application of coaptation splints—convert splints to functional brace and begin range-of-motion exercises for shoulder and elbow 2 weeks after injury.

**Indications for surgery:** Multiply injured patient or extremity, unacceptable reduction, open fractures, nonunion.

**Recommended technique:** 4.5-mm large fragment low-contact dynamic compression plate, explore and protect radial nerve. Alternatively, use an antegrade interlocking humeral nail but expect shoulder pain in 20% to 30% of individuals.

## HCMC Treatment Recommendations

### Distal Humerus Fractures

**Diagnosis:** Anteroposterior and lateral elbow radiographs and physical examinations

**Treatment:** Initial long arm splint after documenting neurocirculatory status

**Indications for surgery:** Any displacement of the joint surface (>2 mm) open fractures

**Recommended technique:** Posterior approach with olecranon osteotomy where articular displacement is severe

## REFERENCES

1. Palvanen M, Kannus P, Niemi S, Parkkari J. Update in the epidemiology of proximal humeral fractures. *Clin Orthop Relat Res.* 2006;442:87-92.
2. Jawa A, Burnikel DL. Treatment of proximal humerus fractures. *JBJS Rev.* 2016;4:1-9.
3. Siebenrock KA, Gerber C. The reproducibility of classification of fractures of the proximal end of the humerus. *J Bone Joint Surg Am.* 1993;75:1751-1755.
4. George M, Kazzam M, Chin P, et al. Reverse shoulder arthroplasty for treatment of proximal humerus fractures. *JBJS Rev.* 2014;2:1-8.
5. Harrison AK, Grison KL, Zmistowski B, et al. Intermediate outcomes following percutaneous fixation of proximal humerus fractures. *JBJS.* 2012;94:1223-1228.
6. Dobbs MB, Luhmann SL, Gordon JE, Strecker WB, Schoenecker PL. Severely displaced proximal humeral epiphyseal fractures. *J Pediatr Orthop.* 2003;23:208-215.
7. Beaty JH. Fractures of the proximal humerus and shaft in children. In: Eibert RE, ed. *AAOS Instructional Course Lectures.* American Academy of Orthopaedic Surgeons; 1992:369-372.
8. Tytherleigh-Strong G, Walls N, McQueen MM. The epidemiology of humeral shaft fractures. *J Bone Joint Surg Br.* 1998;80:249-253.
9. Shao YC, Harwood P, Grotz MR, Limb D, Giannoudis PV. Radial nerve palsy associated with fractures of the shaft of the humerus: a systematic review. *J Bone Joint Surg Br.* 2005;87:1647-1652.
10. Foster RJ, Swiontkowski MR, Bach AW, Sack JT. Radial nerve palsy caused by open humeral shaft fractures. *J Hand Surg Am.* 1993;18:121-124.
11. Wallny T, Westermann K, Sagebiel C, Reimer M, Wagner UA. Functional treatment of humeral shaft fractures: indications and results. *J Orthop Trauma.* 1997;11:283-287.
12. Zagorski JB, Latta LL, Zych GA, Finnieston AR. Diaphyseal fractures of the humerus. Treatment with prefabricated braces. *J Bone Joint Surg Am.* 1988;70:607-610.
13. Basem A, Obremsky W. Treatment of humeral shaft fractures. *JBJS Rev.* 2015;3:1-9.
14. Putti AB, Uppin RB, Putti BB. Locked intramedullary nailing versus dynamic compression plating for humeral shaft fractures. *J Orthop Surg (Hong Kong).* 2009;17:139-141.
15. Moraleda L, Valencia M, Barco R, González-Moran G. Natural history of unreduced Gartland type-II supracondylar fractures of the humerus in children: a two to thirteen-year follow-up study. *J Bone Joint Surg Am.* 2013;95:28-34.
16. Rider CM, Hong VY, Westbrooks TJ, et al. Surgical treatment of supracondylar humeral fractures in a freestanding ambulatory surgery center is as safe as and faster and more cost-effective than in a children's hospital. *J Pediatr Orthop.* 2018;38:e343-e348.
17. Skaggs DL, Hale JM, Bassett J, Kaminsky C, Kay RM, Tolo VT. Operative treatment of supracondylar fractures of the humerus in children. The consequences of pin placement. *J Bone Joint Surg Am.* 2001;83(5):735-740.

18. Ring D, Jupiter JB, Gulotta L. Articular fractures of the distal part of the humerus. *J Bone Joint Surg Am*. 2003;85(2):232-238.
19. Nauth A, McKee MD, Ristevski B, Hall J, Schemitsch EH. Current concepts review: distal humerus fractures in adults. *J Bone Joint Surg Am*. 2011;93:686-700.
20. Song KS, Shin YW, Oh CW, Bae KC, Cho CH. Closed reduction and internal fixation of completely displaced and rotated lateral condyle fractures of the humerus in children. *J Orthop Trauma*. 2010;24:434-438.
21. Lawrence JT, Patel NM, Macknin J, et al. Return to competitive sports after medial epicondyle fractures in adolescent athletes: results of operative and nonoperative treatment. *Am J Sports Med*. 2013;41:1152-1157.

## SELECTED HISTORICAL READINGS

Baumann E. Beiträge zur Kenntnis der Frakturen an Ellbogengellenk unter besonderer Berücksichtigung der Spätfolgen. I. Allgemeines und Fractura supra condylica. *Beitr F Klin Chir*. 1929;146:1-50.
Brown RF, Morgan RG. Intercondylar T-shaped fractures of the humerus. Results in ten cases treated by early mobilization. *J Bone Joint Surg Br*. 1971;53:425-428.
Hardacre JA, Nahigian SH, Froimson AI, Brown JE. Fractures of the lateral condyle of the humerus in children. *J Bone Joint Surg Am*. 1971;53:1083-1095.
Holstein A, Lewis GB. Fractures of the humerus with radial-nerve paralysis. *J Bone Joint Surg Am*. 1963;45:1382-1388.
Nacht JL, Ecker ML, Chung SM, Lotke PA, Das M. Supracondylar fractures of the humerus in children treated by closed reduction and percutaneous pinning. *Clin Orthop Relat Res*. 1983;(177):203-209.
Riseborough EJ, Radin EL. Intercondylar T fractures of the humerus in the adult. A comparison of operative and nonoperative treatment in twenty-nine cases. *J Bone Joint Surg Am*. 1969;51:130-131.
Sarmiento A, Kinman PB, Galvin EG, Schmitt RH, Phillips JG. Functional bracing of fractures of the shaft of the humerus. *J Bone Joint Surg Am*. 1977;59:596-601.
Weiland AJ, Meyer S, Tolo VT, Berg HL, Mueller J. Surgical treatment of displaced supracondylar fractures of the humerus in children. *J Bone Joint Surg Am*. 1978;60:657-661.

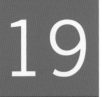

# 19

# Elbow and Forearm Injuries

Ariel A. Williams

## I. Ruptures of the Distal Biceps Brachii

A. **Anatomy.** Rupture of the distal biceps may occur at the muscle–tendon junction or more commonly at its tendinous insertion into the radial tuberosity.

B. **Mechanism of injury.** This injury typically occurs in men aged 30 to 60 years. Most patients report pain or a tearing sensation in the antecubital fossa after elbow flexion against resistance.

C. **Examination.** In a normal elbow, the biceps tendon should be easy to identify and palpate. Inability to "hook" the finger under the lateral edge of the biceps tendon strongly suggests biceps tendon rupture.[1] Because other muscles contribute to elbow flexion, the patient demonstrates minimal elbow flexion weakness, but does have weakness to forearm supination. With an intact biceps tendon, squeezing the biceps muscle belly in the upper arm should produce supination of the forearm. Absence of supination with the "squeeze test" suggests distal biceps tendon rupture.[2]

D. **Radiographs.** Routine elbow radiographs occasionally reveal small bony avulsions from the radial tuberosity, but most often show no abnormalities. If the diagnosis is not clear clinically, a magnetic resonance imaging (MRI) of the elbow can identify biceps tendon rupture (Fig. 19-1).

E. **Treatment.** Treatment of distal tendon tears is controversial. The biceps functions as a weak elbow flexor and a strong forearm supinator, and patients who do not have the tendon repaired do lose some forearm supination strength.[3] They will have easy fatigue with activities requiring repetitive supination, such as turning a screwdriver. Active, otherwise healthy, individuals may wish to undergo surgical repair. Tendon repair is technically easier, and results are better if performed within 3 weeks of the injury. Therefore, patients who may be operative candidates should be referred promptly to an orthopaedic surgeon. Surgeons employ various tendon repair techniques, typically followed by 6 to 8 weeks of rehabilitation.[4] For patients who present in a delayed manner, repair is often impossible because of muscle retraction and atrophy. In such cases, reconstruction with allograft tendon may be an option.

F. **Complications.** Complications of surgical repair include heterotopic ossification and synostosis, loss of forearm rotation, and nerve injury.

## II. Dislocation of the Elbow Joint

Accounts for 20% of all dislocations, second only to glenohumeral and interphalangeal joint dislocations.

A. **Anatomy.** Dislocation of the ulnohumeral joint most commonly occurs in a posterior direction and can result in disruption of the elbow capsule, the medial and collateral ligaments, and the muscles originating from the medial and lateral epicondyles. Associated fractures are also common. O'Driscoll et al.[5] have described the mechanism of the typical elbow dislocation as starting with disruption of the lateral collateral ligament complex, extending through the anterior and posterior capsule, and only disrupting the medial collateral ligament in the most severe cases (Horii circle).

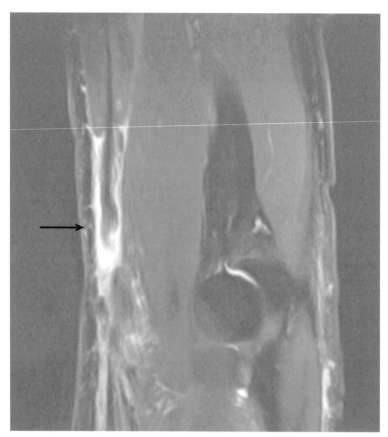

**Figure 19-1.** Sagittal section magnetic resonance imaging of the elbow of a 64-year-old man who had pain and swelling at the elbow after tripping over a treadmill. The *arrow* indicates the distal end of the biceps tendon (*black*) that has retracted surrounded by fluid.

B. **Mechanism of injury.** Elbow dislocation usually results from a fall on an outstretched arm.

C. **Examination.** The elbow typically appears very swollen, and the patient is unable to actively move the joint. In the examination of an injured elbow, there may be confusion about whether the deformity arises from a dislocation of the elbow or from a supracondylar fracture, but this can be resolved clinically by comparing the relative positions of the two epicondyles and the tip of the olecranon by palpation. These **three bony points** form an isosceles triangle. The two sides remain equal in length in a supracondylar fracture. If the elbow is dislocated, however, the two sides become unequal (Fig. 19-2). The position of the proximal radius can be palpated on the lateral surface of the elbow to evaluate for radial head dislocation. The function of the peripheral nerves and the state of the circulation to the hand, including capillary refill and the presence of radial pulse, should be carefully noted. Nerve injuries, most commonly involving the ulnar nerve, occur in 1% to 17% of elbow dislocations.[6]

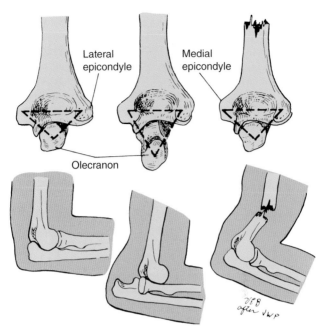

**Figure 19-2.** The two epicondyles and the tip of the olecranon form an isosceles triangle. This triangle is maintained with a supracondylar humeral fracture, but with an elbow dislocation, the two sides of the triangle become unequal or distorted.

Brachial artery injury is rare, but can have devastating consequences if not promptly recognized and treated.

D. **Radiographs.** Radiographs should include anteroposterior (AP) and lateral views of the elbow, an AP view of the humerus, and an AP view of the forearm. Imaging of the elbow demonstrates whether the displacement is directly posterior (Fig. 19-3), posterolateral, or posteromedial. Fractures of the coronoid process have been identified in 10% to 15% of elbow dislocations. Fractures involving the distal humerus, proximal ulna, or radial head signify a more complex injury that typically requires operative intervention.

E. **Treatment.** All elbow dislocations should be initially managed with closed reduction, which can often be performed in the emergency department setting. Sedation is typically necessary for proper muscle relaxation. Reduction can usually be achieved by exerting gentle traction on the slightly flexed elbow while applying countertraction to the humeral shaft. Postreduction AP and lateral elbow radiographs are mandatory to confirm congruent reduction. After reduction, the examiner should move the elbow through a flexion–extension arc to determine whether it is stable. Ideally, this is done with fluoroscopy, the examiner documenting at what degree of extension the joint begins to subluxate. Alternatively, the elbow can be gently taken through flexion and extension, and the patient asked to report when they feel the joint becoming unstable (apprehension). The elbow should be placed in a posterior splint in 80° to 90° of flexion with the forearm in neutral. The patient should be seen within 3 to 5 days with repeat radiographs to confirm reduction and to initiate range of motion (ROM) exercises.[7]

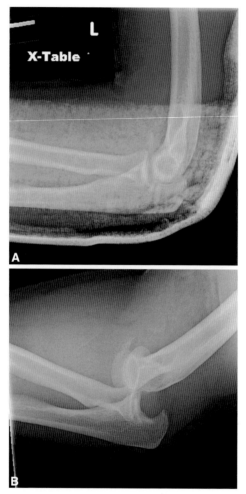

**Figure 19-3. A:** A lateral radiograph of the elbow of a 21-year-old man demonstrating a posterior dislocation of the elbow following a snowboarding injury. **B:** The elbow is concentric following closed reduction. The patient started elbow motion 5 days after injury, and ultimately obtained motion from 0° to 145° of flexion.

If the elbow joint cannot be reduced, there may be interposed soft-tissue or bone fragments, and therefore, prompt open reduction and ligament repair will be necessary. Combination elbow fracture/dislocations almost always require open reduction with internal fixation (ORIF).

**F. Complications**

1. **Limited range of motion.** Early initiation of active ROM (within 5 days) has been shown to improve final ROM.[7]

2. **Heterotopic ossification** can develop, and its treatment should follow the guidelines in **Chapter 3, I.** Posttraumatic elbow stiffness can be

successfully treated by open release.[8] If instability is present following release, a hinged external fixator can be used with good results in motivated patients.[9]

3. **Recurrent instability** can be difficult to diagnose; when recognized, surgical reconstruction can be successful.[5]

## III. Fractures of the Olecranon

A. **Anatomy.** Olecranon fractures may be simple transverse, comminuted, displaced, or nondisplaced. The triceps tendon inserts into the proximal olecranon, and displaced fractures of the olecranon result in inability to actively extend the elbow.

B. **Mechanism of injury.** Olecranon fractures can occur as the result of a fall directly onto the elbow or activation of the triceps against resistance.

C. **Physical examination.** There is often swelling and ecchymosis over the fracture site. If the fracture is not displaced on radiographs and nonoperative treatment is a consideration, the patient's ability to actively extend the elbow should be assessed. Associated neurovascular injuries are uncommon.

D. **Radiographs.** AP and lateral radiographs of the elbow typically demonstrate the fracture.

E. **Treatment**

1. Nondisplaced fractures with intact triceps function should be treated in a posterior splint with the elbow flexed 90°. Pronation and supination movements are started in 2 to 3 days, and flexion–extension movements are started at 2 weeks. Protective splinting or a sling is used until there is evidence of union (usually around 6 weeks). Close clinical and radiographic follow-up is essential to ensure full ROM and identify any displacement.

   Displaced fractures should be reduced anatomically and fixed internally with tension band wiring or plate fixation. Tension band wiring can be used for transvers fractures where plate fixation is the preferred option for comminuted and long oblique fractures.

2. Fixation should be secure enough to allow early motion. In some instances where the proximal fragment is small, fragment excision and triceps advancement can be considered. In elderly, low-demand individuals, nonoperative management of even displaced fractures can yield satisfactory results, although nonunion in these instances is common.[10]

F. **Complications**

1. **Symptomatic hardware.** Regardless of whether a plate or tension band wiring is used for fixation, the hardware is often prominent in the subcutaneous tissue overlying the olecranon.

2. **Loss of motion.** Even patients with simple fractures fixed anatomically often lose 10° to 15° of extension. Functional ROM from 30° to 110° of flexion meets the needs for activities of daily living (ADLs) for most patients.

## IV. Epiphyseal Fractures of the Proximal Radius

A. **Anatomy.** Ossification of the radial head epiphysis typically appears around the age of 5 years.

B. **Mechanism of injury.** These injuries result from a fall on the outstretched hand in children and adolescents aged 6 to 16 years.

C. **Examination.** Pain, occasionally swelling, and tenderness are usually present over the proximal end of the radius. There is also limitation of elbow motion. The wrist should also be carefully examined for evidence of injury to the distal radius and/or distal radioulnar joint (DRUJ).

D. **Radiographs.** AP and lateral radiographs of the elbow often demonstrate the abnormality. Radiographs of the forearm and/or wrist should be obtained in children to rule out any associated injuries. However, owing to the differing appearance of elbow epiphyses as the skeleton matures, images of the contralateral uninjured elbow may be helpful in cases where the diagnosis is not clear.

E. **Treatment**

1. **Fractures with less than 30° of angulation** are immobilized in a long-arm splint for 1 to 2 weeks. Active exercise is then initiated while the arm is protected in a sling.

2. **Angulation of greater than 30°** calls for manipulation under anesthesia. A number of techniques have been described to accomplish this.[11] If this fails, operative reduction is required. These fractures can often be reduced with the aid of an intramedullary wire, as described by Metaizeau et al.[12] After reduction, the intramedullary pin is left in place for about 8 weeks, although active motion exercises for the elbow can begin 2 weeks after surgery. Alternatively, a pin can be used percutaneously as a joystick or lever to reduce the fracture.[13] Open reduction is associated with poorer outcomes and should be avoided if possible.[14] The radial head should never be removed in children.

V. **Fractures of the Radial Head and Neck in Adults**

A. **Anatomy.** The radial head articulates with both the capitellum of the distal humerus and the proximal ulna. It also contributes to elbow stability against valgus loads.

B. **Mechanism of injury.** This common injury should be suspected following a fall on the outstretched hand whenever there is swelling of the elbow joint, tenderness over the head of the radius, and limitation of elbow motion (especially painful pronation and supination).

C. **Physical examination.** Patients with radial head fractures typically present with tenderness directly over the radial head and limited elbow motion. More comminuted or displaced radial head fractures may cause crepitus with pronation and supination. The examiner should document any other areas of elbow tenderness because medial elbow tenderness may indicate a more severe elbow injury with instability. Be careful to also examine the wrist and forearm for tenderness because radial head fractures are associated with Essex-Lopresti injuries (disruption of the interosseous membrane of the forearm).

D. **Radiographs.** If the fracture is not apparent on AP and lateral elbow radiographs, a radial head view may demonstrate the injury. A posterior and/or large anterior fat pad sign, indicative of an elbow effusion, should raise suspicion of a radial head fracture. Fractures are often described using the modified Mason classification.

**Mason 1.** Nondisplaced fracture of the radial head.

**Mason 2.** Partial articular fracture with greater than 2 mm of displacement.

**Mason 3.** Fracture involving the entire radial head, splitting into two or more fragments. In the Hotchkiss's[15] modification of the Mason classification, Type 3 fractures are defined as head fractures too comminuted to allow for ORIF.

**Mason 4.** Fracture of the radial head associated with an elbow dislocation. The Mason 4 is an additional category proposed by Johnston[16] and utilized by some practitioners.

E. **Treatment**

1. Minimally displaced (<1 mm) fractures of the head (Mason 1) or impacted fractures of the radial neck may be placed in a posterior splint for comfort at the time of injury, but elbow motion exercises should be initiated within 3 to 5 days. Early active motion increases the final ROM (particularly elbow extension) and improves outcome.

2. Management of Mason 2 fractures of the radial head depends on the size and number of the fracture fragments, the degree of displacement, associated injuries, and the patient's elbow ROM. Fractures involving less than one-third of the articular surface can be managed with early motion if the

patient is able to move through a full arc of pronation and supination. If the patient cannot pronosupinate because of pain, aspiration of the elbow effusion and injection of 5 mL of 1% lidocaine can relieve pain and allow better assessment of true ROM.

ORIF should be considered for displaced fractures involving more than 30% of the articular surface. Hardware can be placed in a "safe zone" on the radial head that corresponds to the 90° arc between the radial styloid and Lister's tubercle.[17] Fixation should be secure enough to allow early postoperative motion. Results of ORIF of radial head fractures with two or three fragments are superior to results of internal fixation of more comminuted fractures.[18]

3. Comminuted or displaced fractures of the head that involve more than one-third of the articular surface (Mason 3) can be treated by ORIF or excision of the radial head with placement of a metal prosthesis. In most cases, especially if the radial head fracture is part of a more complex injury such as an elbow fracture/dislocation (Mason 4), the radial head should be fixed or replaced and not simply excised. Radial head excision in such cases will lead to recurrent elbow instability. Radial head excision in the setting of an Essex-Lopresti injury (rupture of the interosseous membrane) will lead to proximal migration of the radius and wrist pain.

## VI. Monteggia Fracture–Dislocation of the Elbow

A. **Anatomy.** A Monteggia fracture is a dislocation of the radial head and a fracture of the proximal ulna. There are **four types**, as described by Bado (see Selected Historical Readings), depending on the direction of radial head dislocation and associated ulna fracture. Anterior dislocation of the radial head (Bado Type 1) is the most common pattern.

B. **Mechanism of injury.** This injury typically results from a fall on an outstretched arm, but may also be caused by an anteriorly or posteriorly directed blow.

C. **Physical examination.** The elbow and proximal forearm are often swollen, and the patient has limited active motion. The wrist should also be examined, as distal radius and DRUJ injuries have been reported in conjunction with Monteggia fractures.

D. **Radiographs.** AP and lateral views of the elbow and forearm should be obtained. In a normal elbow film, the center of the radial head should line up with the capitellum on all views (Fig. 19-4). In the case of a Monteggia fracture/dislocation, the line bisecting the radial head does not intersect the capitellum. In children, there may be plastic deformation of the ulna rather than a true fracture, making the injury pattern less obvious on radiographs. The appearance of any "isolated" ulna fracture, especially in a child, should prompt a careful evaluation of radial head alignment.

E. **Treatment**

1. **Children.** Closed reduction of the ulna is carried out. If the radial head has not been indirectly reduced by realigning the ulna, reduction of the radial head is attempted by supination of the forearm and direct pressure on the radial head. When the radial head cannot be anatomically reduced, surgery is undertaken to reduce and fixate the ulna fracture with intramedullary pins or plate fixation. This usually results in reduction of the radial head. If not, opening of the radiocapitellar joint with removal of the interposing joint capsule and repair of the annular ligament is advisable. For Monteggia fractures involving greenstick fractures of the proximal ulna, a stable reduction can most often be obtained without surgery, but close follow-up is necessary to assess for redisplacement.[19]

2. **Adults.** Operative treatment is recommended in all cases.[20] Open reduction with compression plate fixation of the ulna is generally followed by indirect reduction of the radius. If the radial head remains subluxed after

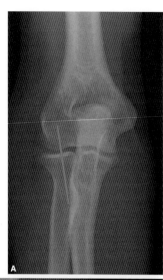

**Figure 19-4.** Normal anteroposterior **(A)** and lateral **(B)** radiographs of the elbow showing the radial head in line with the capitellum on both views.

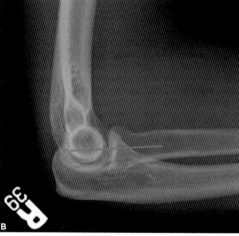

ulnar fixation, the forearm should be supinated while applying pressure over the radial head. If closed reduction of the radial head is unsuccessful, an open reduction must be performed. If the radial head is unstable, cast for approximately 6 weeks in supination, then start active exercises. If the radial head is stable after closed reduction or open repair, start early active motion with a hinged elbow orthosis, maintaining the forearm in supination. Protect the arm until the fracture is healed. With anterior dislocation and an unstable closed reduction, the arm may be immobilized in 100° to 110° of elbow flexion, which relaxes the biceps and helps maintain reduction of the radial head.

**VII. Diaphyseal Fractures of the Radius and Ulna**[21,22]

  **A. Anatomy.** The radius and ulna articulate at the proximal radioulnar joint and the DRUJ and are connected by the strong interosseous membrane throughout the forearm. These structures behave as a ring; thus, a break in one portion of the ring often results in a break elsewhere in the ring.

  **B. Mechanism of injury.** In children, these fractures typically result from a fall on an outstretched arm. In adults, high-energy mechanisms are more common.

  **C. Physical examination.** The forearm is typically swollen, and there is pain and crepitus over the fracture. The wrist and elbow should be examined for tenderness because multilevel injuries are not uncommon. A careful neurologic examination should be documented.

  **D. Radiographs.** AP and lateral radiographs of the wrist, forearm, and elbow should be obtained. Of all upper extremity fractures, this type best exemplifies the need for visualizing the joint above and below fractures of long bones (elbow and wrist), as diaphyseal fractures of the radius and/or ulna can be associated with disruption of the ligaments of the elbow (see Monteggia above) and wrist (see Galeazzi below).

  **E. Treatment**

    1. **Children.** Most both bone forearm fractures in children are successfully managed with closed reduction and casting. Even with considerable displacement of the fracture fragments, a dense periosteal sleeve ordinarily remains. This sleeve is usually sufficient to make satisfactory closed reduction possible. In addition, the bone remodeling that occurs during normal growth allows for correction of some residual deformity. Closed reduction can generally be performed under conscious sedation in the emergency department or with a brief general anesthetic. The remodeling potential for displaced forearm fractures is dependent on the patient's age and fracture location. In general, >15° of deformity is considered unacceptable alignment following closed reduction in patients younger than 10 years and >10° is unacceptable in older patients. Distal both bone forearm fractures can accept more displacement than proximal fractures. Children approaching skeletal maturity, or who have less than 2 years of growth remaining, have less remodeling potential and should be treated as adults.

      Following reduction, the child should be placed in a well-molded long-arm splint or long-arm cast and followed up within 1 week with repeat radiographs. Radiographs should be repeated weekly for the first 3 weeks postinjury. Greenstick fractures (incomplete fractures) tend to redisplace unless the fracture is overreduced, that is, unless the opposite cortex has been fractured with the reduction. Failure to obtain and maintain an adequate reduction is an indication for surgery. For younger children, closed reduction and intramedullary fixation with flexible nails is most common. For older adolescents, ORIF with plates and screws is performed as for the adult.

    2. **Adults.** It is difficult to achieve a satisfactory closed reduction of displaced fractures of the forearm bones, and, if achieved, it is hard to maintain. Unsatisfactory results of closed treatment have been reported to range from 38% to 74%.[23] For this reason, ORIF of both bone forearm fractures is routine in the skeletally mature, except in rare cases of truly undisplaced fractures.[21] ORIF of closed both bone forearm fractures can be performed on a semielective basis. Bone grafting should not be performed routinely.[24] At a minimum, there must be screws engaging six cortices above and below the fracture site. Great care must be exercised to restore the length and curvature of the radius relative to the ulna to prevent the loss of pronation and supination.[22,23] Reliable patients may be placed in a removable splint, and early motion started as soon as wound healing is complete.

**F. Complications**

1. **Loss of motion.** Restoration of the normal anatomy of the radius is associated with better forearm rotation.
2. **Synostosis.** The radius and ulna should be approached through separate incisions to decrease the chance of bone growth across the interosseous membrane.
3. **Refracture.** Plates should not be routinely removed from healed adult diaphyseal forearm fractures, because there is a significant risk of refracture following hardware removal. If removal is to be undertaken, waiting at least 18 months from the time of surgery may lessen the risk of refracture.[25]

## VIII. Galeazzi Fracture–Dislocation of the Radius

**A. Anatomy.** This pattern of injury comprises a fracture of the radial shaft combined with instability of the DRUJ. The classic Galeazzi fracture is a break at the junction of the middle and distal one-third of the radial shaft.

**B. Mechanism of injury.** Galeazzi fractures usually result from a fall on an outstretched hand.

**C. Physical examination.** The patient typically has tenderness directly over the DRUJ, although swelling and deformity in that region may be minimal.

**D. Radiographs.** AP and lateral radiographs of the wrist, forearm, and elbow should be obtained. Identification of an "isolated" radial shaft fracture should raise suspicion of a possible DRUJ disruption. Dorsal dislocation of the ulna (with respect to the radius) is the most common pattern.

**E. Treatment.** Galeazzi fractures should be managed with an ORIF of the radial shaft fracture.[26] Typically, anatomic reduction of the radial shaft results in anatomic reduction of the DRUJ. If the DRUJ is stable in supination (position of stability following dorsal DRUJ dislocation) after radial shaft fixation, the forearm is placed in a sugar tong splint in 45° of supination. If the DRUJ cannot be reduced, there may be interposed soft tissues in the joint, or, more often, the radius has not been anatomically reduced. If an open reduction of the DRUJ is performed, or the DRUJ is unstable in all positions of forearm rotation, soft-tissue repair (triangular fibrocartilage complex [TFCC] repair) or temporary pinning of the DRUJ may be performed.

## IX. Isolated Ulna Fractures

**A. Anatomy.** The subcutaneous location of the ulna makes the bone prone to fracture from a direct impact.

**B. Mechanism.** This fracture frequently occurs as a result of a blow across the subcutaneous border of the bone, thus the term *nightstick fracture*.

**C. Physical examination.** The patient is generally tender directly over the fracture site. Carefully inspect the skin to rule out any opening that may communicate with the fracture. Also examine the elbow and wrist to rule out any associated injury.

**D. Radiographs.** AP and lateral radiographs of the forearm and elbow should be obtained to rule out any associated radial head dislocation (see the section on Monteggia fracture–dislocation of the elbow).

**E. Treatment.** Minimally displaced isolated ulnar shaft fractures can be treated in a short-arm cast or fracture brace. Immobilization in a long-arm cast tends to lead to elbow stiffness and should be avoided. Fractures displaced greater than 50% of the width of the ulnar shaft or angulated more than 10° should be treated with ORIF.[27] Ulnar shaft fractures have the propensity to heal slowly and may take 8 to 12 weeks for complete healing clinically and on radiographs.

## X. Distal Radius Fracture—Adults

**A. Anatomy.** The distal radius typically fractures through the softer metaphyseal bone. The most common pattern is a dorsally angulated extraarticular fracture, also known as a Colles' fracture after Abraham Colles. In his 1814 paper, Colles differentiated this injury from the rare dislocation of the wrist on clinical grounds without the aid of roentgenograms. In more severe injuries, fracture lines may extend into the radiocarpal joint or into the sigmoid notch (the radial articulation of the DRUJ). Associated ulnar styloid fractures are seen in approximately 55% of distal radius fractures, but typically do not require any additional treatment.[28]

B. **Mechanism.** The most common mechanism is a fall from a standing height onto an outstretched hand in a woman older than 55 years.

C. **Examination.** In the classic Colles' fracture, the wrist and hand are displaced dorsally in relation to the shaft of the radius (Fig. 19-5A) to form the classic dinner-fork deformity. The distal radius and distal ulna are tender to palpation. A careful neurologic examination should be performed because these fractures are often associated with median nerve neuropraxia.

D. **Radiographs.** AP and lateral wrist radiographs are essential and should be evaluated for comminution of the dorsal cortex, the degree of angulation of the articular surface, radial shortening, loss of radial inclination, and intraarticular extension of the fracture lines. Normally, the articular surface of the distal radius is tilted volarly 11°, and the radius and ulna are of the same length (ulnar neutral). Radial inclination is usually 19° to 21°. Acceptable alignment criteria are 0° to 20° of volar tilt, 15° to 25° of radial inclination, less than 3 to 5 mm of radial shortening, and no intraarticular step-off more than 1 mm.

**Other patterns.** A **Smith** fracture is an extraarticular metaphyseal distal radius fracture where the distal fragment is displaced volarly (Fig. 19-5B). These fractures are often less stable than their dorsally displaced counterparts. Closed reduction is performed by supinating the forearm and pushing dorsally on the distal fragment. The fracture should be immobilized with the forearm positioned in supination and the wrist in slight extension. Loss of reduction is common, and these fractures are often managed with ORIF.

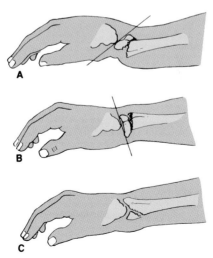

**Figure 19-5. A:** Colles' fracture. **B:** Smith fracture (reversed Colles' fracture). **C:** Barton fracture (causes displacement of the anterior portion of the articular surface).

**Barton** fractures are shear fractures of the articular surface of the distal radius (Fig. 19-5C). There is a coronal fracture line in the articular surface, and the carpus remains attached to and moves with the fracture fragment (usually the volar lip). Alignment may be improved with closed reduction, but these fractures require ORIF to restore joint congruity and function.

E. **Treatment** must be directed as vigorously toward maintaining hand, elbow, and shoulder function as toward obtaining good wrist motion. A patient with a stiff wrist and supple fingers is much more functional than a patient with perfect wrist motion and stiff fingers.

**Reduction**

Fractures that are displaced (do not meet the radiographic criteria above) should initially be managed with closed reduction and placement in a sugar tong splint. Reduction can typically be performed in the emergency department with the combination of a hematoma block and IV pain medication or sedation.

Following hematoma block, the patient's fingers are placed in finger traps, the elbow is bent to 90°, and 5 to 10 lb of weight is hung from a strap over the upper arm. After 5 to 10 minutes in finger trap traction to disimpact the fracture, a manual reduction is then performed. While traction is maintained, pressure is applied to the dorsal aspect of the distal fragment and to the palmar aspect of the proximal fragment to correct dorsal displacement and rotation. Pressure is applied on the radial aspect of the distal fragment to correct radial deviation.

**Immobilization**

The forearm is then placed in a well-molded sugar tong splint that extends just to the distal palmar crease (Fig. 19-6), allowing full motion of the metacarpophalangeal (MP) and proximal interphalangeal (PIP) joints. Extension of splinting material beyond the distal palmar crease limits finger motion and rapidly leads to finger stiffness, especially in elderly patients with underlying osteoarthritis. The wrist may be immobilized in slight flexion (up to 15°), but more severe flexion can cause acute carpal tunnel syndrome and should be avoided. Postreduction radiographs (AP and lateral of the wrist) should be obtained.

**Follow-up care.** If the patient's fracture is well reduced, the patient should be instructed to elevate the affected arm and perform active motion of the digits and gentle pendulum exercises for the shoulder. Repeat radiographs should be obtained on a weekly basis for 3 weeks to confirm that reduction is maintained. Typically, the patient is immobilized in a splint or cast for approximately 6 weeks.

**If the fracture cannot be well reduced**, or the fracture displaces after reduction, the patient may be a candidate for operative intervention. Percutaneous pinning, external fixation, or ORIF with plates may be utilized depending on the fracture characteristics, surgeon experience, and patient demands. Treatment should be tailored to fit the patient's general health and functional level, as distal radius malunions tend to be better tolerated in the elderly population.

F. **Complications**

1. The most frequent complication is **stiffness of the finger joints and shoulder**, which can have devastating effects on hand function. Careful attention to splint/cast placement (see above) and patient instruction on early digital motion and edema control minimizes stiffness.

2. **Acute carpal tunnel syndrome** is rare, but can result in permanent median nerve dysfunction if not identified and treated promptly. It typically occurs within the first 24 to 48 hours following an injury and is marked by progressive pain and loss of median nerve function. Close observation

**Figure 19-6. A:** The plaster is cut at an angle to end in line with the patient's distal palmar crease. **B:** The patient should be able to fully flex all of their metacarpophalangeal joints within the confines of the splint.

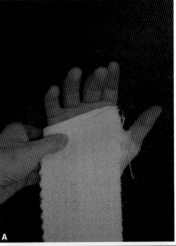

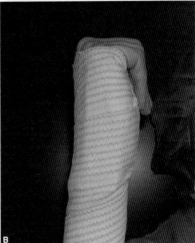

and serial neurologic examinations are warranted for any patient with median nerve dysfunction after distal radius fracture reduction. **Compartment syndrome**, although even less common, often presents with similar symptoms. In addition, the patient will have a tense swollen forearm and pain with passive stretch of the digits.

3. **Extensor pollicis longus rupture** can occur even in minimally displaced fractures. The tendon usually ruptures by attrition in the area around Lister's tubercle 2 to 3 weeks after the initial injury. Tendon transfer (typically of the extensor indicis proprius) restores thumb extension.

**XI. Distal Radial and Ulnar Fractures in Children**

   A. **Anatomy.** These fractures occur in the metaphysis just proximal to the physis in the radius, ulna, or both bones.

**B. Mechanism.** These fractures typically occur after a fall on an outstretched hand.

**C. Radiographs.** AP and lateral radiographs of the wrist and forearm are mandatory. Radiographs of the elbow should also be obtained if there is any swelling, tenderness, or limited motion at the elbow. Be certain that the fracture is not one of the types of epiphyseal slips described below.

**D. Examination.** Tenderness and swelling occurs directly over the fracture site, but the remainder of the extremity, including the elbow, should be carefully examined to rule out other injuries.

**E. Treatment.** Minimally displaced (aka "buckle") fractures do not require reduction. When more significantly displaced, these fractures can be difficult to reduce, particularly when the fracture is 100% displaced and shortened and involves only the radius. Manipulation should be done with the patient anesthetized or under conscious sedation, and the rule "one doctor, one manipulation" applies. Manipulative reduction consists of either.

1. **Traction in line with the deformity** until the bone ends can be "locked on," followed by correction of the deformity.

2. **Increasing the angulation of the distal fragments by manipulation (recreating the deformity)** until the bone ends can be "locked on," followed by alignment of the distal fragment to the proximal fragment to correct the deformity.

   **If reduction can be achieved**, it is usually stable, and treatment then consists of immobilization in a long-arm splint with the elbow at 90°. The patient should be seen within 5 days with repeat radiographs to confirm maintenance of alignment. Radiographs should be repeated weekly for the first 3 weeks. Casting is typically continued for about 6 weeks.

## XII. Distal Radial Epiphyseal Separation

**A. Anatomy.** The distal radius epiphysis first appears around age 14 months and may not fully close until age 19. The distal radius physis contributes about 75% of the total growth of the radius.

**B. Mechanism of injury.** The usual mechanism of injury is a fall on the outstretched hand with a forced rotation of the wrist into dorsiflexion, resulting in dorsal displacement of the distal radius through the epiphyseal plate.

**C. Physical examination.** The patient is usually tender and swollen over the wrist. The elbow and forearm should also be examined to rule out associated injuries.

**D. Radiographs.** AP and lateral radiographs of the wrist and forearm identify the injury. The most common pattern is a Salter-Harris Class 1 or 2 fracture.

**E. Treatment.** The younger the child, the more angulation and displacement can be accepted with assurance of normal subsequent function and cosmesis. In a child of any age, angulation exceeding 25° or displacement exceeding 25% of the radial height should be reduced. A less-than-automatic reduction is preferable to repeated manipulations because multiple reduction attempts can damage the growth plate. The manipulation and postreduction treatment are the same as for a Colles' fracture. If an acceptable reduction cannot be obtained in the emergency department, the surgeon should consider reduction and percutaneous pinning in the operating room. The patient should be immobilized in a long-arm cast for 3 to 4 weeks, followed by a short-arm cast for 2 to 4 weeks.

**F. Complications**

1. **Growth arrest.** As with any fracture involving the growth plate, early physeal arrest can occur.

## HCMC Treatment Recommendations

### Elbow Dislocations

**Diagnosis:** AP and lateral radiographs of the elbow, physical examination.

**Treatment:** Reduction under sedation in the emergency department—longitudinal traction with the elbow slightly flexed—postreduction stability examination and radiographs are essential for planning. If the elbow has good stability, start ROM exercises at 3–5 days.

**Indications for surgery:** Unstable elbow after reduction, intraarticular fragments, associated fractures, especially of the coronoid process or radial head/neck.

## HCMC Treatment Recommendations

### Olecranon Fractures

**Diagnosis:** AP and lateral elbow radiographs, physical examination.

**Treatment:** Splint initially, then generally ORIF.

**Indications for surgery:** Displacement of fracture of more than 2 mm or any persistent angulation, inability to extend elbow.

**Recommended technique:** Posterior approach, ORIF with tension band wire or plate fixation.

## HCMC Treatment Recommendations

### Radial Head Fractures

**Diagnosis:** AP and lateral elbow radiographs, physical examination.

**Treatment:** Early ROM (especially pronation and supination) of the elbow.

**Indications for surgery:** A markedly displaced (>3–4 mm) Mason 2 fracture that inhibits pronation and supination or a Mason 3 fracture.

**Recommended technique:** ORIF wherever technically possible using minifragment screws or plates, or various customized implants. Excision of radial head where reduction is not possible using metallic spacer where there is an associated elbow injury or an ipsilateral wrist injury.

## HCMC Treatment Recommendations

### Forearm Shaft Fractures

**Diagnosis:** AP and lateral radiographs of the forearm, physical examination.

**Treatment:** ORIF with 3.5-mm plates and screws for any displaced forearm shaft fracture in an adult. The exception is the isolated ulna fracture with minimal shortening (<1–2 mm) and at least 50% apposition of bone fragments. Generally, use eight-hole plate length or longer; plates should be left in wherever possible.

- Galeazzi variant—fixation of radius as described, with examination of DRUJ. If stable in supinated position, hold forearm in supinated position for 6 weeks; if joint is unstable, apply temporary K-wire fixation or repair TFCC.
- Monteggia variant—fixation of ulna fracture as described, examination (radiographic and clinical) of radiocapitellar joint. If not reduced, check ulna reduction for anatomicity and, if perfect, undertake ORIF.
- Isolated ulna—ORIF with technique described for fractures with significant displacement and shortening.
- Isolated radius—ORIF with technique described for fractures with significant displacement (>2–3 mm of shortening) or loss of radial bow.

## HCMC Treatment Recommendations

### Distal Radius Fractures

**Diagnosis:** AP and lateral radiographs of the forearm, physical examination. Computed tomography scan can be helpful for intraarticular fractures.

**Treatment:**

- Extraarticular variant—closed reduction under intravenous regional or hematoma block. Follow-up radiographs in 3–7 days to ensure that reduction is maintained. Comminution at the fracture site makes redisplacement likely.
- ORIF or closed reduction with percutaneous pinning for fractures with inadequate reduction.

**Recommended technique:** Percutaneous pinning with K-wires, or ORIF, typically with volar approach and specialized volar distal radius plates.

## REFERENCES

1. O'Driscoll SW, Goncalves LB, Dietz P. The hook test for distal biceps tendon avulsion. *Am J Sports Med*. 2007;35:1865-1869.
2. Ruland RT, Dunbar RP, Bowen JD. The biceps squeeze test for diagnosis of distal biceps tendon ruptures. *Clin Orthop Relat Res*. 2005;437:128-131.
3. Freeman CR, McCormick KR, Mahoney D, Baratz M, Lubahn JD. Nonoperative treatment of distal biceps tendon ruptures compared with a historical control group. *J Bone Joint Surg Am*. 2009;91:2329-2334.
4. Miyamoto RG, Elser F, Millett PJ. Current concepts review: distal biceps tendon injuries. *J Bone Joint Surg Am*. 2010;92:2128-2138.
5. O'Driscoll SW, Morrey BF, Korinek S, An KN. Elbow subluxation and dislocation. A spectrum of instability. *Clin Orthop Relat Res*. 1992;280:186-197.

6. Martin BD, Johansen JA, Edwards SG. Complications related to simple dislocations of the elbow. *Hand Clin.* 2008;24:9-25.
7. Anakwe RE, Middleton SD, Jenkins PJ, McQueen MM, Court-Brown CM. Patient reported outcomes after simple dislocation of the elbow. *J Bone Joint Surg Am.* 2011;93:1220-1226.
8. Husband JB, Hastings H II. The lateral approach for operative release of post-traumatic contracture of the elbow. *J Bone Joint Surg Am.* 1990;72:1353-1358.
9. Morrey BF. Post-traumatic contracture of the elbow. Operative treatment, including distraction arthroplasty. *J Bone Joint Surg Am.* 1990;72:601-618.
10. Duckworth AD, Bugler KE, Clement ND, Court-Brown CM, McQueen MM. Nonoperative management of displaced olecranon fractures in low-demand elderly patients. *J Bone Joint Surg Am.* 2014;96:67-72.
11. Nicholson LT, Skaggs DL. Proximal radius fractures in children. *J Am Acad Orthop Surg.* 2019;27:e876-e886.
12. Metaizeau JP, Lascombes P, Lemelle JL, Finlayson D, Prevot J. Reduction and fixation of displaced radial neck fractures by closed intramedullary pinning. *J Pediatr Orthop.* 1993;13:355-360.
13. Song KS, Kim BS, Lee SW. Percutaneous leverage reduction for severely displaced radial neck fractures in children. *J Pediatr Orthop.* 2015;35:e26-e30.
14. Falciglia F, Giordano M, Aulisa AG, Lazzaro AD, Guzzanti V. Radial neck fractures in children: results when open reduction is indicated. *J Pediatr Orthop.* 2014;34:756-762.
15. Hotchkiss RN. Displaced fractures of the radial head: internal fixation or excision? *J Am Acad Orthop Surg.* 1997;5:1-10.
16. Johnston GW. A follow-up of one hundred cases of fracture of the head of the radius with a review of the literature. *Ulster Med J.* 1962;31:51-56.
17. Caputo AE, Mazzocca AD, Santoro VM. The nonarticulating portion of the radial head: anatomic and clinical correlations for internal fixation. *J Hand Surg Am.* 1998;23:1082-1090.
18. Ring D, Quintero J, Jupiter JB. Open reduction and internal fixation of fractures of the radial head. *J Bone Joint Surg Am.* 2002;84-A:1811-1815.
19. Ramski DE, Hennrikus WP, Bae DS, et al. Pediatric Monteggia fractures: a multicenter examination of treatment strategy and early clinical and radiographic results. *J Pediatr Orthop.* 2015;35:115-120.
20. Ring D, Jupiter JB, Simpson NS. Monteggia fractures in adults. *J Bone Joint Surg Am.* 1998;80:1733-1744.
21. Chapman MW, Gordon JE, Zissimos AG. Compression plate fixation of acute fractures of the diaphysis of the radius and ulna. *J Bone Joint Surg Am.* 1989;71:159-169.
22. Schemitsch EH, Richards RR. The effect of malunion on functional outcome after plate fixation of both bones of the forearm in adults. *J Bone Joint Surg Am.* 1992;74:1068-1078.
23. Sarmiento A, Ebramzaden R, Brys D, Tarr R. Angular deformities and forearm function. *J Orthop Res.* 1992;10:121-133.
24. Wei SY, Born CT, Abene A, Ong A, Hayda R, DeLong WG Jr. Diaphyseal forearm fractures treated with and without bone graft. *J Trauma.* 1999;46:1045-1048.
25. Yao CK, Lin KC, Tarng YW, Chang WN, Renn JH. Removal of forearm plate leads to a high risk of refracture: decision regarding implant removal after fixation of the forearm and analysis of risk factors of refracture. *Arch Orthop Trauma Surg.* 2014;134:1691-1697.
26. Moore TM, Klein JP, Patzakis MJ, Harvey JP Jr. Results of compression plating of closed Galeazzi fractures. *J Bone Joint Surg Am.* 1985;67:1015-1021.
27. Atkin DM, Bohay DR, Slabaugh P, Smith BW. Treatment of ulnar shaft fractures: a prospective, randomized study. *Orthopedics.* 1995;18:543-547.
28. Kim JK, Koh YD, Do NH. Should an ulnar styloid fracture be fixed following volar plate fixation of a distal radius fracture? *J Bone Joint Surg Am.* 2010;92:1-6.

## SELECTED HISTORICAL READINGS

Bado JL. The Monteggia lesion. *Clin Orthop Relat Res.* 1967;50:71-86.
Burwell HN, Charnley AD. Treatment of forearm fractures in adults with reference to plate fixation. *J Bone Joint Surg Br.* 1964;46:404-425.
Fowles JV, Sliman N, Kassab MT. The Monteggia lesion in children. Fracture of the ulna and dislocation of the radial head. *J Bone Joint Surg Am.* 1983;65:1276-1282.
Fuller DJ, McCullough CJ. Malunited fractures of the forearm in children. *J Bone Joint Surg Br.* 1982;64:364-367.
Knirk JL, Jupiter JB. Intraarticular fractures of the distal end of the radius in young adults. *J Bone Joint Surg Am.* 1986;68:647-659.

Linscheid RL, Wheeler DK. Elbow dislocations. *JAMA*. 1965;194:1171-1176.

Mason ML. Some observations on fractures of the head of the radius with a review of one hundred cases. *Br J Surg*. 1954;42:123-132.

Monteggia GB. *Instituzionechirugiche*. 2nd ed. Maspero; 1814.

Morrey BF, Chao EY, Hui FC. Biomechanical study of the elbow following excision of the radial head. *J Bone Joint Surg Am*. 1979;61:63-68.

Taylor TK, O'Connor BT. The effect upon the inferior radio-ulnar joint of excision of the end of the radius in adults. *J Bone Joint Surg Br*. 1964;46:83-88.

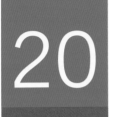

# Acute Wrist and Hand Injuries

Matthew D. Putnam and Julie E. Adams

## I. Basic Principles and Data

Acute injuries to the hand and wrist are common. Obvious reasons for this fact stem from use of the hand as a working tool in sometimes dangerous environments (e.g., as an object holder immediately adjacent to a power tool) and the all-too-frequent use of the arm as brake (fall onto an outstretched arm). A patient's general health characteristics may play an important role in determining the frequency and outcome from such accidents (e.g., diabetics with originally reduced sensation and ongoing reduced blood supply/immune function or osteopenia/osteoporosis with reduced skeletal strength). There are several issues to be considered with all patients.

**A. Date of last tetanus immunization.** One should consider the possibility of skin compromise with injuries to the hand and wrist. Even without obvious laceration, penetration of infectious organisms into the subcutaneous tissue has been known to occur. The effects of infection from one such organism (tetanus) are largely preventable. Consequently, verify the status of tetanus immunization in all patients whom you are treating for hand or wrist trauma. Do not assume that this has been resolved by a prior examiner.

**B. Injury site characteristics.** These may alter your treatment choices. For example, a fracture with a nearby clean laceration from a sharp object can often be managed as though the skin had remained closed, whereas the same fracture associated with a minimal but contaminated (farmyard or sewage) puncture into the fracture hematoma must first be thoroughly irrigated. **Thus,** the first key characteristic is to establish the extent of the skin injury and to specifically determine whether any external injection of organisms deep into the skin surface is likely to have occurred. In the case of burns (cold or hot), knowledge of the depth of the skin injury is important. It is important to be specific when describing wounds. Adjectives used to modify established terminology (e.g., "severe," "bad," or "not bad") should be avoided. Use phrases or classification with known meaning whenever possible.

Helpful adjectives used in characterizing a wound include the following:

1. **Open or closed.** Used most commonly in association with a fracture. **If** the skin is open to a fracture, it is considered open. This same phraseology is important in treating lacerations close to joints and some tendon injuries.

2. **Clean or contaminated.** Generally, a kitchen knife would be considered clean as compared with a saw blade picked up from a farmyard workbench.

3. **Repairable or not repairable.** The margin of a laceration can be so ragged as to prevent repair. In the hand (the same applies to the foot and face), this can preclude tensionless wound closure and thus necessitate advanced wound management methods.

4. The **Gustilo-Anderson classification** specifies soft-tissue injury severity in conjunction with an open fracture and is as follows[1,2]:

**Type I:** represents a low-energy injury with an open lesion of less than 1 cm.

**Type II:** represents an open laceration greater than 1 cm with moderate soft-tissue injury. Generally, the laceration could be closed or closely approximated at the time of initial presentation.

**Type III:** represents an open laceration greater than 1 cm with extensive soft-tissue damage and is further subdivided into three types:

**Type IIIA:** adequate soft-tissue coverage without devitalization of underlying tissue. However, owing to contamination concerns, these wounds are not considered for closure or close approximation as part of initial care.

**Type IIIB:** inadequate soft-tissue coverage. Devitalized bone and/or soft tissue are likely. Extent of debridement needs to be considered per tissue type and ability to move toward reestablishing a skin envelope around clean deep tissues.

**Type IIIC:** associated with arterial injury. Same as IIIB with addition of no arterial in flow.

C. **Patient's habits and addictions.** It is important to be aware of the patient's inclination to follow medical advice. This is particularly important in children (applies to the parents in this instance), and the emergently consulted physician has a responsibility to ensure timely follow-up care. Most hand and wrist injuries requiring consultation from an orthopaedic specialist will need early (2 to 14 days) follow-up, and failure to ensure this care may result in disability. Other habits of importance include the following:

1. **Tobacco use disorder.** In addition to being an established diagnosis (*International Classification of Diseases*, ninth edition [*ICD-9*] = 305.12; *ICD-10* = F17.200), this problem will impact bone healing (known) as well as other tissues (skin, tendon, nerve) (suspected).[3]

2. **Recreational drug use.** Impaired patients will place stresses on casts and dressings such that the surgical repairs (including skin lacerations) may fail. In some circumstances, hospital admission with appropriate consults is required.

D. **Systemic illness.** Illness that compromises immune function is a common reason for delayed recovery after hand/wrist injury. Diseases such as diabetes mellitus, malabsorption syndromes, rheumatoid arthritis, or advanced osteoporosis will impact the result from injury and the type of treatment that can be chosen.

II. **History**

A. **Where and how did the injury occur?** As noted earlier, record the location of the injury and its mechanism. This is important for two basic reasons. First, you need to know the cleanliness of the wound and how much **energy** was applied to the tissues. Second, you need to record the where (work, home, motor vehicle accident, etc.) and how (an allegedly defective tool, a reported assailant, etc.) because the first examining document will be used henceforth as the "truth." *Thus, your written history should contain few adjectives and only known facts.* Always record the source of information/facts you enter in the record.

B. **How did the patient become aware of the injury?** Some injuries will present immediately after the suspected injury occurred. In these instances, recording facts (as previously noted) related to the patient's presentation is important.

A corollary is "what made the patient come in today?" This question is particularly germane when the day of presentation is not the day of injury.

**C. Pain**
1. **Location.** Be specific. Use anatomic descriptors. Try to avoid the use of "medial and lateral" and numbering the digits (because of misinterpretations). The second finger is not the index but the middle. Thus, do not use number references for fingers because too many physicians and most lay people mistake the index for the second finger (which it is not). *Use the following terms: radial and ulnar; dorsal and volar; thumb, index, middle, ring, and small finger.*
2. **Qualities.** Phrases such as "really bad pain" are meaningless. Words such as *burning, radiating, and tingling* may be helpful in detecting/isolating a nerve injury, whereas words such *as deep, constant, and throbbing* may be associated with an infection. Pain upon awakening or that awakens from sleep is important to note because this can be indicative of a deeper ongoing process—such as infection or tumor.

**D. Numbness**
1. **Location** (similar to **C.1**). Describe the anatomic location of the numbness using precise words (e.g., the radial border of the ring finger). These phrases will hopefully be anatomically possible and serve to isolate the nerve difference. Patients describing anatomically unlikely numbness are occasionally seeking secondary gain. In the presence of lacerations or acute injuries, nerve function should be evaluated by assessment of static two-point discrimination and documentation of same.[4] (*Sensation examinations should be performed with standardized tools. Light pressure can be measured using commercially available nonsharp two-point touch at specified distances. A "poor mans" version of this tool can be built with a paper clip Fig. 20-1.*) Patients may not appreciate lack of sensation until later; it is important to document sensory disturbance prior to initial

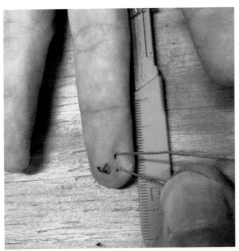

**Figure 20-1.** Tools are manufactured with blunted metal prongs spaced at defined intervals to enable testing and measuring of moving or static 2-point discrimination. A "poor man's" version of this tool can be built with a paper clip set at a specified distance. Such tools enable reasonably precise patient sensory assessment (healthy patients should readily distinguish 2 points 4–6 mm apart).

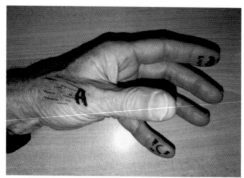

**Figure 20-2.** At the minimum, document sensation over the dorsal aspect of the thumb metacarpal–phalangeal joint (radial sensory nerve [RSN]), pulp tissue of the index finger (median nerve [MN]), and pulp tissue of the small finger (ulnar nerve [UN]).

treatment. Too often "sensation intact" means the examiner did not perform a detailed examination. At the minimum, document sensation over the dorsal aspect of the thumb metacarpophalangeal joint (MCPJ) (radial sensory nerve), pulp tissue of the index finger (median nerve), and pulp tissue of the small finger (ulnar nerve) (Fig. 20-2).

2. **Qualities.** As in **C.2**, specificity is important. In addition, record frequency and inciting factors (e.g., the numbness occurs when I am driving for ### minutes or more).

E. **Range of motion.** Specific ranges to be recorded are demonstrated in Fig. 20-3 and summarized in Table 20-1.

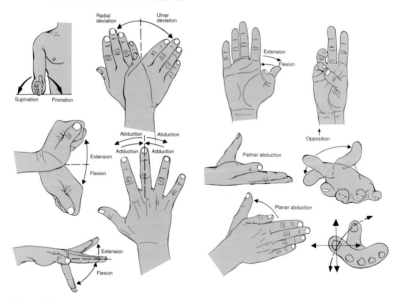

**Figure 20-3.** Terminology for describing forearm, hand, and digital motion. (From Seiler JG III. *Essentials of Hand Surgery.* Lippincott Williams & Wilkins; 2002, with permission.)

| TABLE 20-1. | Normal Hand and Wrist Motion | |
|---|---|---|
| Motion: Active (Passive) | Right | Left |
| Supination (occurs at distal radioulnar joint) | 90 (90) | Same |
| Wrist flexion (occurs at radiocarpal and midcarpal joints) | 70 (90) | Same |
| Wrist extension (occurs at radiocarpal and midcarpal joints) | 70 (90) | Same |
| Wrist radial deviation (occurs at radiocarpal and midcarpal joints) | 20 (30) | Same |
| Wrist ulnar deviation (occurs at radiocarpal and midcarpal joints) | 40 (50) | Same |
| Finger abduction and adduction (occurs at MCPJ, index to small) | 20 (20) | Same |
| Finger base extension and flexion (occurs at MCPJ, index to small) | 10 (30) | Same |
| Thumb and finger individual joint extension and flexion | 0–90 (10, extension to 100, flexion) | Same |
| Thumb palmar abduction | 45 (45) | Same |
| Thumb opposition (how close to small finger base) | 0 cm; able to touch base of small finger | Same |
| Thumb radial (planar) abduction | 45 (45) | Same |

MCPJ, metacarpophalangeal joint.

Idealized numbers are inserted. The key to a successful examination is to measure both sides in the affected areas.

1. **Active.** Active motion helps to document the integrity of tendons and the stability/congruity of joints.
2. **Passive.** Differences and similarities between active and passive motions can help to document/differentiate several conditions, for example, disrupted tendons (active will be absent, and passive will be high/normal) and stiff joints (active will be low, and passive will be low).

F. **Strength.** Generally, the international classification for muscle strength is used. Thus, a muscle can be graded from 0 (flaccid and no evidence of innervation) to 5 (normal). However, specific strengths are often measured in the hand and forearm and compared over time.

1. **Pinch strength.** Measured with a "pinch gauge" and recorded in pounds or kilograms.
   a. **Key.** Thumb to side of index or middle finger (strongest, used for grasp and rotation).
   b. **Chuck.** Thumb to pulp of two fingers (measured as thumb to index and middle) (strong and moderately precise).
   c. **Tip.** Thumb to one finger pulp (weakest and most precise).
2. **Grip strength.** Measured with a "dynamometer" and recorded in pounds or kilograms. Useful to measure recovery of function as healing progresses (Fig. 20-4).
   a. Can be recorded in several setting "diameters" (*diameter here is the width of the device that thereby tests the muscle [sarcomere/internal actin–myosin element] at varying lengths*). Measuring strength at various muscle lengths (dynamometer positions 1 to 5) will produce a curve with the greatest values around the center with the left and right

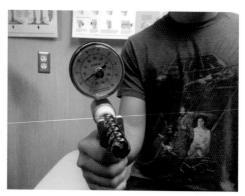

**Figure 20-4.** A Jaymar dynamometer in use to measure a patient's grip strength after stabilization of a malunited distal radius (thin marker indicates the maximum grip [14 kg] and the larger marker the sustained grip [10 kg] obtained at position 2 [positions 1 to 5 with 1 being the smallest]).

sides of the curve being less as a direct result of fewer actin–myosin bonds being available. Normal grip strength is a combination of extrinsic and intrinsic motors. Lack of a "bell-shaped curve" may indicate lack of effort and can indicate the patient is not truly participating in the examination (possible malingering).[5]

## III. Physical Examination

### A. General

The hand has three primary functions: sensation, movement, and cosmesis. Nerves, bones and joints, and tendons and muscles all play an important role in determining the outcome after injury and care.

### B. Region-specific examination (forearm to fingers)

1. **Distal radioulnar joint (DRUJ).** This joint works in combination with the proximal radioulnar joint to guide the rotation of the distal radius around the ulnar head (distal portion of the ulna). Fig. 20-5 demonstrates this important motion.

   a. **Muscle.** The pronator quadratus muscle originates immediately proximal to the DRUJ. It has a deep and superficial head and helps to stabilize and pronate the forearm. The muscle is innervated by the terminal branch of the anterior interosseous nerve. The muscle can be injured in conjunction with distal radius fractures.

   b. **Tendon.** The extensor carpi ulnaris (ECU) (sixth dorsal extensor compartment) and the extensor digiti minimi (fifth dorsal extensor compartment) tendons run alongside and dorsal to the ulnar head. Occasionally, the tendon sheath will tear, and the ECU tendon can become unstable. Also, a lax or irregular DRUJ can damage the extensor tendons, such as in the setting of Vaughan-Jackson ruptures with rheumatoid arthritis. Otherwise, no direct attachment of tendon to the bones occurs.

   c. **Joint/bone.** The DRUJ is a "roll-and-slide" joint. Considerable variance in design occurs. What is universally true is that an unstable DRUJ is uncomfortable or painful. When the joint does not work well, it usually results in a loss of supination. An unusual but possible injury to the joint would be dislocation without fracture in either the volar or the dorsal direction. Ligaments play a larger role than bone shape with respect to the stability of this joint, with one estimate being that only 20% of the stability of the DRUJ is conferred by bony congruency.[6]

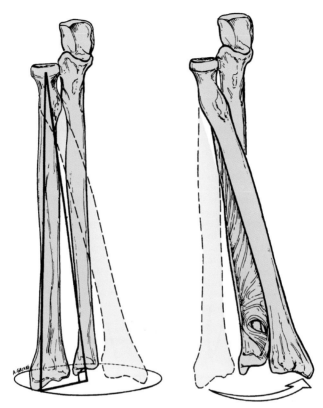

**Figure 20-5.** The axis of rotation of the radius with respect to the ulna, with the center of the axis of rotation being aligned beginning at the center of the radial head and ending near the center of the distal part of the ulna. Rotation is guided by the interosseous membrane and the triangular fibrocartilage. (From Peimer CA, ed. *Surgery of the Hand and Upper Extremity*. McGraw-Hill; 1996, with permission.)

    d. **Triangular fibrocartilage complex (TFCC).** First described in 1981, the TFCC is the major ligamentous stabilizer of the DRUJ and the ulnocarpal joint.[7]

        Within this triangular complex is cartilaginous material that may be injured either acutely (e.g., from a fall onto an outstretched hand) or chronically (e.g., from overuse with the wrist in an ulnar-deviated position, such as with the use of a computer mouse). Patients with ulnar-sided wrist pain that is made worse with compression (analogous to hyperflexion of the knee when assessing for meniscal tears) may have a TFCC injury.

    e. **Nerve and vessel.** A rare but reported injury is entrapment of the ulnar nerve and/or ulnar artery after reduction of a completely dislocated DRUJ. This would generally require a complete separation to occur between the radius and the ulnar head, but could also occur in a young child who fractures through the physeal plate of the radius or ulnar with >100% displacement, thus shifting the soft tissues (tendons, nerves, blood vessels) and, possibly, catching these soft tissues in the bone during reduction of the epiphysis back to the metaphysis. In any event, the important point is to carefully assess nerve function before and after reduction maneuvers and carefully account for any change in function after reduction.

2. **Wrist**

   a. **Muscle.** Indirectly and directly, muscles arise from the wrist. Specifically, the thenar and hypothenar muscles arise from the transverse carpal ligament (thenars) or the hook of hamate and the pisiform (hypothenars). Function of these muscles can be reduced in combination with injuries to their attachments. This would include an indirect injury to the attachments of the transverse carpal ligament such as would occur with a hamate fracture, scaphoid tubercle fracture, or pisiform fracture.

   b. **Tendon.** Tendons do not attach directly to any of the main seven carpal bones (the pisiform is a sesamoid and not a true carpal bone and is surrounded by the flexor carpi ulnaris). However, the flexor carpi radialis does appear to attach indirectly by way of a sheath/pulley to the scaphoid tubercle and consequently transfers a flexion vector to the scaphoid. Also, the wrist and its carpal canal act as a guide for both the flexor and the extensor tendons. Specifically, the carpal canal guides the thumb and finger flexors as well as the median nerve. The extensor retinaculum, anatomically part of the distal forearm (Fig. 20-6, the wrist extensor compartments one to six), stabilizes the finger extensors

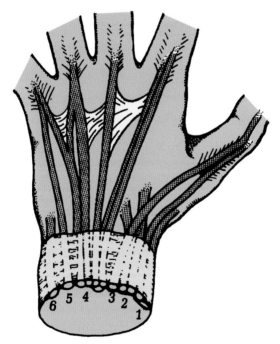

**Figure 20-6.** Arrangement of extensor tendons at the wrist into six compartments: dorsal and cross-sectional views. (From Seiler JG III. *Essentials of Hand Surgery.* Lippincott Williams & Wilkins; 2002, with permission.)

immediately proximal to the radiocarpal joint and acts as a pulley for both these motors in both extension and radial and ulnar deviations. Fractures or lacerations affecting tendons in this area often result in significant stiffness. This may be the result of many structures being injured as well as a consequence of tendons in this area possessing a large excursion. Thus, any loss of tendon glide will be noticeable.

c. **Joint/bone.** Motion of wrist depends upon ligament control of two rows of bones affected by muscles attaching to bones at varying distances distal to the wrist. This arrangement is similar to the ankle. However, nonobvious ligament tears (normal X-rays and nonspecific magnetic resonance imaging [MRI] scans) can significantly disable the normal wrist. This is often the result of a disconnection occurring between the carpal bones with resultant dynamic (under load) instability. This type of disconnection can occur without obvious bone injury. Injury to the scapholunate interosseous ligament is an example of such an injury. However, bone injury can produce the same effect upon the wrist, and the most common fracture causing wrist instability is a scaphoid waist fracture. Finally, although not frequently causing wrist instability, distal radius fractures can cause ligament injury in addition to causing joint surface irregularity and/or poor fit with resultant joint capsular stiffness and/or early posttraumatic arthritis.

d. **Nerve and vessel.** Close proximity of three sensory (radial, median, and ulnar) and two motor (median and ulnar) nerves can result in nerve dysfunction symptoms. Actual direct injury to the nerves is uncommon.

3. **Proximal hand**

a. **Muscle.** The base of the hand is the site of attachment for extrinsic (muscles originating from the forearm) wrist extensors, flexors, and deviators as well as the thumb abductor. Also, the hand base is the origin of the hand intrinsics. Destabilization by fracture of the hand base or metacarpal shafts can be made significantly worse by muscle tone. A debated example of progressive instability secondary to muscle pull/tendon attachment is seen in Bennett's fracture where direct attachment of the abductor pollicis longus (AbPL) to the unstable portion of the first metacarpal results in progressive displacement and joint incongruity. The drawing seen in Fig. 20-7 may represent only a small part of the story related to Bennett's fracture displacement as recent studies (not dynamic) suggest bone positioning and ligaments play an important role as well[8] (Fig. 20-7). Initial splinting attempts to neutralize these forces. In cases such as a Bennett's fracture, splinting may be insufficient, and reduction plus "fixation" may be required. Fig. 20-8 A, B demonstrates highly unstable hand fracture(s) with instability of the first, third, fourth, and fifth metacarpals secondary to muscle forces. This fracture(s) was complicated by being a Type 2 open fracture. Stabilization was achieved using external fixation primarily.

b. **Tendon.** The finger extensors are adjacent to the dorsal metacarpal bone surface. Thus, in addition to acting as a shortening force, the extensors can be injured or entrapped by displaced metacarpal fractures. Tendons overlying dorsally angulated midshaft fractures are the most at risk.

c. **Joint/bone.** Mobile and immobile joints are present in the proximal hand. The thumb base has near-universal motion as compared to the effectively immobile second and third carpometacarpal (CMC) joints. The fourth and fifth proximal joints are intermediate in mobility. The MCPJ distally is remarkable for its unicondylar and multiaxial shape. This multiaxial bone shape allows some radioulnar motion in extension that is reduced to none as the MCPJ moves into flexion and the collateral

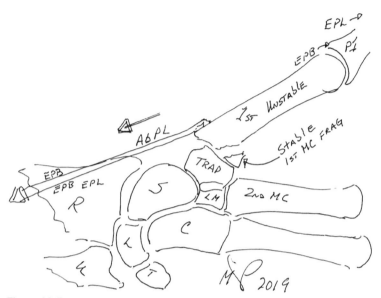

**Figure 20-7.** Bennett's fracture.

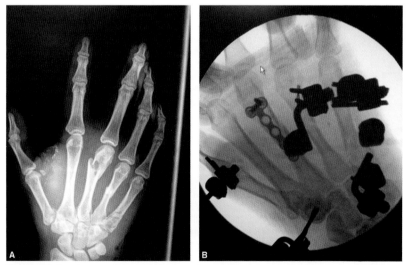

**Figure 20-8.** A highly complex open trauma (4-wheeler rollover) with deforming forces acting at the base of the first metacarpal, the third metacarpal neck, the fourth metacarpal shaft, and the base of the fifth metacarpal. **(A)** illustrates before stabilization and **(B)** illustrates after open reduction internal and external fixation.

ligaments tighten. An interesting note is that the metacarpal epiphyseal plate is distal in the second to fifth fingers and proximal in the thumb.

d. **Nerve and vessel.** Immediately distal to the volar aspect of CMC joints, the ulnar and the median nerve split into its common digital nerve components. In this same region, interconnections between the radial and the ulnar arteries through the deep and superficial arches occur. Significant swelling, displacement, or lacerations can result vascular injury. Depending on vascular anatomy, such injuries can immediately and completely deny blood supply to the digits distally.

4. **Fingers**
   a. **Muscle.** The fingers do not contain any muscle tissue.
   b. **Tendon.** The fingers are balanced by an intricate arrangement of flexor and extensor tendons. Fig. 20-9 depicts the complex balance achieved by the extrinsic and intrinsic extensors. The balance of finger motion

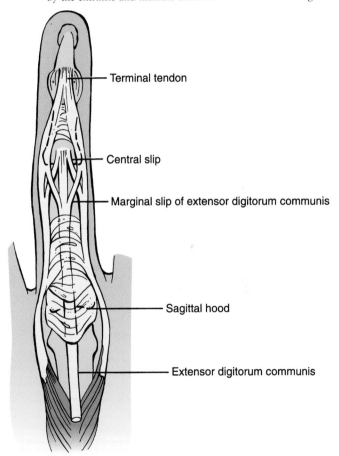

Terminal tendon

Central slip

Marginal slip of extensor digitorum communis

Sagittal hood

Extensor digitorum communis

**Figure 20-9.** Extensor apparatus over the dorsum of the digits. (From Seiler JG III. *Essentials of Hand Surgery*. Lippincott Williams & Wilkins; 2002, with permission.)

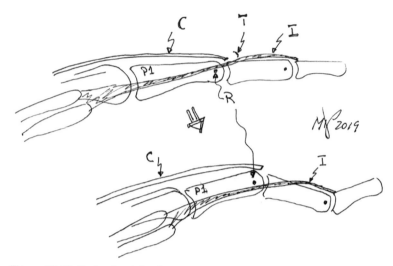

**Figure 20-10.** Boutonniere deformity.

enables one muscle (intrinsic) to serve to directional needs. Specifically, the most proximal joint (MCPJ) can be flexed, whereas the middle (PIPJ) and distal (DIPJ) joints are extended. Essentially, this is the result of the intrinsic tendons transiting from volar to dorsal at the PIPJ. In this location, the tendon (intrinsic) relies upon thin, easily injured, retinacular structures to maintain position. Closed injury to these structures with progressive loss of PIPJ active extension (sometimes accompanied by fixed flexion deformities) and increasing fixed extension at the distal interphalangeal joint (DIPJ) are the hallmarks of the developing boutonniere deformity (Fig. 20-10). The anatomy of the flexor pulleys is critical to normal flexor tendon function (Fig. 20-11).

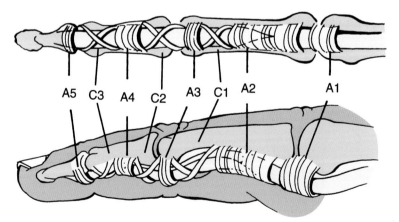

**Figure 20-11.** The annular and cruciate pulleys of the flexor tendon sheath. (From Seiler JG III. *Essentials of Hand Surgery*. Lippincott Williams & Wilkins; 2002, with permission.)

These pulleys guide the flexor tendon and its surrounding tenosynovial sheath during motion of the flexor tendons. Injuries involving the flexor pulleys can result in scarification to the tendons themselves even without tendon laceration. Perhaps more importantly, the pulleys enclose a space that is easily infected after a puncture wound and can serve as a path for infection into the palm and, in the case of the small finger and thumb, into the wrist and forearm.

c. **Joint/bone.** Unlike the more proximal unicondylar MCPJs, the finger IPJs are bicondylar and uniaxial. This configuration results in a joint that is stable throughout the axis of rotation. In practice, this results in a more stable arrangement for pinch-and-grip activities. However, this tight bony fit also means that small changes in bone position from a fracture will interfere with joint function. Ligament injuries to the fingers and thumb are common. These can create unstable and painful joints. One such injury is a "skier's" or "gamekeeper's" thumb. As illustrated in Fig. 20-12, this injury may be a partial sprain or can result

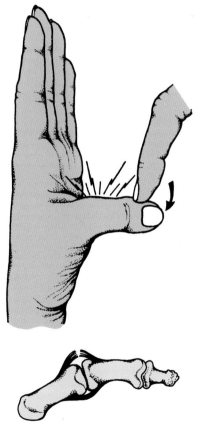

**Figure 20-12.** Rupture of ulnar collateral ligament of the metacarpophalangeal joint of the thumb. (From Seiler JG III. *Essentials of Hand Surgery*. Lippincott Williams & Wilkins; 2002, with permission.)

in complete disruption of the ulnar collateral ligament (UCL) at the MCPJ and require surgical intervention. Critical points to note on the physical examination include the presence or absence of the "Stener lesion" (a palpable mass that represents the detached UCL that has extruded through the aponeurosis) and is unable to heal; the absence of a firm end point suggesting complete tear. Integrity of the proper collateral ligament is assessed in 30° of flexion, whereas the integrity of the accessory collateral ligament is assessed in neutral. Similar injuries can occur at the PIPJ of the fingers and, occasionally, overlap with complete dislocations. In all such patients, three view X-rays of the affected digit (not just hand) should be obtained, and a congruent joint reduction should be present.[9]

d. **Nerve and vessel.** The nerves and blood vessels are situated immediately adjacent to the flexor tendons and maintained in position by dorsal (Cleland) and volar (Grayson) fascial "ligament-like" tissue. Isolated injuries to the nerve and vessel do occur and are sometimes described as cuts with excessive bleeding. Restoring blood flow is almost never an issue because of sufficient redundancy from the remaining blood vessel. Conversely, single nerve injuries can be problematic and often require semielective repair when the injury involves pinch surfaces and/or border digits. For central digits, nerve repair is less clearly indicated and often performed only to manage painful neuromas.

## IV. Specific Injuries
### A. Wrist

**Tendon and nerve.** Nerve and tendon injuries in this region are uncommon in isolation—that is, the lacerations may involve multiple structures (flexor zone 5 sometimes referred to as a "spaghetti wrist").[10] Some of these injuries are self-inflicted. For this reason, the patient's mental and psychological status should **always** be carefully evaluated. As long as blood flow to the hand is adequate, repair of nerve and tendon tissue in this region is urgent, but not emergent. Thus, initial care should focus on wound/tetanus status, skin closure, medical care, and mental health status clearance.

**Joint.** Patients with pain and a history of significant load (e.g., fall from a height or "at speed" or injured in a collision [sports/vehicle/etc.]) whose X-rays are normal can have a **real** ligament injury—unfortunately not visible on static imaging. The most common of these is injury to the scapholunate ligament. Obtaining a posteroanterior (PA) or supinated anteroposterior (AP) X-ray with a "clenched fist" may demonstrate separation of these bones not seen on standard films; however, it is important to compare with the contralateral side films if an injury is suspected. Immobilization and close follow-up must be ensured for suspected injury. Early MRI, MR arthrogram, and even diagnostic arthroscopy are valuable, but should be ordered/performed only by the specialist. A specialist may be able to detect the ligament tear with less expensive tests (e.g., clinical examination, plain radiographs, or fluoroscopic examination). Searching for these ligament injuries is important because it has been documented that early treatment is superior to delayed treatment.[11]

**Bone.** Four bony injuries are noted, including:

1. **Dorsal triquetral avulsion fractures.** Is a common wrist fracture. Fortunately, treatment is symptomatic, and fractures that have not healed and remain painful can be excised. Radiographs should be inspected to ensure that carpal alignment is normal. Patients may be treated symptomatically in a cast or splint for a period (4 weeks) until they become asymptomatic.

2. **Scaphoid fractures.** Many scaphoid fractures are hard to "see" initially. Some of **these** fractures are actually related to serious ligament sprains. Regardless, **all high-energy** wrist injuries, without a clear

diagnosis, should be immobilized, and follow-up should be arranged with a physician in 7 to 14 days. Original X-rays should include four views of the wrist (including a specific "scaphoid" or "navicular view" with the wrist in ulnar deviation to elongate the view of the scaphoid) (Fig. 20-13). Follow-up X-rays would be similar. Continued pain without diagnosis might warrant an MRI. Clinical findings concordant with a scaphoid fracture include pain at the anatomic snuffbox (high sensitivity, low specificity), soft-tissue swelling, pain or tenderness over the scaphoid tubercle, and tenderness with longitudinal compression. Scaphoid waist fractures are the most common, whereas proximal pole fractures have the highest risk of nonunion because of blood supply issues. Immobilization should be in a thumb spica splint or cast. There is continued debate about whether the elbow should be immobilized as well in a long-arm thumb spica splint or cast. In practice, the most important aspects of initial care are high index of suspicion, initial immobilization, and follow-up. There is an increased emphasis on screw fixation of scaphoid fractures displaced greater than 1 mm.[12]

3. **Distal radius fractures.** Most of these fractures are obvious. During initial evaluation, the function of the DRUJ and the median and ulnar nerve should be evaluated, as well as the status of the surrounding skin and soft tissue. Initial care focus is to splint the fracture with sufficient alignment and stability so as to allow comfortable finger, elbow, and shoulder motion. This does not mean that a "formal reduction" is performed on all patients in the urgent setting. It does mean that prior to splint application, the hand to forearm is placed in reasonable alignment. It does mean that sufficient padding is placed so as to protect bony prominences before application of splint. The original splint should immobilize the wrist and the elbow, with the forearm in neutral rotation and the wrist in neutral flexion/extension. The splint should not block finger or thumb flexion/extension and should end at the distal palmar crease. An ideal splint is the "sugar-tong" splint. This is a dorsal and volar splint fabricated with a generally continuous slab of material traversing from the distal palmar crease volarly across the wrist, forearm, around the elbow and extending dorsally across the dorsal forearm and wrist, with opening at the side to allow for swelling. The splint immobilizes the wrist and forearm (pronation and supination), but allows some elbow flexion and extension

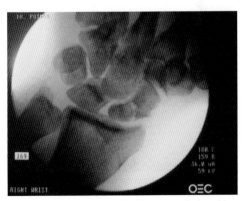

**Figure 20-13.** Scaphoid waist fracture identified by arrow, displaced 1 mm in oblique view. Surgery was chosen by this patient, but casting would be a reasonable initial care.

and full digital range of motion. Critically, this splint does not block full flexion of the finger MCPJ (Fig. 20-14 (A-D)). Patients who remain in marked pain after splinting must be assessed on site by a specialist before discharge to home for compartment syndrome and/or acute carpal tunnel

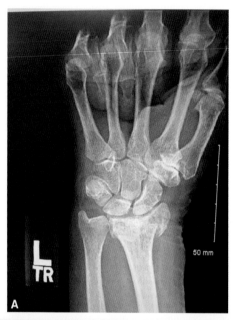

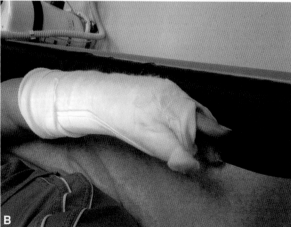

**Figure 20-14.** Distal radius fractures and splint. **(A)** Closed left distal radius fracture in older (>70 years old) patients that demand right-hand dominance. **(B)** Splint applied after initial assessment in ER. Note that volar part of splint is too distal and blocks MCPJ flexion. Blocking the MCPJs will induce stiffness, and the splint does not control the forearms rotation.

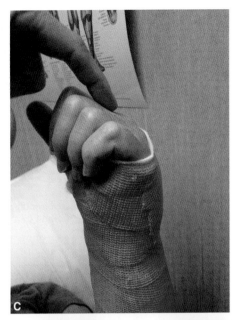

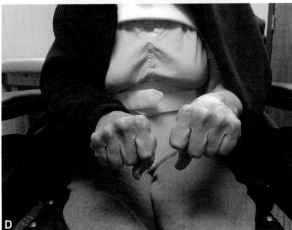

**Figure 20-14.** (*continued*) **(C)** The cast applied in clinic. The MCPJs are free to flex, and the forearm is controlled by interosseous molding. **(D)** At 6 weeks, the patient has regained full finger motion and forearm rotation. The spinal brace is unrelated.

syndrome—especially if they are taking a medication that interferes with normal coagulation. In all patients, early (less than 14 days) follow-up is encouraged. A marked shift in care of this fracture has occurred over the past 20 years, with current treatment favoring open reduction internal fixation (ORIF) for many fractures. However, uncertainties remain.

A horough review of certainties and recommendations was developed by the American Academy of Orthopaedic Surgeons.[13,14]

4. **Galeazzi fracture (fracture of necessity).** A very proximal distal radius fracture may actually be a true Galeazzi fracture. Unlike a distal radius fracture that does automatically impact the DRUJ, all Galeazzi fractures do stress the DRUJ and associated ligamentous tissue (TFCC). The reason this was originally named the "fracture of necessity" was the almost certain malunion of the radius that followed attempts at closed care associated with damage to the DRUJ and consequent loss of normal arm rotation.[15] Thus, it is necessary to operatively repair almost all of these fractures (Fig. 20-15).

**Amputation.** Fortunately, traumatic amputation at the wrist level is rare. Surprisingly, results of replantation at this level are better than those seen at the mid palm or with multiple digits. The keys to successful management are as follows:

a. Place the saline wrapped part in a plastic bag and then float the injured part in ice water. **Do not place the part directly onto ice. Placing the part directly on ice leads to a Frostbite burn.**

b. Antibiotics and tetanus administration

c. Systemic fluid balance

d. EMERGENT transfer to a qualified specialist. It is reasonable to expect that a voice to voice communication will occur between the referring clinician and accepting specialist.

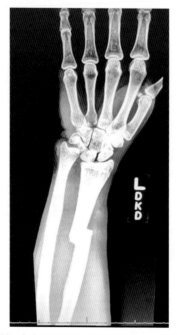

**Figure 20-15.** The white circle surrounds the distal radioulnar joint. Shortening of the radius secondary to the fracture in the distal shaft (marked X) has resulted in the joint being at minimum "subluxed." (Some might say dislocated, but this is somewhat semantics in this instance. The key is noting that the joints alignment is not acceptable.)

**B. Hand**

> **NOTE: Consider absorbable sutures for skin closures on children, nail bed injuries, or fingertip injuries.**

1. **Skin.** Surface burns from cold or heat exposure require tetanus and antibiotic treatment. All blisters should be left intact. In addition to sterile dressings, the hand should be splinted in a functional position. In the case of frostbite, current guidelines recommend rapid rewarming. Evolving guidelines involve antithrombolytic agents, especially for frostbite.

2. **Nail plate and pulp.** Infections are common in the hand and fingernail. Herpetic whitlow and its vesicles are sometimes confused with actual paronychia and associated cellulitis. Differentiation (a history of herpes exposure helps) is important because incision and drainage (I&D) is NOT indicated for herpes, but it is standard treatment for a bacterial paronychia. Drainage of a herpes infection can result in a superinfection with bacteria. When herpes is suspected in an individual in contact with others, the patient must be isolated until the lesions have resolved. Bacterial infection in this region is either around the nail or in the pulp tissues (felon). Felons are hardest to treat. Fig. 20-16 depicts a felon. The need to drain the entire pulp is emphasized. Noninfectious problems in this area include simple subungual hematomas from trauma. Drainage of the hematoma through the nail plate usually results in complete and immediate relief of the pressure pain.

3. **Tendon**

   a. **Flexor.** Flexor tendon lacerations are surgical urgencies. Diagnosis should be made based on functional loss after a trauma. Some important injuries (avulsion of the distal end of the flexor digitorum profundus [FDP]) can occur without a laceration. This may occur when a grasping hand is suddenly pulled away from an object (jersey finger).

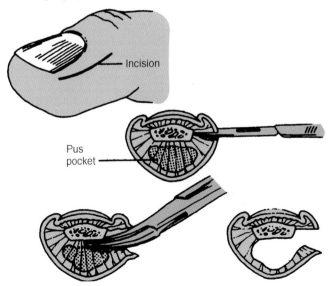

**Figure 20-16.** Drainage of a felon using a midlateral incision. Complete division of the vertical septa should be performed. (From Seiler JG III. *Essentials of Hand Surgery.* Lippincott Williams & Wilkins; 2002, with permission.)

Failure to make an early diagnosis of a flexor tendon injury may preclude a good result. **Thus, after a finger/hand laceration or a sudden pull-away injury, the key diagnostic step is an active motion examination of all fingers at all joint levels and not wound exploration. Wound exploration will not aide in the diagnosis of a flexor tendon laceration needing repair and not only might it create new injury (digital nerve and/or artery), a semi-sterile exploration could contaminate an otherwise sterile flexor sheath and lead to flexor tenosynovitis.** It is essential to test finger flexion with the nonaffected fingers in full extension. Then, test the affected finger without obstruction (flexor digitorum superficialis [FDS]) and with forced extension at the PIP (FDP) so as to isolate the superficialis and profundus tendons. Once a flexor tendon laceration is diagnosed or suspected, immediate referral to a hand specialist is recommended.[16] A flexor repair need not be completed emergently (except in the case of a replant). Almost always, a skin laceration over or near a suspected tendon laceration is closed before the patient is discharged from the emergency department. The patient should be referred to the specialist as soon as possible for planning of the delayed tendon repair. The injured digit and wrist should be splinted in the position of function until the specialist can evaluate the situation.

b. **Extensor.** Extensor tendon lacerations over or into a joint must be urgently managed. Because of the close proximity of the MCPJ, PIPJ, and DIPJ to the tendon, it is possible to contaminate the joint while only partially disrupting the tendon's function. Any laceration that may have contaminated the joint deserves a tourniquet-controlled examination and complete irrigation. Lacerations over joints secondary to any bite (especially human) must be copiously irrigated and should not be primarily closed. In these situations, antibiotics should be considered based upon the flora of the "assailant." Lacerations to extensors not involving joints do not always require direct repair. **Occasionally**, an extensor repair can be completed in the emergency department. Lacerations that can be seen to involve extensor tendon but do not alter active function (partial tendon lacerations) should be cleaned and closed without placement of sutures into tendon. If a definite (at least 10°) active extension loss distal to the observed laceration is documented, consultation with a specialist should be completed or arranged before discharge from the emergency department. A skin laceration over or near a suspected tendon laceration is usually closed before the patient is discharged from the emergency department.

4. **Nerve.** Nerve injuries in the distal arm region are common. Unless they are present in conjunction with a devascularized arm, nerve injuries can be managed on a delayed basis. The most common nerve injury is a digital nerve laceration. When these occur, the ipsilateral digital artery will often be damaged. In this situation, the volume of bleeding is often the immediate concern. **BUT, do not attempt to cauterize or "tie off" the bleeding vessel.** The close proximity of the artery to the nerve makes greater damage to the nerve almost a certainty. Thus, in the case of a finger laceration with bleeding uncontrolled by pressure and time expert, exploration of the wound with proper lighting, instruments, and magnification is appropriate. Experientially, unless the patient has a clotting disorder, pressure and time (30 minutes) are sufficient to control digital bleeding in all but rare circumstances. The keys to satisfactory outcome after nerve injury in the finger are more related to not missing any associated flexor tendon lacerations and not over-managing initial bleeding,

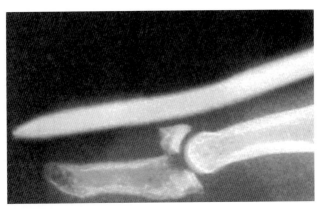

**Figure 20-17.** Bony mallet fracture with joint subluxation that will require reduction and stabilization. (From Seiler JG III. *Essentials of Hand Surgery*. Lippincott Williams & Wilkins; 2002, with permission.)

thereby creating a larger nerve injury. Many digital nerve injuries are never repaired, and yet, the patient functions satisfactorily.

5. **Joint.** An overlap between ligament and joint injuries in the fingers exists. The small size of the joints accounts for this fact. Fig. 20-17 depicts a common fracture pattern in the DIPJ of a finger. However, in this injury, the fracture fragment is large enough so as to destabilize the joint. This destabilization is obvious because a line drawn through the diaphyses of one phalanx on a lateral X-ray no longer bisects the adjacent phalanx. In this example, the fragment must be reduced to achieve a congruent and stable joint. A simple and universal rule is that the joint surface must have equal space between the bony elements at any joint at any location in both a true AP and lateral X-ray. If the distance between bone elements is not equal, the joint is unstable. One common exception to this statement does exist: This is the bony mallet deformity. Such an injury is similar to Fig. 20-17, in that a portion of the distal phalanx is fractured. However, mallet deformities (with or without a bony fragment) differ from Fig. 20-17 because they do not result in volar or dorsal migration of the remainder of the phalanx. Initial treatment of all mallet deformities is a neutral extension splint (Fig. 20-18).

6. **Bone.** Overlap between bone and joint injuries is common as mentioned previously. Four common fracture conditions and one treatment tool follow:
   a. **Boxer's fracture.** Fig. 20-19 depicts a common result of pugilistic activity. The fracture shown is at the proximal margin of the metacarpal neck and is almost a diaphyseal fracture. This is an important point. Because boxer's fractures occur in the neck (immediately proximal to the metacarpal head/joint), significant flexion deformity can be accepted. The exception to this is in the rare cases when the digits involved are the index or middle fingers (typically, the small finger is affected). Thus, open operative treatment is rarely indicated. There are two keys for successful outcome when managing a boxer's fracture:
      i. Do not overlook a puncture wound/open fracture.
      ii. Do not miss a rotational deformity. To exclude rotational deformity, the finger must be gently flexed at the MCPJ, and grip flexion posture must be examined and compared with the adjacent digits and the contralateral hand.

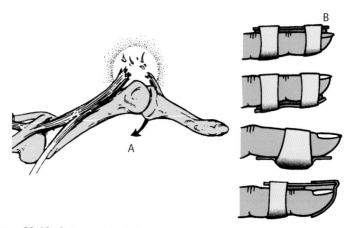

**Figure 20-18. A:** Mechanism. Owing to the extensor apparatus lesion, the distal phalanx flexes by effect of the flexor profundus tendon. The proximal stump of the distal conjoined extensor tendon retracts in a proximal direction, and consequently, the lateral bands are slack initially and later contract and displace dorsally. Owing to the concentration of the extension forces over the middle phalanx, the proximal interphalangeal joint is progressively set in hyper-extension. **B:** Various splints (dorsal padded aluminum splint, volar padded aluminum splint, concave aluminum splint). Dorsal padded aluminum splint allows adjustable fixation of the distal interphalangeal joint. (From Peimer CA, ed. *Surgery of the Hand and Upper Extremity.* McGraw-Hill; 1996, with permission.)

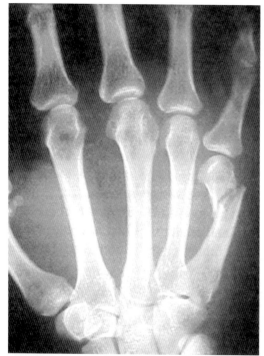

**Figure 20-19.** A "boxer's fracture" that can be treated with closed reduction and splinting in approximately 4 weeks. (From Seiler JG III. *Essentials of Hand Surgery.* Lippincott Williams & Wilkins; 2002, with permission.)

b. **Thumb base fracture and small finger base fracture.** Axial load applied to the border of the hand can result in fracture subluxation at the finger base. Any such fracture is unstable (Fig. 20.7). Almost all such fractures require operative stabilization. The key to successful treatment is early recognition. When treated early, a closed reduction and pinning is usually sufficient. Delay in treatment by as little as 1 week can necessitate open reduction and a more complicated management program. Thus, the first examiner's job is diagnosis. In the case of the thumb, it is easier to obtain a revealing X-ray. Along the ulnar border of the hand, it is usually necessary to obtain several oblique X-rays before a diagnosis can be made or excluded.

c. **Metacarpal fracture(s)**. A majority of metacarpal fractures can be treated closed without special manipulation and simple (supportive) splinting. But, in addition to measuring angular and length differences, it is important to be on guard for rotational deformity. Relatively large difference of length (10 mm) and angle (30°) compared to normal are often tolerated, whereas rotational differences of 10° can be symptomatic because of the affected digit healed in a rotated position that may block normal function of the adjacent digit(s). Fig. 20-20 illustrates the

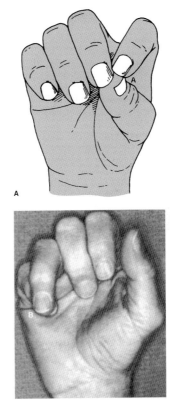

**Figure 20-20. A:** When the digit is flexed, the deformity is quite apparent. **B:** Active finger flexion generates malrotation of ring finger with digital overlapping. (From Seiler JG III. *Essentials of Hand Surgery*. Lippincott Williams & Wilkins; 2002, with permission.)

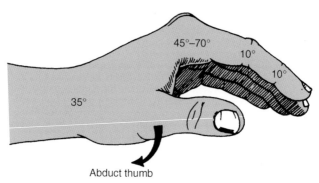

Abduct thumb

**Figure 20-21.** Hand dressing: "safe" position of fingers. (From Seiler JG III. *Essentials of Hand Surgery*. Lippincott Williams & Wilkins; 2002, with permission.)

problem associated with rotational deformity of a finger. Thus, the key deformity to rule out when evaluating a finger fracture is rotational overlap or underlap.

d. **Phalangeal fractures.** Fractures at the base or in the midshaft of the phalanx are tricky. Many of these fractures have significant angular and/or rotational differences. Oblique films in combination with standard AP X-rays are often more helpful than lateral X-rays, which could be confusing because of overlapping digits. Regardless, measurement of rotational difference by clinical examination and shortening of the bony length by X-ray examination are the key facts to be considered when planning for treatment. Unless, the fracture is essentially nondisplaced with **zero** rotational deformity, early referral to a hand specialist is recommended.

e. **Splint placement.** One of the common problems seen after initial hand fracture care by specialist physicians is poor splint technique. The key to good splint placement is maintaining fully lengthened ligaments. In the hand, this is translated to 70° to 80° of MCPJ flexion and no more than 10° of PIPJ and DIPJ flexion. Such a splint is illustrated in Fig. 20-21. By maintaining fully lengthened ligaments, the physician reduces adjacent joint stiffness following fracture care.

7. **Amputation.** Thankfully, amputations have become less common in conjunction with enhanced product safety and public education. Nonetheless, they still do occur. Single digits cut in flexor zone 2 should almost never be replanted. A whole arm might be replanted, but to do so is life-threatening. Guidelines for replantation include the following:

a. Almost any child (not tip injuries as these seem to reform naturally); adolescents are considered adults.

b. Almost any thumb

c. Multiple digits

d. Whole hand

e. Digit in flexor zone 1 with clean bony injury

**V. Pearls and Pitfalls**

A. **Injection injury.** Fig. 20-22 depicts the mechanism of injection injury. This seemingly innocuous original injury should not be overlooked. Failure to treat can result in loss of limb function or life-threatening infection even with emergent care, the outcome of treatment is uncertain. Emergent care by a specialist is mandatory. The keys to diagnosis are as follows:

1. **Injury history.** Use of a high-pressure injector is often revealed.

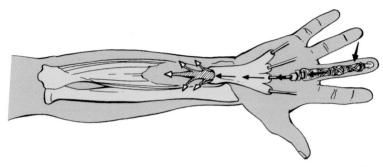

**Figure 20-22.** Palmar wounds at high pressure may spread into the proximal forearm. (From Seiler JG III. *Essentials of Hand Surgery*. Lippincott Williams & Wilkins; 2002, with permission.)

2. **Examination.** One or several small puncture wounds with more proximal tenderness or swelling are evident (Fig. 20-23 A and B).
3. **Pain.** The pain is seemingly greater than the wound would account for.

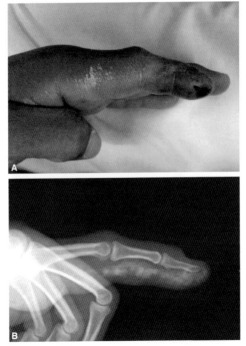

**Figure 20-23. (A)** Approximately 3 hours after high-pressure injection. Already the tip of the finger is ischemic and the patient is beginning to complain of systemic symptoms. **(B)** Injected materials not only entered the subcutaneous space but also tracked via the flexor sheath into the palm. A ray amputation was performed primarily and the wound was loosely closed over a drain, with the patient admitted for analgesia and prophylactic antibiotic coverage for 48 hours.

B. **Fight bites.** This injury is often overlooked. Sometimes, this will occur in conjunction with a boxer's fracture. The patient may not provide an accurate history, and substance abuse in this situation is common. Look for a small laceration overlying the joint that usually communicates to the joint if the finger is brought into a fist position. Flexing the fist during laceration examination is the key to identifying these patients. Treatment includes tetanus immunization or antibodies, antibiotics, complete wound cleansing, placement of a wound drain, and delayed closure.

C. **Compartment syndrome.** In addition to all the normal places, compartment syndrome can occur in the hand. Tight fascial compartments surrounding the hand's intrinsic musculature can swell after injury and cause muscle ischemia. It is important to remember that this ischemia is at the capillary level. Thus, pressures that surpass capillary flow pressures (~30 mm Hg) are all that is needed to begin the process of muscle cell (sarcomere) death (Fig. 20-24). Diagnosis is suspected when pain is increasing and passive motion is becoming more difficult. Sensory change may not occur because of nerve anatomy being outside the pressurized area. Also, wherever compartment syndrome occurs, arterial pulses will remain present, except in the most unusual cases. Pressure measurement may be useful. However, a good foundational rule is **if you think compartment syndrome is present, it is. Release it**.

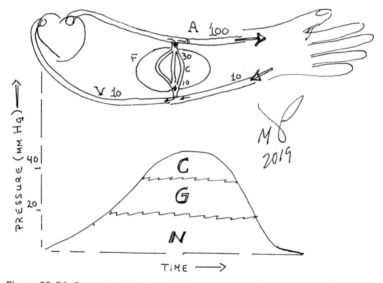

**Figure 20-24.** Compartment syndrome ischemia. A, artery from the heart with MAP 100 mm Hg; V, venous side returning to the heart at 10 mm Hg or less; F, fascia defining a fixed-volume envelope around the muscle; c, capillary network with a front-end pressure of ~30 mm Hg and downstream pressure close to venous (~10 mm Hg); C, compartment syndrome (when the pressure in the compartment precludes capillary flow and muscle sarcomeres experience ischemia). Also, at this greater-than-capillary pressure, nerves are no longer perfused (loose ability to conduct/repolarize); G, a gray zone where, depending on time exposed, muscle cell death may occur; N, normal compartment pressures. It is important to remember that in the absence of flow (from whatever cause) muscle cell death also occurs related to time exposed, and reestablishing the flow will lead to swelling and increased pressure and possible secondary compartment syndrome caused by original limb ischemia.

**D. Fracture and scapholunate ligament tears.** Often, these are diagnoses of suspicion. Almost no patient has been made worse by temporary splinting and early follow-up with a specialist. Whenever a patient presents after a significant injury mechanism (fall onto an outstretched arm), the patient should not be discharged without follow-up even in the face of normal X-rays. Appropriate follow-up does not require a specialist, but does require a high degree of familiarity with the nuances of significant wrist sprains and scaphoid fractures mimicking a mild wrist contusion during the first 4 to 12 weeks of recovery.

## REFERENCES

1. Gustilo RB, Mendoza RM, Williams DN. Problems in the management of type III (severe) open fractures: a new classification of type III open fractures. *J Trauma.* 1984;24(8):742-746.
2. Gustilo RB, Anderson JT. Prevention of infection in the treatment of one thousand and twenty-five open fractures of long bones: retrospective and prospective analyses. *J Bone Joint Surg Am.* 1976;58(4):453-458.
3. Patel R, Wilson R, Patel P, Palmer R. The effect of smoking on bone healing. *Bone Joint Res.* 2013;2(6):102-111.
4. Rowin J, Meriggioli M. *Proprioception, Touch, and Vibratory Sensation. Textbook of Clinical Neurology.* 3rd ed. 2007. doi: 10.1016/B978-141603618-0.10019-0
5. Tredgett M, Pimble L, Davis T. The detection of feigned hand weakness using the five position grip strength test. *J Hand Surg Br Eur Vol.* 1999;24(4):426-428.
6. Stuart PR, Berger RA, Linscheid RL, et al. The dorsopalmar stability of the distal radioulnar joint. *J Hand Surg Am.* 2000;25(4):689-699.
7. Palmer AK, Werner FW. The triangular fibrocartilage complex of the wrist—anatomy and function. *J Hand Surg Am.* 1981;6(2):153-162.
8. Kang JR, Behn AW, Messana J, Ladd AL. Bennett fractures: a biomechanical model and relevant ligamentous anatomy. *J Hand Surg Am.* 2019;44(2):154.e1-154.e5. doi: 10.1016/j.jhsa.2018.04.024
9. Pulos N, Shin AM. Treatment of ulnar collateral ligament injuries of the thumb. *JBJS Rev* 2017;5:1-10.
10. Stefanich RJ, Putnam MD, Peimer CA, Sherwin FS. Flexor tendon lacerations in zone V. (Co-Author, Lead Investigator). *J Hand Surg [Am].* 1992;17(2):284-291.
11. Rohman EM, Agel J, Putnam MD, Adams JE. Scapholunate interosseous ligament injuries: a retrospective review of treatment and outcomes in 82 wrists. *J Hand Surg.* 2014;39(10):2020-2026.
12. Talt MA, Bracey JW, Gaston RG. Acute scaphoid fractures. *JBJS Rev* 2016;4:1-8.
13. Lichtman DM, Bindra RR, Boyer MI, et al. American Academy of Orthopaedic Surgeons clinical practice guideline on: the treatment of distal radius fractures. *J Bone Joint Surg Am.* 2011;93(8):775-778.
14. Patel SP, Rosental T. Management of osteoporotic patients with distal radius fractures. *JBJS Rev* 2014;2:1-9.
15. Wikipedia contributors. (2019). Galeazzi fracture. In *Wikipedia, The Free Encyclopedia.* Retrieved March 2, 2019. https://en.wikipedia.org/w/index.php?title=Galeazzi_fracture&oldid=880602228
16. Morrell NT, Hulvey A, Elsinger J, et al. Team approach: repair and rehabilitation following tendon lacerations. *JBJS Rev* 2017;5:1-7.

## SELECTED HISTORICAL READINGS

Peimer CA, ed. *Surgery of the Hand and Upper Extremity.* McGraw-Hill; 1996:1-1336.
Seiler JG III. *Essentials of Hand Surgery.* Lippincott Williams & Wilkins; 2002:1-276.
Trumble TE, ed. *Hand Surgery Update 3.* Rosemont, IL: American Society for Surgery of the Hand; 2003:1-776.

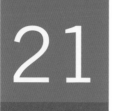

# 21 Nonacute Elbow, Wrist, and Hand Conditions

Matthew D. Putnam and Julie E. Adams

## I. Basic Examination

**A. History.** As with any medical problem, the history leading to the patient visit is critical. Family, social, and personal medical histories as well as infectious disease, and risk behavior history are important to collect and record. Other facts to be recorded include:

1. **Handedness.** Is the patient right- or left-hand dominant?

2. **Work-relatedness.** If the patient believes a problem is related to work or a series of events, it is the physician's job to document the patient's beliefs. The physician can do this by "quoting" the patient exactly. It **is not** the physician's job or duty to question the veracity of a patient's complaint.

3. **Mechanism of onset.** Record the details of the incident or accident as completely as possible. This is particularly relevant for motor vehicle accidents or other such incidents in which there may at some point be controversy over the extent of injury or the cause of injury. Record details such as whether the patient was in the car, the patient's position in the vehicle, whether patient was belted, if the air bags were deployed, whether the steering wheel was bent (particularly if the injured person was the driver), and the amount of damage done to the car (e.g., drivable after the accident, dollars to repair?). Additional factors include if the patient had loss of consciousness, if the patient was ambulatory at the scene or required assistance with extraction from the vehicle, and the presentation to medical care (taken by ambulance to an emergency center vs. sought care as outpatient via private vehicle, etc.).

4. **Date of most recent tetanus booster.** This is important with any direct trauma. **Do not** assume that another first examiner has resolved this issue. Obviously, if the trauma was in the past, this issue is not urgent.

**B. Physical examination**

1. **General.** At first glance, the upper extremity is a mirror of the lower. But several key differences are obvious as follows:

a. The **shoulder** has more freedom of motion and is consequently less stable than the hip.

b. The "patella" of the elbow is fused to the ulna as the **olecranon**. However, it performs a similar function to the patella in that it increases the "lever arm" for the attached muscle (triceps in the arm, quadriceps in the leg).

c. The **elbow and wrist** participate equally in guiding forearm rotation (supination and pronation). A similar motion is not available in the lower extremity.

d. The **wrist** has more motion and less bony stability than the ankle.

e. The **fingers** are longer in proportion to the palm than the toes in relationship to the midfoot.

f. The **thumb** is opposable to the digits.

2. **Region specifics**
   a. **Elbow**
      i. The elbow joint moves in a hinge manner at its articulation between the humerus and the ulna. Thus, the ulnar–humeral articulation is uniaxial related to flexion and extension. Forearm rotation is a different issue as its control is shared between the elbow and wrist (proximal radioulnar joint [PRUJ] and distal radioulnar joint [DRUJ], respectively). The radio-capitellar joint participates in forearm rotation and the radius can transmit load to the humerus in "high-strength" situations. This issue of load transfer/support is even more important if the elbow ligaments are injured. In general, the elbow gains least stability from muscle support and is reliant on ligament support to guide joint motion.
      ii. Examination of this joint should document the active and passive arcs of flexion and extension. Varus (lateral ligament loading) and valgus (medial ligament loading) should be assessed.
      iii. Standard radiographs include anteroposterior (AP) and lateral views centered on the humeral-ulna articulation.
   b. **Forearm**
      i. Rotation of the forearm is guided by bone support at the PRUJ and DRUJ. Additional stability and guidance for this motion is provided by the interosseous membrane.
      ii. Examination should record the active and passive arcs of supination and pronation. Crepitance or pain at the PRUJ or DRUJ should be noted. Pain or swelling in the mid-forearm should be assessed.
      iii. Standard radiographs include AP and lateral views.
   c. **Wrist**
      i. The **wrist moves in a multiaxial manner.** The carpus is divided into proximal (scaphoid, lunate, and triquetrum) and distal (hamate, capitate, trapezoid, and trapezium) rows. (*Note: the "eighth" carpal bone, the pisiform, is actually a sesamoid bone surrounded by the flexor carpi ulnaris [FCU] tendon and it articulates with the triquetrum. The offset of the FCU increases its flexion moment arm.*) Some of the key intercarpal articulations have more easily described relationships (the scaphoid moves relative to the lunate in flexion and extension). However, taken as a whole, the wrist is multiaxial and its motion is highly dependent on ligament function. There is no direct attachment of an extrinsic (forearm based) muscle or tendon to the bones of the proximal wrist. Thus, these bones (scaphoid, lunate, and triquetrum) are 100% dependent on ligament integrity for function.
      ii. **Examination** should record passive and active arcs of flexion, extension, radial deviation, and ulnar deviation. Obvious pain or crepitance should be recorded as specifically as possible.
      iii. **Standard radiographs** include posteroanterior (PA) or AP and lateral views. If the scaphoid is the focus of attention, AP and lateral views of the scaphoid should be specifically requested. The AP view should be obtained with the wrist in ulnar deviation to capture the scaphoid in full profile. These are oblique to the normal PA and lateral views of the wrist. Fig. 21-1 shows an x-ray AP view of a wrist with joint space narrowing between the distal scaphoid, trapezoid, and trapezium often referred to as scaphotrapeziotrapezoid (STT) arthritis. Because all the joint space is lost this would be graded as advanced or Stage 3 arthritis.

d. **Hand**

   i. The **hand** contains uniaxial (interphalangeal), multiaxial-stabilized (metacarpal phalangeal), and multiaxial-unstabilized (first and fifth carpometacarpal [CMC]) articulations (Fig. 20-1). Thus, these joints have varying degrees of ligamentous or muscle stability requirements. For example, all finger proximal interphalangeal joints depend on ligament support. Whereas, the index finger's metacarpophalangeal joint can be partially stabilized by hand intrinsic muscle support (mostly 1st dorsal and 1st volar interosseous as related to radial and ulnar support, respectively).

   ii. **Examination** should record active and passive arcs of flexion and extension for all joints. Thumb examination should additionally include ability to abduct (palmar and radial), adduct, retropulse (extend), and oppose. Joint stability should be tested and any laxity, tenderness, or other abnormality noted.

   iii. **Standard radiographs** include PA and lateral views. Note: To obtain a lateral view of a finger, the adjacent digits need to be moved aside. Similar to the scaphoid, "normal" thumb views are oblique to the hand. It is important to request specific images to address pathology. For example, if the patient complains of finger pain, specific radiographs of that digit are appropriate, rather than three views of the "hand."

   iv. **Note:** Always examine the opposite or unaffected side. This is particularly important when assessing stability.

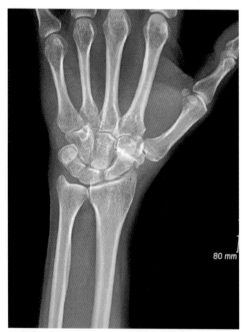

**Figure 21-1.** An x-ray AP view of a wrist with joint space narrowing between the distal scaphoid, trapezoid, and trapezium, often referred to as STT arthritis. Because all the joint space is lost, this would be graded as advanced or stage 3 arthritis.

## II. Developmental Differences

### A. Developmental birth conditions (one recent general review[1])

1. **Radial agenesis.** The absence of the radius can be full or complete. Occasionally, this longitudinal deficiency is accompanied by thumb agenesis. An even more rare condition is presence of the radius and absence of the ulna. In either event, stability of the wrist is compromised. The deformity is often characterized as a "club hand." The absence of the radius would then be termed a *radial club hand*. Full assessment of this condition requires complete assessment of the child to include renal, cardiovascular, neural, and other musculoskeletal regions (shoulder, elbow, and hand). If the child has associated anomalies, correction of the deformity at the forearm carpal articulation may actually compromise function. Thus, any direct treatment must consider the whole forearm and carpal articulation. Fig. 21-2A, B is an example of a child with absent radius and thumb clinically and radiographically. Fortunately, there were no other differences.

2. **Syndactyly**

   a. This is the most common congenital hand condition (1 in 2,000 live births). The cause is not known. It is divided into **simple** (soft-tissue joining of two or more digits with no associated bone or joint anomaly)

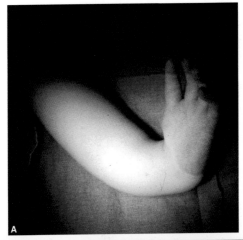

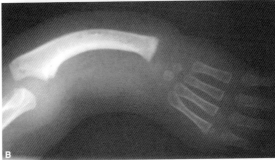

**Figure 21-2.** Clinical appearance and x-ray of a child with absent radius and thumb.

and **complex** (joining of two or more digits to include soft tissue and bones or joints) categories. Further subdivision is possible on the basis of the length of the syndactyly. **Complete** syndactyly involves the whole length of the finger, whereas **incomplete** syndactyly does not. Simple syndactyly is often completely correctable. The complex differences, however, can occur in combination with other congenital differences (Apert's syndrome) (Fig. 21-3A–C). Apert's syndrome before and after resection of bony block and soft-tissue release plus skin grafting.

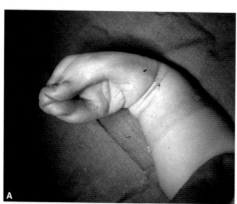

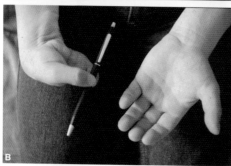

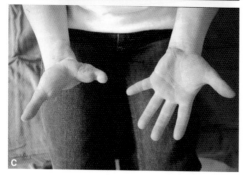

**Figure 21-3.** Child with Apert's bony syndactyly. The central digits were "fused" together with insufficient blood supply to allow separation into multiple fingers, so a decision was made to retain a working thumb and small finger enabling some "pinch" and gross grasp.

Improved (not normal) function obtained. Initial care of this child was substantially delayed because issues related to physical location.

b. In general, surgical correction of this difference should be performed as soon as is anesthetically feasible. Correction of a multiple finger difference is done in stages. Limitations of correction are often related to digital blood supply; usually, full-thickness skin grafts are required at surgery. One interesting note is that deepening of new "clefts" between fingers is less limited by nerves because they can be longitudinally dissected/separated whereas the blood vessel cannot. Thus, the proximal vascular bifurcation defines the depth of the new web space.

3. **Polydactyly**

a. This difference is classified into **preaxial duplication** (involvement of the thumb), central duplication (index, middle, or ring involvement), and postaxial duplication (small finger involvement). **Postaxial duplication** has a clear genetic component and is seen in as many as 1 in 300 live births. Correction of this difference usually involves excision. The degree of duplication and joint involvement determines the complexity of the procedure.

b. **Treatment methods** for thumb duplication generally focus on excision of an unstable duplicate thumb. Duplication of the thumb has been characterized to occur in at least seven different patterns. The outcome of thumb reconstruction depends on the ability to create a thumb of appropriate length, rotation, stability, and mobility and to integrate the thumb into the child's daily routine. It is on this basis that earlier correction is generally recommended.

4. **Madelung deformity.** First described by Malgaigne in 1855 and later by Madelung in 1878, this difference of growth related to the distal epiphysis of the radius is believed to be congenital in nature, although it is usually not noted before adolescence. It is a rare, genetic condition transmitted in an autosomal dominant pattern. Because of incomplete growth of the radius, the clinical presentation may be prominence of the ulnar head (distal ulna). Alternatively, abnormal forearm rotation may be the presenting complaint; pain may not be a component. The method of surgical correction (shortening of the ulna vs. lengthening of the radius) is less important than the goal of obtaining or maintaining stable, painless forearm rotation with unrestricted use of the wrist.

5. **Brachial plexus**

a. The brachial plexus comprises a coalescence of cervical and upper thoracic spine nerve roots. It traverses the space between the neural foramina and the infraclavicular regions where it again separates into individual nerves. Injuries relating to the brachial plexus can occur at any age and generally represent an avulsion (roots) or stretch (trunks and/or cords) event. In birth injuries of plexus two main types are seen: upper (**Erb**), lower (**Klumpke**), or both aspects (combined). These injuries occur generally in the process of vaginal delivery of the child. Fig. 21-4 depicts the plexus and its various regions. Note the position of the clavicle overlies the cords as they descend into the arm as terminal/proper nerves.

b. Critical to the **examination** of any child with a presumed brachial plexus lesion is verification of normal shoulder bony anatomy. The physician should document this by way of physical examination, and shoulder radiographs confirming the shoulder (glenohumeral joint) is located.

c. Occasionally, a child with nothing more than **a fractured clavicle (noted at birth)** will be mistaken to have a brachial plexus injury.

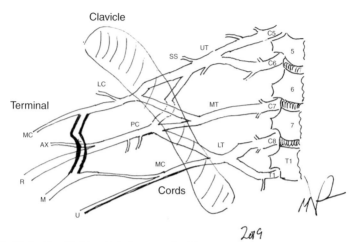

**Figure 21-4.** Simplified brachial plexus emphasizing roots, trunks, cords, and terminal branches. Structures moving anterior are bold and those moving posterior are dotted. Roots are labeled C5 to T1. Upper, middle, and lower trunks are UT, MT, and LT, respectively. Similarly, lateral, posterior, and medial cords are LC, PC, and MC, respectively. Terminal branches are as follows: SS = suprascapular; MC = musculocutaneous; AX = axillary; R = radial; M = median; and U = ulnar.

Thus, it is important to include the clavicle in the physical examination of the infant. Generally, a single AP chest radiograph suffices to detect such a fracture in the neonate.

d. **Management** of brachial plexus injuries at birth should include the following:

   i. Documentation that the glenohumeral joint is located (usually requires an x-ray).

   ii. Documentation of passive mobility of all upper extremity joints, including cervical spine mobility.

   iii. Documentation of observed active motion in shoulder, upper arm, elbow, forearm, wrist, and hand using a 0 to 5 muscle grading system assessing shoulder to fingers.

   iv. Initiation of twice-daily active-assisted "whole-arm" mobilization program to be completed by the **care team** or parents.

   v. Plan for follow-up examination at frequent intervals to verify understanding and completion of passive- and active-assisted exercises and available joint motion (both passive and active—looking for change or improvement).

e. The **prognosis** for many brachial plexus injuries is for complete or near complete recovery. Children whose function remains compromised are evaluated and occasionally operated upon within the first 6 to 18 months of age. The treating physician who cannot document substantial improvement early (<6 months of age) should arrange further evaluation by an upper extremity specialist.

**B.** Delayed presentation of developmental differences

1. **Cerebral palsy**

a. Patients with cerebral palsy constitute the largest group of pediatric patients with neuromuscular disorders. The frequency varies from 0.6 to 5.9 patients per 1,000 live births. Difficulties related to this problem persist into adulthood. However, unlike many neuromuscular disorders, this condition does not progress. Relative progression of the disorder may occur in relation to growth, weight gain, or onset of degenerative change. However, any real progression should cause review of the original diagnosis. Generally, the problem relates to prenatal, natal, or early postnatal brain injury (temporary $O_2$ deprivation is the most common cause of this injury). The injury can express itself in a wide pattern, ranging from single limb to whole body involvement.[2] Two clinical types of injury are seen:

    i. **Spastic type**—represents an injury to pyramidal tracts in the brain. Exaggerated muscle stretch reflex and increased tone are seen.

    ii. **Athetoid type**—probably a lesion in the basal ganglia. Continuous motion of the affected part is present; this type is more rare.

b. **Diagnosis** is the first component of treatment. In cases with lesser involvement, diagnosis may not be obvious until the child fails to reach normal motor milestones or has difficulty with coordinated tasks. In some cases, the diagnosis is suspected because of early "under-use" of a part. For example, a child demonstrating a strong hand preference before 18 months of age should be watched carefully. If this preference continues, a diagnosis of cerebral palsy should be considered.

c. **Treatment** of cerebral palsy should always focus on functional improvement. Generally, surgery has a cosmetic benefit, but the initial goal should be to improve a specific function. Intelligence and sensory awareness of the child are the two biggest determinants for functional improvement after surgery.[3] Improvements of arm function are possible by improvement in the position of the shoulder, elbow, forearm, wrist, hand, and thumb. Three of the more successful surgeries are as follows:

    i. release of an internal rotation/adduction spastic contracture involving the shoulder;

    ii. release/rebalancing of a flexed and pronated spastic wrist/forearm;

    iii. release/rebalancing of a thumb into palm deformity.

III. **Acquired Nonacute Dysfunction of the Elbow, Wrist, and Hand**

A. **Nerve.** Nerve tissue is responsible for communication in two directions between the brain and the periphery. Like the brain, nerve function is highly dependent on oxygen. Depolarization of a single axon takes advantage of an energy gradient. But repolarization of the axon is dependent on adenosine triphosphate to run the $Na^+/K^+$ pump to "recharge" the axon potential. Thus, although local loss of $O_2$ will not cause death of the peripheral axon cell body (located proximally), local loss of $O_2$ will affect the ability of the axon to conduct information. This change in conduction is generally transient, depending on $O_2$ availability. However, frequent episodes of reduced $O_2$ can produce permanent change in function. Common sites for nerve dysfunction to occur in the arm are the carpal canal (wrist, median nerve), the cubital tunnel (elbow, ulnar nerve), and the arcade of Frohse (elbow, posterior interosseous [PIN] branch of the radial nerve).

1. **Carpal tunnel syndrome**

a. Fig. 21-5 depicts the carpal tunnel as seen from end on. The carpal tunnel is seen to be formed by the three bony borders of the carpus (trapezium, lunate, and hook of hamate) and the transverse carpal ligament. As such, it is a defined space with a fixed volume. Changes in the fixed volume can occur as a result of actual changes in the bony outline resulting from late effects of trauma or arthritis. Also, relative change in volume available can be the result of mass effect occurring from tendon or muscle swelling or synovitis, presence of an anomalous

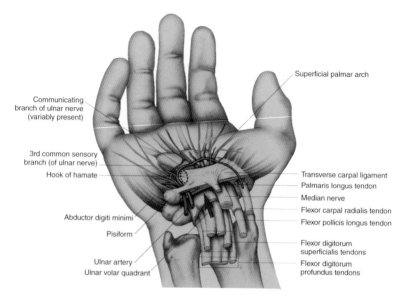

**Figure 21-5.** The carpal tunnel is bounded by bone on three sides and by the ligament (transverse carpal) on one side. Guyon canal overlies the ulnar side of the carpal tunnel. The median nerve lies in the radial volar quadrant of the carpal canal. Generally, it is immediately below or slightly radial to the palmaris longus.

muscle, or presence of an actual mass (e.g., lipoma). The patient with reduction in available volume is less able to tolerate or accommodate increases in pressure within the carpal canal. Thus, in patients with reduced carpal canal volume (relative or real), provocative maneuvers such as Tinel's (tapping or percussion of a nerve in a specific location), Phalen's (flexion of the wrist causing indirect nerve pressurization), or Durkin's compression test (manual pressure by examiner on the median nerve) are more likely to be positive.

b. Presenting complaint is most commonly pain in the median nerve distribution. Pain is often exacerbated at night or by specific activities.[4] As the syndrome advances, numbness occurs in the distribution of the median nerve. Weakness of the thenar muscles with associated wasting is a late stage event.

c. **Laboratory testing.** Radiographs to check for degenerative joint disease (DJD) or old fractures are occasionally of benefit. The most widely accepted diagnostic method is electrodiagnostic testing (electromyogram/nerve conduction velocity [EMG/NCV]). This test can document slowing of nerve conduction and later muscle denervation. The EMG/NCV is most sensitive test if the symptoms have been present for at least 1 month. Given the association of hypothyroidism and rheumatologic disorders, testing of the thyroid stimulating hormone and rheumatoid factor (RF) should be strongly considered. Finally, carpal tunnel syndrome (CTS) is very common in pregnancy, and symptoms frequently resolve after delivery.

d. **Treatment** of CTS focuses on relief of pain. Initial therapy can include medication to relieve pain and swelling (nonsteroidal anti-inflammatory drugs [NSAIDs]), splint support, and exercises to increase mobility. No test or study has shown definite value for NSAIDs in the management of CTS, except as they are related to relief of pain. An injection of corticosteroid into the carpal tunnel may be effective as a treatment when swelling is a transient event. There is some benefit from vitamin $B_6$ and C oral therapy.

    e. Surgery for relief of CTS symptoms is very successful, with patient satisfaction exceeding 95% and complications less than 1%.[5] The surgery can be completed by various methods (open surgery vs. percutaneous or arthroscopic-assisted release) without a clear benefit to one method versus another method, as long as complete longitudinal division of the transverse carpal ligament is achieved along the ulnar half.[4,6-8] Return to unrestricted activity after CTS surgery requires 4 to 8 weeks.

2. **Cubital tunnel syndrome**

    a. The **cubital tunnel** is formed by the bony borders of the medial epicondyle and medial ulna and overlying soft-tissue constraints including the entrance between the ulnar and the humeral head of the two origins of the FCU. Like the carpal canal, it is a defined space with a fixed volume. Changes in the fixed volume can occur as a result of actual changes in the bony outline as a result of late effects of trauma or arthritis (osteoarthritis or rheumatoid arthritis). Relative change in volume available can be the result of mass effect occurring from tendon and muscle swelling or synovitis. Laxity of the soft-tissue supporting structures can allow the ulnar nerve to migrate out of the cubital tunnel and over the medial epicondyle during flexion. This motion is often referred to as subluxation of the ulnar nerve and produces a "Tinel-like" distal sensory disturbance.

    b. **Presenting complaint** is most commonly pain in the distribution of the ulnar nerve distribution.[9] Pain is often exacerbated at night or by specific activities including those with the elbow in flexion. As the syndrome advances, numbness occurs in the distribution nerve. Weakness or atrophy of the hypothenar muscles and the first dorsal interosseous is a late stage event. In some patients, this later stage weakness is their first complaint.

    c. **Laboratory testing** (thyroid function tests and RF) and radiographs (elbow arthritis, old fractures) are occasionally of benefit. The most widely accepted diagnostic test method is electrodiagnostic testing (EMG/NCV). This test can document slowing of nerve conduction and early muscle denervation (FCU and Hand Intrinsics). Again, the EMG/NCV is most sensitive if symptoms have been present for at least 1 month; it is not uncommonly normal even in the presence of profoundly bother some symptoms and positive provocative testing on clinical examination.

    d. Treatment of cubital tunnel syndrome focuses on relief of pain.[10] Initial therapy can include medication (NSAIDs) to relieve pain and swelling, provision of antielbow flexion splint support or pad, and exercises to increase mobility. It is often helpful to have the patient avoid elbow flexion particularly at night (a rolled up towel may be placed in the antecubital fossa). No test or study has shown definite value for NSAIDs in the management of cubital tunnel syndrome, except as related to relief of pain.

    e. Surgery for relief of cubital tunnel symptoms is an option. The surgery can be completed by various methods (small vs. large surgical exposure vs. endoscopic release; in situ decompression vs. transposition—subcutaneous, submuscular, intramuscular). In situ decompression seems to result in symptomatic relief for most patients with a lower rate of complications compared to transposition; however, if the nerve subluxates following decompression, it may be transposed. Patients who fail initial in situ decompression or have recurrent symptoms or who have an unfavorable local milieu may benefit from transposition of the nerve.[11] The patient returns to unrestricted activity within days to weeks after in situ decompression.

3. **PIN compression/others**

   a. The **PIN** branch of the radial nerve travels through a defined space with a fixed volume. The tightest region of this space is formed by a fascial connection at the proximal margin of the two heads of the supinator muscle in the proximal forearm (arcade of Frohse). Changes in the fixed volume can occur as a result of actual changes in the bony outline that result from late effects of trauma or arthritis. Relative change in volume available can be the result of mass effect occurring from tendon and muscle swelling or synovitis, presence of an anomalous muscle, or presence of an actual mass (e.g., lipoma). The most common cause of a change in nerve function in this region is believed to be the result of thickening of the facial margin in response to time (age) and stress (speculative). Two different clinical entities are thought to exist: PIN syndrome and radial tunnel syndrome.

   b. **Presenting complaint** of radial tunnel syndrome is most commonly pain in the general region of the supinator muscle and the proximal forearm. Pain is often exacerbated at night or by specific activities. Numbness does not occur. The presenting complaint of PIN syndrome is weakness of the PIN innervated muscles; associated wasting is a later stage development. Pain is generally absent.

   c. The most widely accepted **diagnostic test** method for PIN syndrome is electrodiagnostic testing (EMG/NCV). However, testing is substantially less sensitive when compared with other nerve compression syndromes. Nonetheless, it shows muscle denervation in some cases and in these cases the test is specific and useful. In addition, magnetic resonance imaging (MRI) may show evidence of nerve compression and or denervation of PIN innervated muscles.

   d. In terms of **diagnostic testing** for radial tunnel syndrome, MRI and electrodiagnostic tests are often ordered but typically normal. Radial tunnel syndrome is a clinical diagnosis.

   e. **Treatment** of PIN syndrome focuses on relief of nerve compression, typically with surgical decompression of the nerve. Dependent on time from loss of muscle innervation, this surgery can be successful. Surgery for definite PIN compression appears to be much more useful than surgery for radial tunnel syndrome.

   f. Treatment of radial tunnel syndrome focuses on pain relief. Initial therapy can include medication to relieve pain or swelling (NSAIDs), activity modulation, and exercises to increase mobility. Splints may exacerbate the problem if placed over the nerve. Wrist splints to reduce load on wrist extensors (the wrist extensors cross over the supinator) are occasionally helpful. As with the other nerve compression syndromes, no test or study has shown a definite value for NSAIDs in management of radial tunnel syndrome. A corticosteroid injection is not recommended by these authors, although some surgeons do use injection as a diagnostic (relief of pain) and therapeutic (relief of pain by reduction of "swelling") maneuver. The authors know of no data to support this option.

   g. **Surgery** for relief of radial tunnel symptoms is substantially less successful than surgery for relief of CTS and is controversial. Some surgeons perform this commonly, others reluctantly and occasionally and still others do not offer surgery for this condition. Various surgical approaches have been described. The arcade of Frohse is identified and released. Return to unrestricted activity after surgery requires days to weeks.

4. **Others.** Nerve compression can occur wherever a nerve exits or enters a fascial plane/transition zone. The foregoing are the most common sites. Knowledge of extremity anatomy will aid the student in assessing other sites of suspected nerve entrapment.

B. **Muscle and tendon.** Muscles and tendons work together to generate and transmit force. The effect of load transfer depends on stable points of origin and insertion. **Three locations of function failure** are apparent[4]: bone-muscle origin,[12] muscle-tendon junction,[13] and tendon–bone insertion. An example of each is provided.

1. **Bone-muscle origin interface failure.** lateral epicondylitis (Fig. 21-6)

a. **Failure of the muscle origin** of forearm extensors (lateral) or flexors (medial) is a common condition. The condition is uncommon in youths

**Figure 21-6. A:** The path of the extensor carpi radialis brevis (ECRB) from lateral epicondyle to the base of the third metacarpal. **B:** The center of the epicondyle is the usual pain foci. **C:** Injection of lidocaine at the painful site. This should eliminate the pain. The injection is into the muscle origin, below the fascia. **D:** Postinjection strength testing usually reveals greater strength after pain is eliminated (successful injection). (From Putnam MD, Cohen M. Painful conditions around the elbow. *Orthop Clin North Am.* 1999;30(1):109-118, with permission.)

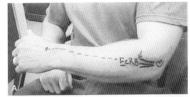

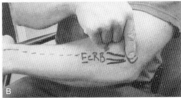

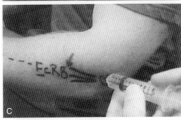

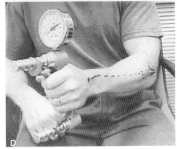

or persons of advanced age. It is occasionally seen in conjunction with working activities.

b. **Presenting complaint** is usually pain focused at the muscle origin. Resisted use of the muscle aggravates the condition. The pain usually subsides with rest. Swelling is rarely present; no mass is seen with this condition. Range of motion may be uncomfortable, but a full active or active-assisted range of motion should be possible.

c. **Laboratory testing** is of no particular value. Screening roentgenograms may be obtained but are generally normal for age. An injection test may be of confirmatory benefit.[13] This is performed as outlined in Fig. 21-6. In this situation, the hope is that a precise injection of lidocaine with or without steroid into the area of extensor origin will eliminate or significantly alleviate the pain (at least temporarily to aide diagnosis).

d. **Treatment** of epicondylitis focuses on reducing the stress at the muscle origin. Although the name implies inflammation, studies have shown actual tendon macro- and microfiber failure with little in the way of inflammatory cells—thus not an inflammatory condition. Theoretically, if the stress is low enough, the healing process can succeed in healing the injured interface. Thus, use of splints to reduce the load on the injured muscle origin, massage to increase the blood supply for healing, and stretching exercises to increase muscle excursion are all measures that are likely to provide success. The value of injections versus oral NSAIDs, rest, and splint support has not been clarified, and in one study, corticosteroid injection has been suggested to be deleterious.[14]

2. **Muscle-tendon pathway failure** results in trigger finger, trigger thumb, and de Quervain's tenosynovitis.

a. The **junction** between a specific muscle and its tendon is a potential site of failure. However, failure or pain at this location is uncommon in the upper extremity. Achilles tendinitis represents a condition occurring in the lower extremity. A similar condition does not occur in the upper extremity with any frequency. Problems along the tendon pathway, however, do occur.

b. Commonly referred to as **trigger digits**, snapping of flexor tendon function caused by bunching of the flexor synovium at the annular one (A1) pulley does occur. This condition is seen more often in older patients, although a congenital version also occurs (the pathology is not the same). The condition occurs more often in patients with diabetes. Patients with active tenosynovitis (rheumatoid arthritis) may have a condition that is often confused for tendon triggering. But rheumatoid arthritis and synovitis in other patients can be distinguished from true trigger digit by the inability to obtain complete active flexion. This is the result of too much synovium "blocking" the active flexion of the digit (the excursion of the flexor tendon is blocked). In the case of de Quervain's tenosynovitis, the problem is focused within the first dorsal extensor compartment of the wrist. The pathophysiology is the same, but this condition results in pain and crepitus along the tendon rather than triggering. The problem and degree of discomfort varies with time of day and activity.

c. **Clinical diagnosis** of trigger dysfunction is made on the basis of pain or tenderness, crepitance, and locking focused at the A1 pulley of a specific digit.

d. **Laboratory studies** are essentially within normal limits. Radiographic studies are not generally useful. In the case of de Quervain's tenosynovitis, a special clinical test (Finkelstein) is routinely performed.

Finkelstein test is positive if ulnar wrist deviation combined with thumb adduction and flexion of the metacarpal phalangeal joint reproduces the patient's complaint of pain.

e. **Treatment** of trigger digit and de Quervain's synovitis includes rest, stretching exercises, steroid injection into the tendon sheath, and surgical release of the tendon sheath.[7-12,15] If nonsurgical care fails, response to supportive modalities is variable. In up to 60% of patients, the condition resolves after steroid injection.[16] Surgical release of the sheath is thought to be 95% effective in those who fail to respond to lesser treatments.[17]

3. **Tendon–bone insertion failure** results in mallet finger and distal biceps rupture.

a. **Failure** at the distal point of muscle action can occur as a result of attrition or age-related change, or excessive load. Occasionally, all methods are involved. Patients are usually seen for diagnosis soon after the failure occurs. Pain is usually less an issue than is weakness or dysfunction.

b. These conditions are **diagnosed** on the basis of findings observed on clinical examination. Laboratory studies and roentgenographic findings are usually normal, the exception being when the extensor tendon involved with a mallet finger pulls off a piece of the proximal aspect of the distal phalanx (thus, a "bony mallet"). Larger tendon ruptures can be further clarified using MRI if there are unclear physical findings.

c. **Treatment** is based on the ability to reposition the specific insertion and maintain this in a tension-free position. For the terminal extensor-mallet finger, 6 weeks of a conservative distal interphalangeal (DIP) extension splint treatment is generally successful.[12,18] Conversely, distal biceps ruptures will not heal without surgery because the tendon cannot be reliably positioned. However, because the muscle is a supporting elbow flexor (not the only elbow flexor), patients who do not require forceful supination (the biceps is the prime supinator) may choose to forego repair (and tolerate the functional limitations).

C. **Joint.** Painless, stable joint function is maintained by a combination of healthy cartilage, retained shape of the joint surface, ligamentous integrity, and muscle/tendon strength. Change in any of these four factors begins a process of increasing joint wear and dysfunction. Aging alone causes changes in the surface of the joint that accelerate wear. Most **arthritic conditions** of the arm are a combination of load, genetics, and history. However, it is occasionally possible to point to a single event many years earlier that has gradually led to joint dysfunction. Processes such as rheumatoid arthritis are usually the sole cause of dysfunction. Even in these diseases, isolated or cumulative trauma can play a role.

1. **Thumb CMC DJD** may be the most common site of arthritic presentation. In any of the upper extremity sites, the most common presenting complaint is pain. To the degree that a specific joint is unstable, incongruous, or both, motion and stress aggravate symptoms. Certain activities and prior injury may predispose to arthritis, but underlying genetics is likely the most predominant cause.

2. **Diagnosis** is a combination of history, examination, laboratory study, and plain radiographs. MRI or computed tomography (CT) methodology is less useful. Most patients complain of pain after activity that is relieved by rest. Oral NSAIDs are of some benefit. Care must always be taken with long-term administration of these medications, particularly in elderly patients.

3. **Treatment** begins with supportive splints and hot/cold modalities, proprioception, and pain relieving measures. Hand- or forearm-based rigid or flexible splints are particularly helpful for thumb CMC. Selective

strengthening programs focusing upon strengthening of the thumb supporting muscles may be beneficial in some patients.[19]

4. Corticosteroid injections are used in many patients. At some point, many patients can no longer "tolerate" the pain. This is the time to consider **surgery**. Unlike the lower extremity, upper extremity arthritic surgery can offer patients reliable joint rebuilding procedures without resorting to joint replacements. An example of such an excisional arthroplasty is shown in Fig. 21-7. Such procedures report greater than 90% success rate relative to pain relief.[20]

5. In the event that first-stage arthritic procedures do not work, newer and increasingly durable total **joint replacement** options are becoming available for the elbow, wrist, and the proximal interphalangeal joints.

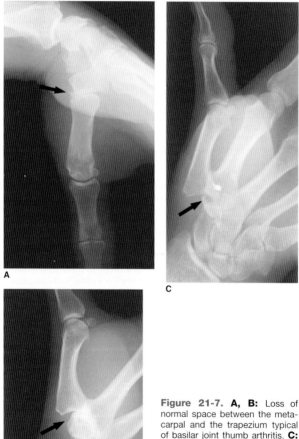

**Figure 21-7. A, B:** Loss of normal space between the metacarpal and the trapezium typical of basilar joint thumb arthritis. **C:** After trapezial resection and stabilization of the first to second metacarpal, a new space for thumb carpometacarpal motion has been "created."

**D. Bone.** Skeletal support is essential for function of the legs and arms. As such, immediate change (fracture) or gradual change (e.g., avascular necrosis and tumor) will alter the function of the arm or leg. Gradual change is rarely as painful as acute or fracture change in bone support. This may explain the late presentation for treatment of patients whose slow change process has progressed to the point at which curative or reconstructive treatment is no longer an option. Avascular necrosis of bone is a condition in which presentation and diagnosis are often delayed. As such, it is a good model to discuss the evaluation of bone pain.

1. **Avascular necrosis, Kienböck (lunate)** (Fig. 21-8), **Preiser (scaphoid), and Panner (humeral capitellum)** are more common focal avascular lesions of bone seen in the upper extremity. Genetics, overload, endocrine and systemic illness, and steroid use may play contributory roles. Patients usually have pain in the focal area and, on testing, it is usually possible to document a reduction in motion. Age of presentation varies from adolescence to late adulthood. Plain radiographs may reveal a change in bone

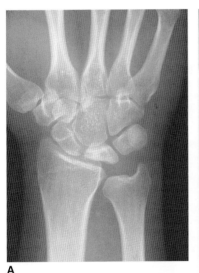

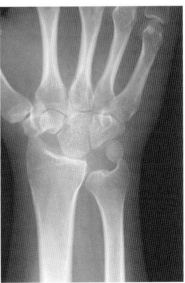

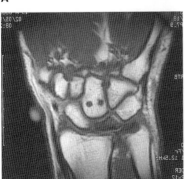

**A**

**B**

**C**

**Figure 21-8. A:** Posteroanterior (PA) wrist radiograph showing "collapse" of the lunate. **B:** Magnetic resonance imaging study of the same wrist from the same point in time showing essentially no vascular signal within the lunate marrow. **C:** PA wrist radiograph showing the capitate "seated" in the lunate fossae after excision of the lunate.

density. In more advanced cases, the shape of the bone is altered. Change in shape is a precursor to diffuse arthritis.

a. **Treatment** starts with making a definite diagnosis. This is true for any unexplained pain in bone. If the diagnosis confirms a focal change in bone vascularity without change in bone shape, initial treatment may focus on joint support. However, many patients, particularly those with Kienböck's disease, do not gain sufficient pain relief from splints, and other joint "unloading" treatments are sought.

b. **Surgical treatments** for these processes can be broken down into treatments that reduce load on the injured bone segment, debride the injured bone segment, or replace/excise the injured bone segment. These treatments are likely to relieve pain in a majority of patients; however, full functional recovery rarely occurs. Fig. 21-9A, B shows an MRI of the elbow in an adolescent with progressive pain and locking of his elbow. A loose flap of bony cartilage measuring 12 × 12 mm was removed and his motion recovered with time.

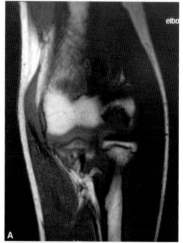

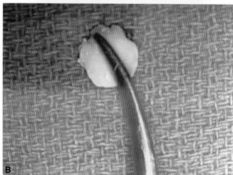

**Figure 21-9.** An MRI of the elbow in an adolescent with progressive pain and locking of his elbow. A loose flap of bony cartilage measuring 12 by 12 mm was removed, and his motion recovered with time.

E. **Tumors.** The upper extremity is the site of various tumors, many of which are rare, some appearing almost exclusively on the hand and the arm, and still others are common to all regions of the body. Although most tumors of the upper extremity are benign, few present simple therapeutic problems. The close anatomic relation of the tumor to the nerves, vessels, and muscles in the upper extremity presents a great challenge to the treating surgeon.

1. Surgeons who treat hand and upper extremity tumors must be familiar with the wide range of **possible diagnoses**. Tumors that look innocent may not be; every mass should be considered potentially dangerous.

2. **Symptomatic tumors**, especially those that have increased in size, must be diagnosed and then classified as to stage. The patient's clinical and family history, the physical characteristics of the lesion, and diagnostic images provide information to determine whether the growth is aggressive and should be "staged."

3. **Diagnostic strategies** to accurately stage the lesion should be pursued before obtaining a biopsy. Appropriate evaluation includes a detailed history and proficient physical examination, imaging, and laboratory studies. The history should determine the length of time a lesion has been present, associated symptoms, and any incidence of family history. Physical examination requires detailed evaluation of the entire limb and testing, especially for sensibility, erythema, fluctuance, range of motion, tenderness, and adenopathy.

4. There are a few lesions that have significant associated **blood chemistry changes**. These include the elevated sedimentation rate of Ewing's sarcoma and the serum protein changes in multiple myeloma. Serum alkaline phosphatase is elevated in metabolic bone disease and in some malignancies. A serum immunoelectrophoresis determines whether multiple myeloma is present.

5. **Imaging** further aids in determining the location of the tumor and the presence or absence of tumor metastasis. There are various imaging techniques that are useful tools.

   a. **Plain films and tomography.** Radiographs are of great importance in the diagnosis of bone tumors. Plain films are the benchmark in predicting presence and location of bone involvement. Tomography or CT affords improved resolution.

   b. **MRI** has developed as one of the more important tools for diagnosing bone tumors. It offers excellent delineation of soft-tissue contrast as well as the ability to obtain images in axial, coronal, and sagittal planes. In addition, MRI can visualize nerve, tendon, and vessels, and with advanced protocols, cartilage can also be evaluated. In tumors, such as osteosarcoma, an MRI can detect a "skip lesion" in the same bone before x-rays will detect the same change. This finding will definitely change management.

6. **Classification of lesions.** Correct treatment must always take into consideration the location and size of the tumor, the histologic grade and clinical behavior, and the potential for metastasis. If a lesion increases in size or becomes symptomatic, or if the physical or radiographic appearance suggests an aggressive lesion, appropriate staging studies including a tissue diagnosis (biopsy) must be obtained.

7. **Specific tumors**

   a. **Benign**

      i. **Ganglion.** Not a true tumor. However, it is worth mentioning because the patient will see this lesion as a growth and be worried for that reason. Also, in cases where a ganglion is removed it is occasionally so obvious a ganglion that no diagnostic tissue needs to be sent to pathology. However, in cases where any doubt exists as to tissue type—gross and microscopic pathologic review should be pursued.

ii. **Lipoma.** This common tumor occasionally presents in the hand or wrist as a firm mass within a nerve or vascular passageway. As such, it may be associated with CTS. Its nature may be suspected on the basis of clinical examination alone (mass). To understand its dimensions and relationship to adjacent tissues, an MRI scan is usually only obtained when there is concern regarding relationships to nerve and blood vessels. Excision (marginal) is the treatment of choice.

iii. **Enchondromas** (Fig. 21-10) of the hand are common; they are sometimes multiple and often present after a fracture. Initial treatment in this circumstance is aimed at satisfactory fracture healing. They can clinically be confused with osteochondromas. Radiographic examination easily differentiates the two processes, as the enchondroma is contained within the bone and can create an expansile deformity while the osteochondroma is contiguous with a portion of the surface of the bone. Most randomly identified lesions can be observed; any lesion associated with pain or increasing size in adulthood should be more carefully studied. Treatment is

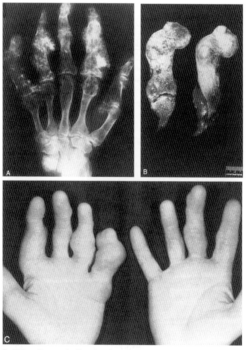

**Figure 21-10. A:** PA radiograph showing bone changes consistent with multiple enchondromas. **B:** Longitudinal section of the small finger. Pathology seen was consistent with low-grade chondrosarcoma. **C:** Preoperative clinical photo showing multiple digit enlargements. In this case, the patient noted rapid enlargement of the small finger during several months before surgery. (From Putnam MD, Cohen M. Malignant bony tumors of the upper extremity. *Hand Clin.* 1995;11(2):265-286, with permission.)

either observation or intralesional excision. Occasionally, previously benign lesions recur or undergo malignant transformation (Fig. 21-10). Any such lesion should be biopsied and carefully considered for wide excision.

b. **Malignant (extensive review of this subject are available)**[21]
   i. **Melanoma.** The hand, wrist, and forearm are common sites of melanoma. Any change in a pigmented lesion warrants biopsy.
   ii. **Osteosarcoma and chondrosarcoma.** Malignant bone lesions do occur in the arm. Most distal lesions are likely to represent degenerative change of benign processes (Fig. 21-10). Any bone or enlarging soft-tissue mass must always receive a complete evaluation (staging and biopsy) leading to a definitive diagnosis.

8. **Metastasis.** Lesions from elsewhere appearing as metastasis are the most common form of malignancy in the hand. This should be kept in mind, particularly for the patient who is not known to have a malignancy and whose lesion is not in keeping with local origin. A search for the primary tumor is appropriate. Perhaps, the most common example to keep in mind is the older adult patient presenting with a new uncomfortable swelling of the distal phalanx and no history of trauma. In many cases, this represents metastatic carcinoma (often lung).[22]

F. **Other factors: workmen's compensation.** The hand is often the first tool in and last tool out of a dangerous situation. As such, it is the frequent site of workplace injuries.[23] Not all injuries are clearly documented. It is the physician's responsibility to remain the patient's advocate while at the same time remaining an objective observer. Occasionally, these tasks are in conflict. Three simple rules apply in these situations:
   1. Remain a dispassionate recorder of medical facts.
   2. Search for an accurate diagnosis.
   3. Offer no treatment without a specific diagnosis.

## REFERENCES

1. Ragati-Haghi Y, Noorbakhsh F, Taghinia AH. Congenital hand differences: a review. *Iran J Pediatr.* 2018;28(5):e62240. doi:10.5812/ijp.62240
2. Mohammed M. Cerebral palsy: comprehensive review and update. *Ann Saudi Med.* 2006;26(2):123–132. doi:10.5144/02564947.2006.123
3. Van Heest AE, House J, Putnam M. Sensibility deficiencies in the hands of children with spastic hemiplegia (Secondary Author). *J Hand Surg [Am].* 1993;18(2):278-281.
4. D'Arcy CA, McGee S. The rational clinical examination. Does this patient have carpal tunnel syndrome? *JAMA.* 2000;283:3110-3117.
5. Ingram J, Mauck BM, Thompson NB, Calandruccio JH. Cost, value, and patient satisfaction in carpal tunnel surgery. *Orthop Clin North Am.* 2018;49(4):503-507. doi:10.1016/j.ocl.2018.06.005
6. Paryoivi E, Zimmerman RM, Means KR. Endoscopic compared with open operative treatment of carpal tunnel syndrome. *JBJS Rev.* 2016;4:1-7.
7. Kay NR. De Quervain's disease. Changing pathology or changing perception. *J Hand Surg Br.* 2000;25:65-69.
8. Khin-Kyemon A, Wu WK, Tokumi A, et al. Outcomes of open carpal tunnel release at a minimum of 10 years. *J Bone Joint Surg Am.* 2013;95:1067-1073.
9. Posner MA. Compressive neuropathies of the ulnar nerve at the elbow and wrist. *Instr Course Lect.* 2000;49:305-317.
10. Mowlavi A, Andrews K, Lille S, Verhulst S, Zook EG, Milner S. The management of cubital tunnel syndrome: a meta-analysis of clinical studies. *Plast Reconstr Surg.* 2000;106:327-334.
11. Kleinman WB. Cubital tunnel syndrome: anterior transposition as a logical approach to complete nerve decompression. *J Hand Surg Am.* 1999;24:886-897.
12. Foucher G, Binhamer P, Cange S, et al. Long-term results of splintage for mallet finger. *Int Orthop.* 1996;20:129-131.

13. Smidt N, Assendelft WJ, van der Windt DA, et al. Corticosteroid injections for lateral epicondylitis: a systematic review. *Pain.* 2002;96(1–2):23-40.
14. Olaussen M, Holmedal O, Lindbaek M, Brage S, Solvang H. Treating lateral epicondylitis with corticosteroid injections or non-electrotherapeutical physiotherapy: a systematic review. *BMJ Open.* 2013;3(10):e003564. doi:10.1136/bmjopen-2013-003564
15. Blood T, Morrell N, Weiss A-P. Tenosynovitis of the hand and wrist. *JBJS Rev.* 2016;4:1-8.
16. Zingas C, Failla JM, Van Holsbeeck M. Injection accuracy and clinical relief of de Quervain's tendinitis. *J Hand Surg Am.* 1998;23:89-96.
17. Ta KT, Eidelman D, Thomson JG. Patient satisfaction and outcomes of surgery for de Quervain's tenosynovitis. *J Hand Surg Am.* 1999;24:1071-1077.
18. Geyman JP, Fink K, Sullivan SD. Conservative versus surgical treatment of mallet finger: a pooled quantitative literature evaluation. *J Am Board Fam Pract.* 1998;11:382-390.
19. O'Brien VH, Giveans MR. Effects of a dynamic stability approach in conservative intervention of the carpometacarpal joint of the thumb: a retrospective study. *J Hand Ther.* 2013;26(1):44-51; quiz 52. doi:10.1016/j.jht.2012.10.005
20. Putnam MD, Meyer NJ, Baker D, Brehmer J, Carlson BD. Trapezium excision and suture suspensionplasty (TESS) for the treatment of thumb carpometacarpal arthritis. *Tech Hand Up Extrem Surg.* 2014;18(2):102-108.
21. Putnam M, Cohen M. Malignant bony tumors of the upper extremity. *Hand Clin.* 1995;11(2):265-286.
22. Flynn C, Danjoux C, Wong J, et al. Two cases of acrometastasis to the hands and review of the literature. *Curr Oncol.* 2008;15(5):51-58.
23. Piligian G, Herbert R, Hearns M, Dropkin J, Landsbergis P, Cherniack M. Evaluation and management of chronic work-related musculoskeletal disorders of the distal upper extremity. *Am J Ind Med.* 2000;37:75-93.

## SELECTED HISTORICAL READINGS

deQuervain F. On a form of chronic tendovaginitis by Dr. Fritz de Quervain in la Chaux-de-Fonds. 1895. Illgen R, Shortkroffs, trans-ed. *Am J Orthop (Belle Mead NJ).* 1997;26:641-644.

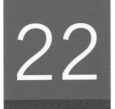

# 22 Fractures of the Pelvis

Thuan V. Ly and David C. Templeman

## I. Pelvic Ring Disruptions
### Key Points
Pelvic ring disruption can range from stable to unstable injuries. Stable pelvic fractures are often seen in the elderly patient from a low-energy mechanism such as a fall from standing height. Pubic rami fractures are the most common pattern often with an impaction injury of the sacral ala; a stable lateral compression (LC) pattern. They are isolated injury and majorities are treated nonoperatively with protected weight bearing (toe touch or partial weight bear <50% with assisted device) and early mobilization with weight bearing as tolerated. However, they frequently need to be admitted because of their comorbidities that will require medical management and disposition. Unstable pelvic fractures are often seen in younger patients from a high-energy mechanism such as motor vehicle accident or fall from significant height. Early management will require multidisciplinary approach with the acute care general surgeon and emergency physician following the Advanced Trauma Life Support (ATLS) protocol. These unstable pelvic ring disruptions are commonly associated with head, chest, abdomen, and extremity injuries.[1-3] The fatality rate from pelvic hemorrhage despite advancements in trauma life support ranges from 5% to 20%.[4,5] If a patient presents with signs and symptoms consistent with shock, the mortality rate increases to 57%.[6] In the acute setting, early mortality in patients with pelvic fractures occurs as a result of hemorrhage. Multisystem organ failure is the more common cause of death in the subacute setting (after 24 hours).[7] Pelvic ring injuries may require early temporary stabilization with a circumferential pelvic sheet or commercial binder as part of patients' early supportive care.[4,8] These life-saving measures limit the volume of the unstable bony pelvis and can contain intrapelvic hemorrhage.
This allows for better bleeding control and appropriate resuscitation prior to definitive surgical fixation for pelvic ring stability.

## II. Pelvic Anatomy and Stability
The pelvis is a ring that consists of the bony architecture (sacrum, ilium, ischium, and pubic) and ligaments that provide rotational and vertical stability. The pelvis contents are surrounded by muscles, nerves, vessels, genitourinary, and intestinal structures that can easily be damaged when the pelvic ring is disrupted. The anterior pelvic ring provides approximately 40% of the stability. Disruption of the pubis symphysis and the pelvic floor (sacrospinous, sacrotuberous) ligaments will result in rotational instability. The posterior pelvic ring provides 60% of the stability. Disruption of the posterior bone–ligamentous complex can result in vertical instability. A stable pelvis can be defined as one that will withstand normal physiologic forces without abnormal deformation (mobilization without significant displacement or deformation).[2] Owing to the innate ring structure, it is rare to have an isolated anterior or posterior pelvic ring injury.

## III. Classification of Pelvic Fractures
The two most commonly used classifications are the Young–Burgess[1,2] and the Tile[9] classification systems. The Young–Burgess classification is based on the mechanism of injury and is useful in acute management (predicting blood loss and

resuscitative requirement) in the trauma bay. This system has four categories: LC, anterior–posterior compression (APC), vertical shear (VS), and combined mechanism (CM). The LC and APC are further subdivided into LC-1, LC-2, and LC-3 and APC-1, APC-2, and APC-3. There is increasing instability and correlation with hemorrhage with higher stages.

**A.** LC—transverse fracture of pubic rami with ipsilateral or contralateral posterior ring injury (Fig. 22-1)

  1. LC-1 sacral fracture on the side of impact (can be incomplete or complete)
  2. LC-2 typical small posterior iliac wing (crescent) with or without sacroiliac (SI) joint involvement
  3. LC-3 can be a LC-1 or LC-2 with a contralateral SI joint diastasis (Windswept)

**B.** APC—anterior pelvic ring disruption (pubic symphysis diastasis) with or without posterior involvement (Fig. 22-2)

  1. APC-1 pubic symphysis diastasis <2.5 cm
  2. APC-2 pubic symphysis diastasis >2.5 cm with anterior SI joint widening but intact posterior SI ligaments (rotationally unstable but vertically stable)
  3. APC-3 anterior pelvic ring disruption with complete posterior SI joint disruption (rotationally and vertically unstable)

**C.** VS—anterior and posterior pelvic ring disrupted with significant vertical instability (fall from significant height) (Fig. 22-3)

**D.** CM—combination of other LC, APC, and VS

  The Tile classification is based on stability of the pattern (Table 22-1). Below is the Tiles classification when compared with the Young–Burgess classification.

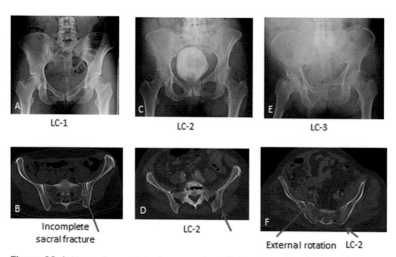

**Figure 22-1.** Young–Burgess lateral compression (LC) type I, type II, and type III. **A:** Anteroposterior (AP) pelvis shows superior and inferior rami fractures on the left with internal rotation deformity of left hemipelvis. **B:** Computed tomography (CT) scan shows sacral ala fracture that is buckled or incomplete. This is consistent with an LC-1 injury. **C:** AP pelvis shows left rami fracture with internal rotation deformity. **D:** CT scan shows complete sacroiliac (SI) joint disruption crescent fracture/dislocation. **E:** AP pelvis shows LC-2 on left side. **F:** CT scan shows LC-2 on left side with SI joint distances on right side (windswept mechanism).

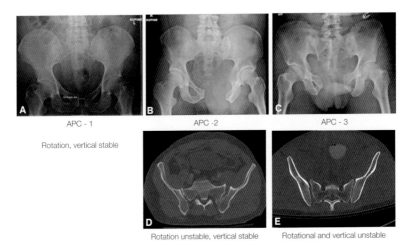

APC - 1  APC -2  APC - 3

Rotation, vertical stable

Rotation unstable, vertical stable    Rotational and vertical unstable

**Figure 22-2.** Young–Burgess anterior–posterior compression type I, type II, and type III. **A:** Anteroposterior (AP) pelvis shows pubis symphysis widening less than 2.5 cm (19.8 mm). Posterior sacroiliac joints are not wide. **B:** AP pelvis shows pubis symphysis diameter >2.5 cm with left SI joint widening. **C:** Computed tomography (CT) scan shows the anterior SI joint widening but posterior SI joint still intact. **D:** AP pelvis shows pubis symphysis diameter > 2.5 cm. There is a complete SI joint disruption with vertical instability on the right side and a SI diastasis on the left side. **E:** CT scan shows complete SI disruption on the right side and anterior SI joint widening but posterior SI joint still intact on the left side.

**E. Tiles classification: types**
1. Type **A:** stable
   a. Young–Burgess analogous APC-1 and most LC-1
2. Type **B:** rotationally unstable, but **vertically** and **posteriorly** stable
   a. Young–Burgess analogous APC-2, some LC-1, some LC-2
3. Type **C: rotationally** and **vertically unstable**
   a. Young–Burgess analogous APC-3, LC-3, most LC-2, some complete LC-1

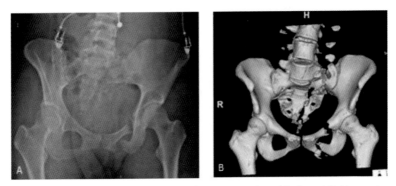

**Figure 22-3.** Young–Burgess vertical shear. **A:** Anteroposterior pelvis shows left side superior and inferior rami fractures with disruption of left posterior SI joint involvement. **B:** 3D images from computed tomography scan shows comminuted sacral fracture on the left side with anterior rami fracture.

| TABLE 22-1 | Substances of Pelvic Fractures |
|---|---|

**Type A: Stable**
A1 Fractures not involving ring; avulsion injuries
- A1.1 Anterior superior spine
- A1.2 Anterior inferior spine
- A1.3 Ischial tuberosity

A2 Stable, minimal displacement
- A2.1 Iliac wing fractures
- A2.2 Isolated anterior ring injuries (four-pillar)
- A2.3 Stable, undisplaced, or minimally displaced fractures of the pelvic ring

A3 Transverse fractures of sacrum and coccyx
- A3.1 Undisplaced transverse sacral fractures
- A3.2 Displaced transverse sacral fractures
- A3.3 Coccygeal fracture

**Type B: Rotationally unstable; vertically and posteriorly stable**
B1 External rotation instability; open-book injury
- B1.1 Unilateral injury
- B1.2 <2.5 cm displacement

B2 Internal rotation instability; lateral compression injury
- B2.1 Ipsilateral anterior and posterior injury
- B2.2 Contralateral anterior and posterior injury; bucket-handle fracture

B3 Bilateral rotationally unstable injury

**Type C: Rotationally, posteriorly, and vertically unstable**
C1 Unilateral injury
- C1.1 Fracture through ilium
- C1.2 Sacroiliac dislocation or fracture–dislocation
- C1.3 Sacral fracture

C2 Bilateral injury, with one side rotationally unstable and one side vertically unstable
C3 Bilateral injury, with both sides completely unstable

F. **Fractures of the acetabulum** are discussed in **Chapter 23**.

G. Note for historical purposes that a **Malgaigne fracture** is a vertical fracture or dislocation of the posterior SI joint complex involving one side of the pelvis.

### IV. Assessment and Emergency Management

A. Pelvic ring disruptions in a hemodynamically unstable patient require assessment per the ATLS protocol. It is important to identify life-threatening injuries, specifically ruling out other sources of hemorrhage. A multidisciplinary team approach has been shown to decrease mortality.[10-14] Often, it will be a combination of acute surgery service and the emergency department doctors leading the ATLS and consulting other subspecialties (orthopaedic surgery, neurosurgery, urology, etc.) as needed. The main objectives in assessing and evaluating patient with pelvic fracture are to (1) identify pelvic instability via physical examination and imaging studies; (2) identify high-risk injury for bleeding to avoid delay in resuscitative efforts; and (3) early intervention to control hemorrhage.

  1. Physical Examination

    a. Pelvic fractures are suspected in patients presenting with pain, swelling, crepitus, or **tenderness over the symphysis pubis, anterior iliac**

**spines, iliac crest, or sacrum**, but a good roentgenographic examination is essential for diagnosis. Correlation of the mechanism of injury with evaluation of the anteroposterior (AP) pelvis radiographs can help determine whether there is a stable or unstable pelvic fracture at risk of hemorrhage. Patients with these injuries are often unconscious or intubated; thus, the examination for pelvis or lower extremity injuries is critical. Historically, manual stress examination for stability was recommended; however, recent studies identify poor sensitivity for identifying unstable pelvic fractures with stress examination.[15]

b. Mandatory physical examination should include assessing the perineal region and performing a rectal, vaginal, and neurologic evaluation. Despite the difficulties involved, a pelvic and/or rectal examination should be performed to identify fresh blood, open wounds, perineal sensation, an unstable prostate, and sphincter tone. Open pelvic fractures historically have had high mortality rates up to 50%.[2] In a recent review article, however, the rate has been reduced owing to improved treatments that reduce hemorrhage, local infection, and sepsis.[16] Pelvic fractures are frequently associated with neurologic damage; thus, a careful neurologic evaluation and documentation should be performed in all patients.

c. Signs of significant pelvic trauma include perineal ecchymosis, lacerations, scrotal/labial swelling, flank ecchymosis, or Morel-Lavallee lesions (soft-tissue degloving injuries).[17,18] Beware of associated injuries that include extremity fractures, neurologic deficits, urologic injuries such as ureteral tears, gynecologic injuries such as vaginal lacerations, or intraabdominal trauma.[2]

B. **Radiographs. An AP view of the pelvis** is taken routinely in all patients who have suffered severe trauma or who complain of pain in and around the pelvic region.

Information gathered from the emergency medical service (EMS) and review of the AP pelvis can assist with predicting blood loss and associated injuries.

C. **Other specific studies.** Most trauma patients should have an indwelling urinary catheter to measure urine output, to determine adequate volume resuscitation and to potentially investigate bladder trauma. Urethral and bladder disruptions can be missed in up to 23% of pelvic fracture patients upon initial evaluation.[19] If there is blood at the penile meatus, a retrograde urethrogram should be performed by a consulting urologist before passage of the catheter.[2,19] A cystogram should be performed if there is concern for bladder rupture (gross hematuria or increased red blood cells in the urinalysis).

V. **Initial Management**

A. **Resuscitation.** Most causes of hemorrhage are adequately handled by rapid replacement and maintenance of blood volume, followed by reduction (when appropriate) and stabilization of the fractures. Adequate blood replacement is the first priority, and its effectiveness is monitored by the patient's pulse, blood pressure, central venous pressure, and urine output. Blood loss of 2,500 mL is common, and blood replacement is usually necessary even without evidence of active hemorrhage. Diagnostic peritoneal lavage is a useful test to rule out intraabdominal injury at the site of hemorrhage if imaging studies are unavailable.[20] Abdominal computed tomography (CT) scan and abdominal ultrasound are effective initial screening tests for this condition. Other sources of bleeding or shock (thoracic, abdominal, open fractures, cardiogenic and spinal shock, and hypothermia) should also be considered.[2,5,21] In addition to resuscitating patients with 2 L of crystalloid and packed red blood cells, it is important to correct the impending coagulopathy with fresh frozen plasma and platelets. ATLS recommends transfusion of red blood cells, plasma, and platelets in a 1:1:1 ratio.[14,22,23]

**B. Hemorrhage control and temporary pelvic stabilization.** Early intervention in patient with an unstable pelvis and hemorrhage can be managed with (1) circumferential pelvic wrapping (sheets and towel clamps or pelvic binder), (2) pelvic external fixator, (3) traction pin, (4) angiography with selective embolization, and (5) pelvic packing.[2,8,14]

**C. Hemorrhage control** and pelvic compression (especially in the open-book pelvis) can temporarily be achieved with circumferential sheets and towel clamps or commercially made pelvic binders.[4,8,24,25] The key is to apply the sheet over the greater trochanteric region at the level of the pubis symphysis to maximize its effectiveness. The sheet should be as smooth as possible and reassessed often to avoid soft-tissue complications.[4,8,24,25] Pelvic external fixator placement can help decrease the pelvic volume (tamponade) and minimize gross motion while allowing venous clots to stabilize. External fixation also allows access to the abdomen and groin region by the general surgeon and improves comfort for patient transfer. Pins can be placed in the iliac crests or supra-acetabular regions through percutaneous or open techniques, depending on the surgeon's experience and preference.[2,26,27] A pelvic C-clamp is ideal for posterior unstable fractures of the pelvic ring because of the compression gained across the SI joints. It requires skill, familiarity with the device, and fluoroscopic guidance.[28,29] For vertically unstable pelvic ring injuries, placement of distal femoral skeletal traction can be beneficial to help with gross realignment of the pelvic ring.[30]

**D. Angiography with selective embolization and pelvic packing.** The three major sources of pelvic bleeding are venous, arterial, and skeletal fractures. Both angiography with selective embolization and pelvic packing have successfully decreased mortality.[2,10,11,14,31-34] However, utilization of these two methods varies among institutions because of the availability of angiography and the comfort level of the general and orthopaedic surgeons for performing the pelvic packing. Pelvic angiography with selective embolization of distal arterial bleeding with blood clot, Gelfoam, or coils has also been useful.[10,11,14,31] Drawbacks to these methods include excessive time requirements (which can inhibit resuscitative efforts), acute renal failure, gluteal muscle necrosis, and postsurgical wound complication. Pelvic packing is more popular in European centers and is being more commonly used in selective institutions in the United States. Pelvic packing provides a tamponade effect for venous and bony bleeding. It is often performed in conjunction with exploratory laparotomy and placement of a pelvic external fixator. The operating surgeon must be experienced in the Pfannenstiel approach to the anterior pelvic ring to place sponges in the paravesical and parasacral space to tamponade the bleed. The patient should return to the operating room within 24 to 48 hours for packing removal and definitive fixation of the pelvic ring at that time.[8,10,11,31]

**VI. Imaging Studies**

**A. Radiographs (AP pelvis, inlet and outlet views).** After the patient is fully resuscitated and hemodynamically stable, dedicated pelvic films are indicated, including inlet and outlet pelvic radiographs. The inlet view is obtained with a 40° cephalad tilt of the x-ray beam from vertical. The outlet view is obtained with a caudad tilt of the x-ray beam from 40° from vertical. The inlet view provides information regarding anterior or posterior displacement of the hemipelvis and rotational deformity. The outlet view allows for assessment of superior or inferior displacement of the hemipelvis. The sacrum and its foramina are best visualized with the outlet view.[2,9,27]

**B. CT scans** can be most useful in defining posterior ring injuries.[1,2,27,35] Fifty percent of sacral fractures are missed on plain radiographs, but they are well visualized on CT scans. These advanced images assist with delineating partial versus complete disruption of the SI joint, defining the zone of sacral fracture, and identifying associated acetabular fractures. In addition, CT scan with contrast can reveal an active bleed if a blush is seen. These pelvic blushes are common and clinical signs of active hemorrhage should consider before proceeding with pelvic angiography and embolization.[21]

## VII. Treatment

A. **Tile type A fractures, Young and Burgess APC-1, and most LC-1 (incomplete sacral fracture) are stable** pelvic ring fracture patterns. These stable fracture patterns are treated nonoperatively. Bruce et al.[36] reported that LC-1 with a complete sacral fracture that is associated with ipsilateral rami fractures will not displace. Physical therapy should be consulted to assist with mobilization and to prevent complications of prolonged bed rest. As soon as the patient can move comfortably in bed, he or she can ambulate with a walker and progress to walking with crutches. The fractures are through cancellous bone with a robust blood supply, and stability of the fracture is usually present in 6 weeks. Excellent healing is expected within 3 months. The ability to perform a straight leg raise on the affected side correlates with independent ambulation, healing, and weaning off of assistive walking devices. Some patients can expect to have lingering lower back pain because of the dense plexus of nerves about the sacrum and coccyx that can be injured or irritated. Injuries to this area may produce chronic low back pain that may take 6 months to 1 year to improve.[31]

B. **Tile type B fractures (rotationally unstable, but vertically and posteriorly stable), Young and Burgess APC-2, and some LC-1 (complete sacral fracture)** must be treated on an individual basis. Fracture displacements, associated injuries, age of the patient, and functional demands should be taken into account.[1,5,27,35] In open-book fractures, disruption of the anterior SI joints and sacrospinous ligaments occurs if there is displacement of more than 2.5 cm in the pubis symphysis joint. These may be reduced and stabilized by external fixation or plate fixation across the symphysis.[27,37,38] The authors generally prefer plate fixation because of patient comfort as well as the complications associated with pin tract infection, pin loosening, and loss of reduction with external fixation.[5,26,39] External fixation can be beneficial in situations where the patient is hemodynamically unstable and requires rapid temporary fixation to decrease the pelvic volume and assist with resuscitation. Minimally displaced B1, B2, and B3 injuries may be treated conservatively with bed to wheelchair mobilization for 6 to 8 weeks, followed by crutch ambulation with weight bearing to tolerance on the side of the pelvis where the posterior ring is uninjured or more stable. Internal fixation is used for more widely displaced and unstable injuries.[27,35,37] Traction is not recommended because of the complications (decubitus ulcer, urinary tract infection, DVT, etc.) that may occur with prolong bed rest as well as the limited ability to improve fracture alignment indirectly. LC-1 pelvic fractures with a complete sacral fracture and displacement (>5 mm) should be reduced and stabilized with iliosacral screws. LC-1 that has a complete sacral fracture but <5 mm displacement that is associated with anterior rami fracture can be unstable. Bruce et al.[36] found that these complete sacral fractures that are associated with unilateral and bilateral rami fractures displaced at a rate of 33% and 66%, respectively. Thus, discussion should be done with the patient about the risks and benefits of surgery.

C. **Type C (rotationally and vertically unstable), Young and Burgess APC-3, most LC-2, and some complete and displaced LC-1** should undergo surgical fixation. Displaced anterior pelvic ring fractures are best stabilized with open reduction and internal fixation with plates and screws. Posterior pelvic ring disruptions (fractures of the sacrum and SI joints) can be managed with closed reduction and percutaneous iliosacral screw fixation. Occasionally, open reduction with plate fixation or percutaneous iliosacral screw fixation may be necessary because of the wide displacement of the fracture. Definitive management of pelvic ring fractures is complex and has the potential for high morbidity because of close vicinity of adjacent neurovascular structures. Thus, patients with type C injuries should be referred to an experienced pelvic and acetabular surgeon.[27,35]

**VIII. Complications**

**A.** Complications from **associated injuries** (e.g., of the bladder, cranium, chest, and abdomen)

**B. Persistent symptoms from SI joint instability**, including pain and leg length inequality

**C. Chronic pain patterns** from injuries around the coccyx and sacrum and SI joint,[30,40] including dyspareunia

**D. Persistent neurologic deficit** from nerve root injury with L5, S1, and distal sacral root injuries are possible with erectile dysfunction being most common in men

**E.** Pulmonary and fat emboli

**F.** Infection from bacterial seeding of the large hematomas or from open pelvic fractures.[18] Injuries to the large bowel are common.

## Authors Treatment Recommendations

### Pelvic Ring Fractures

**Diagnosis:** Good thorough history and physical examination, AP pelvic radiograph, inlet–outlet views, and CT scan.

**Treatment:** Management of hemorrhage if high-energy mechanism. Stable pelvic fracture pattern (most LC-1 and APC-1): protected weight bearing (6 to 8 weeks), followed by progressive weight bearing as tolerated and follow-up radiographs to check for late instability.

**Indications for surgery:** Ongoing hemorrhage (external fixation or posterior pelvic clamp). Unstable pelvic fracture pattern: some LC-1 (complete sacral fractures that are displaced or nondisplaced sacral fracture with bilateral rami fractures), most LC-1, all LC-3, APC-2, and APC-3.

**What do you fix?** Rotational unstable: fix the front or the back. Rotational and vertically unstable: fix the front and the back.

**Recommended technique:** Symphysis plating for anterior pelvic ring disruption, posterior iliosacral screws for sacral or SI disruption. Percutaneous iliosacral screws if there is anatomic reduction otherwise will require open reduction and internal fixation with iliosacral screw or plates and screws. Occasionally, anterior SI joint fixation is performed if posterior skin is tenuous or if the injury is associated with an ipsilateral acetabular fracture.

# REFERENCES

1. Burgess AR, Eastridge BJ, Young JW, et al. Pelvic ring disruptions: effective classification system and treatment protocols. *J Trauma*. 1990;30(7):848-856.
2. Langford JR, Burgess AR, Liporace FA, Haidukewych GJ. Pelvic fractures: part 1. Evaluation, classification, and resuscitation. *J Am Acad Orthop Surg*. 2013;21(8):448-457.
3. Dalal SA, Burgess AR, Siegel JH, et al. Pelvic fracture in multiple trauma: classification by mechanism is key to pattern of organ injury, resuscitative requirements, and outcome. *J Trauma*. 1989;29(7):981-1000; discussion 1000-1002.
4. Bottlang M, Krieg JC, Mohr M, Simpson TS, Madey SM. Emergent management of pelvic ring fractures with use of circumferential compression. *J Bone Joint Surg Am*. 2002;84-A(Suppl 2):43-47.
5. Failinger MS, McGanity PL. Unstable fractures of the pelvic ring. *J Bone Joint Surg Am*. 1992;74(5):781-791.
6. Starr AJ, Griffin DR, Reinert CM, et al. Pelvic ring disruptions: prediction of associated injuries, transfusion requirement, pelvic arteriography, complications, and mortality. *J Orthop Trauma*. 2002;16(8):553-561.
7. Smith W, Williams A, Agudelo J, et al. Early predictors of mortality in hemodynamically unstable pelvis fractures. *J Orthop Trauma*. 2007;21(1):31-37.
8. Bonner TJ, Eardley WGP, Newell N, et al. Accurate placement of a pelvic binder improves reduction of unstable fractures of the pelvic ring. *J Bone Joint Surg Br*. 2011;93(11):1524-1528.
9. Tile M. Pelvic ring fractures: should they be fixed? *J Bone Joint Surg Br*. 1988;70(1):1-12.
10. Olson SA, Burgess A. Classification and initial management of patients with unstable pelvic ring injuries. *Instr Course Lect*. 2005;54:383-393.
11. Giannoudis PV, Pape HC. Damage control orthopaedics in unstable pelvic ring injuries. *Injury*. 2004;35(7):671-677.
12. Balogh Z, Caldwell E, Heetveld M, et al. Institutional practice guidelines on management of pelvic fracture-related hemodynamic instability: do they make a difference? *J Trauma*. 2005;58(4):778-782.
13. Hak DJ, Smith WR, Suzuki T. Management of hemorrhage in life-threatening pelvic fracture. *J Am Acad Orthop Surg*. 2009;17(7):447-457.
14. Mauffrey C, Cuellar DO 3rd, Pieracci F, et al. Strategies for the management of haemorrhage following pelvic fractures and associated trauma-induced coagulopathy. *Bone Joint J*. 2014;96-B(9):1143-1154.
15. Shlamovitz GZ, Mower WR, Bergman J, et al. How (un)useful is the pelvic ring stability examination in diagnosing mechanically unstable pelvic fractures in blunt trauma patients? *J Trauma*. 2009;66(3):815-820.
16. Grotz MRW, Allami MK, Harwood P, Pape HC, Krettek C, Giannoudis PV. Open pelvic fractures: epidemiology, current concepts of management and outcome. *Injury*. 2005;36(1):1-13.
17. Tseng S, Tornetta P 3rd. Percutaneous management of Morel-Lavallee lesions. *J Bone Joint Surg Am*. 2006;88(1):92-96.
18. Hak DJ, Olson SA, Matta JM. Diagnosis and management of closed internal degloving injuries associated with pelvic and acetabular fractures: the Morel-Lavallee lesion. *J Trauma*. 1997;42(6):1046-1051.
19. Ziran BH, Chamberlin E, Shuler FD, Shah M. Delays and difficulties in the diagnosis of lower urologic injuries in the context of pelvic fractures. *J Trauma*. 2005;58(3):533-537.
20. Mendez C, Gubler KD, Maier RV. Diagnostic accuracy of peritoneal lavage in patients with pelvic fractures. *Arch Surg*. 1994;129(5):477-481; discussion 481-482.
21. Verbeek DO, Zijlstra IAJ, van der Leij C, Ponsen KJ, van Delden OM, Goslings JC. Management of pelvic ring fracture patients with a pelvic "blush" on early computed tomography. *J Trauma Acute Care Surg*. 2014;76(2):374-379.
22. Sperry JL, Ochoa JB, Gunn SR, et al. An FFP:PRBC transfusion ratio>/=1:1.5 is associated with a lower risk of mortality after massive transfusion. *J Trauma*. 2008;65(5):986-993.
23. Holcomb JB, Tilley BC, Baraniuk S, et al. Transfusion of plasma, platelets, and red blood cells in a 1:1:1 vs a 1:1:2 ratio and mortality in patients with severe trauma: the PROPPR randomized clinical trial. *JAMA*. 2015;313(5):471-482.
24. Krieg JC, Mohr M, Ellis TJ, Simpson TS, Madey SM, Bottlang M. Emergent stabilization of pelvic ring injuries by controlled circumferential compression: a clinical trial. *J Trauma*. 2005;59(3):659-664.

25. Spanjersberg WR, Knops SP, Schep NWL, van Lieshout EMM, Patka P, Schipper IB. Effectiveness and complications of pelvic circumferential compression devices in patients with unstable pelvic fractures: a systematic review of literature. *Injury.* 2009;40(10): 1031-1035.

26. Hupel TM, McKee MD, Waddell JP, Schemitsch EH. Primary external fixation of rotationally unstable pelvic fractures in obese patients. *J Trauma.* 1998;45(1):111-115.

27. Langford JR, Burgess AR, Liporace FA, Haidukewych GJ. Pelvic fractures: part 2. Contemporary indications and techniques for definitive surgical management. *J Am Acad Orthop Surg.* 2013;21(8):458-468.

28. Ganz R, Krushell RJ, Jakob RP, Küffer J. The antishock pelvic clamp. *Clin Orthop Relat Res.* 1991;267:71-78.

29. Richard MJ, Tornetta P 3rd. Emergent management of APC-2 pelvic ring injuries with an anteriorly placed C-clamp. *J Orthop Trauma.* 2009;23(5):322-326.

30. Nepola JV, Trenhaile SW, Miranda MA, Butterfield SL, Fredericks DC, Riemer BL. Vertical shear injuries: is there a relationship between residual displacement and functional outcome? *J Trauma.* 1999;46(6):1024-1029; discussion 1029-1030.

31. Starr AJ. Re: Miller, PR et al. External fixation or arteriogram in bleeding pelvic fracture: initial therapy guided by markers of arterial hemorrhage. *J Trauma.* 2003;55(2):389; author reply 389-390.

32. Cothren CC, Osborn PM, Moore EE, Morgan SJ, Johnson JL, Smith WR. Preperitoneal pelvic packing for hemodynamically unstable pelvic fractures: a paradigm shift. *J Trauma.* 2007;62(4):834-839; discussion 839-842.

33. Vaidya R, Waldron J, Scott A, Nasr K. Angiography and embolization in the management of bleeding pelvic fractures. *J Am Acad Orthop Surg.* 2018;26(4):e68-e76.

34. Matityahu A, Marmor M, Elson JK, et al. Acute complications of patients with pelvic fractures after pelvic angiographic embolization. *Clin Orthop Relat Res.* 2013;471(9):2906-2911.

35. Routt ML Jr, Kregor PJ, Simonian PT, Mayo KA. Early results of percutaneous iliosacral screws placed with the patient in the supine position. *J Orthop Trauma.* 1995;9(3):207-214.

36. Bruce B, Reilly M, Sims S. OTA highlight paper predicting future displacement of nonoperatively managed lateral compression sacral fractures: can it be done? *J Orthop Trauma.* 2011;25(9):523-527.

37. Matta JM, Saucedo T. Internal fixation of pelvic ring fractures. *Clin Orthop Relat Res.* 1989;242:83-97.

38. Kellam JF. The role of external fixation in pelvic disruptions. *Clin Orthop Relat Res.* 1989;241:66-82.

39. Lindahl J, Hirvensalo E, Böstman O, Santavirta S. Failure of reduction with an external fixator in the management of injuries of the pelvic ring. Long-term evaluation of 110 patients. *J Bone Joint Surg Br.* 1999;81(6):955-962.

40. Copeland CE, Bosse MJ, McCarthy ML, et al. Effect of trauma and pelvic fracture on female genitourinary, sexual, and reproductive function. *J Orthop Trauma.* 1997;11(2):73-81.

# Hip Dislocations, Femoral Head Fractures, and Acetabular Fractures

Thuan V. Ly and David C. Templeman

## I. Hip Dislocation

Hip dislocations can be simple (without fracture) or complex (associated with femoral head, femoral neck, and/or acetabular fractures). Posterior hip dislocations are much more common than anterior hip dislocation. High-energy traumas such as motor vehicle accidents or pedestrian-automobile accidents are often the mechanism of injury due to the inherent stability of this ball and socket joint. The stability comes from the bony anatomy and the soft-tissue constraints, such as the capsule, labrum, and ligamentum teres. Advance Trauma Life Support (ATLS) protocols should be followed because of the high association of fractures and other systemic injuries (head, thoracic, and abdomen).[1,2] A fracture or fracture–dislocation at the hip can easily be missed when associated with a distracting, ipsilateral extremity injury. Such an injury emphasizes the rule: always visualize the joint above and below the diaphyseal fracture. Because injuries about the pelvis can be missed in a critically traumatized patient, ATLS protocol includes a routine pelvic roentgenogram for all patients involved in severe blunt trauma. Native hip dislocations are an orthopaedic emergency. In general, the earlier the reduction is achieved, the better the patient outcome.[1-5] The goals are to minimize the complications (femoral head avascular necrosis [AVN], posttraumatic arthritis, sciatic nerve palsy) that are associated with this injury.[1,2]

## II. Classification of Dislocations

Hip dislocations are described based on the (1) direction of the femoral head dislocation relative to the acetabulum (anterior or posterior) and (2) whether or not there is an associated fracture.[1,2] Thompson and Epstein is a commonly used classification.[1,6,7]

Type I: Dislocation with or without a small fracture
Type II: Dislocation with a large posterior wall fragment
Type III: Dislocation with comminuted posterior wall fragment
Type IV: Dislocation with fracture involving the acetabular floor
Type V: Dislocation with fracture of the femoral head

Stewart–Milford system is another commonly used classification for hip dislocations that include associated fractures.[8]

### A. Anterior dislocations (Thompson and Epstein)[1,7] (Fig. 23-1A, B)
1. **Obturator**
2. **Iliac**
3. **Pubic**
4. **Associated femoral head fractures** (see **V**)

## III. Anterior Dislocations

A. Anterior hip dislocations are rare, occurring in approximately 10% of hip dislocations. The **mechanism of injury** usually occurs in an automobile accident, in a severe fall, or from a blow to the back while squatting.[1,2,5] The mechanism of injury is forced abduction with an externally rotated hip. The neck of the femur or trochanter impinges on the rim of the acetabulum and levers the femoral head out through a tear in the anterior capsule. If in relative extension, an iliac or pubic dislocation occurs or if the hip is in flexion, an

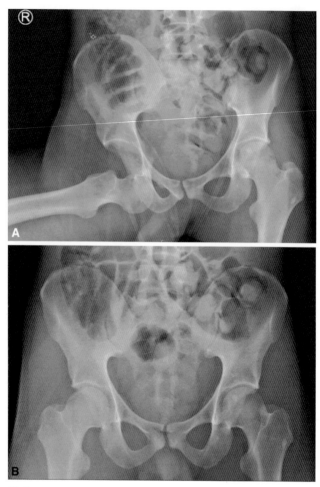

**Figure 23-1. A:** An anteroposterior (AP) pelvis showing a right anterior hip dislocation. **B:** An AP pelvis showing a right hip dislocation.

obturator dislocation occurs. In many instances, there is an associated impaction or shear fracture of the superior articular surface of femoral head as the head passes superiorly over the anteroinferior rim of the acetabulum. These injuries are associated with poor long-term results.[1,2,5,9,10]

**B. Physical examination.** The initial key examination should include the following: the ATLS protocol to evaluate other injuries, visualizing the position or deformity of the leg (anterior or posterior dislocation), documenting the neurologic examination (peroneal nerve deficit is most common) before reduction, and obtaining an anteroposterior (AP) pelvis radiograph. On examination with an obturator dislocation, the hip is abducted, externally rotated, and flexed; however, in the iliac or pubic dislocation, the hip may be extended. The femoral head can usually be palpated near the anterior iliac spine in an iliac dislocation or in the groin in a pubic dislocation. In all patients, one must carefully assess the vascular and neurologic status of the patient before attempting a reduction. The diagnosis is readily apparent on roentgenogram, which shows the femoral head dislocated out of the acetabulum in an inferior and medial position.

C. **Treatment.** Early closed reduction is the treatment of choice, but open reduction may be necessary.[1,2] Reduction is optimally attempted under spinal or general anesthesia, which ensures complete muscle relaxation. In the polytrauma patient, reduction may be attempted in the emergency department with sedation or pharmacologic paralysis. After the airway is controlled, initiate strong but gentle traction along the axis of the femur while an assistant applies stabilization of the pelvis by pressure on the anterior iliac crests. For the **obturator dislocation**, the traction is continued while the hip is gently flexed, and the reduction is accomplished usually by gentle internal rotation. A final maneuver of adduction completes the reduction, but should not be attempted until the head has cleared the rim of the acetabulum with traction in the flexed position. For the **iliac or pubic dislocation**, the head should be pulled distal to the acetabulum. The hip is gently flexed and internally rotated. No adduction is necessary. If the hip does not reduce easily, forceful attempts are not indicated. Failure to obtain easy reduction with the above maneuvers usually indicates that traction is increasing the tension on the iliopsoas or closing a rent in the anterior capsule, producing a "buttonhole" effect. Forced maneuvers only increase the risk for iatrogenic damage. Because the closed reduction may fail, the patient is initially prepared for an open procedure. The open reduction can be accomplished through a muscle-splitting incision, using the distal portion of the standard anterior Smith-Peterson approach. The structures preventing the reduction are released. The postreduction treatment is similar to a posterior dislocation of the hip, except it is important to avoid excessive abduction and external rotation, which are positions that place the extremity at risk for redislocation.

D. **Prognosis and complications.** Excellent reviews of hip dislocations have been published. Anterior dislocations occur in approximately 13% of hip dislocations. Early reduction is necessary for satisfactory results, and although the end result is frequently excellent in the child, traumatic arthrosis and, occasionally, AVN make the prognosis guarded in the adult. Recurrent dislocation is rare in an adult.[3,4,9] Bastian et al. reported a more recent series that anterior hip dislocation occurred in 10 of 100 patients with traumatic dislocation. Associated fractures (femoral head, anterior wall) were seen in six of the patients. These additional fractures correlated with inferior clinical and radiographic results.[5]

IV. **Posterior Dislocations** (Fig. 23-2)

A. The **mechanism of injury** is usually a force applied against the flexed knee with the hip in flexion, as occurs most commonly when the knee strikes the dashboard of an automobile during a head-on impact. If the hip is in neutral or adduction at the time of impact, a simple dislocation is likely, but if the hip is in slight abduction, an associated fracture of the posterior or posterosuperior acetabulum can result. As the degree of hip flexion increases, it is more probable that a simple dislocation is produced.[1,2]

B. **Physical examination** reveals that the leg is shortened, internally rotated, and adducted. A careful physical examination should be performed prior to reduction, including a sensory examination and muscle group motor strength grading. Sciatic nerve injury is associated with 10% to 13% of these injuries.[1,11] Associated bony or ligamentous injury to the ipsilateral knee, femoral head, or femoral shaft is not uncommon.[12] When associated with a femoral shaft fracture, a dislocation may go unrecognized because the classic position

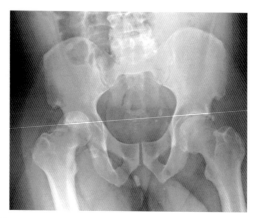

**Figure 23-2.** An anteroposterior pelvis showing a right hip posterior dislocation.

of flexion, internal rotation, and adduction is not apparent. In this situation, the diagnosis is confirmed by a single AP roentgenogram of the pelvis as part of the initial trauma roentgenographic series.

C. **Imaging.** A single AP pelvis does not allow adequate assessment of any associated acetabular fracture. Therefore, additional roentgenograms are needed for treatment planning before performing a reduction if an acetabular fracture is identified. The patient, not the X-ray beam, is moved to obtain the following films: the AP, obturator oblique, and the iliac oblique view.[13-16] This is best accomplished by keeping the patient on a backboard and using foam blocks to support the oblique position of the board (Fig. 23-3). If necessary, computed tomography (CT) scanning can also be performed; optimally, this is completed after the closed reduction of the hip joint to reestablish femoral head circulation. Although some authors question its routine use after uneventful closed reduction, a postreduction CT scan can evaluate for loose bodies or intraarticular fragments (Fig. 23-3).[1,16-18]

D. **Treatment**

1. **Posterior dislocation without fracture.** A dislocated hip is an orthopaedic emergency. This dislocation should be reduced as soon as possible to reduce the risk of femoral head osteonecrosis. The most common reduction technique is the Allis maneuver (Fig. 23-4).

   The reduction can be performed in the emergency department with conscious sedation, but may require general anesthesia with muscle relaxation if unsuccessful with just analgesia. The essential step in a reduction is traction in the line of the deformity, followed by gentle flexion of the hip to 90°, while an assistant stabilizes the pelvis with pressure on the iliac spines. With continued traction, the hip is then gently rotated into internal and external rotation, which usually brings about a prompt restoration of position. Although considerable traction is necessary, under no circumstances, should rough or sudden manipulative movement be attempted. If closed reduction is unsuccessful despite general anesthesia and complete paralysis, then the surgeon should proceed to open reduction. The surgical approach is determined by the direction of the dislocation (anterior or posterior). Kocher-Langenbeck approach is used for posterior hip dislocation. Smith-Peterson approach is used for anterior hip dislocation. Postreduction stability should be confirmed on physical examination, including

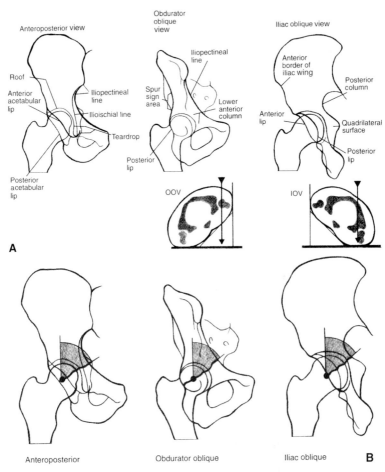

**Figure 23-3.** Radiographic assessment of acetabular fractures. **A:** The anteroposterior, obturator oblique, and iliac views are essential for evaluating the fracture. **B:** The "roof arc" measurement is made between a vertical line and the angle of the fracture. Angles greater than 45° on all three views indicate a fracture, which may be treated nonoperatively. (From Hansen ST, Swiontkowski MF. *Orthopaedic Trauma Protocols.* Raven; 1993, with permission.)

a confirmation of symmetric limb lengths as well as a fluid log roll without mechanical block to motion. A roentgenogram should be obtained in the operating room to ensure that there are no fractures around the femoral head or neck.

a. **Postreduction treatment.** Complete AP pelvis and Judet views should be obtained after reduction to confirm concentric reduction and evaluate for other injuries, such as acetabular, femoral head, and neck fractures. A CT scan is recommended if a nonconcentric joint is seen on plain films to evaluate for chondral or bony loose bodies. Frick and Sims[17] reported that a CT scan is not necessary if the hip joint is concentric on all

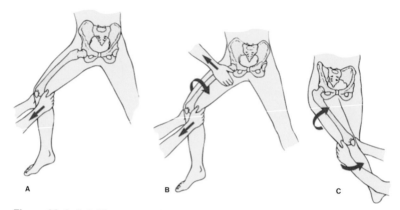

**Figure 23-4. A–C** Allis maneuvers for reduction of a posterior hip dislocation.

three pelvic views (AP, Judets). Mullis and Dahners found loose bodies in seven of nine patients who underwent hip arthroscopy after traumatic dislocations despite postreduction imaging that showed concentric reduction without loose bodies.[19] However, further studies are needed to determine whether removal of these loose bodies in an already concentric joint makes a clinical difference in long-term outcomes. Beware of possible ipsilateral knee injuries. There is a high incidence of meniscal and collateral ligament injury to the knee, and a magnetic resonance imaging (MRI) is warranted if there is clinical suspicion.[12]

b. **Rehabilitation.** Nonoperative treatment is recommended with a stable and congruent hip joint after reduction. Posterior hip precaution includes avoiding hip flexion greater than 60°, adduction, and internal rotation past midline. Toe-touch weight bearing (TTWB) with assistive devices is recommended for 4 to 6 weeks. Isometric exercises for the hip musculature are instituted as soon as pain subsides sufficiently. Continuous passive motion (CPM) may be useful to maintain joint motion, but is not essential.

c. **Prognosis and complications**

   i. Sciatic nerve injuries are discussed in the next section under posterior dislocation with associated acetabular fracture.

   ii. **AVN of the femoral head** is the most feared delayed complication from a simple posterior dislocation of the hip. It occurs late, but various authors have noted an average time of 17 to 24 months from injury to the time of diagnosis. Rates of approximately 6% to 27% are reported, and figures show an incidence of 15.5% for early closed reductions, increasing to 48% if reduction is delayed. There are poor results if the reduction is delayed more than 48 hours. In Epstein's classic study of 426 cases, better results were obtained with open reduction and internal fixation (ORIF) in patients who had associated fractures.

   iii. Epstein also reported an overall rate of **traumatic osteoarthritis** of 23% following posterior hip dislocations, with a rate of 35% in dislocations treated by closed means and a rate of 17% in those treated by open means. In another series, after 12 to 14 years of follow-up, 16% of patients had posttraumatic arthritis, and arthritis developed in an additional 8% as a result of AVN.[3] Similar results have been reported from other centers.[2-4]

2. **Posterior dislocation with associated acetabular fracture**
   a. As previously noted, the **dislocation is reduced as soon as possible, considering the patient's other injuries.** If the patient requires a lengthy trauma evaluation, an attempt can be made in the emergency department to reduce the hip with sedation. In the intubated patient, chemical paralysis completely eliminates muscle spasm and aids reduction. If reduction attempts fail, the urgency for hip reduction must be relayed to the trauma team leader who can expedite care quickly to the operating room. An alternative to standard closed reduction maneuvers involves inserting a 5-mm Schanz pin into the ipsilateral proximal femur at the level of the lesser trochanter. This allows more focused lateral and distal traction by a second assistant to accompany the reduction maneuver. If this maneuver fails, open reduction is preferred through a posterior approach. A posterior wall fracture is internally fixed with lag screws and a buttress plate after joint lavage. If a more complex acetabular fracture is present, an experienced acetabular and pelvic surgeon should be consulted.[20] If the basic posterior acetabular anatomy appears intact and the joint debridement is complete, a CT scan should be obtained to check on the adequacy of debridement and to evaluate for associated fractures.[1,2] Posterior wall fragments measuring less than 20% are likely indicative of a stable hip.[21] However, intraoperative dynamic stress views should be performed to confirm that the hip is concentric and stable, and the posterior wall does not require surgical fixation. Using an obturator view with the fluoroscopic radiograph, the hip is assessed for concentricity: (1) hip in neutral extension, (2) hip flexed to 90°, internally rotated, and adducted, (3) #2 with axial load applied.[21,22]
   b. **Postoperative treatment.** With stable internal fixation, early motion is advised starting with CPM. Flexion is generally limited to 60° for the first 6 weeks postoperatively for large posterior wall fractures. TTWB with crutches are used for 10 to 12 weeks.[13-16]
   c. **Sciatic nerve injury.** Direct contusion, partial laceration by bone fragments, a traction injury, or occasionally an iatrogenic injury resulting from improper placement of retractors during open reduction can cause this injury. Nerve injury should be evaluated early by a careful motor and sensory examination before reduction. If the nerve function is normal before reduction and is abnormal after reduction, this may represent sciatic nerve entrapment in a fracture line. Emergent open reduction and nerve exploration are indicated.[13-16] The peroneal portion of the sciatic nerve is most commonly injured because it lies against the bone in the sciatic notch and tethered over the proximal fibula. When the entire distal sciatic nerve function is abnormal, the tibial portion of function returns nearly 100% of the time. The peroneal portion of function is regained in 60% to 70% of cases: The denser the motor injury, the less likely it is to return to good function.[11] Electromyography (EMG) and nerve conduction studies should be considered for persistent neuropraxias that remain for 3 to 6 months after the injury. The postinjury foot drop is generally managed by a plastic ankle–foot orthotic. Tendon transfers to restore dorsiflexion of the ankle at a later date remain an option.
   d. **Prognosis and complications.** Late traumatic arthritis and femoral head AVN can result in 20% to 30% of cases.[13-16,23] Of all acetabular fractures, the posterior wall injury, despite its being the simplest pattern, has the worst prognosis with regard to these complications.[24-26] Total hip arthroplasty is the most acceptable reconstruction option

when these complications occur. Long-term results in this situation are not as predictable as with total hip arthroplasty for arthritis.[4,25] Rarely, total hip arthroplasty is indicated as the initial surgical therapy in elderly patients with complex fracture patterns.[27,28] Most patients who sustain these injuries are younger than 50 years, and loosening of the components over the patient's lifetime is a real concern.[26]

## V. Fractures of the Femoral Head

**A. Diagnosis.** Fractures of the femoral head generally occur with an associated hip dislocation (posterior more common than anterior). Clinical examination will help diagnose the direction of dislocation if there is significant deformity. The leg will be shortened, flexed, adducted, and internally rotated with posterior hip dislocation. If there is an anterior hip dislocation, the limb will often be abducted and externally rotated. The initial AP pelvis X-ray will show either as indentation fractures of the superior aspect of the head in association with an anterior dislocation or as shear fractures of the inferior aspect of the head in association with a posterior dislocation. Comminuted head fractures occasionally occur with severe trauma. Femoral neck or acetabular fractures may be involved. The diagnosis is established by roentgenograms and CT scan.[10,29,30] The Pipkin classification is the most commonly used system to describe the location of the femoral head and any associated fractures (femoral neck, acetabular).[31]

**B. Classification (Pipkin)** (Fig. 23-5)
1. Type I. Hip dislocation with fracture line of the femoral head inferior to ligamentum teres
2. Type II. Hip dislocation with fracture line of the femoral head superior to ligamentum teres
3. Type III. Type I or II with an associated femoral neck fracture
4. Type IV. Type I or II with an associated acetabular fracture

**C. Treatment**
1. **Initial management.** Early treatment must focus on reducing the hip dislocation and diagnosing the fracture pattern. It is imperative to evaluate the roentgenograms before reducing the hip because occult, nondisplaced femoral neck fractures may become displaced with the reduction maneuver. For Pipkin I and II, gentle closed reduction is recommended in the emergency department. If an occult femoral neck fracture is identified (Pipkin III), the reduction should be performed in the operating room under fluoroscopy and complete muscle relaxation. This allows the surgeon to proceed with an open reduction should the femoral neck fracture displace with the reduction maneuver. If the closed reduction is successful, a repeat AP pelvis is obtained to confirm the reduction. Additional studies should include Judet views and a CT scan to evaluate the concentricity of the hip joint, other associated fractures (femoral neck, acetabular), loose bodies, and size of the femoral head and acetabular posterior wall fracture. This useful information will assist the surgeon with treatment recommendation and pre-op planning.[29,30,32]
2. **Definitive management.** Goals are anatomic reduction, stable and concentric hip joint. If the femoral head fracture is an indentation fracture associated with an anterior dislocation, early CPM and mobilization with crutches (partial weight bearing) are indicated. The prognosis regarding degenerative joint disease is poor, however.[9,10,32,33]
   a. **Pipkin Type I, infrafoveal.** Nonoperative treatment is recommended if it is a small fragment, there is <1 mm of displacement, concentric, and stable hip joint after reduction. Early mobilization, TTWB × 8 to 10 weeks, and close follow-up with serial radiographs are encouraged. Indications for surgery include a displaced and noncongruent hip joint

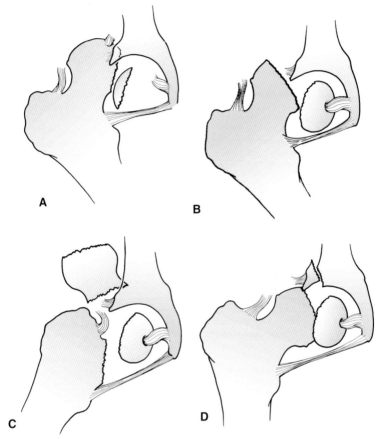

**Figure 23-5.** Pipkin classification of dislocations with femoral head fractures. **A:** Type I. **B:** Type II. **C:** Type III. **D:** Type IV. (From Koval KJ, Bucholz RW, Heckman JD, Court-Brown C, Tornetta P, eds. *Rockwood and Green's Fractures in Adults.* 6th ed. Lippincott Williams & Wilkins; 2006, with permission.)

(often an incarcerated fragment is present) and multiple associated injuries where fixation can assist with early mobilization.[34] The fracture should be approached anteriorly through a Smith-Peterson approach for best visualization and fixation.[32,33] Hip arthroscopy with fragment excision has been shown to be successful.[35]

b. **Pipkin Type II, suprafoveal.** The reduction should be anatomic or within 1 mm on the postreduction CT to proceed with conservative treatment as outlined earlier. If it is displaced, ORIF with well-recessed (countersunk) screws (2.0-, 2.4-, or 2.7-mm screws) or headless compression screws using an anterior approach is indicated.[32,33] Other common approach is the Kocher-Langenbeck with the surgical hip dislocation via trochanteric osteotomy. Though more extensile, the surgical hip dislocation provides better visualization of the hip socket for debridement and fixation of the femoral head.[36-39]

    c. **Pipkin Type III.** Both the femoral head and neck fractures should be internally fixed through an anterior approach. The prognosis for this combination injury is not as favorable as with isolated femoral head fractures because of the higher incidence of posttraumatic osteonecrosis associated with the neck fracture. Thus, in the physiologically older patient with multiple medical problems, consideration should be made for immediate total hip arthroplasty.

    d. **Pipkin Type IV.** These fractures should be operated on in conjunction with the acetabular fracture. Generally, this is accomplished operatively by an experienced pelvic/acetabular surgeon.[13-15] The surgical approach is determined by the acetabular fracture, and the femoral head should be fixed to allow early motion. The Kocher-Langenbeck approach with surgical hip dislocation surgery provides excellent exposures for access to the femoral head and acetabular posterior wall fractures. This has been shown to provide better visualization and removal of bony and chondral joint debris, fixation of the femoral head, and fixation of the posterior wall or repair of capsular/labral tears.[36-39]

**D. Prognosis and complications.** Giannoudis et al.[30] reported a systemic review on 453 femoral head fracture with a mean follow-up of 55.6 months. Major complications included osteonecrosis (11.9%), posttraumatic arthritis (20%), and heterotopic ossification (HO) (16.8%).

## VI. Acetabular Fractures without Posterior Dislocation

**A. Mechanism of injury.** These fractures result from a blow on the greater trochanter or with axial loading of the thigh with the limb in an abducted position.

**B. Physical examination.** These patients often have multiple injuries, and there is a relationship between the acetabular fracture patterns and the associated injuries.[40] The management of the patient is the same as outlined in **Chapter 2**. A careful examination of the sciatic nerve function must be conducted with detailed sensory examination to light touch and motor grading of all distal muscle groups. The muscles innervated by the femoral and obturator nerves must also be examined because they can occasionally be injured with complex anterior column fractures. The AP pelvis admission trauma film and the two 45° pelvic oblique views described by Letournel and Judet[41] (Fig. 23-3), as well as a CT scan of the pelvis, are used to evaluate the fracture pattern.[13-16] The scan is helpful in determining the presence of intraarticular bone fragments, femoral head fractures, size of the posterior wall fracture, and displacement in the weight-bearing region of the acetabulum.[18] Roof arc measurements are useful for treatment planning (Fig. 23-3).[13-15]

**C. Diagnosis.** Management of acetabular fracture can be challenging, but it is imperative to have a clear understanding of the anatomy, radiographic interpretation, and common fracture patterns that comprise of the classification. Letournel and Judet characterized the acetabulum as an inverted "Y" two-column concept.[41] The anterior column (longer) and the posterior column are connected to the sacroiliac joint by a strong sciatic buttress. Radiographic interpretation relies on evaluating the six radiographic lines and their relationship with the structural anatomy on the AP pelvis radiograph.

    1. Iliopectineal line. Anterior column
    2. Ilioischial line. Posterior column
    3. Anterior rim. Anterior wall
    4. Posterior rim. Posterior wall
    5. Roof. Dome of the acetabulum
    6. Tear drop. Medial wall

Additional radiographs with the Judet views will assist with correctly classifying the acetabular fracture. There are 10 common fractures in the Letournel classification that are separated into elementary types and associated types[41] (Fig. 23-6). CT scan should always be obtained for surgical planning, but it does not improve the interobserver or intraobserver reliability of the classification in the experienced surgeons.[42] There are several publications that describe systematic approach that rely on pattern recognition[43] and algorithm[44] (Fig. 23-7) to improve the accuracy with the Letournel classification.

**D. Treatment.** Nonoperative versus operative treatments for acetabular fractures should be made by experienced trauma fellowship trained orthopaedic surgeons who have clear knowledge in radiographic interpretation, surgical approaches, and fracture reduction and fixation.[13-16,18] Many of these factors include patient's medical history, age, fracture pattern, hip stability, hip congruency, amount of fracture displacement, institutional resources (radiologist technician, operating room table, etc.), and surgeon's experiences. Thus, most of these acetabular fractures will need to be transferred to at least a Level II if not a Level I trauma center.

1. **Nonoperative.** The goals of treatment are to obtain a stable and congruent hip joint to decrease the risk of posttraumatic arthritis. Nonoperative treatment is reserved for nondisplaced acetabular fracture, minimal displaced (<2 mm) in the weight-bearing dome of the acetabulum, or displaced fractures in the non–weight-bearing dome of the acetabulum. The weight-bearing dome or surface of the acetabulum can be defined using the "roof arc angle" measurement (Fig. 23-3). Roof arc angle greater than 45° in all three views (AP pelvis, Judet views) indicated that the fracture does not involve the significant weight-bearing surface of the acetabulum. Thus, nonoperative treatment should be considered because it is less likely to develop posttraumatic arthritis. As definitive therapy, traction is no longer generally recommended, with the exception of elderly patients with multiple medical comorbidities. It is generally reserved for temporary treatment of displaced, complex acetabular fractures, patterns

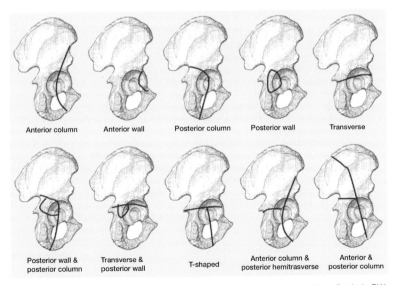

Anterior column    Anterior wall    Posterior column    Posterior wall    Transverse

Posterior wall & posterior column    Transverse & posterior wall    T-shaped    Anterior column & posterior hemitrasverse    Anterior & posterior column

**Figure 23-6.** Letournel and Judet classification of acetabular fractures. (From Bucholz RW, Heckman JD, eds. *Rockwood & Green's Fractures in Adults.* 5th ed. Lippincott, Williams & Wilkins; 2001.)

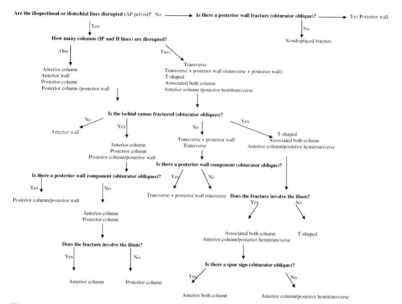

**Figure 23-7.** Algorithm for classifying acetabular fractures. (From Clinical Orthopaedics and Related Research.) Ly TV, Stover MD, Sims SH, Reilly MC. The use of an algorithm for classifying acetabular fractures: a role for resident education? *Clin Orthop Relat Res.* 2011;469(8):2371-2376.

in which the femoral head is articulating on the ridge of the fracture edge on the lateral portion of the joint. Traction prevents further cartilage injury and femoral head indentation; however, it must be heavy (35 to 50 lb) and with a distal femoral pin. If nonoperative management is selected, bed-to-chair mobilization with TTWB × 8 to 10 weeks is recommended. If patient does develop posttraumatic arthritis, total hip arthroplasty is an effective salvage technique.[25,26] Prophylactic pharmacologic agent should be given for at least 4 weeks to prevent deep venous thrombosis (DVT) in these patients.

2. **Operative.** With modern techniques, nearly all significantly displaced acetabular fractures can be fixed safely and effectively, even in elderly individuals.[13-16,23,45] In young patients, displacement of 2 to 3 mm in the major weight-bearing portions of the acetabulum is an indication for open reduction.[13-16] If there is any concern about hip stability or congruency, a stress examination of the hip under general anesthesia is recommended.[22] The two most common surgical approaches for reduction and fixation of these operative acetabular fractures are the Kocher-Langenbeck approach (posterior base fracture pattern) and the ilioinguinal approach (anterior base fracture pattern). Other surgical approaches that can provide more exposure but are less commonly used are the extended iliofemoral and combined approaches. Postoperatively, patients are mobilized with 10 to 12 weeks of TTWB with crutches. If posterior wall involvement is significant, flexion is restricted to 60° for the first 6 weeks.

3. **Complications.** This my include infection (1% to 2%), HO (4% to 6% functionally limiting), AVN (5%), DVT (10% to 20%), pulmonary embolus (1% fatal), degenerative arthritis (20% to 30%, generally associated with posterior wall fractures), and sciatic nerve injury (2% to 5%).[23,24,45-48] HO is most commonly associated with extended posterior (the extended iliofemoral) and combined approaches.[46] These complications occur more often when surgeons are inexperienced. The use and relative benefits of radiation therapy versus indomethacin remain controversial for HO prophylaxis. However, a recent systemic review by Blokhuis and Frolke. supports the use of radiation therapy (700 to 800 cGy) for prevention of HO formation.[49]

## Author's Treatment Recommendations

### Hip Dislocations

**Diagnosis:** AP pelvis radiograph and physical examination. Leg is shortened and internally rotated for posterior dislocation and flexed and externally rotated for anterior dislocation. Judet views and CT scan are obtained after reduction.

**Treatment:** Reduction in emergency department with deep sedation and muscle relaxation; reduction in operating room if other injuries so require.

**Indications for surgery:** Irreducible dislocation, intraarticular loose bodies diagnosed on postreduction radiographs or CT scan.

**Recommended technique:** Hip arthroscopy for small loose bodies, arthrotomy with posterior approach for irreducible dislocation.

## Author's Treatment Recommendations

### Femoral Head Fractures

**Diagnosis:** AP pelvis radiograph and physical examination—these nearly always accompany a hip dislocation, 90% of which are posterior dislocations.

**Treatment:** Closed reduction of the hip followed by CT scan to assess size and reduction of fragment. If reduction is anatomic, TTWB with crutches for 8 to 10 weeks will be necessary.

**Indications for surgery:** Displaced large head fragment (Pipkin II, >2-mm displaced) or displaced Type III or IV fracture.

**Recommended technique:** ORIF through anterior Smith-Peterson approach or posterior Kocher-Langenbeck with surgical hip dislocation, fixation with countersunk lag screws.

## Author's Treatment Recommendations

### Acetabular Fractures

**Diagnosis:** Physical examination, AP pelvis and Judet views, CT scan.

**Treatment:** Nonoperative for nondisplaced fracture, congruent and stable hip joint. 8 to 10 weeks TTWB.

**Indications for surgery:** Displaced fracture (>2-mm) in weight-bearing surface (roof arc angle <45° on all three views), unstable and noncongruent hip joint.

**Recommended technique:** Surgical approaches include ilioinguinal for anterior-based fracture pattern and Kocher-Langenbeck for posterior-based fracture pattern. Fixation with lag screws and reconstruction plates. TTWB for 10 to 12 weeks postoperative.

## REFERENCES

1. Foulk DM, Mullis BH. Hip dislocation: evaluation and management. *J Am Acad Orthop Surg.* 2010;18(4):199-209.
2. Clegg TE, Roberts CS, Greene JW, Prather BA. Hip dislocations—epidemiology, treatment, and outcomes. *Injury.* 2010;41(4):329-334.
3. Dreinhofer KE, Schwarzkopf SR, Haas NP, Tscherne H. Isolated traumatic dislocation of the hip. Long-term results in 50 patients. *J Bone Joint Surg Br.* 1994;76(1):6-12.
4. Upadhyay SS, Moulton A, Srikrishnamurthy K. An analysis of the late effects of traumatic posterior dislocation of the hip without fractures. *J Bone Joint Surg Br.* 1983;65(2):150-152.
5. Bastian JD, Turina M, Siebenrock KA, Keel MJB. Long-term outcome after traumatic anterior dislocation of the hip. *Arch Orthop Trauma Surg.* 2011;131(9):1273-1278.
6. Thompson VP, Epstein HC. Traumatic dislocation of the hip; a survey of two hundred and four cases covering a period of twenty-one years. *J Bone Joint Surg Am.* 1951;33-A(3): 746-778; passim.
7. Epstein HC. Traumatic dislocations of the hip. *Clin Orthop Relat Res.* 1973;92:116-142.
8. Stewart MJ, Milford LW. Fracture-dislocation of the hip: an end-result study. *J Bone Joint Surg Am.* 1954;36(2):315-342.
9. DeLee JC, Evans JA, Thomas J. Anterior dislocation of the hip and associated femoral-head fractures. *J Bone Joint Surg Am.* 1980;62(6):960-964.
10. Konrath GA, Hamel AJ, Guerin J, Olson SA, Bay B, Sharkey NA. Biomechanical evaluation of impaction fractures of the femoral head. *J Orthop Trauma.* 1999;13(6):407-413.
11. Birch R. *Surgical Disorders of the Peripheral Nerves.* Springer Science & Business Media; 2011.
12. Schmidt GL, Sciulli R, Altman GT. Knee injury in patients experiencing a high-energy traumatic ipsilateral hip dislocation. *J Bone Joint Surg Am.* 2005;87(6):1200-1204.
13. Matta JM. Fractures of the acetabulum: accuracy of reduction and clinical results in patients managed operatively within three weeks after the injury. *J Bone Joint Surg Am.* 1996;78(11):1632-1645.
14. Matta JM, Anderson LM, Epstein HC, Hendricks P. Fractures of the acetabulum. A retrospective analysis. *Clin Orthop Relat Res.* 1986;(205):230-240.
15. Manson T, Schmidt AH. Acetabular fractures in the elderly. *JBJS Rev.* 2016;4:1-14.
16. Mayo KA. Fractures of the acetabulum. *Orthop Clin North Am.* 1987;18(1):43-57.
17. Frick SL, Sims SH. Is computed tomography useful after simple posterior hip dislocation? *J Orthop Trauma.* 1995;9(5):388-391.
18. St Pierre RK, Oliver T, Somoygi J, Whitesides T, Fleming LL. Computerized tomography in the evaluation and classification of fractures of the acetabulum. *Clin Orthop Relat Res.* 1984;(188):234-237.
19. Mullis BH, Dahners LE. Hip arthroscopy to remove loose bodies after traumatic dislocation. *J Orthop Trauma.* 2006;20:22-26.

20. Morshed S, Knops S, Jurkovich GJ, Wang J, MacKenzie E, Rivara FP. The impact of trauma-center care on mortality and function following pelvic ring and acetabular injuries. *J Bone Joint Surg Am.* 2015;97(4):265-272.
21. Moed BR, Ajibade DA, Israel H. Computed tomography as a predictor of hip stability status in posterior wall fractures of the acetabulum. *J Orthop Trauma.* 2009;23(1):7-15.
22. Tornetta P 3rd. Non-operative management of acetabular fractures. The use of dynamic stress views. *J Bone Joint Surg Br.* 1999;81(1):67-70.
23. Kaempffe FA, Bone LB, Border JR. Open reduction and internal fixation of acetabular fractures: heterotopic ossification and other complications of treatment. *J Orthop Trauma.* 1991;5(4):439-445.
24. Moed BR, Willson Carr SE, Gruson KI, Watson JT, Craig JG. Computed tomographic assessment of fractures of the posterior wall of the acetabulum after operative treatment. *J Bone Joint Surg Am.* 2003;85(3):512-522.
25. Romness DW, Lewallen DG. Total hip arthroplasty after fracture of the acetabulum. Long-term results. *J Bone Joint Surg Br.* 1990;72(5):761-764.
26. Weber M, Berry DJ, Harmsen WS. Total hip arthroplasty after operative treatment of an acetabular fracture. *J Bone Joint Surg Am.* 1998;80(9):1295-1305.
27. Mears DC, Velyvis JH. Acute total hip arthroplasty for selected displaced acetabular fractures: two to twelve-year results. *J Bone Joint Surg Am.* 2002;84(1):1-9.
28. Lin C, Caron J, Schmidt AH, Torchia M, Templeman D. Functional outcomes after total hip arthroplasty for the acute management of acetabular fractures: 1-to 14-year follow-up. *J Orthop Trauma.* 2015;29(3):151-159.
29. Droll KP, Broekhuyse H, O'Brien P. Fracture of the femoral head. *J Am Acad Orthop Surg.* 2007;15(12):716-727.
30. Giannoudis PV, Kontakis G, Christoforakis Z, Akula M, Tosounidis T, Koutras C. Management, complications and clinical results of femoral head fractures. *Injury.* 2009;40(12):1245-1251.
31. Pipkin G. Treatment of grade IV fracture-dislocation of the hip: a review. *J Bone Joint Surg Am.* 1957;39(5):1027-1197.
32. Marecek GS, Scolaro JA, Routt ML. Femoral head fractures. *JBJS Rev.* 2015;3:1-7.
33. Swiontkowski MF, Thorpe M, Seiler JG, Hansen ST. Operative management of displaced femoral head fractures: case-matched comparison of anterior versus posterior approaches for Pipkin I and Pipkin II fractures. *J Orthop Trauma.* 1992;6(4):437-442.
34. Chen ZW, Lin B, Zhai WL, et al. Conservative versus surgical management of Pipkin type I fractures associated with posterior dislocation of the hip: a randomised controlled trial. *Int Orthop.* 2011;35(7):1077-1081.
35. Park MS, Yoon SJ, Choi SM. Arthroscopic reduction and internal fixation of femoral head fractures. *J Orthop Trauma.* 2014;28(7):e164-e168.
36. Gardner MJ, Suk M, Pearle A, Buly RL, Helfet DL, Lorich DG. Surgical dislocation of the hip for fractures of the femoral head. *J Orthop Trauma.* 2005;19(5):334-342.
37. Ganz R, Gill TJ, Gautier E, Ganz K, Krügel N, Berlemann U. Surgical dislocation of the adult hip a technique with full access to the femoral head and acetabulum without the risk of avascular necrosis. *J Bone Joint Surg Br.* 2001;83(8):1119-1124.
38. Solberg BD, Moon CN, Franco DP. Use of a trochanteric flip osteotomy improves outcomes in Pipkin IV fractures. *Clin Orthop Relat Res.* 2009;467(4):929-933.
39. Siebenrock KA, Gautier E, Woo AKH, Ganz R. Surgical dislocation of the femoral head for joint debridement and accurate reduction of fractures of the acetabulum. *J Orthop Trauma.* 2002;16(8):543-552.
40. Porter SE, Schroeder AC, Dzugan SS, Graves ML, Zhang L, Russell GV. Acetabular fracture patterns and their associated injuries. *J Orthop Trauma.* 2008;22(3):165-170.
41. Letournel E, Judet R. *Fractures of the Acetabulum.* Springer Science & Business Media; 2012.
42. Beaule PE, Dorey FJ, Matta JM. Letournel classification for acetabular fractures. Assessment of interobserver and intraobserver reliability. *J Bone Joint Surg Am.* 2003;85(9):1704-1709.
43. Saterbak AM, Marsh JL, Turbett T, Brandser E. Acetabular fractures classification of Letournel and Judet—a systematic approach. *Iowa Orthop J.* 1995;15:184-196.
44. Ly TV, Stover MD, Sims SH, Reilly MC. The use of an algorithm for classifying acetabular fractures: a role for resident education? *Clin Orthop Relat Res.* 2011;469(8):2371-2376.
45. Helfet DL, Borrelli J Jr, DiPasquale T, Sanders R. Stabilization of acetabular fractures in elderly patients. *J Bone Joint Surg Am.* 1992;74(5):753-765.
46. Ghalambor N, Matta JM, Bernstein L. Heterotopic ossification following operative treatment of acetabular fracture. An analysis of risk factors. *Clin Orthop Relat Res.* 1994;(305):96-105.

47. McLaren AC. Prophylaxis with indomethacin for heterotopic bone. After open reduction of fractures of the acetabulum. *J Bone Joint Surg Am*. 1990;72(2):245-247.

48. Webb LX, Rush PT, Fuller SB, Meredith JW. Greenfield filter prophylaxis of pulmonary embolism in patients undergoing surgery for acetabular fracture. *J Orthop Trauma*. 1992;6(2): 139-145.

49. Blokhuis TJ, Frolke JP. Is radiation superior to indomethacin to prevent heterotopic ossification in acetabular fractures?: a systematic review. *Clin Orthop Relat Res*. 2009;467(2):526-530.

# Fractures of the Femur

Emily A. Wagstrom

## ADULT FRACTURES

### I. Fractures of the Femoral Neck

A. **Epidemiology.** Femoral neck fractures account for just over half of all proximal femoral fractures and are most common in patients older than 50 years, with elderly patients accounting for approximately 95% of the total number of cases.[1,2] Recent Medicaid data show that there is an overall increase in the total number of fractures in the elderly.[3] These fractures become more common with increasing age because of the combination of osteoporosis and an increasing propensity for falls. Besides osteoporosis, other factors associated with an increased risk of femoral neck fracture are early menopause (or low estrogen state), alcoholism, smoking, low body weight, steroid therapy, history of stroke, phenytoin treatment, and lack of exercise. Excessive use of sedative drugs has also been implicated.[4] Typical patients are female, fair, and thin.

Femoral neck fractures in younger patients usually result from high-energy trauma. In addition to traumatic injuries, stress fractures of the femoral neck may occur in active patients. Stress fractures that occur along the superior aspect of the femoral neck are called tension fractures and have a high propensity to progress to complete fractures. The compression stress fracture, which occurs at the base of the femoral neck, is less likely to displace.

B. **Classification of fractures.** From the clinical standpoint, femoral neck fractures consist of four basic types: stress, impacted, nondisplaced, and displaced fractures. Radiographs readily distinguish these patterns, although some nondisplaced fractures may be difficult to visualize on plain radiographs. If there is a high suspicion for fracture but negative plain radiographs, magnetic resonance imaging (MRI) is the imaging modality of choice to assess for occult fracture.[5] Approximately two-thirds of femoral neck fractures are displaced.[2]

C. **Symptoms and signs of injury.** Patients with stress fractures, nondisplaced fractures, or impacted fractures may complain only of pain in the groin or sometimes pain in the ipsilateral knee. Patients with stress fractures often have a history of a recent increase in activity and may believe themselves to have a "groin" strain. In contrast, patients with nondisplaced or impacted fractures typically have a history of trauma. They generally have a higher intensity of pain, can associate the onset with a traumatic event, and are seen early for medical treatment. In all three groups of patients, there is no obvious deformity on physical examination, but there is generally pain with internal rotation. A high index of suspicion must be maintained to avoid delay in diagnosis. Patients with displaced femoral neck fractures complain of pain in the entire hip region and lie with the affected limb shortened and externally rotated. Anteroposterior (AP) and high-quality cross-table lateral (obtained by flexing the uninjured hip) radiographs of the hip are necessary to diagnose displaced, nondisplaced, and impacted fractures and for planning treatment. Traction, internal rotation AP view of the affected hip in displaced fractures allows for better classification of the fracture and for appropriate choice of implant needed for operative fixation.[6] Pending treatment, patients should be non–weight-bearing and allowed to rest with the limbs in the most comfortable position, which is generally in slight flexion on a pillow. Traction is not necessary and may increase pain.[5]

**D. Treatment**

1. **Stress fractures.** These fractures commonly occur in young, vigorous individuals and require careful evaluation. A high index of suspicion for this injury should be kept for active patients presenting with groin pain.[7] Patients with femoral neck stress fractures often have decreased bone density compared with age-matched controls.[8] Femoral neck stress fractures may heal uneventfully but have the potential to displace, especially if on tension side. Upon diagnosis, patients should be treated by restricted weight bearing. Use of crutches or a walker is mandatory, and patients should also be cautioned not to attempt straight-leg raising exercises and not to use the leg for leverage in rising or in changing positions, particularly getting up out of a chair. Partial weight bearing is safe within 6 weeks, with full weight bearing in 12 weeks, as long as the fracture shows roentgenographic evidence of healing, which is evidenced by sclerosis at the superior femoral neck. Because of the potentially severe complications of displacement (nonunion, osteonecrosis, need for surgery), in situ pinning should be considered in active or unreliable patients or any patient with a tension side fracture. Compression types of fractures in elderly individuals generally do well with limiting activity as outlined above. Functional complaints may persist for years in patients with femoral neck stress fractures.[9]

2. **Impacted fractures.** These can be treated either nonoperatively or operatively, and the decision is made after discussion with the patient.[1,10] With nonoperative treatment, pain is controlled with oral medications and/or a fascia iliaca block with a goal of mobilizing the patient early to prevent complications, such as bed sores or pneumonia. Protected ambulation with a walker is then initiated. In a series of over 300 patients with impacted femoral neck fractures treated nonoperatively, displacement only occurred in 5% of younger, healthy patients.[10] When displacement occurred in these patients, operative treatment led to a successful outcome in all cases.[10] However, operative treatment should be strongly considered to prevent displacement from occurring. Internal fixation of impacted fractures has many advantages over nonoperative methods, especially using percutaneous technique. Although the rate of avascular necrosis (AVN) may not be different, a union rate of 100% in operative cases has been reported, compared with 88% with closed management. A matched-pair study compared internal fixation of nondisplaced fractures with hemiarthroplasty in displaced fractures, showing dramatic benefits in the internal fixation group and suggesting that hemiarthroplasty should not be done in nondisplaced fractures.[11]

3. **Displaced fractures.** The management of displaced femoral neck fractures is surgical by either internal fixation or arthroplasty. Patients must be treated with an understanding of their physical and mental abilities. It is important to rapidly arrange family discussions and explain the risks and benefits of the various surgical interventions to the patient's family. The goal is to perform surgical intervention within 48 hours as it is associated with better outcomes. It is recommended that patients older than 65 years should be treated with arthroplasty,[5] with an increasing incidence of arthroplasty in even younger patients. Knowing your patient and their physical function will help decide if you perform a hemiarthroplasty or a total hip arthroplasty (THA). If internal fixation is chosen, anatomic reduction is mandatory. This can be achieved by either closed or open

methods. The FAITH trial compared surgical fixation with either multiple cancellous screws or a dynamic hip screw. The results did not show any difference between the use of multiple cancellous screws versus dynamic hip screw, except in the following specific subgroups: displaced fractures, fractures at the base of the femoral neck, and in those who are current smokers. Therefore, in displaced femoral neck fractures, a dynamic hip screw should be used.[12]

The most difficult situation is the active patient with a displaced femoral neck fracture. Fractures in healthy younger patients, with or without slight comminution, should be **reduced, impacted**, and **internally fixed**. Although the literature is not definitive, there is consensus that surgery should be undertaken as quickly as possible.[13-15] Intracapsular tamponade from fracture hematoma has an unfavorable effect on femoral head blood flow, as does nonanatomic position, so there is a rationale for proceeding with urgency.[1,16,17] There is consensus that accurate reduction and impaction at the fracture site are essential to a good end result. Anatomic reduction allows the maximum opportunity for reestablishment of the vascular supply. Any stretch or kinking of the vessels of the ligamentum teres or retinaculum is avoided, while stability of the fracture is optimized.[16] Internal fixation is clearly associated with an increased risk of reoperation compared with arthroplasty.[18-20] There is also evidence that too much shortening of the femoral neck at the time of final healing leads to a poor outcome.[21] A reliable method to surgically repair femoral neck fractures without loss of fixation or some collapse of the femoral neck remains an elusive goal. Anatomic reduction can be obtained via closed or open means. If attempts at closed reduction are unsuccessful, open reduction should be undertaken.

4. **Failed fixation.** The most frequent complications following internal fixation of displaced femoral neck fracture are loss of reduction, protrusion of the screw or pins into the acetabulum, and collapse with symptomatic AVN. These complications are reliably salvaged by THA.

5. **Postoperative care and rehabilitation in elderly.** The aim of treatment is to return the patient to preoperative status by the quickest, safest method. Therefore, rehabilitation planning should begin at the time of admission because most patients are elderly and do not tolerate prolonged periods away from familiar environments. Surgery is carried out as soon as possible, and the procedure should be one that allows immediate weight bearing to tolerance, the first step in rehabilitation. As long as stable internal fixation is achieved, gains from early weight bearing far outweigh the risks. Patients are encouraged to ambulate and to apply as much weight as is comfortable. Initially, a walker is used, and then gradual progress is made to crutches, if practical, and eventually a cane. In the case of the patient with balance problems, the walker or cane may be used indefinitely to help prevent more falls.

## II. Intertrochanteric Femur Fractures

A. **Epidemiology.** The fracture occurs primarily in the elderly, the average age reported being 66 to 76 years, which is slightly older than for femoral neck fractures. There is a predominance of women, with a ratio of women to men of around 3:1.[22]

B. **Classification of fractures.** Classic intertrochanteric fractures occur in a line between the greater and lesser trochanters and are considered extracapsular fractures. Several classifications and subclassifications have been proposed.[23-25] From the standpoint of treatment and prognosis, a simple classification into stable or unstable fractures is most satisfactory. A stable intertrochanteric fracture is one in which it is possible for the medial cortex of the femur to butt against the medial cortex of the calcar of the femoral neck fragment. Not uncommonly, the lesser trochanter is fractured off as a small secondary fragment, but this does not interfere with the basic stability of the fracture. The unstable intertrochanteric fracture is one in which there is comminution of the posteromedial–medial cortex (along the calcar femorale), involvement of the lateral wall,[26,27] or an associated fracture of the femoral neck.[25] In the most common unstable pattern, a large posteromedial fragment encompasses the lesser trochanter, with or without a fracture, through the greater trochanter (four-part fracture). A fracture with high obliquity may be considered unstable because of the high shearing force at the fracture site, despite anatomic reduction and internal fixation. Lateral wall integrity is important to analyze as it may change the implant you choose for operative fixation.[26,27] In fractures where a fracture line exits lateral to the tip of the greater trochanter, intraoperative fracture of the lateral wall can be expected to occur when using a sliding hip screw, which, in turn, predictably leads to maximal collapse, shortening, and a poor outcome.[27]

**C. Symptoms and signs of injury.** The leg is shortened and lies in marked external rotation. Any movement of the extremity is painful and should not be attempted. Both AP and lateral radiographs should be made to confirm the diagnosis and to delineate the fracture pattern. The lateral film is obtained as a cross-table view, which can be obtained by flexing the uninjured hip. In many cases, an internal rotation view in traction is very helpful and may even change the apparent classification of the fracture and, therefore, the recommended treatment.[6]

**D. Treatment.** Operative treatment is the procedure of choice for all but the most debilitated patients. The goal of treatment is to restore the patient to his/her preoperative status as early as possible, which is best achieved by reduction and internal fixation in a stable manner that allows immediate ambulation. In stable intertrochanteric femur fractures, a sliding hip screw or cephalomedullary device may be used.[5,28] In unstable fractures, intramedullary fixation is recommended.[5,29]

1. **Sliding hip screw.** When using a sliding hip screw, the fracture should ideally be intrinsically stable, or it must be reduced to a stable position; that is, the medial cortices about each other anatomically. The reduction is accomplished on a fracture table by direct traction, slight abduction, and external rotation. If these maneuvers do not produce an anatomic reduction, the fracture site should be opened to ensure stability of the reduction. Not infrequently, there is some posterior displacement at the fracture site that requires the femur shaft to be lifted anteriorly to secure an anatomic reduction at the time of fixation. Regardless of the internal fixation used, in the elderly osteoporotic patient, the neck itself might be little more than a hollow tube; to gain purchase, it is essential to insert the nail or screw into the head. The position should be in the center of the femoral head on both views. The "tip–apex distance" (TAD), defined by Baumgaertner et al.[30,31] as the sum of the distances from the tip of the implant to the apex of the femoral head on both AP and lateral radiographs, is used to determine appropriate position of the implant within the femoral head. The risk of complications increases dramatically when the TAD exceeds 25 mm.[31] The sideplate should be securely fixed across both femoral cortices by two to four screws (Fig. 24-1). When a compression hip screw is used in unstable fracture patterns, a trochanteric side plate may be used to prevent excessive collapse.[28]

2. Cephalomedullary devices are now commonly used for intertrochanteric fractures, and there is consensus that they are the most appropriate implant for unstable fracture patterns. One must be careful to adequately ream and insert the nail by hand to avoid intraoperative femoral shaft

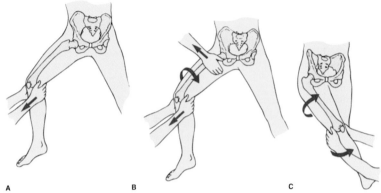

**Figure 24-1.** Technique for closed reduction of a posterior hip dislocation. **A:** Apply longitudinal traction. **B:** An assistant stabilizes the pelvis and pushes posteriorly on the upper thigh to unlock the femoral head from the posterior aspect of the acetabulum. **C:** Linear traction is increased with gentle internal rotation and adduction of the thigh until the femoral head reduces within the acetabulum.

fracture. Many authors use the same TAD criteria for cephalomedullary devices. Cephalomedullary nails are best inserted with the patient on a fracture table, in either the supine or lateral position. It is important to note that the fracture must be reduced prior to insertion of the nail; in some fracture patterns, pointed reduction clamps or threaded Schanz pins are needed to assist with obtaining and maintaining fracture reduction during nail insertion. The use of short or long intramedullary nails is up to the surgeon because there has shown to be equal outcomes and complication rates between the two.[32]

3. **Postoperative care and rehabilitation in elderly.** Just like femoral neck fractures in the elderly, patients should be mobilized as quickly as possible.

### III. Greater Trochanteric Fractures

Isolated avulsion or comminuted fractures of the greater trochanter occasionally are seen. Unless displacement of the fragment is greater than 1 cm, the fracture is treated as a soft-tissue injury with protected weight bearing until the patient is asymptomatic. Several days of bed rest are usually required, followed by walker or crutch ambulation for 3 to 4 weeks. In elderly patients, even with separation greater than 1 cm, operative treatment with internal fixation is rarely indicated.

In the younger patient, when displacement is greater than 1 cm, it is advisable to fix the fracture fragment internally with either two cancellous screws or a wire loop to secure fragments. This maneuver reconstitutes the functional integrity of the abductor mechanism. Postoperatively, the extremity is protected until soft-tissue healing is secured. Then, the patient is allowed to ambulate without weight bearing for 3 to 4 weeks, followed by partial weight bearing for another 3 to 4 weeks until limp-free walking can be achieved.

### IV. Lesser Trochanteric Fractures

These fractures are seen mainly in children and athletic young adults. If they occur in an older patient, one must consider the possibility of metastatic disease. Unless displacement is greater than 2 cm, operative fixation is not indicated, and the end result is excellent.

With displacement greater than 2 cm, it is advisable to stabilize the avulsed fragment with a cancellous screw or a cortical screw, securing it to the opposite cortex. This procedure is most readily accomplished through a medial approach to the hip. Complications are minimal, and the end result is most satisfactory.

## V. Subtrochanteric Femur Fractures

A. **Epidemiology.** The subtrochanteric region of the femur extends from the inferior portion of the lesser trochanter to 5 cm distal to this point. The fracture may extend outside this zone.

B. **Classification of fractures.** There are several fracture classifications for subtrochanteric femur fractures, but the most practical classification is the system of Russel and Taylor.[33] This system divides such injuries into high and low fractures and has direct implications for the most appropriate type of internal fixation. High fractures occur above the lesser trochanter and may or may not involve the greater trochanter and piriformis fossa of the proximal femur. Fractures that involve the piriformis fossa require plate fixation or trochanteric nailing. High fractures not involving the piriformis fossa may be treated by second-generation reconstruction nailing. Low fractures occur below the lesser trochanter, may or not be comminuted, and have varying degrees of extension down the femoral shaft. These fractures, regardless of pattern, are readily treated with standard intramedullary nails.

Atypical subtrochanteric fractures are not included in this system. They are seen in patients treated with bisphosphonates in the setting of osteoporosis. They have a typical lateral breaking appearance.

C. **Symptoms and signs of injury.** Because the forces required to produce the fracture are substantial, other injuries in the same extremity and elsewhere in the body often occur. Emergency traction splinting is generally required with eventual conversion to skeletal traction. Hemorrhage in the thigh may be significant, so the patient should be monitored for hypovolemic shock, and blood replacement may be necessary. Good AP and lateral radiographs are necessary to clearly assess the extent of the fracture.

D. **Treatment.** Operative stabilization to allow early rehabilitation is the treatment of choice. These fractures have a characteristic deformity that should be understood in order to facilitate fracture reduction. If the lesser trochanteric fragment remains attached to the head and neck fragment, it causes a pronounced flexion deformity. In addition, the strong adductors attached to the femoral shaft tend to cause varus angulation. These deformities must be corrected during the surgical procedure either through the use of the fracture table and/or open reduction.

1. **High fractures.** Care must be taken to understand the involvement of the piriformis fossa. If it is involved, a trochanteric intramedullary nail or fixed-angle device can be used based on surgeon preference. Care should be taken when using an intramedullary device to avoid insertion through the fracture site. If the piriformis fossa is not involved, intramedullary fixation is recommended.

2. **Low fractures.** Intramedullary devices are typically used in such fracture patterns. Care must be taken to obtain the appropriate starting point for the nail chosen to avoid varus alignment.

3. **Postoperative care.** Stable subtrochanteric fractures or those that can be rendered stable by operative treatment can be managed much as intertrochanteric fractures. The unstable subtrochanteric fracture must be supported and protected from weight bearing until the union is secure.

## VI. Diaphyseal Femur Fractures

A. **Epidemiology.** Femur fractures are seen in a bimodal distribution. Young adult fractures are often seen in high-energy accidents, whereas older adult fractures are often the result of low-energy trauma.

B. **Signs and symptoms of injury.** Diaphyseal fractures of the femur are the result of significant trauma and are usually associated with considerable soft-tissue damage. Blood loss of 2 to 3 units is common. Advanced Trauma Life Support protocol should be used at initial presentation. Patients may present with obvious deformity or may have been placed in a traction splint by first responders. In addition, these fractures have a high incidence of associated injury in the same extremity, including fractures of the femoral neck,[34] posterior fracture–dislocations of the hip, tears of the collateral ligaments of the knee, and osteochondral fractures involving the distal femur or patella and fractures of the tibia. High-quality AP and lateral X-rays of the femur should be obtained. With a high incidence of ipsilateral femoral neck fractures in these injuries, fine-cut computed tomography (CT) images through the femoral neck should be part of the imaging protocol.[34]

C. **Classification.** Winquist classification has been most commonly used in the past and is based on comminution of the fracture.[35] However, the AO Orthopaedic Trauma Association (AO OTA) classification has been used more recently and describes various fracture patterns.[36]

D. **Treatment.** Emergency treatment consists of the immediate application of a traction splint. Unless there is gross comminution or the patient is not a surgical candidate, fractures of the shaft of the femur from the lesser trochanter to approximately 10 cm above the knee joint should be treated by interlocking nailing, with reaming of the canal using flexible reamers.[35,37] Currently, both antegrade and retrograde nails are acceptable, with similar complication rates and outcomes. Specific indications for retrograde nailing include severe obesity, pregnancy, bilateral fractures, and ipsilateral tibia, patella, or acetabular fractures (that require repair via a posterior hip approach).[38] Femoral nailing by either technique is accomplished as soon as the patient is adequately resuscitated, as indicated by serum bicarbonate or base deficit.[39,40] Immediate fixation is appropriate for most isolated fractures. In polytrauma patients, the more severely injured the patient, the more critical stable fixation of the femur fracture becomes. Early fixation has been shown to be associated with decreased narcotic use, reduced pulmonary complications (e.g., adult respiratory distress syndrome), and decreased mortality rate.[41] Even patients with isolated femoral shaft fractures, including elderly patients, benefit from urgent (within 24 hours of admission) stabilization of the femur with an interlocking nail.[41-43] When the patient is severely traumatized, especially those with traumatic brain injuries at risk for secondary brain insults, provisional fracture stability can be achieved with external fixation or plates much more rapidly on a standard table. The fixator is generally exchanged for an interlocking nail within the first 5 to 7 days when the patient's condition has stabilized. Primary interlocking nailing immediately following debridement is the procedure of choice for most open femoral shaft fractures.[44]

## VII. Supracondylar Fractures

A. **Epidemiology.** In older individuals, these fractures are sustained with minimal trauma. In young people, these fractures are generally caused by massive trauma and are often associated with vascular and other soft-tissue injuries. This fracture has a bimodal age distribution as well.

B. **Signs and symptoms of injury.** A careful assessment of nerve and vascular status distal to the fracture is critical here as with any fracture. Care must be taken to ascertain any injuries to the soft tissues about the knee and whether the fracture extends into the joint. AP, lateral, and, occasionally, oblique radiographic views are necessary. CT is helpful to evaluate intraarticular involvement; especially coronal plane (Hoffa) fractures of either condyle.

C. **Classification.** There have been several classification systems; however, the AO OTA classification system is currently the most widely used and accepted.[36]

D. **Treatment.** Nondisplaced supracondylar fractures or fractures may be treated with either a lateral submuscular plate or a retrograde nail to reduce the risk of loss of reduction. In patients, a hinged knee brace or cast brace may be used, but frequent radiographs must be obtained. In either case, early motion must be initiated to optimize results. Inferior results with nonoperative management for these fractures have been documented.[45]

Displaced supracondylar fractures are managed by open reduction and internal fixation.[46-48] The fracture requires open anatomic reduction of the joint surface via a lateral or anterolateral approach if intraarticular extension is noted. Stripping of the soft-tissue attachments to the extraarticular fragments is avoided. This speeds union and decreases the need for bone grafting while minimizing infection.[49] Locking periarticular plates are often chosen, but retrograde femoral nails with four distal screw options can also be used depending on the fracture pattern. Newer techniques have involved nailplate constructs to allow for immediate weight bearing in elderly individuals.[50]

## PEDIATRIC FRACTURES

### I. Femoral Neck Fractures

A. **Epidemiology.** Pediatric femoral neck fractures are rare injuries. However, there is a risk of long-term complications significantly decreasing their physical function. There is an estimated incidence of 0.3% to 0.5% of fractures in children annually. The peak incidence is 10 to 13 years and a 1.3 to 1.7:1 ratio of boys to girls.[51-56]

B. **Signs and symptoms of injury.** Most of these injuries are the result of high-energy trauma. Therefore, advanced trauma life support should be initiated. The presentation is similar to adults, with the leg held in a shortened and externally rotated position. They have pain in the groin, and sometimes referred pain to the knee, with manipulation of the limb. High-quality AP and lateral X-rays of the affected hip are obtained.

C. **Classification.** The Delbet classification is most commonly used.[57] The classification is based on fracture location and is prognostic of long-term outcomes.

D. **Treatment.** Transepiphyseal fractures are uncommon, and there is no series of sufficient size to make any conclusions about the treatment of choice. The authors recommend reduction with capsulotomy and fixation.[58]

Undisplaced and minimally displaced cervicotrochanteric fractures carry a risk of AVN. The pathophysiology may involve intracapsular tamponade of the vessels supplying the femoral head.[58] The authors recommend capsulotomy, reduction if necessary, and fixation with lag screws short of the femoral head epiphysis. The screws are generally sufficient because of the density of the bone. In children aged 8 years and younger, postoperative spica cast immobilization can also be used for 6 to 12 weeks. Displaced fractures are treated in the same way. These fractures must be treated emergently to minimize the complication of AVN.

E. **Complications**
   1. **Coxa vara.** Although this complication is commonly reported, it is generally associated with nonoperative management.
   2. **Avascular necrosis.** Fracture classification and patient age are predictive factors for the development of AVN, which ranges from 5% to 35%.[59] The long-term consequence is generally degenerative arthritis, which requires THA in patients in their 40s to 60s.
   3. **Premature closure of the epiphysis** occurs in less than 10% of cases and is not a significant long-term problem, except when it occurs in children younger than 8 years.

### II. Diaphyseal Femur Fractures

A. **Epidemiology.** Fractures of the femur in children account for 1.4% to 1.7% of all pediatric fractures.[60,61] Boys have a higher risk of fractures than girls.[62,63] The etiology of the fracture varies by age but includes falls, sports injuries, motor vehicle accidents, and abuse.[62,64]

B. **Signs and symptoms of injury.** Similar to adults, femur fractures in children can be associated with high-energy trauma. Appropriate evaluation and management for pediatric trauma should be undertaken. The patient complains of pain if verbal or may avoid moving or using the leg if nonverbal. Care should be taken to assess the skin for signs of open injury or bruising from nonaccidental trauma. High-quality AP and lateral X-rays of the femur should be taken.

C. **Classification.** The classification for pediatric femur fractures typical involves location and pattern of the fracture. They can be broadly classified as stable, with transverse and short oblique fracture patterns, or unstable, with long oblique, spiral, or comminuted fracture patterns.

D. **Treatment.** Treatment recommendations for pediatric femur fractures are based on the age of the child. The American Academy of Orthopaedic Surgeons (AAOS) updated their treatment recommendations in 2015 and are provided below.[65] In patients under the age of 36 months with a femur fracture, it is recommended that the patient be evaluated for child abuse.

**For children under 6 months of age**, treatment can be with either a Pavlik harness or spica cast. Both result with good outcomes. However, there are more skin complications with the use of hip spica cast.

**For children between the ages of 6 months and 5 years** with an uncomplicated, isolated femoral shaft fracture, a spica cast can be used for primary treatment. Spica placement can be placed immediately or after a short period of traction.

**Children aged 5 to 11 years** are too large and heavy to be managed with spica casts and usually receive some sort of operative fixation. Antegrade interlocking nails, as used in adults, are not appropriate in skeletally immature patients because of the risk of osteonecrosis of the hip. For transverse, length stable fractures, retrograde flexible nailing has gained increased acceptance.[66] There is an increased risk of fixation failure with flexible nails in patients weighing more than 49 kg.[67] Other options for fixation include submuscular plating and external fixation.

**Children older than 11 years have multiple options for fixation.** Trochanteric nails may be considered for the teenage child with fractures of the diaphysis of the femur. The starting point for the nail should be moved laterally to decrease the risk of AVN. Piriformis entry nails should not be used (AAOS). Compression plating remains a very good option[68]; percutaneous submuscular plating is an ideal technique in this age group. Flexible nails also remain an option in this age group, depending on the fracture pattern and patient size.

**Children with head injuries** or multiple trauma should be managed with operative stabilization. In patients younger than 12 years, this should involve plates, retrograde flexible nails, or external fixators. Children older than 11 years may undergo treatment with intramedullary nails.

E. **Complications.** Complications from femur fracture treatment include nonunion, delayed union, malunion, leg length discrepancy, knee stiffness, compartment syndrome, and neurovascular injuries.

## REFERENCES

1. Swiontkowski MF. Intracapsular fractures of the hip: current concepts review. *J Bone Joint Surg Am.* 1994;76:129-138.
2. Thorngren KG, Hommel A, Norrman PO, Thorngren J, Wingstrand H. Epidemiology of femoral neck fractures. *Injury.* 2002;33(suppl 3):C1-C7.
3. Sundaram K, Culler S, Simon A, Jevsevar DS, Gitajn IL, Schlosser MJ. Hip fracture admissions among medicare beneficiaries 2010-2015-rising hospital costs and falling reimbursements. *Int J Musculoskelet Disord.* 2018;10. doi: 10.29011/IJMD-107.000007

4. Ray WA, Griffin MR, Downey W. Benzodiazepines of long and short elimination half-life and the risk of hip fracture. *JAMA*. 1989;262:3303-3307.
5. American Academy of Orthopaedic Surgeons. Management of hip fractures in the elderly. Published September 5, 2014. Accessed February 21, 2020. http://www.aaos.org/research/guidelines/HipFxGuideline.pdf
6. Koval KJ, Oh CK, Egol KA. Does a traction-internal rotation radiograph help to better evaluate fractures of the proximal femur? *Bull NYU Hosp Jt Dis*. 2008;66:102-106.
7. Clough TM. Femoral neck stress fracture: the importance of clinical suspicion and early review. *Br J Sports Med*. 2002;36:308-309.
8. Muldoon MP, Padgett DE, Sweet DE, Deuster PA, Mack GR. Femoral neck stress fractures and metabolic bone disease. *J Orthop Trauma*. 2001;15:181-185.
9. Weistroffer JK, Muldoon MP, Duncan DD, Fletcher EH, Padgett DE. Femoral neck stress fractures: outcome analysis at minimum five-year follow-up. *J Orthop Trauma*. 2003;17:334-337.
10. Raaymakers EL. The non-operative treatment of impacted femoral neck fractures. *Injury*. 2002;33(suppl 3):C8-C14.
11. Parker MJ, White A, Boyle A. Fixation versus hemiarthroplasty for undisplaced intracapsular hip fractures. *Injury*. 2008;39:791-795.
12. Nauth A, Creek AT, Zellar A, et al. Fracture fixation in the operative management of hip fractures (FAITH): an international, multicentre, randomised controlled trial. *Lancet*. 2017;389(10078):1519-1527.
13. Al-Ani AN, Samuelsson B, Tidermark J, et al. Early operation on patients with a hip fracture improved the ability to return to independent living. A prospective study of 850 patients. *J Bone Joint Surg Am*. 2008;90:1436-1442.
14. Holt G, Smith R, Duncan K, McKeown DW. Does a delay to theatre for medical reasons affect the peri-operative mortality in patients with a fracture of the hip? *J Bone Joint Surg Br*. 2010;92:835-841.
15. Simunovic N, Devereaux PJ, Sprague S, et al. Effect of early surgery after hip fracture on mortality and complications: systematic review and meta-analysis. *CMAJ*. 2010;182:1609-1616.
16. Ort PJ, LaMont T. Treatment of femoral neck fractures with a sliding hip screw and the Knowles pins. *Clin Orthop Relat Res*. 1984;(190):158-162.
17. Swiontkowski MF, Winquist RA. Displaced hip fractures in children and adolescents. *J Trauma*. 1986;26:384-388.
18. Gjertsen JE, Vinje T, Engesæter LB, et al. Internal screw fixation compared with bipolar hemiarthroplasty for treatment of displaced femoral neck fractures in elderly patients. *J Bone Joint Surg Am*. 2010;92:619-628.
19. Leonardsson O, Sernbo I, Carlsson Å, Akesson K, Rogmark C. Long-term follow up of replacement compared with internal fixation for displaced femoral neck fractures: results at ten years in a randomised study of 450 patients. *J Bone Joint Surg Br*. 2010;92:406-412.
20. Parker MJ, Pryor G, Gurusamy K. Hemiarthroplasty versus internal fixation for displaced intracapsular hip fractures: a long-term follow-up of a randomised trial. *Injury*. 2010;41:370-373.
21. Zlowodzki M, Brink O, Switzer J, et al. The effect of shortening and varus collapse of the femoral neck on function after fixation of intracapsular fracture of the hip: a multi-centre cohort study. *J Bone Joint Surg Br*. 2008;90:1487-1494.
22. Löfman O, Berglund K, Larsson L, Toss G. Changes in hip fracture epidemiology: redistribution between ages, genders and fracture types. *Osteoporos Int*. 2002;13(1):18-25.
23. Bannister GC, Gibson GF, Ackrund CE, Newman JH. The fixation and prognosis of trochanteric fractures. A randomized, prospective controlled trial. *Clin Orthop Relat Res*. 1990;254:242-246.
24. Larsson S, Friberg S, Hansson LI. Trochanteric fractures; influence of reduction and implant position in impaction and complications. *Clin Orthop Relat Res*. 1990;259:130-138.
25. Kyle RF, Ellis TJ, Templeman DC. Surgical treatment of intertrochanteric hip fractures with associated femoral neck fractures using a sliding hip screw. *J Orthop Trauma*. 2005;19:1-4.
26. Gotfried Y. The lateral trochanteric wall. A key element in the reconstruction of unstable pertrochanteric hip fractures. *Clin Orthop Relat Res*. 2004;425:82-86.
27. Palm H, Jacobsen S, Sonne-Holm S, Gebuhr P; Hip Fracture Study Group. Integrity of the lateral femoral wall in intertrochanteric hip fractures: an important predictor of a reoperation. *J Bone Joint Surg Am*. 2007;89-A:470-475.
28. Lindskog DM, Baumgaertner MR. Unstable intertrochanteric hip fractures in the elderly. *J Am Acad Orthop Surg*. 2004;12:179-190.
29. Platzer P, Thalhammer G, Wozasek GE, Vécsei V. Femoral shortening after surgical treatment of trochanteric fractures in nongeriatric patients. *J Trauma*. 2008;64:982-989.

30. Baumgaertner MR, Curtin SL, Lindskog DM, et al. The value of the tip-apex distance in predicting failure of fixation of peritrochanteric fractures of the hip. *J Bone Joint Surg Am.* 1995;77:1058-1064.

31. Baumgaertner MR, Solberg BD. Awareness of tip-apex distance reduces failure of fixation of trochanteric fractures of the hip. *J Bone Joint Surg Br.* 1992;79:969-971.

32. Boone C, Carlberg KN, Koueiter DM, et al. Short versus long intramedullary nails for treatment of intertrochanteric femur fractures (OTA 31-A1 and A2). *J Orthop Trauma.* 2014 ;28(5):e96-e100.

33. Russell TA, Taylor JC. Subtrochanteric fractures of the femur. In: Browner BD, Jupiter JB, Levine AM, et al, eds. *Skeletal Trauma.* 2nd ed. Saunders; 1992.

34. Tornetta P III, Kain MSH, Creevy WR. Diagnosis of femoral neck fractures in patients with a femoral shaft fracture. Improvement with a standard protocol. *J Bone Joint Surg Am.* 2007;89-A:39-48.

35. Winquist RA, Hansen ST, Clawson DK. Closed intramedullary nailing of femoral fractures. *J Bone Joint Surg Am.* 1984;66:529-539.

36. Meinberg EG, Agel J, Roberts CS, Karam MD, Kellam JF. Fracture and dislocation classification compendium—2018. *J Orthop Trauma.* 2018;32:S1-S170.

37. Wolinsky PR, McCarty E, Shyr Y, Johnson K. Reamed intramedullary nailing of the femur: 551 cases. *J Trauma.* 1999;46:392-399.

38. Patterson BM, Routt ML Jr, Benirschke SK, Karlbauer A, Wagner M. Retrograde nailing of femoral shaft fractures. *J Trauma.* 1995;38:38-43.

39. Crowl AC, Young JS, Kahler DM, Claridge JA, Chrzanowski DS, Pomphrey M. Occult hypoperfusion is associated with increased morbidity in patients undergoing early femur fracture fixation. *J Trauma.* 2000;48:260-267.

40. Nahm NJ, Como JJ, Wilber JH, Vallier HA. Early appropriate care: definitive stabilization of femoral fractures within 24 hours of injury is safe in most patients with multiple injuries. *J Trauma Acute Care Surg.* 2011;71(1):175-185.

41. Bone LB, Johnson KD, Weigelt J, Scheinberg R. Early versus delayed stabilization of femoral fractures: a prospective randomized study. *J Bone Joint Surg Am.* 1989;71:336-340.

42. Cameron CD, Meek RN, Blachut PA, O'Brien PJ, Pate GC. Intramedullary nailing of the femoral shaft: a prospective, randomized study. *J Orthop Trauma.* 1992;6:448-451.

43. Morgan CG, Gibson MJ, Cross AE. Intramedullary locking nails for femoral shaft fractures in elderly patients. *J Bone Joint Surg Br.* 1989;72:19-22.

44. O'Brien PJ, Meek RN, Powell JN, Blachut PA. Primary intramedullary nailing of open femoral shaft fractures. *J Trauma.* 1991;31:113-116.

45. Butt MS, Krikler SJ, Ali MS. Displaced fractures of the distal femur in elderly patients; operative vs. non-operative treatment. *J Bone Joint Surg Br.* 1995;77:110-114.

46. Bolhofner BR, Carmen B, Clifford P. The results of open reduction and internal fixation of distal femur fractures using a biologic (indirect) reduction technique. *J Orthop Trauma.* 1996;6:372-377.

47. Ostrum RF, DiCiccio J, Lakatis R, et al. Retrograde intramedullary nailing of femoral diaphyseal fractures. *J Orthop Trauma.* 1998;12:464-468.

48. Kregor PJ. Distal femur fractures with complex articular involvement: management by articular exposure and submuscular fixation. *Orthop Clin North Am.* 2002;33:153-175.

49. Ostrum RF, Geel C. Indirect reduction and internal fixation of supracondylar femur fractures without bone graft. *J Orthop Trauma.* 1995;9:278-284.

50. Liporace FA, Yoon RS. Nail plate combination technique for native and periprosthetic distal femur fractures. *J Orthop Trauma.* 2019;33(2):e64-e68.

51. Leung PC, Lam SF. Long-term follow-up of children with femoral neck fractures. *J Bone Joint Surg Br.* 1986;68(4):537-540.

52. Davison BL, Weinstein SL. Hip fractures in children: a long-term follow-up study. *J Pediatr Orthop.* 1992;12(3):355-358.

53. Mirdad T. Fractures of the neck of femur in children: an experience at the Aseer Central Hospital, Abha, Saudi Arabia. *Injury.* 2002;33(9):823-827.

54. Bimmel R, Bakker A, Bosma B, Michielsen J. Paediatric hip fractures: a systematic review of incidence, treatment options and complications. *Acta Orthop Belg.* 2010;76(1):7-13.

55. Ratliff A. Fractures of the neck of the femur in children. *Age (Omaha).* 1962;3579:15.

56. Azouz EM, Karamitsos C, Reed MH, Baker L, Kozlowski K, Hoeffel JC. Types and complications of femoral neck fractures in children. *Pediatr Radiol.* 1993;23(6):415-420.

57. Delbet MP. Fractures de col de femur. *Bull Mem Soc Chir.* 1907;33:387-389.

58. Swiontkowski MF, Winquist RA, Hansen ST. Fractures of the femoral neck in patients between the ages of twelve and forty-nine years. *J Bone Joint Surg Am.* 1984;66:837-846.

59. Moon ES, Mehlman CT. Risk factors for avascular necrosis after femoral neck fractures in children: 25 Cincinnati cases and meta-analysis of 360 cases. *J Orthop Trauma*. 2006;20(5):323-329.
60. Sahlin Y. Occurrence of fractures in a defined population: a 1-year study. *Injury*. 1990;21:158-160.
61. McCartney D, Hinton A, Heinrich SD. Operative stabilization of pediatric femur fractures. *Orthop Clin North Am*. 1994;25:635-650.
62. Hinton RY, Lincoln A, Crockett MM, Sponseller P, Smith G. Fractures of the femoral shaft in children. Incidence, mechanisms, and sociodemographic risk factors. *J Bone Joint Surg Am*. 1999;81:500-509.
63. Rewers A, Hedegaard H, Lezotte D, et al. Childhood femur fractures, associated injuries, and sociodemographic risk factors: a population-based study. *Pediatrics*. 2005;115:e543-e552.
64. Femoral Shaft Fractures Guideline Team. Evidence-based care guideline for medical management of Femoral Shaft Fractures. *Guideline*. 2006;22:1-19. Cincinnati Children's Hospital Medical Center.
65. American Academy of Orthopaedic Surgeons. Treatment of pediatric diaphyseal femur fractures. Accessed February 21, 2020. Published June 12, 2015. https://www.aaos.org/globalassets/quality-and-practice-resources/pdff/pdff-cpg-update-final-2015-4-23-19.pdf
66. Greisberg J, Bliss MJ, Eberson CP, Solga P, d'Amato C. Social and economic benefits of flexible intramedullary nails in the treatment of pediatric femoral shaft fractures. *Orthopedics*. 2002;25:1067-1070.
67. Moroz LA, Launay F, Kocher MS, et al. Titanium elastic nailing of fractures of the femur in children: predictors of complications and poor outcome. *Bone Joint J Br Vol*. 2006;88(10):1361-1366.
68. Caird MS, Mueller KA, Puryear A, Farley FA. Compression plating of pediatric femoral shaft fractures. *J Pediatr Orthop*. 2003;23:448-452.

# 25 Knee Injuries: Acute and Overuse

Caitlin C. Chambers and Bradley J. Nelson

## I. Foundation of Injury Diagnosis

Knee injuries are common in active individuals. Both acute and overuse injuries occur, and they require different investigative processes to diagnose and treat them properly.

### A. Subdivision of clinical categories

1. Acute injury is an injury that happens where a single application of force creates the musculoskeletal damage. This is common in athletics, motor vehicle trauma, and so on.

2. Acute on chronic injury is an injury that results in a disabled state that can be quiescent over time and result in a new injury episode at a later time. This new injury would represent an acute injury. However, this new injury typically involves less force than the original acute injury, as there was preexisting damage to the musculoskeletal tissue. Common examples might be recurrent patella instability or recurrent shoulder subluxation.

3. Overuse injury is an injury that is characterized by the absence of a traumatic event. This kind of injury results from repetitive submaximal or subclinical trauma that results in macroscopic or microscopic damage to a structural unit and/or its blood supply. This overuse pattern can be seen in all musculoskeletal tissue but is most common in bone (overuse pattern resulting in stress fracture), bursal tissues (overuse pattern resulting in bursitis), and tendon (overuse pattern resulting in tendinosis).

### B. Clinical correlation.
The clinical approach to a knee injury (acute/chronic/overuse) depends on four cornerstones:

1. History
2. Physical examination
3. Tests and their interpretations
4. Treatment

## II. Approach to the Acutely Injured Knee

### A. History

1. **Mechanism of injury.** This helps to identify potential structures that may have been damaged by the application of force, either direct (contact) or indirect (noncontact, i.e., a twisting mechanism, deceleration mechanism). If the injury was a contact injury, one should look for external signs at the point of force application and what structures might have been injured as that force continues. For instance, a blow to the anterior tibia might create upper tibial bruising. This force creates a posterior displacement of the tibia on the femur, potentially injuring the posterior cruciate ligament (PCL). Noncontact injuries frequently involve rotatory twisting motion; the lower limb remains fixed as the upper body twists around the knee.

2. **Was a pop heard or felt?** A pop is frequently associated with tearing of a ligament, most commonly the anterior cruciate ligament (ACL), or a bone bruise.

3. **Return to play.** The degree of pain and/or disability cannot be used as a reliable indicator of the seriousness of an injury. However, continued play

with little or no impairment in performance diminishes the likelihood of a serious knee injury.

4. **Has the joint been previously injured?** Frequently, this question uncovers an acute on chronic injury. Two common examples are recurrent patellar dislocation and recurrent subluxation after initial ACL injury.

5. **Joint swelling.** A knee joint effusion or swelling within 12 hours after an injury is, by definition, blood within the joint. An effusion that occurs after 12 hours suggests synovial fluid accumulation due to reactive synovitis, often due to cartilage or meniscus damage.

6. In an acute knee injury, bloody effusion or hemarthrosis is indicative of a significant intraarticular injury.[1] The **differential diagnosis** is as follows:

   a. **Ligament injury.** The ACL and PCL are intraarticular, although the PCL is extrasynovial. Rupture of the ACL is the most common cause of an acute hemarthrosis (70%). Injury to the PCL may result in a hemarthrosis, but the posterior capsule is often injured and blood does not remain within the knee joint. An injury to the deep medial collateral ligament (MCL) may result in interarticular bleeding, but this is less common. The lateral collateral ligament (LCL) is extraarticular, and injury to this ligament does not result in hemarthrosis.

   b. **Peripheral meniscus tear.** The outer, or peripheral, one-third of the meniscus is vascular, and a tear in this region results in a hemarthrosis. Meniscus tears in this zone have the potential for healing and are repairable. Tears in the inner two-thirds of the meniscus are more often associated with synovial irritation, leading to a serous effusion that arises later (e.g., 24 to 48 h) after the initial injury.

   c. **Fractures.** Any fracture that involves the joint surface results in a joint hemarthrosis. In addition to obvious condylar/patellar fractures, occult osteochondral fractures can be a source of hemarthrosis. These can include avulsion fractures of the PCL and ACL (more common in developing adolescents) and fractures secondary to patella dislocation.

   d. **Synovial/capsular tears.** Patella dislocations, even in the absence of fractures, are a source of hemarthrosis as the medial patellofemoral ligament (MPFL) and medial retinacular restraints are torn. Also, a significant contusion without a frank fracture or ligament/meniscus injury can create synovial bleeding. This is often considered a diagnosis of exclusion.

**B. Physical examination**

1. **Inspection**

   a. **Effusion (joint swelling).** An effusion usually indicates an intraarticular injury. The absence of a joint effusion often indicates an extraarticular injury. However, it is possible that a significant intraarticular knee injury results in capsular disruption and extravasation of fluid into the soft tissue.

   b. **Localized bruises and abrasions.** These can be useful to identify the point of application of force in a contact injury. These can indicate the direction of the force that helps to indicate what structures may be injured.

2. **Palpation**

   a. **Careful palpation** of the injured area can often result in an accurate diagnosis. The medial and lateral joint lines can be palpated and may indicate injury to the menisci. Palpation of the LCL and MCL can indicate the presence and anatomic location of the injury. Tenderness along the medial retinaculum or at the adductor tubercle on the femur may indicate a patellar dislocation. Careful palpation of the medial plica and pes anserine tendons can indicate overuse injury to these soft-tissue structures.

**Lateral patella dislocation.** This is associated with tenderness along the patella retinaculum, especially at the medial epicondyle where the MPFL inserts and/or along the superior medial portion of the patella. Note that although the patella dislocates laterally, it is the medial-based structures that are injured and thus are painful when palpated. A large hemarthrosis and "locking up" of the knee with range of motion (ROM) often indicates that an osteochondral lesion may have broken off during the traumatic dislocation.

3. **Range of motion.** ROM is best assessed with the patient in the supine position. It should be compared with the contralateral knee. Lack of symmetrical hyperextension or full flexion compared with the contralateral knee would indicate loss of motion. When the knee has an effusion, the knee's resting position is around 30° of flexion (where potential capsular distention is largest).

   a. A **locked knee** is defined as the inability to obtain full passive motion of the joint secondary to a mechanical block. This does not mean that the knee is in one position, but rather that there is an inability to obtain full motion, typically full extension. Common causes are a displaced meniscus tear or loose body.

   b. A **pseudo-locked knee** is defined as the inability to obtain full ROM secondary to pain or intraarticular knee swelling. A torn meniscus without displacement can result in pain at the limits of flexion and/or extension. If the patient's knee "locks" in full extension and does not want to bend, the most common reason is an injury to the extensor mechanism, resulting in pain when the patient attempts to engage the kneecap in the trochlear groove.

   c. **Active ROM** assesses the integrity of the motor units surrounding a joint. Even in a severely injured knee, the patient typically retains the ability to lift his/her leg. Therefore, active straight leg **raising** and ROM should be assessed. Frequently missed acute knee injuries are disruptions of the extensor mechanism, which include quadriceps tendon and patella tendon injuries. In this instance, the patient will generally be incapable of a straight leg raise, or the leg is raised with a notable extensor lag.

   d. An **extensor lag** is the difference between active and passive ROM and signifies a disrupted extensor mechanism, muscular weakness, nerve injury, or muscular guarding due to pain.

4. **Stability testing.** The *sine qua non* of a ligament disruption is the presence of pathologic joint motion.

   a. **Single-plane instabilities** are the easiest to test. The tibia is moved in relation to the femur in four known planes. The amount of instability is graded according to the American Medical Association (AMA) classification: Grade 1, less than 5 mm of translation or opening; Grade 2, 5 to 10 mm; and Grade 3, more than 10 mm of translation or opening.[2]

      i. **Medial instability** or valgus opening is associated with injury to the MCL.
         The main **clinical motion test** for providing an analysis of the severity of MCL complex injuries is a valgus stress test with the knee flexed at 30°.

      ii. **Lateral instability** or varus opening is associated with injury to the LCL. The main **clinical motion test** for providing an analysis of the severity of LCL is a varus stress on the knee with the knee flexed at 30°. Typically, injuries to the LCL also involve injury to the **posterolateral complex**. Motion tests to determine the amount of injury to the posterolateral complex of the knee are the most complex of all knee examinations.[3]

iii. **Anterior instability** is associated with injury to ACL. The main clinical motion test for an analysis of ACL injuries is the **Lachman test** (Fig. 25-1). This is performed with the knee in approximately 20° of flexion, with the leg in neutral rotation. Grading of displacement of the tibia anteriorly on the femur is along the AMA guidelines. The anterior drawer test (done at 90° of knee flexion), although historically cited, has low reliability in the acute setting.[4,5]

iv. **Posterior instability** is associated with injury to the PCL. The main clinical motion test to detect injuries of the PCL is the **posterior**

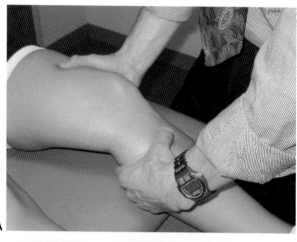

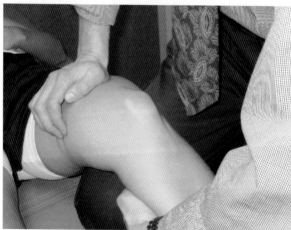

**Figure 25-1.** Lachman examination of the knee: This is a test for deciding the degree of anterior translation of the tibia under the femur. The knee is held firmly in place at 20° to 30° of flexion by the examiner's hand **(A)** or by resting the patient's leg over the examiner's knee **(B)**. With a firm hold of the proximal tibia, the examiner places an upward or anteriorly directed force on the tibia, judging both the distance of translation and the firmness of the endpoint.

**drawer test**. This is performed by placing the knee at 70° to 90° of flexion. The key to this test is accurately assessing the starting point of the tibia, with the medial tibial plateau resting 1 cm anterior to the medial femoral condyle at 90° of knee flexion in a ligamentously intact knee.[6] Failure to test sagittal stability with the tibia in this normal starting point can result in misinterpretation of a posteriorly translated tibia reducing forward into its normal position as a positive anterior drawer test.

v. **Medial or lateral opening** with the knee in full extension indicates injury to the collateral ligament as well as injury to either one or both of the cruciate ligaments.

(**Note:** If you have straight plane pathologic motion of the knee in full extension, that is, knee opens to valgus stressing, it signifies injury to one or both central posts, for example, the cruciate ligaments.)

b. **Rotary instabilities.** This refers to the rotation of the tibia around its vertical or longitudinal axis (Fig. 25-2).

i. **Anterolateral instability** is associated with ACL injury. The test to determine anterolateral instability is the **pivot shift test** or Losee maneuver.[7] This test is performed by beginning with the knee in extension, applying a valgus force with axial load as the examiner brings the knee into flexion. A positive test results in a "clunk" as the tibia reduces from its anteriorly subluxated position. This test is challenging to perform in acutely injured patients due to muscular guarding, but is highly specific for ACL injury.

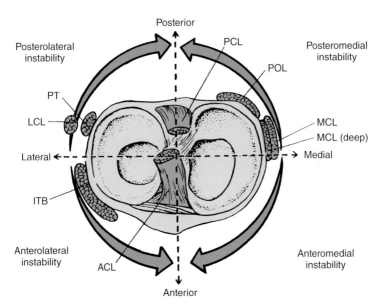

**Figure 25-2.** Rotatory instability of the knee. ACL, anterior cruciate ligament; ITB, iliotibial band; LCL, lateral collateral ligament; MCL, medial collateral ligament; PCL, posterior cruciate ligament; POL, posterior oblique ligament; PT, popliteal tendon. (From Arendt EA. Assessment of the athlete with a painful knee. In: Griffin LY, ed. *Rehabilitation of the Injured Knee*. 2nd ed. Mosby; 1990, with permission.)

    ii. **Posterolateral instability** is associated with injury to the postero-lateral corner (LCL, popliteal fibular ligament, popliteus tendon). Concomitant ACL or PCL injury is common with posterolateral instability. These are frequently associated with PCL and/or ACL injuries. The **dial test** assesses for asymmetry in passive external rotation indicative of posterolateral corner injury. This is best performed by placing the patient prone and having an assistant hold the patient's flexed knees together. Both tibiae are simultaneously passively externally rotated through the feet with the knees flexed to 90°, then at 30° of flexion. A positive test with more than 10° increase in passive external rotation compared to the contralateral side at 30° knee flexion is consistent with a posterolateral corner injury, whereas more than 10° asymmetry with the knees flexed to 90° indicates posterolateral corner and PCL injury.

    iii. **Posteromedial injuries.** These injuries are rare and involve injury to the PCL as well as the MCL.

    iv. **Anteromedial injuries** are associated with ACL/MCL injuries.

  c. **Extensor mechanism instability**

    i. **Apprehension sign.** Passive lateral movement of the patella causing pain and/or quadriceps contraction is suggestive of patellofemoral (PF) subluxation/dislocation. This maneuver is typically done with the leg in full extension, quadriceps muscles relaxed.

    ii. **Straight leg raising against gravity** confirms integrity of the extensor mechanism, including quadriceps tendon, patella, and patella tendon. A "lag" sign represents the difference between passive and active extension of the knee, with an inability to actively maintain full extension against gravity. A lag signifies disruption and/or weakness of the extensor mechanism.

    iii. **Medial/lateral patella restraints.** Stability testing of the PF joint involves assessing the amount of passive patella motion in a medial and lateral direction of the patella. This is typically measured against an imaginary midline of the patella in the resting position (Fig. 25-3). This maneuver tests the static restraints of the medial and lateral extensor retinaculum complex. Any change from the patient's "normal" measured against their uninjured contralateral knee is suggestive of extensor mechanism retinacular injury. Most particularly, an increase in lateral patella translation represents laxity or incompetence of the MPFL and medial retinacular structures associated with lateral patella dislocation.

**C. Imaging**

  1. **Plain radiographs.** The primary utility of plain radiographs is to evaluate the knee for bony injury. In addition, the presence of osteoarthrosis can be determined by looking at the cartilage space at the tibial–femoral articulation as well as the PF articulation.

    a. **Anterior/posterior view.** This radiograph is obtained in the coronal plane. Standing views are preferred because they best assess tibial femoral joint space as well as knee alignment under the influence of the patient's body weight. If pain/swelling limits full extension and/or full weight bearing (WB), supine views are performed but provide less information.

    b. **Lateral view** is obtained in the sagittal plane. The lateral view allows evaluation of the caudad/cephalad position of the patella. Patella alta or increase in the cephalad position of the patella suggests a patellar tendon injury if it is asymmetric. Avulsion fractures of the ACL and PCL can often be identified on a lateral radiograph. Trochlear

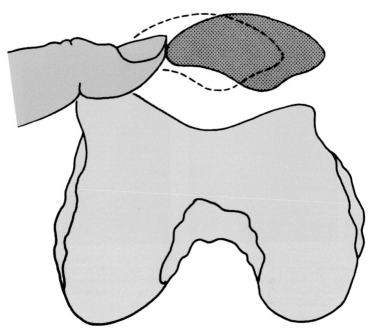

**Figure 25-3.** A quadrant medial "glide." The patella is divided visually into four quadrants. Holding the patella between the examiner's thumb and index finger, the limits of medial and lateral motion are assessed and recorded as "quadrants" of motion. (From Halbrecht JL, Jackson DW. Acute dislocation of the patella. In: Fox JM, Pizzo WD, eds. *The Patellofemoral Joint*. McGraw-Hill; 1993, with permission.)

dysplasia, which predisposes to recurrent patellar instability, is best viewed on the true lateral radiograph and is suggested by the presence of a crossing sign and supratrochlear spur (Fig. 25-4).

c. **Axial view** evaluates the position of the patella in its relationship to the femoral trochlear groove. Often, osteochondral fractures following a patella dislocation can be visualized on this view. Typically, one would see fragmentation of the medial patella facet and/or lateral femoral condyle (LFC) in an acute patella dislocation (Fig. 25-5). Different axial views have been established (Laurin's, Merchant's).[8] The clinician should become familiar with one technique. Axial views are a must for complete evaluation of all acute knee injuries.

d. **Rosenberg or posteroanterior (PA) view** with a flexed knee is taken at 45° of flexion.[9] This view is useful in determining early cartilage space narrowing secondary to osteoarthrosis. This view is not typically obtained for an acute knee injury.

2. **Magnetic resonance imaging (MRI)** of the knee. MRI has its largest application in evaluating meniscus and cruciate ligament injury. The overall accuracy is greater than 90%.[10,11] An MRI is typically an adjunct test in the evaluation of an acutely injured knee. It should be performed only if it will alter the treatment protocol and should be recommended by the physician or physician assistant who will be giving definitive treatment. It should never be used in the absence of a thorough and knowledgeable

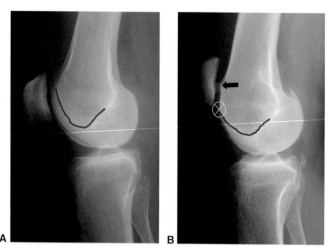

**Figure 25-4.** Lateral knee radiograph demonstrating **(A)** normal trochlear morphology and depth, with the floor of the trochlea delineated by the *red line* and **(B)** trochlear dysplasia with a crossing sign (x) and supratrochlear spur (arrow). Obtaining a high-quality lateral radiograph, with the posterior femoral condyles aligned without overlap, is crucial to appropriate determination of trochlear morphology.

history and physical examination. Posterolateral knee structures are not well visualized in the standard MRI sequences and often require special technique for accurate assessment. In addition, articular cartilage integrity is not well assessed with standard MRI. However, recent techniques (e.g., gadolinium-enhanced, T2 mapping) and the use of more powerful magnets (3 Tesla) improve the accuracy of assessing articular cartilage injury.

3. **Computed tomography (CT)** is useful in the evaluation of complex fractures about the knee. Tibial plateau fractures, certain patella fractures, and unusual femoral condyle fractures are best visualized with CT. Three-dimensional reconstructions can add additional information about complex fractures.

4. **Stress radiographs** can be extremely helpful in evaluating knee ligament injuries. They are often difficult to perform in the acute setting when patients have significant pain. However, in the subacute setting, they are

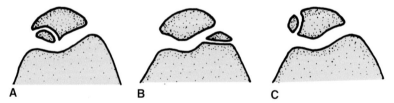

**Figure 25-5.** Three types of fractures associated with patella dislocation. **A:** Osteochondral fracture of the medial patella facet. **B:** Osteochondral fracture of the lateral femoral condylar. **C:** Avulsion fragment of medial patella femoral ligament of medial epicondyle (osseous-nonarticular). (From Halbrecht JL, Jackson DW. Acute dislocation of the patella. In: Fox JM, Pizzo WD, eds. *The Patellofemoral Joint*. McGraw-Hill; 1993, with permission.)

useful to evaluate the degree of fibular collateral ligament (FCL) and MCL injury. In addition, they can help evaluate the degree of PCL injury. In adolescence, stress radiographs may allow the diagnosis of physeal injury.

5. **Tc-MDP bone scans** are most useful in occult infections and to rule out stress fractures. Their usefulness in diagnosing reflex sympathetic dystrophy is variable. This is not a common diagnostic test prescribed for acute knee injuries.

## D. General treatment

1. **Joint aspiration can be used to help evaluate and treat an acute knee injury. Aspiration or removal of a tense knee joint effusion can reduce pain and improve motion.** In addition, the presence of fat droplets within the hemarthrosis can make the diagnosis of an intraarticular fracture. Aspiration also tends to be used in nontraumatic knee joint effusions to evaluate for infection, rheumatologic diseases, and crystalline deposit diseases.

2. **Immobilization/crutches. Knee joint** immobilization with a brace or knee immobilizer is recommended until definitive diagnosis can be made. In addition, protected WB with crutches should be utilized until a definitive diagnosis can be made. Care should be taken to avoid prolonged knee joint immobilization because this can result in muscle atrophy and knee joint adhesions and stiffness.

3. **Reduction of swelling.** Strategies to reduce swelling should be included in the initial treatment recommendation. These include activity reduction; ice; gentle, passive, or active assisted range of knee motion; elevation; and compression.

4. **Repeat examination** is helpful in establishing a more firm diagnosis, especially when pain, swelling, and/or apprehension limit the initial examination.

5. **Medication.** Tylenol should be the first-line medication to relieve pain in acute knee injuries. Nonsteroidal anti-inflammatory drugs (NSAIDs) are commonly used to control pain and reduce swelling. However, NSAIDs do alter platelet function and may increase bleeding at the site of injury. In addition, NSAIDs may slow tissue healing by interfering with the normal inflammatory process. It is recommended that this class of medication be used judiciously and for short periods only.

## III. Specific Acute Knee Injuries

### A. Fractures of the patella

1. **Anatomic considerations.** The patella is a sesamoid bone that is contained within the extensor mechanism. Its main function is to provide a lever arm for superior mechanical functioning of the extensor mechanism and to help stabilize the limb in deceleration. The strong quadriceps muscle tendon complex attaches to the superior pole of the patella and the stout patellar ligament connects the inferior pole of the patella to the anterior tibia.

2. Common types of **fractures**

   a. **Transverse fractures**, with or without comminution. These can be caused by direct or indirect trauma. They are frequently associated with disruption of the extensor mechanism and when displaced need to be surgically stabilized in order to regain the mechanical function of the extensor mechanism.

   **Vertical fractures** of the patella are frequently because of a direct injury; infrequently, they represent an overuse injury of the patella. When they are associated with no or minimal displacement, they do not constitute a disruption of the extensor mechanism and can be treated nonoperatively. Vertical patella fractures may be subtle and missed on anteroposterior (AP) and lateral radiographs. A merchant view radiograph may be the only view a vertical fracture is seen. A bipartite patella is an unfused ossification center at the superior lateral patella and can be confused with a vertical patella fracture.

b. **Chip fractures** of the medial border are commonly seen with a patella dislocation; infrequently, they can be associated with direct trauma. This variety will be more thoroughly discussed under patella dislocation.

3. **Treatment**

a. **Nondisplaced or minimally displaced fractures** may be treated symptomatically without surgery. However, they must be protected from further damage. Immobilization of the knee in extension with an immobilizer for 2 to 4 weeks is sufficient with WB as tolerated. Quadriceps isometric exercises can be performed during this time. Gentle, passive ROM as per the patient's comfort level is recommended.

b. **Displaced fractures** involving the articular surface or compromising the extensor mechanism should be treated with open reduction and internal fixation. A tension band wire technique through cannulated lag screws is the treatment of choice.[12]

c. **Comminuted fractures** usually require surgical treatment. A partial patellectomy is necessary if reduction and internal fixation of the fragments are not possible. If more than half of the patella remain intact, the comminuted pieces may be excised, and the tendon sutured just above the subchondral bone into the remaining pole of the patella. Occasionally, fragments are large enough to fix with tension band wiring or 2.7-mm cortical lag screws.[12]

d. **Osteochondral fractures often require** arthroscopy for evaluation of the osteochondral fragment. These injuries are usually the result of a patellar dislocation. Large osteochondral fragments with viable bone should be fixed with careful reduction and internal fixation. Cartilage injuries are ominous for the future health of the joint; their treatment is beyond the scope of this text.[13,14]

e. **Postoperative treatment** must be individualized according to the type of fracture and the security of the repair. Most knees are initially placed in a compressive dressing with a posterior splint or knee immobilizer. If rigid internal fixation is achieved and the patient is trustworthy, early protective passive ROM is initiated, progressing to active motion. Typically, 6 weeks of some form of immobilization is necessary for healing of the fracture(s). Quadriceps muscle strengthening exercises, within the limits of the allowed knee motion, should be encouraged throughout this time.

f. The **prognosis** of patella fractures depends on the ability to reestablish a congruent articular surface as well as a well-functioning extensor mechanism. If articular damage is minimal and good extensor mechanism strength can be restored, the prognosis for patella fractures is excellent.

B. **Patellofemoral dislocations**

1. **Anatomic considerations.** The MPFL is the main patella stabilizer against lateral patellar dislocation.[15] Lateral patella dislocations are associated with MPFL disruption, but to date, there is no evidence that laxity of this ligament is a risk factor for PF dislocation. There are anatomic risk factors for lateral PF dislocation, including patella alta, increased quadriceps vector, and trochlear dysplasia.[16]

2. **Mechanism of injury.** This injury can result from a direct blow but is more commonly associated with a noncontact twisting injury involving

an externally rotated tibia combined with a forceful quadriceps contraction. The patella is dislocated laterally, thus disrupting the MPFL and medial retinaculum. Spontaneous reduction frequently occurs when the patient instinctively tries to straighten his/her leg. When the patella relocates, osteochondral injury can occur as the medial patella facet abuts the LFC. These two areas, in particular, should be scrutinized for osteochondral damage (Fig. 25-5).

**Medial** patellar dislocations are rare in knees that have not had previous surgery. It is most often associated with iatrogenic causes, in particular an overzealous lateral retinacular release.[17]

3. **Physical examination.** The patient will invariably have medial retinacular tenderness, especially at the medial femoral condylar region. If an attempt is made to displace the patella laterally, the patient resists this by reporting pain and/or contracting their quadriceps muscle, thus limiting patella excursion (patella apprehension test). A straight leg raise test should be attempted. This may result in patient discomfort but should be possible with only a minimal extensor lag (the difference between passive and active extension).

**In the acute setting, passive patella mobility is hard to judge secondary to pain.** In the subacute or chronic setting, increased passive patella lateral translation is a necessary component to make the diagnosis of lateral patella dislocation by physical examination.

4. **Radiographs.** AP lateral and *axial* view radiographs are necessary for a complete evaluation of PF dislocations. If the patient is seen prior to spontaneous reduction of the patella, axial views will reveal the dislocated patella. Once reduced, the axial view may reveal residual tilt and/or subluxation as well as the presence of osteochondral fragmentation. Axial views taken in lower degrees of flexion (Laurin's 20° views[18] or Merchant's 30° views)[19] will be more likely to show minor degrees of continued increased lateral translation.

5. **Treatment**
   a. If the patella **remains dislocated**, a reduction should be performed without delay to relieve pain. Achieve intravenous analgesia with morphine sulfate and a hypnotic before reduction is attempted. Once the patient's muscles are relaxed, the knee is placed in full extension, and the patella is reduced into place by a gentle, medially directed pressure. Slight elevation of the medial border of the patella during this maneuver is ideal. On occasion, the kneecap can be "trapped" by the condyle, and reduction can be difficult. After appropriate prep of the skin, grabbing the kneecap with a large towel clip and using it to gently unlever the kneecap can be a useful maneuver for difficult reductions. Owing to large hematomas frequently associated with patella dislocations, and the fact that there is a large retinacular tear medially, the use of local intraarticular anesthetic is not particularly helpful for the reduction. General or regional block anesthetic is rarely required.
   b. If a large associated **hemarthrosis** is present, aspiration of the knee joint is suggested for pain relief.
   c. There is no consensus in **surgical treatment** for patellar dislocations. It is recommended that arthroscopy with removal or repair be undertaken in patients with osteochondral fractures. It is unclear whether concomitant surgical repair of the injured medial retinacular structures is necessary in this situation.[20,21]
   d. When **acute surgical repair** is performed, it is directed at the medial retinacular structures with repair or reconstruction of the MPFL. The results of acute repair of the MPFL in primary patella dislocation

have not shown improved results over nonoperative management.[22] Whether associated risk factors such as patella alta should be corrected at the time of surgery continues to be debated.

    e. If there is no evidence of a fracture or continued radiographic evidence of increased lateral translation and/ortilt, **nonoperative treatment** can be elected. Nonsurgical treatment is directed at providing an environment where the patella does not dislocate, and restoring joint motion and strength. There is agreement on the goals of such treatment; however, there is no consensus on the degree of knee flexion when immobilized, or length of knee immobilization.[23] One accepted protocol is for the patient to be treated initially with crutches and a knee sleeve, encouraging gentle motion and WB ambulation. In the presence of a significant hemarthrosis, a compression dressing and immobilization in extension is appropriate until early motion and WB are comfortable. The patient increases WB and independent knee motion as their knee pain and strength allow. The knee sleeve is used for 4 to 6 weeks, whereas an aggressive strengthening program is pursued, directed at CORE and those muscles that control limb rotation, in addition to the quadriceps muscles. Typically, 6 weeks of monitored activities, keeping the knee out of pivoting and twisting activities, is recommended. The most important thing to accomplish in the first 6 weeks postinjury is return of normal quadriceps strength. Hamstring stretching and vastus medialis oblique (VMO) muscle strengthening are the primary focus of physical therapy for rehabbing lateral patella instability return to full functional activities should be based on functional strength rather than a specific period from the original injury.[24]

6. **Complications**

    a. **Recurrent dislocation.** The main physical examination feature associated with recurrent dislocation is continued quadriceps weakness. Recurrent dislocators who have not successfully accomplished strength comparable with their other side will likely need surgical reconstruction to stabilize their patella and often have risk factors of patella alta and/or trochlear dysplasia. Recurrent patella dislocations are frequently associated with recurrent effusions at the time that the patient dislocates; a history that "my knee gives out" following an initial patella dislocation may represent quad weakness and not necessarily a redislocation.

    b. **Degenerative joint changes** of the PF joint may occur **when** significant cartilage trauma is present from the initial/recurrent patella dislocation.

C. **Meniscus injuries**

1. **Anatomic concerns.** The menisci are C-shaped structures consisting of type I collagen that rests on the medial and lateral tibial plateau. The primary function of the meniscus is to distribute force and protect the articular cartilage. In addition, the medial meniscus provides stability to the knee. This is particularly important when the ACL has been compromised.

2. **History**

    a. **Mechanism of injury.** Most isolated injuries of the meniscus are secondary to rotatory stress on a WB knee. In young patients, this is usually associated with a traumatic event. However, in older patients, the meniscus may tear with repetitive activities of daily living.

    b. Patients often complain of sharp pain along the medial or lateral joint line. They may also complain of locking or catching.

3. **Physical examination**[25]
   a. Joint line tenderness is typically present along the medial (medial meniscus tear) or lateral (lateral meniscus tear) joint lines. This joint line pain increases with attempts at full extension or full flexion.
   b. The **McMurray test**. An audible, palpable, and often painful clunk is produced when the knee is extended from the full flexed position, while the tibia is forcefully externally rotated (medial meniscus) or internally rotated (lateral meniscus). This sign is associated with a torn meniscus. Crepitus or pain along the joint line, even in the absence of an audible clunk, is also suggestive of a meniscus tear. Although this test is classically discussed in most text books, the reliability is low.[26]
   c. Typically, the normal knee has less than 15 mL of fluid and is not detectable on physical examination. Small amounts of fluid can be detected by "milking" the suprapatellar pouch, looking for a fluid wave as one tries to push the fluid from the lateral side of the knee to the medial side of the knee. This maneuver is the best way to detect small amounts of swelling. The presence of an **effusion** often limits complete ROM and can result in pain with attempts at full extension or full flexion.

4. **Radiographs**
   a. Although a meniscus tear is not visible on **plain radiographs, these studies should be obtained on patients with suspected meniscal pathology**. The presence of osteoarthrosis on X-ray evaluation is an important factor to consider when developing a treatment plan for a meniscal tear.

5. **MRI** is frequently performed to confirm the presence of a meniscus tear. It has a high accuracy rate in diagnosing meniscus tears (>93%).[10,11]

6. **Treatment**
   a. The surgical treatment of an **isolated meniscus tear** depends on the location and morphology of the tear. The outer one-third of the meniscus (red-red zone) has a vascular supply and is amenable to repair. The central one-third of the meniscus (red-white zone) has a less robust blood supply, but studies have demonstrated acceptable healing rates as compared to the inner third (white-white zone), which is not typically appropriate for repair due to avascularity and low healing potential.[27] Tears of the inner third are best treated with partial meniscectomy in most patients.
   b. There are multiple meniscal repair techniques with generally similar healing rates. Optimal repair technique is decided by the surgeon based on tear location, morphology, and size.
   c. **Inside-out meniscus repair** is the gold-standard technique for meniscal repair and involves making an open incision to allow retraction and protection of adjacent neurovascular structures. Sutures are then passed from the arthroscopic portals through the meniscus and capsule, then retrieved through the open incision by an assistant and tied down directly on top of the joint capsule.
   d. **All-inside meniscus repair** utilizes special devices that allow repair of the meniscus through the arthroscopic incisions with no requirement for an open approach. This technique improves ease and speed of repair and eliminates the morbidity of an open incision, but does typically carry a higher financial burden. There does also exist a small potential for neurovascular penetrative injury, so careful attention should be paid to trajectory of the devices relative to expected neurovascular bundle location.

e. **Outside-in meniscus repair** is less commonly utilized, but involves creating a longitudinal incision and passing sutures from this incision into the joint, retrieving the sutures through the arthroscopic portals. This is generally most useful for anterior horn meniscal tears, which have a difficult trajectory for other repair techniques.

f. **Transosseous pull-out suture repair** is used for repair of meniscal root avulsions. The meniscus root is reduced to its anatomic bony insertion point by passing sutures through the meniscus and pulling these through a transosseous tunnel spanning from the root attachment point out through the anterior tibia.[28]

g. A **symptomatic meniscus tear in the nonrepairable zone** and/or a complex meniscus tear that persists despite conservative management should be arthroscopically debrided. However, in the older age group, consideration must be given to the fact that the symptoms may be the result of osteoarthritis and cartilage wear and not from the meniscal tear.[28,29]

h. In the **older age group**, where one suspects a degenerative meniscus tear, the meniscus tear is a reflection of generalized early arthritis of the knee joint. This "tear" should be treated symptomatically according to the patient and physician's discussion. The presence of a degenerative meniscus tear on MRI is not an indication to operate. If the symptoms associated with a degenerative meniscus tear can be resolved with rest, relative rest, and/or medication, surgical treatment may not be necessary.[30]

**D. Ligamentous injuries** of the knee

1. **Anatomic considerations.** The ACL resists anterior translation of the tibia relative to the femur. In addition, the ACL resists rotation of the tibia on the femur. The ligament has two distinct bundles: the anteromedial that controls anterior translation and the posterolateral that primarily controls rotation. The PCL functions to resist posterior translation of the tibia on the femur. This ligament also has two bundles: the anterolateral that functions in more flexion and the posteromedial that functions in more extension. The LCL or FCL limits varus opening and is part of the posterolateral complex. The MCL or tibial collateral ligament (TCL) has a superficial and a deep component. The deep component is essentially a thickening of the joint capsule, with the superficial component providing a greater degree of varus stability.

2. **Mechanism of injury**

   a. **Ligamentous injuries** can be the result of a direct or indirect trauma. Indirect trauma frequently occurs when the body rotates around a relatively fixed foot/leg. Direct injuries are a consequence of force directed to the knee or limb. Typically, the ligament opposite to the area of contact is the ligament that is the most vulnerable. For instance, a blow to the lateral side of the knee usually results in injury to the MCL.

   b. As mentioned above, MCL injuries result from a valgus stress to the knee. In addition, the MCL can be injured along with the ACL or PCL in higher energy mechanisms. In an **isolated tear of the MCL**, palpable discomfort can be detected anywhere along the ligament from its origin on the medial femoral condyle to its insertion on the tibia (approximately three finger breadths below the joint line). The deep capsular ligament is a thickening at the joint line. Medial joint line tenderness is also associated with medial meniscal injuries. However, different from a meniscal injury, an MCL injury would create pain to stressing the knee in a valgus direction, as well as externally rotating the leg with the knee flexed. Although attached to the medial meniscus, the incidence of an in-substance medical meniscus tears in an isolated tear of the MCL is low.[31]

c. **Isolated injuries of the LCL** are rare and occur with varus stress. These seem to be more prevalent in wrestling. The LCL is more frequently injured as part of a complex ligamentous injury pattern involving the ACL and/or the PCL. These injuries tend to be associated with a high-energy mechanism and may result in peroneal nerve injury. These injuries require urgent evaluation by an orthopaedic surgeon.

d. **Isolated tears of the PCL** are most commonly caused by a direct posterior blow to the proximal tibia. This occurs when the knee strikes the dashboard in a motor vehicle crash or when a flexed knee strikes the ground in a collision sport, such as football. Isolated PCL tears can also occur from a hyperextension mechanism; however, this mechanism usually results in additional injury to the medial or lateral structures.

e. **Isolated ACL injuries** occur either through noncontact deceleration mechanisms or via direct contact. Noncontact injuries are much more common. Risk factors for noncontact ACL injuries have been studied intensely.[32] Deficits in neuromuscular control have been implicated as a primary cause of noncontact ACL injuries, particularly in female athletes. Jump-landing training may improve this control and prevent injury.[33,34]

3. **Physical examination.** The *sine qua non* of a knee ligament injury is pathologic joint motion. The specific ligament tests were discussed previously.

a. An acute knee examination should include **all major ligamentous structures** within the knee. Significant AP translation (>10 mm) with the drawer or Lachman test may suggest an injury to both the ACL and the PCL.

4. **Treatment**

a. **Isolated tears** of ligamentous injuries

i. **MCL.** Most isolated tears of the MCL can be treated nonoperatively.[31] Grade 3 injuries require protective bracing and early ROM. Complete recovery after isolated MCL injuries is expected. Proximal injuries tend to heal more reliably than distal MCL injuries. For complete tears, progressive WB on crutches, in a brace-limiting valgus stress for 4 to 6 weeks, is recommended for the best outcome of restored joint stability. In the absence of a complete tear of the MCL, one can bear weight as pain and motion permits.

ii. **Isolated PCL injuries** are usually Grade 1 or Grade 2 injuries and can be treated nonoperatively. In the rehabilitation process, special emphasis on quad strength is important to maintain a muscular support to limit posterior displacement of the tibia.

iii. **Isolated tears of the ACL** are prone to subluxation events when jumping and pivoting activities are performed. In young active patients, or middle-aged patients who have a high demand job or recreational aspirations, ACL reconstruction is typically advised. The goal of ACL reconstruction is to prevent future subluxation events that can be associated with meniscus and/or articular cartilage damage.

iv. **Multiligamentous knee injuries** range from relatively common ACL and MCL injuries to much more complex knee dislocations. The MCL will often heal spontaneously when associated with ACL reconstruction. Subsequent ACL reconstruction is all that is required. MCL injuries associated with PCL tears are more controversial. Surgical reconstruction of both ligaments is frequently required. ACL or PCL injuries associated with an LCL injury usually require surgical reconstruction of all involved ligaments.

**E.** Knee dislocations

1. **Evaluation and treatment.** Knee dislocations are relatively uncommon and are often associated with high-energy mechanism of injury. Immediate reduction is required. A reduction under anesthesia is sometimes necessary. Careful neurovascular evaluation is required following reduction of a knee dislocation.[35]

   The preferred test is to obtain ankle–brachial indices (ABIs). If the ABIs are asymmetric, arteriography should be performed. Careful monitoring for compartment syndrome is essential, and prophylactic fasciotomy may be necessary. An external fixator may be required to stabilize the knee joint in cases of severe instability or when a vascular repair is required.

2. Ligament **reconstruction following knee dislocation is a complex decision-making process.**[36]

   The condition of the skin and soft tissues, the presence of bony fractures, and the status of all involved ligaments must be taken into account to develop a treatment plan.[37]

   In general, ACL and PCL injuries associated with lateral-sided injuries are best reconstructed within 6 weeks of injury. LCL reconstruction is preferred over a direct repair. Injuries involving the MCL are more controversial. It is often advisable to achieve full ROM prior to reconstructing the ACL, PCL, and MCL.

3. **Extensor mechanism disruptions**

   a. **Anatomic considerations.** The extensor mechanism consists of the quadriceps muscle complex, quadriceps tendon, patella, patella tendon, and patella tendon insertion into the tibial tubercle. Disruption of the extensor mechanism along any one of its parts can result in failure of the patient to perform a straight leg–raising effort. A partial tear frequently results in the patient's ability to lift his/her leg, but with a considerable lag (difference between passive and active extension of the leg).

   b. **Clinical considerations**

      i. A **quadriceps tendon disruption** is difficult to assess on physical examination unless one requests a straight leg–raising effort by the patient. Quadriceps tendon ruptures are a frequently missed after acute knee injury. A routine knee MRI does not always scan proximal enough to accurately diagnose this injury; therefore, this must be requested when ordering an MRI.

      ii. **Patella tendon disruptions** are often associated with an indirect trauma consisting of a forceful quadriceps contraction against a relatively fixed lower limb. These can be subtle injuries.

         If the rupture is below the inferior border of the patella (i.e., in the patella tendon or at the tibial tubercle), patella alta would be present and best seen on lateral knee X-rays.

      iii. **Extensor mechanism disruptions,** especially quadriceps ruptures, commonly occur in patients with systemic illness such as diabetes or renal failure, or with the use of exogenous steroids (prednisone or anabolic steroids). Cortical steroid injections for treatment of patella tendinosis have been associated with an increased incidence of rupture.

   c. **Treatment.** The goal of treatment is to restore a functioning extensor mechanism to the knee. This is **best** accomplished surgically.

**IV. Special Concerns in the Growing Adolescent**

**A. Physeal injuries.** Acute knee trauma in a growing adolescent can result in injury to the physis (growth plate).

1. A **distal femur physeal injury** can be confused with an MCL injury. This is particularly true if the physeal injury is nondisplaced. Stress radiographs

should be performed if there is any suspicion for a physeal injury. Surgical reduction and stabilization for unstable physeal injuries are required. Stable (nondisplaced) injuries may be treated nonoperatively.[38]

2. The **tibial apophysis** can avulse in the adolescent with closing growth plates. The tibial growth plate fuses from posterior to anterior, and an avulsion of the tibial tubercle frequently involves an intraarticular fracture. This injury is associated with a strong quadriceps contraction, such as landing from a jump. Radiographs may reveal patellar alta as well as the displaced tibial tubercle. Surgical reduction and fixation are preferred for displaced injuries.

**B. Ligament avulsion.** Cruciate ligament avulsions can occur in the growing adolescent. Tibial eminence avulsions at the insertion of the ACL are the most common. Displaced injuries require surgical reduction and fixation. Associated stretch injury to the ligament may result in residual laxity.

## V. Overuse Syndromes

**A. Definition.** Repetitive submaximal or subclinical trauma that results in macroscopic and/or microscopic damage to a tissue's structural unit can result in pain and/or dysfunction. Although clinicians refer to it as an "itis," an inflammatory response is not seen histologically. It is thought that damage to a tissue's structural unit and/or blood supply is a frequent cause of overuse injuries.

The most common form of overuse injury is from an endogenous source, that being, mechanical circumstances in which the musculoskeletal tissue is subjected to greater tensile force or stress than the tissue can effectively absorb.

**B. History.** Overuse injuries are characterized by the absence of an acute injury, or at least no injury significant enough to explain the current clinical situation. The most important feature to look for in the patient's history is a "change" in functional demand. A transitional athlete/worker, defined as a person with a change in his/her internal or external environment, is at high risk for development of overuse injuries. These include the following:

1. Change in intensity of repetitive activity (distance/time)
2. Change in frequency or duration of repetitive activity
3. Changes in equipment (footwear/surface changes, including material composition and/or slope)
4. Changes in competitive climate/work climate/activity level
5. Changes in weather
6. Changes in lifestyle (puberty, aging, significant weight gain, and, for women, pregnancy and menopause)

**C. Physical examination**

1. **Inspection**

   a. **Alignment** of the limb is a must in evaluating any overuse injury of the lower extremity. This includes tilt of the pelvis, rotation of the femur, varus or valgus alignment of the knee, and pronation or supination at the foot. Any change in "normal alignment" can cause tissue overload anywhere along the kinetic chain. Some limb alignment features are constitutional and cannot be changed short of surgery; others can be modified. The two most common forms of modification are as follows:

      i. An **orthotic** may change the position of a flexible foot and thus can affect the entire kinematic chain. Particularly, a flexible pronated foot can be restored to normal alignment with the use of an orthotic.

      ii. An anteriorly tilted pelvis is associated with **increased internal femoral rotation** and functional **knee valgus**. This can frequently be altered by appropriate hip abductor and extensor strengthening exercises.[39]

   b. **Redness or warmth** is not common in overuse injuries but may indicate the presence of an injured bursa or tendon.

    c. **Joint effusion** is not common in overuse injuries. It indicates an intraarticular source of pathology.

    d. **Investigation tests**

      i. **Strength tests.** These can include the following:

        (a) **Weakness** compared with the contralateral limb

        (b) **Concentric** (muscle shortens while contracting) muscle strength versus eccentric (muscle lengthens while contracting) muscle strength in same muscle group

        (c) **Agonist** (joint motion in one plane due to muscle contraction) versus antagonist (the muscle group opposing or resisting joint motion caused by agonist muscle) strength in same limb (i.e., quad to hamstring strength)

        (d) **Absolute strength** and **peak torque** to body weight ratio compared with population norms

        (e) **Endurance strength** with a measure of muscle fatigability

      ii. Evaluation of **flexibility**, especially in key muscle groups, including quadriceps, hamstring, hip flexors, and Achilles tendon

**D. Radiographs**

  1. **Plain radiographs** are infrequently necessary for evaluation of overuse injuries. Radiographic views of the PF joint, in particular, axial views, may be helpful to assess patella position. Standing knee views show arthritic changes, including bone spurs and joint space narrowing.

  2. **MRI.** The main advantage of an MRI is its ability to view intraarticular versus extraarticular pathology. Routine use of an MRI to diagnose overuse injuries is not advantageous. Although significant tendinosis and bursal edema can be visualized by MRI, these entities tend to also be identifiable on clinical examination.

**E. Blood work/Knee aspiration**

  1. When there is a knee effusion that arises spontaneously or is associated with other complaints (e.g., rash or fatigue), it is important to consider systemic diseases. Evaluate for **systemic disease**, including collagen vascular disease and Lyme's disease.

    These patients require laboratory evaluation, including complete blood count with differential, erythrocyte sedimentation rate, C-reactive protein, rheumatoid factor, fluorescent antinuclear antibody test, and Lyme titer.

    When there is a knee effusion without trauma, aspiration is done to rule out infection versus inflammatory conditions; the fluid should be sent for culture, cell count, and crystalline analysis.

**F. Treatment**

  1. **Reduce tissue irritation and pain with:**

    a. **Analgesic** non-narcotic medications (NSAIDs, acetaminophen)

    b. **Physical therapy** modalities (ultrasound, E-stim, massage) as well as strengthening and gait training

    c. **Rest or relative rest** of the injured part (reduce activities, substitute activities, and protect the injured part)

    d. **Ice**

    e. **Elevation** and **compression** if swelling is present

  2. **Correct anatomic problems** when possible (patella sleeves, orthotics, braces, taping, rarely surgery)

  3. **Correct biomechanical errors** when possible (training sequence, sport style and form, strengthening and stretching of musculoskeletal units, evaluation of workplace station)

  4. **Correct environmental concerns** when possible (new shoes, change to a more absorbent surface, adequate clothing)

G. **Sports-specific rehabilitation**
   1. **Recovery** of strength
      a. **Closed chain exercises** of the lower extremity are those exercises where the foot is supported or planted during the exercise, thus "closing the loop." Leg press or stand-up exercises such as partial squats are examples of closed chain lower leg exercises. For **lower extremity activities**, closed chained techniques are more functional and can obtain comparable gains in quadriceps strength with less overuse of the PF joint.[39]
      b. **Concentric/eccentric** muscle strength. **Concentric** muscle contractions occur when a muscle shortens as it contracts. In an eccentric contraction, the muscle lengthens as contraction occurs.

      **Eccentric** strengthening has long been favored for recovery of strength in the treatment of tendinosis. For the PF joint, eccentric muscle activity is an important part of functional use of the joint. Eccentric strength is the main decelerator of the body, an important function of the quadriceps complex.

H. **The physician.** The **physician's** role in managing overuse injuries is to make the appropriate diagnosis, recommend treatment, and educate the patient. Patient education is the best treatment for the prevention of future overuse injuries.

I. **The patient.** The patient's role is to understand the causative **factors** in the injury and the progression from injury to wellness. This includes activity modifications and their role in modifying their activities. The patient needs to implement a paced return to full activities.

VI. **Specific Overuse Injuries about the Knee**
   A. **Patellar tendinosis**
      1. Patellar tendinosis is a common overuse injury that more typically affects the proximal attachment of the patella ligament to the inferior pole of the patella, but can also affect the distal end of the tendon. Patellar tendinosis is also called jumper's knee because it frequently occurs in athletes who require repetitive eccentric quadriceps contractions (landing from a jump). In addition, athletes who participate in frequent heavy weight training commonly develop patellar tendinosis.
      2. The cause of **patellar tendinosis** is generally considered to be chronic stress overloading, resulting in microscopic tears of the tendon with incomplete healing.
      3. **Treatment** is most commonly nonoperative. In addition to the general scheme of treatment of overuse syndromes outlined previously, the primary treatment emphasizes maximizing quad strength and knee joint flexibility, reducing repetitive eccentric quadriceps contraction exercises, and readding them in a paced manner.[40]

         An ultrasound can be used to define the area of the tendon affected by chronic tearing and subsequent degeneration, and this area can be injected with various nonsteroid substances.[41]

         Infrequently, surgery is necessary for the patient with recalcitrant disease.[42]
      4. **Iliotibial band syndrome**
         a. **Iliotibial band (ITB) syndrome (also known as ITB tendinosis)** is caused by excessive friction between the ITB and the distal LFC. The ITB functions as a weak extender of the knee in near full extension, and a more powerful knee flexor after 30° of knee flexion. The ITB is most stretched over the LFC at 30° of knee flexion. This condition is common in runners and cyclists.

b. **Anatomic factors** have been implicated in ITB syndrome and include excessive foot pronation, genu varum at the knee, tight lateral patella retinacular structures, and an anterior tipped pelvis. Treatment is directed at modification of the initiating causative factors and reducing the excessive friction. Stretching of the ITB, treating foot pronation with an orthotic, treating a tight lateral patella retinaculum with manual therapy, and repositioning of an anterior tilted pelvis all can be useful interventions when the patient has these physical examination features.

## B. Patellofemoral pain syndrome

1. **Definition.** PF pain syndrome is used to describe a constellation of symptoms that is related to the PF joint. Typically, this type of pain is considered an overuse syndrome, although the exact etiology and nature of pain continues to be poorly understood. PF pain syndrome is that pain which originates in the anterior knee structures, in the absence of an identifiable acute injury (blunt trauma, dislocating or subluxating patella).

   *Chondromalacia patella* (CMP) is a term often used to describe anterior knee pain, although the use of this term to describe clinical symptoms is not appropriate. It should be used only to describe the pathologic entity of cartilage softening on the underneath side of the kneecap. Typically, this could only be diagnosed by surgical observation or MRI. The presence of cartilage softening does not always result in the clinical symptom of pain.

   **Preexisting conditions.** Anatomic factors that can predispose a patient to PF pain can include flexibility deficits of the limb, malalignment of the lower limbs including excessive femoral anteversion, high Q-angle, rotation variations of the tibia, genu valgum at the knee, hindfoot valgus, and pes planus. **Kneecap malalignment**, both static and functional, has been implicated in the etiology of PF pain. However, there are a few population-based studies to support the "malalignment theory kneecap pain." Any one abnormality may be trivial as a single entity. However, in combination with other anatomic variables and associated with overtraining and overuse, they frequently can lead to overuse injury.

   The role of **malalignment** and the etiology of PF pain continue to be debated. Radiographic imaging studies can reveal a patella that is malaligned within the trochlear groove, as evidenced by a patella excessive lateral patella tilt and/or translation. Some malalignment syndromes of the patella are residual from previous subluxating or dislocating events. However, other malalignment syndromes can be present in the absence of an acute event and frequently are similar in both knees of the same person. It is felt that patella malalignment, when constitutional in a person, can become an overuse syndrome more readily and become a painful problem. In patients who have pain and swelling as their primary presenting symptoms, evaluation of their cartilage integrity is advised, typically with an MRI. A series of axial CT scans taken in various degrees of flexion and extension is a valuable study to quantify abnormal patellar tracking and osseous malalignment. This CT series, often referred as a Fulkerson study, measures the lateral offset of the tibial tuberosity from the deepest point in the trochlear groove. Increased lateral offset of the tibial tubercle contributes to lateral instability and is an indication for an anterior medialization (AMZ) procedure.[43]

2. **Clinical presentation.** The most common clinical presentation of a PF pain syndrome patient is pain on the anterior aspect of the knee that is aggravated by prolonged sitting and stair climbing. Because the retinacular structures of the patella extend both medially and laterally from the patella, pain can also be associated with either medial- or lateral-sided

knee pain; therefore, it can create a very confusing clinical presentation. It is infrequently associated with swelling. Giving-way episodes can be reported; typically, the giving-way episode is with straight-ahead activities or stair climbing, when one tries to engage the quad and the quad "fatigues." This should not be confused with giving-way episodes associated with ligamentous instability, which typically occur with planting, pivoting, or jumping activities. Patients can also present with catching or clicking phenomena. This can occur because of irritation of the kneecap as it tracks in the trochlear groove. Another common patient complaint is that the knee "locks." If the knee "locks" in full extension, this is a manifestation of PF pain. The patient does not want to engage the knee cap in the groove because of pain and, therefore, keeps his/her leg straight. If the knee is locked secondary to a loose body or torn meniscus, it is always locked in some degree of flexion.

3. **Treatment.** Nonsurgical treatment is the cornerstone for most PF pain disorders. The primary goal of PF rehabilitation is to reduce the symptoms of pain. This is done by a combination of physical therapy exercises and modalities, improving quadriceps strength, and endurance. Other tools such as orthotics, knee sleeves, and McConnell taping can be used.[44] Pelvic muscle strength, especially hip abductor and hip extensor strength, is essential for rotational control of the limb.[39,45]

**C. Pes anserinus bursitis**

1. **Definition.** The "pes" tendons are terminal insertions of three long thigh muscles, one from each muscle group. These tendons come together to insert on the anteromedial aspect of the proximal tibia, between the tibial tubercle and the distal (tibial) attachment of the medial (tibial) collateral ligament. The three tendons are sartorius (femoral innervation), gracilis (obturator innervation), and semitendinosus (sciatic innervation). They are powerful internal rotators of the leg (tibia) and also aide in knee flexion.

2. **Clinical presentation.** The patient will present with soreness just below the medial knee, which can be reproduced by direct palpation or resisted internal rotation of the leg. In middle age, it can represent a **referred** pain pattern from the knee due to medial knee arthritis.

3. **Treatment.** In addition to the rest, ice, compression, and **elevation** (RICE) principle and physical therapy with modalities of stretching and strengthening, a steroid injection at the bursa site can be helpful.

**VII. Specific Concerns of Overuse Injuries in the Adolescent Athlete**

**A. Osteochondritis dissecans**

1. **Definition.** Osteochondritis dissecans (OCD) is injury to the subchondral bone that most often begins in the skeletally immature athlete. Although the etiology of this subchondral bony injury is unknown, the most common theory is repetitive stress loading of the bone. Other commonly accepted theories include abnormal ossification within the epiphysis, ischemia, or endocrine abnormalities. Approximately 40% of patients with OCD have a history of prior knee trauma. The medial condyle is involved 85% of the time with less frequent involvement of the LFC, patella, and trochlear. Fifty percent of loose bodies in the knee are associated with OCD.[46,47]

2. **Natural history.** Most OCD lesions diagnosed in the skeletally immature knee will heal spontaneously with activity modification. Lesions that have not healed by physeal closure will usually persist into adulthood. These lesions may occasionally separate away from the health bone and form a loose body. Juvenile OCD lesions can be treated nonsurgically with activity modifications. The use of cast immobilization is controversial. The use

of crutches or an unloader brace may be helpful in aiding the resolution of juvenile OCD lesion. Failure of the lesion to heal within 6 months is an indication for surgical intervention. Arthroscopic drilling with or without internal fixation has been shown to provide good results.

3. **Treatment**

   a. **Juvenile osteochondral** lesions can generally be treated nonsurgically with rest or reduction from high-impact activities and repetitive deep knee bending. The goal is to have the knee become pain free. The presence of an effusion is indicative of possible disruption of the articular surface, signifying the need for surgical evaluation. The patient and their family should be informed to return to the doctor if recurrent effusions are present. Following these patients in regular intervals (6 to 12 months) until resolution of the lesion on X-ray is advised.

   b. **The treatment of symptomatic OCD lesions in the adult usually requires surgical management. Arthroscopically assisted or open internal fixation of the lesion can save the patient's native articular cartilage. Cartilage restoration procedures may be required if the articular cartilage is not viable and the patient remains symptomatic.**[13,14,47]

   c. **Tibial tubercle apophysitis (Osgood–Schlatter disease)**

      i. **Clinical diagnosis.** Osgood–Schlatter disease is an irritation of the insertion site of the patellar tendon into the tibial tubercle. It is frequently seen in the rapidly growing adolescent athletic with open growth plates. Chronic irritation results in bony overgrowth at the tibial tubercle. Radiographs may demonstrate a prominent or irregular tibial tubercle apophysis. There may be a free bony ossicle anterior and superior to the tibial tubercle.

      ii. **Treatment.** Symptoms tend to resolve with fusion of the tibial tubercle apophysis. Therefore, treatment is aimed at symptom control until skeletal maturity. Activity modification, icing, and physical therapy can be helpful. Surgical treatment is rarely indicated. Aggressive treatment might occasionally involve limited use of a knee immobilizer in recalcitrant cases where the patient is dysfunctional in day-to-day activities or noncompliant in activity reduction.

   d. **Inferior pole of patella apophysitis (Sinding-Larsen-Johansson disease)**

      i. **Clinical diagnosis.** Sinding-Larsen-Johansson disease is a traction apophysitis with irritation of the proximal patellar tendon attachment on the inferior pole of the patella. It is less common than Osgood–Schlatter disease, but has similar pathogenesis.

      ii. **Treatment.** Sinding-Larsen-Johansson disease is generally self-limited. Treatment is primarily symptomatic, utilizing NSAIDs, antiinflammatory medications, and strengthening exercises. In rare cases, surgery for debridement of inflammatory tissue to stimulate local healing is undertaken.

## REFERENCES

1. Arendt EA. Assessment of the athlete with an acutely injured knee. In: Griffin LU, ed. *Rehabilitation of the Injured Knee*. Mosby; 1990:20-33.
2. AMA. *Standard Nomenclature of Athletic Injuries*. American Medical Association; 1966.
3. LaPrade RF, Terry GC. Injuries to the posterolateral aspect of the knee. Association of anatomic injury patterns with clinical instability. *Am J Sports Med*. 1997;25:433-437.
4. Benjaminse A, Gokeler A, van der Schans CP. Clinical diagnosis of an anterior cruciate ligament rupture: a meta-analysis. *J Orthop Sports Phys Ther*. 2006;36:267-288.

5. Katz JW, Fingeroth RJ. The diagnostic accuracy of ruptures of the anterior cruciate ligament comparing the Lachman test, the anterior drawer sign, and the pivot shift test in acute and chronic knee injuries. *Am J Sports Med.* 1986;14:88-91.

6. Secrist ES, Frederick RW, Tjoumakaris FP, et al. A comparison of operative and nonoperative treatment of ACL injuries. *JBJS Rev.* 2016;4:1-9.

7. Losee RR, Johnson TR, Southwick WO. Anterior subluxation of the lateral tibial plateau. *J Bone Joint Surg Am.* 1978;60:1015-1030.

8. Duerr RA, Chauhan A, Frank DA, DeMeo PJ, Akhavan S. An algorithm for diagnosing and treating primary and recurrent patellar instability. *JBJS Rev.* 2016;4:1-11.

9. Rosenberg TD, Paulos LE, Parker RD, Coward DB, Scott SM. The forty-five-degree posteroanterior flexion weight-bearing radiograph of the knee. *J Bone Joint Surg Am.* 1988;70:1479-1483.

10. Cheung LP, Li KC, Hollett MD, Bergman AG, Herfkens RJ. Meniscal tears of the knee: accuracy of detection with fast spin-echo MR imaging and arthroscopic correlation in 293 patients. *Radiology.* 1997;203:508-512.

11. Rappeport ED, Wieslander SB, Stephensen S, Lausten GS, Thomsen HS. MRI preferable to diagnostic arthroscopy in knee joint injuries. A double-blind comparison of 47 patients. *Acta Orthop Scand.* 1997;68:277-281.

12. Muller ME, Allgöwer M, Schneider R, Willenegger H. *Manual of Internal Fixation.* 3rd ed. Springer-Verlag; 1991.

13. Gomoll AH, Farr J, Gillogly SD, Kercher JS, Minas T. Surgical management of articular cartilage defects of the knee. *Instr Course Lect.* 2011;60:461-483.

14. Løken S, Heir S, Holme I, Engebretsen L, Årøen A. 6-year follow-up of 84 patients with cartilage defects in the knee. Knee scores improved but recovery was incomplete. *Acta Orthop.* 2010;81:611-618.

15. Conlan T, Garth WP Jr, Lemons JE. Evaluation of the medial soft-tissue restraints of the extensor mechanism of the knee. *J Bone Joint Surg Am.* 1993;75:682-693.

16. Dejour H, Walch G, Nove-Josserand L, Guier C. Factors of patellar instability: an anatomic radiographic study. *Knee Surg Sports Traumatol Arthrosc.* 1994;2:19-26.

17. Hughston JC, Deese M. Medial subluxation of the patella as a complication of lateral retinacular release. *Am J Sports Med.* 1988;16:383-388.

18. Laurin CA, Dussault R, Levesque HP. The tangential x-ray investigation of the patellofemoral joint: x-ray technique, diagnostic criteria and their interpretation. *Clin Orthop Relat Res.* 1979;(144):16-26.

19. Merchant AC, Mercer RL, Jacobsen RH, Cool CR. Roentgenographic analysis of patellofemoral congruence. *J Bone Joint Surg Am.* 1974;56:1391-1396.

20. Arendt EA, Lind M, Van Der Merwe W. Indications for MPFL reconstruction after patellar dislocation. *ISAKOS Newsl.* 2009;13(2):29-31. http://www.isakos.com/assets/newsletter/sum09.pdf.

21. Amin NH, Lynch TS, Patel R, Patel N, Saluan P. Medial patellofemoral ligament reconstruction. *JBJS Rev.* 2015;3:1-9.

22. Christiansen SE, Jakobsen BW, Lund B, Lind M. Isolated repair of the medial patellofemoral ligament in primary dislocation of the patella: a prospective randomized study. *Arthroscopy.* 2008;24:881-887.

23. Stefancin JJ, Parker RD. First-time traumatic patellar dislocation: a systematic review. *Clin Orthop Relat Res.* 2007;455:93-101.

24. Arendt EA, Fithian DC, Cohen E. Current concepts of lateral patella dislocation. *Clin Sports Med.* 2002;21:499-519.

25. Nickinson R, Darrah C, Donell S. Accuracy of clinical diagnosis in patients undergoing knee arthroscopy. *Int Orthop.* 2010;34:39-44.

26. Solomon DH, Simel DL, Bates DW, Katz JN, Schaffer JL. The rational clinical examination. Does this patient have a torn meniscus or ligament of the knee? Value of the physical examination. *JAMA.* 2001;286:1610-1620.

27. Barber-Westin SD, Noyes FR. Clinical healing rates of meniscus repairs of tears in the central-third (red-white) zone. *Arthroscopy.* 2014;30(1):134-146.

28. Strauss EJ, Day MS, Ryan M, Jazrawi L. Evaluation, treatment and outcomes of meniscal root tears. *JBJS Rev.* 2016;4:1-10.

29. Lau BC, Conway D, Mulvihill J, Zhang AL, Feeley BT. Biomechanical consequences of meniscal tear, partial meniscectomy and meniscal repair in the knee. *JBJS Rev.* 2016;4:1-10.

30. Bhattacharyya T, Gale D, Dewire P, et al. The clinical importance of meniscal tears demonstrated in magnetic resonance imaging in osteoarthritis of the knee. *J Bone Joint Surg Am.* 2003;85A:4-9.

31. Indelicato PA. Non-operative treatment of complete tears of the medial collateral ligament of the knee. *J Bone Joint Surg Am.* 1983;65:323-329.
32. Arendt EA, Dick R. Knee injury patterns among men and women in collegiate basketball and soccer: NCAA data and review of literature. *Am J Sports Med.* 1995;23(6):694-701.
33. Griffin LY, Albohm MJ, Arendt EA, et al. Understanding and preventing noncontact anterior cruciate ligament injuries: a review of the Hunt Valley II meeting, January 2005. *Am J Sports Med.* 2006;34:1512-1532.
34. Renstrom P, Ljungqvist A, Arendt E, et al. Non-contact ACL injuries in female athletes: an International Olympic Committee current concepts statement. *Br J Sports Med.* 2008;42:394-412.
35. Gray JL, Cindric M. Management of arterial and venous injuries in the dislocated knee. *Sports Med Arthrosc.* 2011;19:131-138.
36. Howells NR, Brunton LR, Robinson J, Porteus AJ, Eldridge JD, Murray JR. Acute knee dislocation: an evidence based approach to the management of the multiligament injured knee [epublished ahead of print December 12, 2010]. *Injury.* doi: 10.1016/j.injury.2010.11.018
37. Levy BA, Boyd JL, Stuart MJ. Surgical treatment of acute and chronic anterior and posterior cruciate ligament and lateral side injuries of the knee. *Sports Med Arthrosc.* 2011;19:110-119.
38. Edwards PH Jr, Grana WA. Physeal fractures about the knee. *J Am Acad Orthop Surg.* 1995;3:63-69.
39. Powers CM. Rehabilitation of patellofemoral joint disorders: a critical review. *J Orthop Sports Phys Ther.* 1998;28:345-354.
40. Lorenzen J, Krämer R, Vogt PM, Knobloch K. Systematic review about eccentric training in chronic patella tendinopathy. *Sportverletz Sportschaden.* 2010;24:198-203.
41. van Ark M, Zwerver J, van den Akker-Scheek I. Injection treatments for patellar tendinopathy [published ahead of print May 3, 2011]. *Br J Sports Med.* 2011. doi: 10.1136/bjsm.2010.078824
42. Santander J, Zarba E, Iraporda H, Puleo S. Can arthroscopically assisted treatment of chronic patellar tendinopathy reduce pain and restore function? [published ahead of print April 2, 2011]. *Clin Orthop Relat Res.* 2011. doi: 10.1007/s11999-011-1886-y
43. Image quiz: patellofemoral instability and pain. *JBJS J Orthop Phys Assist.* 2017;5(2):e12.
44. McConnell J. The management of chondromalacia patellae: a long-term solution. *Aust J Physiother.* 1986;32:215-223.
45. McConnell EJ. The physical therapist's approach to patellofemoral disorders. *Clin Sports Med.* 2002;21(3):363-387.
46. Chambers HG, Shea KG, Anderson AF, et al. Diagnosis and treatment of osteochondritis dissecans. *J Am Acad Orthop Surg.* 2011;19:297-306.
47. Heyworth BE, Kocher MS. Osteochondritis of the knee. *JBJS Rev.* 2015;3:1-12.

## SELECTED HISTORICAL READINGS

Green NE, Allen BL. Vascular injuries associated with dislocation of the knee. *J Bone Joint Surg Am.* 1977;59:236-239.
Torg JS, Conrad W, Kalen V. Clinical diagnosis of anterior cruciate ligament instability in the athlete. *Am J Sports Med.* 1976;4:84-93.

# 26 Fractures of the Tibia

Mohit Bhandari and Marc F. Swiontkowski

**I. Fractures of the Tibial Plateau**[1-4]

  **A.** For practical purposes, fractures of the tibial plateau are classified as follows:

    1. **Undisplaced** (a vertical fracture of the plateau)

    2. **Split** (a split fracture with displacement, with or without slight comminution)

    3. **Depressed** (centrally depressed fracture)

    4. **Split and depressed** with an intact tibial rim

    5. **Any of one through four with metaphyseal or even diaphyseal extension.** The elements of these descriptions are contained within **Schatzker system** (Fig. 26-1).

  **B.** **Examination** is different from that for other knee injuries. It is wise to carry out a definitive examination only after roentgenographs have been obtained. Differential diagnosis includes a major ligamentous injury or knee dislocation.[5-7] The examination should include inspection for wounds and evaluation of the distal circulation (pulses and capillary refill) and neurologic (motor or sensory) function. Motion and stability should not routinely be assessed in these injuries; however, this type of injury can be associated with ligamentous or meniscal damage.[1]

  **C.** **Radiographs.** Oblique films in addition to the routine anteroposterior and lateral radiographs are often helpful in identifying fracture lines and articular displacement. Computed tomography demonstrates minor fractures and accurately depicts the degree of depression of the tibial plateau; axial cuts with sagittal reconstruction are the routine.

  **D.** Magnetic resonance imaging (MRI) can be helpful when there is clinical concern for associated ligamentous injury. The incidence of complete ligamentous or meniscal disruption associated with operative tibial plateau fractures on MRI has been reported as high as 99% in one follow-up study. In split-depressed fractures, depression was greater than 6 mm and widening was greater than 5 mm, predicted lateral meniscal injury in 83% of fractures, compared with 50% of fractures with less displacement ($P < .05$). Increasing displacement can also be associated with cruciate ligament injuries and lateral collateral ligament injuries in almost 30% of patients.

    1. **Undisplaced fractures.** In some settings, especially when multiple injuries are involved, fixation with two percutaneous cannulated cancellous lag screws is advisable to ensure maintenance of reduction. For isolated injuries, generally, nonoperative management is selected. A splint is applied, and the leg is elevated for the first 24 to 48 hours. Knee aspiration is carried out if a significant hemarthrosis is present, and knee motion may be started with continuous passive motion (CPM) if available. As soon as the patient is comfortable and the range of motion is increasing, he/she can be followed up as an outpatient. Follow-up radiographs should be obtained shortly after motion is instituted to ensure that the fracture remains nondisplaced. Touch-down weight bearing should be maintained for 8 weeks to prevent displacement from shear forces. The typical treatment

411

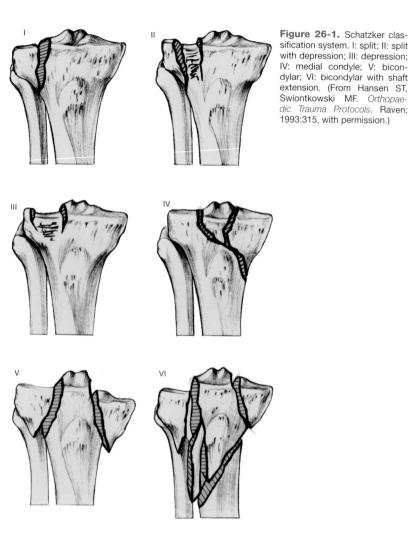

**Figure 26-1.** Schatzker classification system. I: split; II: split with depression; III: depression; IV: medial condyle; V: bicondylar; VI: bicondylar with shaft extension. (From Hansen ST, Swiontkowski MF. *Orthopaedic Trauma Protocols*. Raven; 1993:315, with permission.)

for nondisplaced tibial plateau fractures includes non–weight bearing with the knee locked in extension with gait. Non–weight-bearing range of motion is usually started when the pain and swelling subside. Weight bearing is initiated when pain subsides and with radiographic signs of healing.

2. **Displaced fractures**

   a. **Split fracture.** Open reduction and fixation is generally done if there is a significant widening (lateral or medial displacement of more than 3 to 5 mm) of the plateau.[8,9] The internal fixation must be rigid enough to allow movement of the joint as soon as there is soft-tissue healing. In this situation, the authors prefer to use the Association for the Study of Internal Fixation (ASIF) buttress plate or a dynamic compression or locking plate when the patient is osteoporotic.[4] Recently, there has been a move toward the use of smaller implants for all tibial plateau fixation. Specialized 3.5-mm T- and L-buttress plates allow the placement of more screws under the articular surface. If the patient is young and has dense bone, multiple percutaneous cannulated lag screws can be inserted under fluoroscopic and/or arthroscopic control. Percutaneous placement of a large reduction clamp is often successful in providing reduction of the fracture. If open reduction and internal fixation is not feasible, treatment should be as for comminuted fractures.

b. **Central depression of the plateau.** If depression is greater than 3 to 5 mm, especially with valgus stress instability of the knee greater than 10° in full extension, most authors currently recommend elevation with bone grafting and fixation.[2,3,9,10] More recently, articular reductions have been done with arthroscopic visualization with percutaneous technique for elevation of the segment. Autogenous bone graft has typically been the treatment of choice, but allograft and cancellous substitutes, such as coralline hydroxyapatite and calcium phosphate cements, have been successfully used.[9] Randomized trials comparing calcium phosphate cements and to controls have suggested that the use of calcium phosphate bone cement for the treatment of fractures in adult patients is associated with a lower prevalence of pain at the fracture site in comparison with the rate in controls (patients managed with no graft material). Loss of fracture reduction is also decreased in comparison with that in patients managed with autogenous bone graft. Generally, percutaneous lag screws are adequate for support of the elevated joint surface and bone graft or graft substitute material.

c. **Split-depressed fractures** with a displacement/depression of more than 3 to 4 mm are treated with reduction, fixation, and early motion in most young patients. Generally, this reduction is done with an open technique, with an anterior or anterolateral approach, elevation, and bone grafting using buttress or locked buttress plates for older patients (Fig. 26-2) and lag screws or 3.5-mm small fragment T- or L-plates or one-third tubular plates (as washers) in younger patients (Fig. 26-3). These fractures may be managed with arthroscopic reduction in skilled hands. Secure fixation is critical so that early motion with or without CPM can be initiated. Patients are generally limited to touch-down weight bearing for 12 weeks to prevent late fracture settling. If the patient's limb is stable to varus and valgus stress in an examination under anesthesia shortly after injury, traction treatment with a tibial pin and early motion is an option.[10,11] The patient is placed in a cast brace (as described in Chapter 8, III.H) or a hinged knee brace after 3 to 4 weeks.[1] This treatment is not currently recommended on a routine basis. If the instability exceeds 10°, reduction and fixation as described earlier is indicated.[11]

d. **Fractures with metaphyseal/diaphyseal extension** are treated similarly to split-depressed fractures if the joint extension is significant. Generally, buttress plate fixation and bone grafting are required. When the injury is bicondylar, stripping the soft tissues off both condyles from an anterior approach should be avoided; this results in a high incidence of nonunion and deep infection. Instead, the most unstable condyle (usually lateral) is selected for the buttress fixation via an anterolateral approach, and the other condyle is stabilized by percutaneous screw fixation, fixation with a posterior medial incision and small buttress plate, or neutralization with an external fixator for 4 to 6 weeks while motion is limited. With all tibial plateau fractures

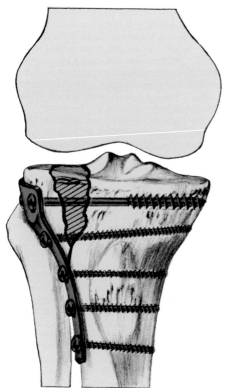

**Figure 26-2.** Internal fixation of a split depression fracture of the tibial plateau using L-buttress plate fixation with bone grafting of the elevated segment. (From Hansen ST, Swiontkowski MF. *Orthopaedic Trauma Protocols.* Raven; 1993:318, with permission.)

treated with operative stabilization, it is important to examine the knee for ligamentous stability after completing the fixation in the operating room to rule out ligamentous injury (see II.B).[1] The functional results of **treatment** are often better than the routine radiographs seem to predict. Early motion of the knee joint and delayed full weight bearing are the keys to the maximum restoration of joint function.[2-4]

    i. Apply self-hinged knee braces, which are lightweight and limit varus and valgus stress and are widely used. The same ambulation protocol, touch-down weight bearing, is followed.

    ii. In special situations, the patient is placed in a **long-leg cast** until the fracture is healed. Then, the patient is placed in a rehabilitation program to regain full extension and flexion of the knee to beyond 90°. The patient is kept on protected weight bearing for at least 3 to 4 months. This treatment is generally limited to patients with a severe neurologic condition or significant osteopenia.

**E. Complications**

  1. Significant **loss of range of motion** may occur, particularly if early movement is not instituted.

  2. **Early degenerative joint changes** with pain can occur, regardless of the degree of joint reconstruction. In some instances, the pain may be severe enough to require arthroplasty or arthrodesis.[8]

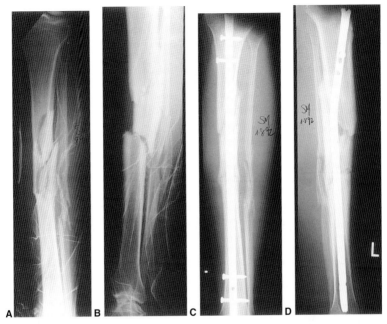

**Figure 26-3.** Displaced closed fractures of the tibia shaft, when shortened more than 1 cm or considered to be unstable, are best treated with interlocking nails. **A,B:** Preoperative radiographs of a shortened, unstable segmental fracture of the tibia shaft. **C,D:** The interlocking nail in place. The screws placed through the holes in the nail proximal and distal to the fracture provide length and rotational stability for the fracture. Nearly all fractures of the femoral shaft in skeletally mature individuals are treated with similar interlocking nails, allowing mobilization of the patient and early range of motion of adjacent joints.

3. The **infection rate** following operative treatment is reduced in experienced hands. Most infections occur because of excessive soft-tissue stripping.

4. **Nerve and vascular injuries** that occur at the time of injury or subsequent to treatment are not uncommon.[12] Nerve injuries are usually traction injuries, and recovery is unpredictable. Compartment syndrome may be present and should be treated as described in Chapter 3, III.

## II. Extraarticular Proximal Tibial Fractures

A. **Classification.** Proximal tibial fractures are classified similar to diaphyseal fractures (see III.C).

B. **Examination.** Initial examination should be comprehensive, including inspection, palpation, and lower extremity neurovascular assessment. The integrity and condition of the soft tissues should be carefully inspected. The alignment of the lower extremity should also be noted. The compartments of the leg should be palpated, and passive flexion and extension of the toes performed to assess for pain and possible compartment syndrome. Distal pulses may be palpable despite ischemia from increased compartment pressure. Definitive diagnosis may require measurement of intracompartmental pressures (see Chapter 3, III). The diagnosis of a compartment syndrome is a surgical emergency and requires prompt release of pressure to preserve muscle and nerve viability. A careful examination of the extremity pulses is imperative to rule out potential vascular injury.

C. **Radiographs.** Although a tibial diaphyseal fracture may be obvious from clinical examination, anteroposterior and lateral radiographs of the tibia (including the knee and ankle joints) are needed to plan management. Radiographs should be carefully reviewed to ensure fracture lines do not reveal intraarticular extension. Computed tomograms or plain tomograms can be helpful to identify intraarticular extension when plain X-rays are difficult to interpret.

D. **Treatment.** Extraarticular proximal tibial fractures are often the result of high-energy trauma with displacement and comminution. Most authors agree that operative management of such fractures is warranted to optimize patient outcomes. However, it remains unclear which surgical option (plate, nail, external fixator, or combination) is preferable. The rates of nonunion between implants did not appear to differ between treatment options (Table 26-1). Infection rates were significantly lower with intramedullary nails than with plates or external fixators $(P < .05)$.[13] A trend toward increased rates of malunion with intramedullary nails was identified $(P = .062)$. Pooled results across studies may be limited by heterogeneity between studies. Results should be interpreted with caution.

E. **Complications.** Extraarticular fractures of the tibia are prone to infection, malunion (i.e., valgus and procurvatum deformities), nonunion, compartment syndrome, and implant failure (Table 26-1).[13]
   1. **Infection:** Range 8% to 14% (deep infection rates 3% to 5%)
   2. **Malunion:** Range 2.4% to 20%
   3. **Nonunion:** Range 2% to 8%
   4. **Compartment syndrome:** Range 2% to 6%
   5. **Implant failure:** 8%

III. **Diaphyseal Fractures**
   A. **Epidemiology.** Tibial fractures are the most common long bone fracture. They occur commonly in the third decade of life at a rate of 26 diaphyseal fractures per 100,000 populations annually.

| TABLE 26-1 | Proximal Extraarticular Tibial Fractures | | | | |
|---|---|---|---|---|---|
| Point Estimates and 95% Confidence Intervals | | | | | |
| | Infection (%) | Nonunion (%) | Malunion (%) | CS (%) | Implant Failure (%) |
| Plate | 14 (8–3) | 2 (0.3–8) | 10 (5–18) | 2 (0.3–8) | – |
| IM nail | 2.5 (0.1–3)[a] | 3.5 (1.7–7) | 20 (1.5–26)[b] | 5.5 (3.1–9.6) | 7.5 (5–12) |
| Ex-flx | 8 (4–15) | 8 (4–15) | 4 (1.5–10) | – | – |
| | DI: 3 (1–8) | | | | |
| Ex-flx | +12 (5–26) | – | 2.4 (0.4–13) | – | – |
| Plate | DI: 5 (1–16) | | | | |

[a]$P > .05$ when compared with plate.
[b]$P = .06$ when compared with plate.
CS, compartment syndrome; DI, deep infection; Ex-flx, external fixation; IM, intramedullary.
From Busse J, Bhandari M, Kulkarni A, et al. The effect of low intensity, pulsed ultrasound on time to fracture healing: a meta-analysis. *CMAJ.* 2002;166:437-441, with permission.

B. **Mechanism of injury.** Five causes of injury include falls, sports related, direct blunt trauma, motor vehicle accidents, and penetrating injuries (e.g., gunshots).

C. **Classification.** The most comprehensive classification for tibial fractures is the AO ASIF/Orthopaedic Trauma Association system that divides injury patterns into three broad categories: unifocal, wedge, and complex fractures.

   1. Unifocal fractures are further described as spiral, oblique, and transverse fractures (A).
   2. Wedge fractures are further described as intact spiral, intact bending, and comminuted wedge fractures (B).
   3. Complex fractures (i.e., multiple fragments) can be described as spiral wedge, segmental, and comminuted fractures (C).

D. **Examination.** Initial examination should be comprehensive, including inspection, palpation, and lower extremity neurovascular assessment. The integrity and condition of the soft tissues should be carefully inspected. The alignment of the lower extremity should also be noted. The compartments of the leg should be palpated, and passive flexion and extension of the toes performed to assess for pain and possible compartment syndrome. The diagnosis of a compartment syndrome is a surgical emergency and requires prompt release of pressure to preserve muscle and nerve viability (see Chapter 3, III).

E. **Radiographs.** Although a tibial diaphyseal fracture may be obvious from clinical examination, anteroposterior and lateral radiographs of the tibia (including the knee and ankle joints) are needed to plan management. Radiographs can provide information about fracture morphology, quality of the bone (i.e., osteopenia, osteoporosis), and gas in the tissues, suggesting an open wound.

F. **Treatment.** The selection of nonoperative or operative management must involve the consideration of many factors, including associated skeletal and ligamentous injuries, the degree of soft-tissue injury, injuries to other organ systems, the general condition of the patient, the skill and experience of the treating physician, and the resources of the facility. Options for treatment include casting/functional bracing (nonoperative), external fixation, plate fixation, and intramedullary nailing.

   1. **Nonoperative management** is commonly reserved for closed tibial diaphyseal fractures with less than 1.5 cm of shortening, axially stable transverse fractures, spiral oblique of comminuted fractures with less than 12 mm of initial shortening, angulations less than degrees initially, and less than 50% displacement.[15] However, acceptable degrees of fracture shortening and translation are highly variable among surgeons (<5 to >15 mm). Patients who desire early weight bearing or cannot tolerate 8 to 12 weeks of non–weight bearing with conservative treatment may consider intramedullary fixation. With a stable reduction, intramedullary fixation allows for early weight bearing as tolerated; this treatment decision-making falls into the category of shared decision-making where patient preferences play a major role. Surgeons' definitions of acceptable angular malunions (rotational, varus/valgus, and procurvatum/recurvatum) range from less than 5° to 20°.[16] Sarmiento et al.[17,18] developed a below-the-knee cast (patellar tendon bearing [PTB]) and prefabricated functional brace that allows knee motion while maintaining stability and length in the affected leg. This PTB cast is generally applied after 2 to 3 weeks in the long-leg bent knee cast that is applied following a closed reduction. Prefabricated braces are the most widely used. One of these two treatment methods should be chosen, and the particular technique should be strictly adhered to if the same excellent results reported in the literature are to be expected. These cast techniques are described in detail in Chapter 8. It must be reemphasized that a below-the-knee total contact

cast may not be applied immediately after the fracture; one must wait until the swelling has diminished. The authors suggest using a modified Robert Jones compression long-leg splint during the period of acute swelling. When the patient is ready for casting and following an appropriate spinal or general anesthetic, nearly all tibial fractures can be reduced by placing the leg over the end of the table. Adequate reduction and alignment are maintained in this position, while the cast is applied. If shortening is minimal, analgesia may suffice. The average healing time with closed treatment is approximately 18 weeks (range from 14.5 to 21.0 weeks). One of Sarmiento's principles is that, in general, the amount of final shortening is demonstrated on the initial radiograph, and the patient should be so informed. Good functional outcomes can be expected in 90% of cases.[19-21] Closed treatment is recommended for children's fractures, except when the physis or joint is involved.[22]

2. **Operative management** is reserved for those fractures deemed unacceptable for nonoperative treatment. Most surgeons prefer intramedullary nails in the treatment of closed low-energy fractures (95.5%), high-energy fractures (96%), and those closed fractures with associated compartment syndrome (80.4%).[23] Most surgeons prefer intramedullary nails in the treatment of open tibial shaft fractures; however, there is a decline in the use of intramedullary nails as the severity of the soft-tissue injury increases from Types I to IIIB (Type I, 95.5%; Type II, 88.1%; Type IIIA, 68.4%; Type IIIB, 48.4%).[23]

   a. **Closed fractures.** There have been three published meta-analyses evaluating treatment alternatives for closed tibial shaft fractures: two pooling data from primarily observational studies and one pooling data from on-use randomized trials.[21,24,25] Littenberg and colleagues,[21] in a comprehensive review of the available literature, identified 2,005 patients treated with a cast or brace, 474 patients treated with a plate and screws, and 407 patients treated with intramedullary nails. Pooled infection rates were lower with casts (0%) and intramedullary nails (0% to 1%) when compared with plates (0% to 15%). Although plate fixation achieved the fastest time to fracture union (median = 13 weeks) when compared with either casts (median = 13.7 weeks) or intramedullary nails (median = 20 weeks), there were no differences in the ultimate rates of nonunion between the groups. Rates of deep infection were lower with casts and intramedullary nails than with plates (ranges: 0% to 2%, 0% to 1%, and 0% to 15%, respectively).

   In a review of prospective studies (eight observational and five randomized trials) evaluating treatment alternatives for tibial shaft fractures, Coles and Gross[24] found plate fixation to result in the lowest nonunion rates (2.6%) and highest infection rates (9%) compared with other treatment alternatives. Despite the apparent benefits of plate fixation in decreasing the time to fracture healing, only 2.1% to 7.4% of surgeon respondents to a survey preferred them in the treatment of closed tibial shaft fractures (low energy, high energy, and those with associated compartment syndrome). This likely reflects an assessment that the high risk of infection with plates outweighs their relative benefit in decreasing time to fracture union. It remains unclear whether surgeons from less industrialized countries, who prefer plate fixation in closed tibial shaft fractures, have similar access to intramedullary nails as those surgeons in developed nations.

   A substantial proportion of respondents chose external fixation for high-energy tibial shaft fractures and those associated with compartment syndrome. The role of external fixation in closed tibial shaft fractures has been evaluated in an observational study.[26] Turen and colleagues,[26] in a review of 68 closed fractures, identified a longer fracture healing time in fractures with compartment syndrome than those without (30.2 weeks vs. 17.2 weeks). Moreover, fracture healing times for closed fractures with compartment syndrome were similar to open fractures.

There remains considerable variability in their preference to ream the intramedullary canal or not. The evidence favoring reamed or nonreamed nail insertion is suggestive, but not definitive. Bhandari and colleagues[25] conducted a systematic review and found nine randomized trials ($n$ = 646 patients) comparing reamed and nonreamed intramedullary nail insertion in tibial and femoral fractures. Reamed nailing resulted in a 56% reduction in the relative risk (RR) of nonunion compared with nonreamed nailing (95% confidence interval 7% to 79%). The largest study comparing alternative nail insertion approaches in tibial shaft fractures (SPRINT) was multicenter, blinded randomized trial enrolling 1,319 adults. In patients with closed fractures, 45 (11%) of 416 in the reamed nailing group and 68 (17%) of 410 in the unreamed nailing group experienced a reoperation within 1 year (RR 0.67; 95% confidence interval 0.47 to 0.96; $P$ = .03). This difference was largely due to higher rates of nail dynamization in the nonreamed group. SPRINT's treatment effect was much less than that expected based on the previous meta-analysis, suggesting that differences between both techniques are less dramatic than previously reported. This is likely because interventions to gain fracture union in the SPRINT trial were prohibited until 6 months from surgery. The valuable message here is that one should be patient and wait before intervening surgically until at least 6 months as radiographic healing often lags behind clinical fracture union.

b. **Open fractures.** An international survey suggests a progressive decline in the use of intramedullary nails as the severity of the soft-tissue injury increases from Type I to Type IIIB.[14] This is related to an increased use of external fixation with increasing soft-tissue injury (3% to 51%).[27] Surgeons rarely prefer plates in the treatment of open fractures (0.8% to 1.1%). One study ($n$ = 56) suggests external fixators that significantly decrease the risk of reoperation relative to plates (RR 0.13; 95% confidence interval 0.03 to 0.54; $P$ < .01).[15] A meta-analysis found that nonreamed nails, in comparison to external fixators (five studies, $n$ = 396 patients), reduced the risk of reoperation (RR 0.51; 95% confidence interval 0.31 to 0.69).[28] Nonreamed nails also offered advantages in decreasing the RR of malunion (RR 0.42; 95% confidence interval 0.25 to 0.71) and superficial infection (RR 0.24; 95% confidence interval 0.08 to 0.73). Although these studies shared methodologic limitations of lack of concealment, blinding, and loss to follow-up, the narrow confidence intervals make the results more definitive than those of the studies comparing reamed versus unreamed nailing. In the open tibial fracture trials, reamed nails, when compared with nonreamed nails, showed a trend toward decreasing the risk of reoperation (two studies, $n$ = 132; RR 0.75; 95% confidence interval 0.43 to 1.32).[6] Because the confidence interval is very wide, the relative effect of reamed and unreamed nails in open tibial fractures remains unresolved. The SPRINT study did not identify any significant difference between reamed and undreamed nailing in terms of revision surgery to gain union for open fractures of the tibial shaft (SPRINT investigators). However, it did trend in the direction that favored nonreamed intramedullary nail insertion.[33]

**G. Complications.** Most patients experience some residual disability after a tibial fracture.[21,24]

1. **Compartment syndrome** has been discussed previously (see Chapter 3, III).
2. **Joint stiffness** can be largely prevented by aggressive treatment to achieve early union. Flexion and extension exercises to the toes must not be neglected because these joints frequently stiffen and produce considerable postcasting dysfunction.
3. **Complex regional pain syndrome** (reflex sympathetic dystrophy) can occur in 30% of patients with tibial diaphyseal fractures.[29] Vigorous physical therapy and sympathetic nerve blocks may be required (see Chapter 3).
4. **Delayed union and nonunion**[30]
   a. **The following factors are related to delayed union or nonunion:**
      i. **Severe initial displacement** of the fracture fragments (probably indicating significant soft-tissue injury)
      ii. **Significant comminution**
      iii. **Associated soft-tissue injuries or open fractures**
      iv. **Infection**
      v. **Open management with inadequate stability**
      vi. These complications can be minimized by adequate immobilization, early weight bearing (which is often delayed for 2 months if a dynamic compression plate is used), and early bone grafting where delayed union appears certain.
   b. Adjunctive therapies. **Low-intensity pulsed ultrasound** (30 mW/cm$^2$) given at 20 minutes/day has shown potential **benefits** in improving time to healing. A meta-analysis identified 138 potentially eligible studies, of which six randomized trials met inclusion criteria.[31] Three trials, representing 158 fractures, were of sufficient homogeneity for pooling. The pooled results showed that time to fracture healing was significantly shorter in the groups receiving low-intensity ultrasound therapy than in the control groups. The weighted average effect size was 6.41 (95% confidence interval 1.01 to 11.81), which converts to a mean difference in healing time of 64 days between the treatment and control groups. Lack of clinical and functional evidence in previous trials has led to further study evaluating the evidence for use of bone stimulators in routine clinical practice. Recent trials and additional analyses (from a meta-analysis of 13 randomized controlled trails) suggest that evidence for the effect of low-intensity pulsed ultrasonography on healing of fractures is moderate to very low in quality and provides conflicting results. The lack of functional outcome data is a key limitation to translating the positive radiographic findings.
5. **Infection** is a complication of open fractures or the opening of a closed fracture. The risk of infection is minimized by efficient **surgical** technique, by the proper use of antibiotics, and by a delayed primary closure for open fractures. For the most severe soft-tissue injuries, aggressive debridement and coverage with free or rotational muscle flaps minimizes this complication. Pin tract infection is common with the use of external fixators.
6. **Revision surgery.** An observational study of 192 patients with tibial shaft fractures identified three simple predictors of the need for reoperation within 1 year.[32] Three variables predicted reoperation: the presence of an open fracture wound (RR 4.32; 95% confidence interval 1.76 to 11.26), lack of cortical continuity between the fracture ends following fixation (RR 8.33; 95% confidence interval 3.03 to 25.0), and the presence of a transverse fracture (RR 20.0; 95% confidence interval 4.34 to 142.86).

## HCMC Treatment Recommendations

### Tibial Plateau Fractures

**Diagnosis:** Anteroposterior and lateral radiographs and physical examination. Computed tomography scans are helpful for the assessment of displacement and for surgical planning.

**Treatment:** Open reduction and internal fixation or percutaneous reduction with lag screw fixation aided by arthroscopy for fractures displaced more than 2 mm (depression or gapping). Knees that remain stable to varus/valgus stress in full extension may be treated nonoperatively.

**Indications for surgery:** Knees with more than 10° of instability in extension and/or joint displacement of >2 mm.

**Recommended technique:** Joint visualization via open reduction or arthroscopy, reduction and fixation with lag screws and/or low-profile plates and bone graft or bone-graft substitute, early range of motion therapy, and limited weight bearing for 8 to 12 weeks.

## HCMC Treatment Recommendations

### Tib-Fib Fractures

**Diagnosis:** Anteroposterior and lateral radiographs of the leg and clinical examination. In 10% to 20% cases, there is an open wound communicating with the fracture.

**Treatment:** Nonoperative care for fractures that are isolated and not shortened more than 1 cm on initial radiographs, long-leg splint for 2 to 3 weeks followed by fracture brace until fracture is united, operative stabilization for length unstable and/or open fractures. Interlocking nail, inserted with reaming, is the procedure of choice.

**Indications for surgery:** Fractures close to the joint or shortened on initial radiographs >1 cm or failure to control angulation with nonoperative technique or open fracture.

**Recommended technique:** Interlocking nailing, statically locked. Insert with reaming: more reaming for larger diameter nails with closed fractures, less reaming for open fractures.

## REFERENCES

1. Delamarter RB, Hohl M, Hopp E Jr. Ligament injuries associated with tibial plateau fractures. *Clin Orthop Relat Res*. 1990;250:226-233.
2. Honkonen SE. Degenerative arthritis after tibial plateau fractures. *J Orthop Trauma*. 1995;9:273-277.
3. Honkonen SE. Indicators for surgical treatment of tibial condyle fractures. *Clin Orthop Relat Res*. 1994;302:199-205.
4. Keating JF. Tibial plateau fractures in the older patient. *Bull Hosp Jt Dis*. 1999;58:19-23.

5. Burrus MT, Werner BL, Griffin JW, Winston Gwathmey F, Miller MD. Diagnostic and management strategies for multiligament injuries. *JBJS Rev.* 2016;4:1-9.
6. Rasul AT Jr, Fischer DA. Primary repair of quadriceps tendon rupture. Results of treatment. *Clin Orthop Relat Res.* 1993;289:205-207.
7. Rougraff BT, Reeck CC, Essenmacher J. Complete quadriceps tendon ruptures. *Orthopedics.* 1996;19:509-514.
8. Volpin G, Dowd GS, Stein H, Bentley G. Degenerative arthritis after intraarticular fractures of the knee: long-term results. *J Bone Joint Surg Br.* 1990;72:634-638.
9. Lee AK, Cooper SA, Collinge C. Bicondylar tibial plateau fractures. *JBJS Rev.* 2018;6:1-12.
10. Jensen DB, Rude C, Duus B, Bjerg-Nielsen A. Tibial plateau fractures. A comparison of conservative and surgical treatment. *J Bone Joint Surg Br.* 1990;72:49-52.
11. Rasmussen PS. Tibial condyle fractures: impairment of knee joint stability as an indication for surgical treatment. *J Bone Joint Surg Am.* 1973;55:1331-1350.
12. Dennis JW, Jagger C, Butcher JL, Menawat SS, Neel M, Frykberg ER. Reassessing the role of arteriograms in the management of posterior knee dislocations. *J Trauma.* 1993;35:692-697.
13. Bhandari M, Audige L, Ellis T, Hanson B; Evidence-Based Orthopaedic Trauma Working Group. Operative treatment of extra-articular proximal tibial fractures. *J Orthop Trauma.* 2003;17:591-595.
14. Gustilo RB, Anderson JT. Prevention of infection in the treatment of one thousand and twenty-five open fractures of long bones: retrospective and prospective analyses. *J Bone Joint Surg Am.* 1976;58:453-458.
15. Sarmiento A, Sharpe FE, Ebramzadeh E, Normand P, Shankwiler J. Factors influencing outcome of closed tibial fractures treated with functional bracing. *Clin Orthop Relat Res.* 1995;315:8-24.
16. Bhandari M, Guyatt GH, Swiontkowski MF, Tornetta P 3rd, Sprague S, Schemitsch EH. A lack of consensus in the assessment of fracture healing among orthopaedic surgeons. *J Orthop Trauma.* 2002;16:562-566.
17. Sarmiento A, Gersten LM, Sobol PA, Shankwiler JA, Vangsness CT. Tibial shaft fractures treated with functional braces. Experience with 780 fractures. *J Bone Joint Surg Br.* 1989;71:602-609.
18. Sarmiento A, McKellop HA, Llinas A, et al. Effect of loading and fracture motion in diaphyseal tibial fractures. *J Orthop Res.* 1996;14:80-84.
19. Faergemann C, Frandsen PA, Röck ND. Expected long-term outcome after a tibial shaft fracture. *J Trauma.* 1999;46:683-686.
20. Schemitsch EH, Bhandari M, Guyatt G, et al. Prognostic factors for predicting outcomes after intramedullary nailing of the tibia. *J Bone Joint Surg Am.* 2012;94:1786-1793.
21. Littenberg B, Weinstein LP, McCarren M, et al. Closed fractures of the tibial shaft. A meta-analysis of three methods of treatment. *J Bone Joint Surg Am.* 1998;80:174-183.
22. Spiegel PG, Cooperman DR, Laros GS. Epiphyseal fractures of the distal ends of the tibia and fibula. *J Bone Joint Surg Am.* 1978;60:1046-1050.
23. Bhandari M, Guyatt GH, Swiontkowski MF, et al. Surgeons' preferences in the operative treatment of tibial shaft fractures: an international survey. *J Bone Joint Surg Am.* 2001;83-A:1746-1752.
24. Coles CP, Gross M. Closed tibial shaft fractures: management and treatment complications. A review of the prospective literature. *Can J Surg.* 2000;43:256-262.
25. Bhandari M, Guyatt GH, Tong D, Adili A, Shaughnessy SG. Reamed versus non-reamed intramedullary nailing of lower extremity long bone fractures: a systematic overview and meta-analysis. *J Orthop Trauma.* 2000;2:9.
26. Turen CH, Burgess AR, Vanco B. Skeletal stabilization for tibial fractures associated with acute compartment syndrome. *Clin Orthop Relat Res.* 1995;315:163-168.
27. Bach AW, Hansen ST Jr. Plate versus external fixation in severe open tibial shaft fractures. A randomized trial. *Clin Orthop Relat Res.* 1989;241:89-94.
28. Bhandari M, Guyatt GH, Swiontkowski MF, Schemitsch EH. Treatment of open fractures of the shaft of the tibia. *J Bone Joint Surg Br.* 2001;83:62-68.
29. Sarangi PP, Ward AJ, Smth EJ. Algodystrophy and osteoporosis after tibial fractures. *J Bone Joint Surg Br.* 1993;75:450-452.

30. Blick SS, Brumback RJ, Lakatos R, Poka A, Burgess AR. Early prophylactic bone grafting of high-energy tibial fractures. *Clin Orthop Relat Res*. 1989;240:21-41.

31. Busse JW, Bhandari M, Kulkarni AV, Tunks E. The effect of low intensity, pulsed ultrasound on time to fracture healing: a meta-analysis. *CMAJ*. 2002;166:437-441.

32. Bhandari M, Tornetta P III, Sprague S, et al. Predictors of re-operation following operative management of fractures of the tibial shaft. *J Orthop Trauma*. 2003;17:353-361.

33. SPRINT investigators. Randomized trial of reamed and undreamed intramedullary nailing of tibial shaft fractures. *J Bone Joint Surg Am*. 2008;90A:2567-2578.

## SELECTED HISTORICAL READINGS

Burwell HN. Plate fixation of tibial shaft fractures. A survey of 181 injuries. *J Bone Joint Surg Br*. 1971;53:258-271.

Clancey GJ, Hansen ST Jr. Open fractures of the tibia: a review of one hundred and two cases. *J Bone Joint Surg Am*. 1978;60:118-122.

Dehne E. Treatment of fractures of the tibial shaft fractures. *Clin Orthop Relat Res*. 1969;66:159-173.

Fernandez-Palazzi F. Fibular resection in delayed union of tibial fractures. *Acta Orthop Scand*. 1969;40:105-118.

Karlström G, Olerud S. External fixation of severe open tibial fractures with the Hoffmann frame. *Clin Orthop Relat Res*. 1983;180:68-77.

Lottes JO. Medullary nailing of the tibial with the triflange nail. *Clin Orthop Relat Res*. 1974;105:53-66.

Nicoll EA. Fractures of the tibial shaft. *J Bone Joint Surg Br*. 1964;46:373-387.

Olerud S, Karlström G. Secondary intramedullary nailing of tibial fractures. *J Bone Joint Surg Am*. 1972;54:1419-1428.

Pare A. Compound fracture of leg. Pare's personal care (Mil, 328). In: Hamby WB, ed. *The Case Reports and Autopsy Records of Ambrose Pare*. Charles C Thomas Publisher; 1960:82-87.

Sarmiento A. Functional bracing of tibial fractures. *Clin Orthop Relat Res*. 1974;105:202-219.

Schatzker J, McBroom R, Bruce D. The tibial plateau fractures. The Toronto experience 1968–1975. *Clin Orthop Relat Res*. 1979;138:94-104.

Sorensen KH. Treatment of delayed union and nonunion of the tibia by fibular resection. *Acta Orthop Scand*. 1969;40:92-104.

# Ankle Injuries

Fernando A. Pena

## I. Ankle Sprains

The approach to ankle sprains should distinguish between the acute and chronic ankle sprains. The most common **ankle sprain** consists of an inversion injury of the foot with some degree of plantar flexion. Overall, the period of recovery is relatively short and uneventful. A more significant injury with a completely different period of recovery is the injury while the foot is in eversion, the so-called **high-ankle sprain (ankle syndesmotic sprain)**. It accounts for 1% to 15% of the total ankle sprains.[1] Therefore, it is important to identify the mechanism of injury to direct the examination correctly. Given the possibility of fractures, it is often recommended to obtain the history and do a brief examination using only palpation and, if suspicion for a fracture is present, obtain X-rays prior to performing a thorough physical examination.

### A. Acute presentation

1. **Inversion injuries.** With inversion ligamentous injuries, there is tearing of the lateral ligaments usually from anterior to posterior. Thus, the anterior talofibular ligament (ATFL) is the most commonly injured ligament followed by the calcaneofibular ligament and, in very rare instances, the posterior talofibular ligament.

   Fig. 27-1 shows the anatomic location of the ligaments. Fractures can occur with simple inversion injuries. The most common sites are the distal fibula and the base of the fifth metatarsal. More rarely, the lateral process of the talus and the anterior process of the calcaneus may fracture as well.

   a. **Examination.** Palpation of the bones around the ankle is key to examining ankle injuries. Special attention should be drawn to the distal fibula, distal tibia, and the base of the fifth metatarsal as per the Ottawa criteria (Table 27-1). If there is a component of blunt trauma to the ankle/lower leg, the fibula should be palpated looking for a fracture. All ankle ligaments should be palpated looking for tenderness. In the acute setting, pain can be quite limiting. In the absence of fractures, soft-tissue swelling and pain will dictate the treatment.

   b. **Radiographic imaging.** The need for X-rays can be dictated by the Ottawa ankle rules (Table 27-1). It is important to note that the rules do not apply to a pediatric population with open growth plates (to be safe, it is recommended to X-ray those under age 18). Although not specifically listed, we recommend a low threshold to obtain X-rays on people over the age of 50, especially women over the age of 50 because of lower bone mass and subsequent higher fracture rates. X-rays should include anteroposterior (AP), lateral, and mortise views of the ankle in a weight bearing status if pain allows.

   c. **Treatment.** If there is no medial tenderness, the ankle joint should be considered a **stable joint**. The traditional principles of rest, minimal immobilization, compression, elevation, and icing should be applied. A functional return to activities will be recommended and can be managed by a physical therapist. Commercially available ankle braces can

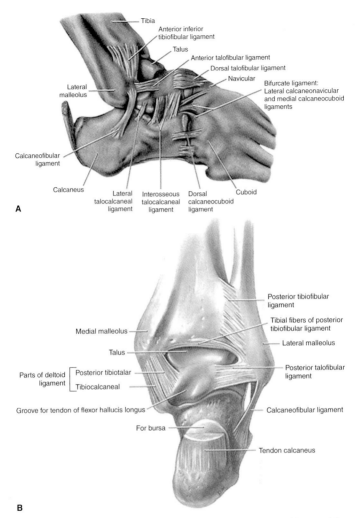

**Figure 27-1.** Anatomic description of the most significant ligaments and bones of the ankle and midfoot area.

be utilized until the pain allows proper muscle contraction of the dynamic stabilizers of the ankle (peroneal and deep compartment muscles of the lower leg). In rare occasions, owing to pain with weight bearing, the patient will have to be protected with crutches for a short period of time.

If there is medial or anterior capsule tenderness, the possibility of developing **long-term ankle instability** may be higher. If suspected, the ankle could be immobilized in a walking cast or boot for as long

| TABLE 27-1 | Ottawa Criteria to Perform Radiographic Examination |
|---|---|

**Ankle Injuries**
- Pain along the **posterior** margin of the most distal 6 cm of the fibula
- Pain along the **posterior** margin of the medial malleolus
- Unable to bear weight immediately after the injury or to take four steps in the Emergency Department (even with a limp)
- Age <18

**Midfoot Injuries**
- Pain along the base of the fifth metatarsal
- Pain along the navicular
- Unable to bear weight immediately after the injury or to take four steps in the Emergency Department (even with a limp)
- Age <18

as 6 to 8 weeks until the medial and anterior tenderness disappear. Activity-related ankle pain and swelling after 2 to 3 months of injury may signal resolving bony edema or an osteochondral lesion of the talus, which is diagnosed on magnetic resonance imaging (MRI). Bone edema or "bone bruising" may take up to 4 months to resolve before high-impact activities, such as running and jumping, are pain free.

Deep vein thrombosis (DVT) prophylaxis should be considered if range-of-motion exercises are not encouraged. At that time, it can be treated as a stable injury depending on the remaining discomfort within the ankle joint.

2. **Eversion injuries**
   a. **Examination.** The examination will show some tenderness along the most anterior and distal aspects of the syndesmosis of the ankle. Some tenderness along the lateral ligament complex may be present, although to a much lesser degree than with true inversion ankle sprain. Any degree of external rotation, which stresses the ankle mortise, will increase or reproduce the pain. The external rotation can be applied directly by the examiner holding the lower leg with one hand and torquing on the foot with the opposite hand while keeping the ankle in a neutral position, so the talus is locked in the ankle mortise. If a fracture has been ruled out, a "squeeze test" (using both hands to push the mid-fibula and tibia together, noting pain distal to the area of compression) can be performed to assess syndesmotic injuries. If the patient can tolerate weight bearing, a more sensitive test for a syndesmosis injury consists of standing on the injured leg and applying an external rotation force to the ankle with an internal turn of the pelvis with the knee fully extended. If the patient can stand and perform some degree of external rotation, the suspicion for an unstable mortise should be low. If there is any tenderness in the proximal lower leg, full-length tibia and fibula radiographs should be obtained to evaluate for a proximal fibula fracture (Maisonneuve fracture) or an unstable syndesmosis. The best projection to assess ankle syndesmosis instability is the mortise view of the ankle. This projection is taken as an AP view with 30° of internal rotation (when both malleolus are equidistant from the X-ray beam). A noncompetent syndesmosis is defined as one that presents on an AP view of the ankle with more than 6 mm of clear space between the tibia and the fibula measured 10 mm proximal from the joint line[2]

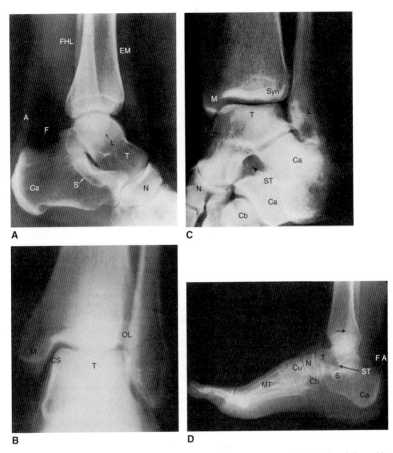

**Figure 27-2.** Radiographic appearance of the most common bony landmarks of the ankle and foot. **A:** Medial view of ankle region. **B:** Anterior view of ankle region. **C:** Mortise view of ankle region. **D:** Lateral view of foot. A, Achilles tendon; Ca, calcaneus; Cb, cuboid; CS, tibiofibular clear space; Cu, cuneiforms; EM, extensor muscles; F, fat; arrowhead, superimposed tibia, and fibula; FHL, flexor hallucis longus; L, lateral malleolus; M, medial malleolus; MT, metatarsal; N, navicular; OL, tibiofibular overlap; S, sustentaculum tali; ST, sinus tarsi; Syn, syndesmosis; T, talus.

(Fig. 27-2). When it comes to X-ray measurements, the clear space in between the tibia and the fibula has been shown to be more reliable and less subjective to rotation than the overlap in between the tibia and fibula (<5 mm). If the syndesmosis appears intact on a static radiograph, but suspicion for syndesmotic instability remains high, consider stressing the ankle (ideally under fluoroscopic dynamic examination) while applying external rotation to the foot for final assessment. For subtle cases, ankle arthroscopy will increase the sensitivity of the diagnosis by direct visualization of the intraarticular gap in between the fibula and the tibia. The patient may need to be either sedated or injected with local anesthetic along the syndesmosis prior to stressing the syndesmosis for evaluation under fluoroscopic examination. A total of 5 to 15 mL of lidocaine 1% with epinephrine should suffice to anesthetize the syndesmosis. The injection is performed using a 25G or 22G needle along the anterior aspect of the syndesmosis, starting immediately proximal to the joint line level and always "walking" along the lateral cortex of the tibia from distal to proximal. Special attention has to be paid to not angle the needle too posteriorly, never posterior to the plane of the fibula, to avoid damage into vital structures of the posterior compartment of the leg.

b. **Treatment.** If the syndesmosis is **stable** and has no fractures, the patient should follow a functional return to activities. If the syndesmosis is **unstable** or has a proximal fibula fracture, the patient will require fixation of the syndesmosis followed by immobilization for 6 to 8 weeks. The fixation method is variable, with some devices recently gaining popularity without the need for removal or second surgeries (unlike more traditional fixation with screws). A residual wide syndesmosis because of a misdiagnosis or improper treatment is a devastating sequelae that will often lead to posttraumatic osteoarthritis of the ankle joint within 1 to 2 years.

B. **Subacute–chronic presentation**

1. **Inversion injuries.** The patient presents with some residual discomfort in areas where there may still be some healing taking place or where an injury has been missed. The physician has to evaluate for any residual instability, reported to be present in 20% to 40% of ankle sprains, or a chondral injury of the talus, present in 6.5% of ankle sprains.[3] If the patient continues to report instability after a period of physical therapy, one may consider stress views of the ankle. Although they are not absolutely necessary to confirm the diagnosis, they help to document the degree of instability. The patient may require having the ankle anesthetized to allow a reliable radiographic evaluation. A total of 5 mL of lidocaine 2% with epinephrine should be enough to anesthetize the ankle joint. The injection is performed with a 25G or 22G needle along the most medial border of the ankle joint immediately distal to the medial shoulder of the tibial plafond and medial to the anterior tibialis tendon. The needle has to be angled at 45° from the coronal plane (see Chapter 30). The ankle can also be approached through the lateral aspect over the **"soft spot,"** which is defined as the junction of the tibia and fibula at the level of the joint line. However, the chances of damaging the dorsal cutaneous branch from the superficial peroneal nerve are not low. The best chance to identify the nerve branch is with gentle palpation of the skin, looking for a cord-like structure, when both the ankle and fourth toe are forced into plantar flexion.

The stress views are obtained with a lateral radiograph while the foot is pulled forward (an anterior drawer test) in slight plantar flexion. The most commonly injured ligament, the ATFL, is stressed during this maneuver. A 10-mm difference of anterior displacement between the stress view and the resting view or a 3-mm difference of anterior displacement compared with the stressed opposite side is indicative of ankle instability. Treatment options for chronic instability include a formal physiotherapy program; if that fails, the next reasonable step is a surgical repair/reconstruction of the lateral ligament complex of the ankle. Best results are obtained with an anatomic repair of the ligaments with reinforcement by the extensor retinaculum (modified Brostrom technique). In the absence of an obvious chondral injury of the talus on plain X-rays, an MRI scan is necessary for evaluation. A symptomatic chondral injury most likely will require some surgical treatment (i.e., arthroscopic debridement and/ or subchondral drilling) to improve the symptoms.

2. **Eversion injuries.** The most common reason to present with residual pain after a syndesmosis sprain will be some degree of remaining instability. A careful and detailed evaluation of the patient has to be performed as surgical fixation of the syndesmosis will be the most likely treatment recommendation.

## II. Ankle Fractures

**A. Classification.** Ankle fractures are intraarticular injuries, and accurate reduction as well as maintenance of the reduction is required for a satisfactory long-term result. To achieve reduction by closed manipulation, it is necessary to know the direction of the forces producing the fractures. It must be emphasized that fractures about the ankle usually are not isolated injuries and more likely than not will have associated ligamentous injuries. Ankle fractures may be classified by the Lauge–Hansen scheme (Fig. 27-3). This classification is useful because of the method used for its description. The first term makes reference to the position of the foot at the time of injury and the second term to the direction of the force applied to produce the fracture. That information is extremely valuable in planning closed reduction maneuvers.

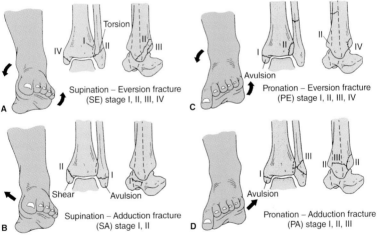

**Figure 27-3.** The Lauge–Hansen classification of ankle fractures. **A:** The supination–eversion fracture. Stage I: The avulsion of the anterior talofibular ligament (ATFL) from the fibula or simple rupture of the ligament. Stage II: The classic oblique fracture of the distal fibula, beginning anteriorly at the joint line and extending obliquely and posteriorly toward the shaft of the bone. Stage III: Avulsion or rupture of the posterior tibiofibular ligament. Stage IV: Avulsion fracture of the medial malleolus. **B:** The supination–adduction fracture. Stage I: Avulsion of the tip of the lateral malleolus or rupture of the associated ligaments. Stage II: Vertical fracture of the medial malleolus, usually beginning at the plafond. **C:** The pronation–eversion fracture. Stage I: Avulsion of the medial malleolus or ruptured deltoid ligament. Stage II: Rupture of the anterior tibiofibular ligament. Stage III: A high short oblique fracture of the fibula. Stage IV: A posterior lip fracture of the tibia. **D:** The pronation–abduction fracture. Stage I: Avulsion of the medial malleolus or ruptured deltoid ligament. Stage II: Rupture or avulsion of the syndesmotic ligaments. Stage III: A short, oblique fracture of the distal fibula at about the level of the ankle joint. (From Weber MJ. Ankle fractures and dislocations. In: Chapman MW, Madison M, eds. *Operative Orthopaedics.* 2nd ed. JB Lippincott; 1993:731-745, with permission.)

The Danis–Weber or AO Association of Osteosynthesis classification system concentrates on the pattern of the fibular fracture (Fig. 27-4). Type A fracture is distal to the level of the syndesmosis and frequently transverse, type B fracture is a spiral oblique fracture at the level of the syndesmosis, and type C fracture is proximal to the syndesmosis level.

**B. Examination.** The ankle has to be palpated for tender areas. The Ottawa criteria (Table 27-1) for the evaluation and management of ankle injuries have been proven to be a practical way to approach these injuries. One study found a sensitivity of 99.6% for detecting fractures.[4] However, in spite of

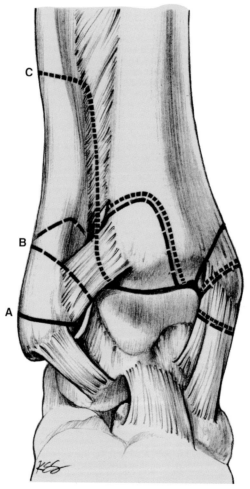

**Figure 27-4.** Diagrammatic representation of the Danis–Weber classification system. **A:** Transverse fracture of the distal malleolus. **B:** Spiral fracture at the level of the mortise. **C:** Fractures above the mortise with disruption of the syndesmosis. (From Hansen ST, Swiontkowski MF. *Orthopaedic Trauma Protocols.* Raven; 1993, with permission.)

these reports, it does not seem to be used routinely for fear of missing ankle fractures and the potential legal consequences associated with it. The lack of soft-tissue swelling in some situations may be misleading, especially in the elderly population.

C. **Radiographs.** AP, lateral, and oblique (the mortise view) films are essential for evaluating any ankle injury. A clearer delineation of the medial malleolar fracture may be achieved by an additional view obtained with the foot in 45° of internal rotation. A lateral radiograph obtained at 50° of external rotation is the best way to visualize the posterior malleolus.[5]

D. **Treatment.** The main feature that determines the treatment plan is whether the ankle fracture is a stable or unstable injury.

1. **Stable injuries.** A stable ankle fracture is defined as one that presents with no widening of the medial or lateral mortise joint space. A fracture distal to the syndesmosis with a ruptured deltoid ligament, which is suspected if there is significant medial tenderness, will represent an unstable ankle fracture with a stable syndesmosis. Therefore, the definition of stability should be an ankle joint where the fracture is distal to the syndesmosis with no injury to the medial stabilizers and consequently with no widening of the medial mortise. The immediate treatment consists of elevation, reduction of the fracture, and immobilization as soon as possible to reduce soft-tissue swelling. If the fracture is merely a small avulsion off of the distal tip of the fibula without any involvement of the mortise, treatment can be similar to a ligament sprain. For stable fractures that are larger and with minimal displacement, a closed reduction maneuver can be attempted. For most oblique fractures of the fibula, the reduction is via plantar flexion and internal rotation. This can often be achieved by lifting the patient's limb (with the patient in the supine position) by the great toe. Immobilize the patient's leg in a short-leg splint in this position. For long-term treatment (more than 4 to 6 weeks), the ankle must be maintained in a neutral position (90° from the long axis of the lower leg) to prevent any Achilles contracture and a longer than expected recovery time. The patient should be instructed in toe-touch weight bearing until there are radiographic signs of callus and lack of tenderness to pressure over the lateral malleolus (around 6 to 8 weeks). Do not be misled by the patient with peripheral neuropathy and his/her inability to feel pain and protect the ankle. In those situations, extend by two times the regular timelines for recovery from an injury. The acceptable amount of fracture displacement continues to decrease as more reports are coming out with less than ideal long-term outcomes for ankle fractures treated by nonsurgical means.

2. **Unstable injuries**

   a. These fractures should be reduced and internally fixed as an urgent procedure if the patient is seen **before significant swelling is apparent**.[7,8] Prophylactic preoperative antibiotics should be utilized.[9] Preoperative planning is essential to minimize soft-tissue stripping and maximize fixation. Patients with open fractures should be managed with wound debridement and internal fixation; the results are generally equivalent to those for closed fractures.[10] Significant improvement can be expected to continue 6 to 12 months after the fracture occurred.[11,12]

      i. **Medial malleolar fragments** should be reattached with screws for larger fragments and with Kirschner wires with supplemental tension band wires for smaller fragments. With screw fixation, a length of 40 to 50 mm is appropriate so that the metaphyseal bone is engaged and the medullary canal is avoided where there is no purchase of the screws. The rate of nonunion with surgical treatment is reported to be as low as 1% compared with 15% with conservative treatment.[13]

ii. **Posterior malleolar fragments** are stabilized with screw fixation if they involve more than one-fourth of the articular surface. Generally, these fragments are reduced by reduction of the associated distal fibula fracture. The lag screw placement can be done from the anterior to posterior direction (frequently percutaneously). Formal open reduction, if required, must be done before definitive fixation of the lateral malleolus, which may limit the surgical exposure; the incision must be well posterior to the fibula. This generally requires alternative patient positioning to the usual supine position.

iii. **Lateral malleolar fractures** below the ankle joint (Danis–Weber A) may be reduced as medial malleolar fractures. If possible, an attempt should first be made to reduce and fix the fracture with a lag screw. Spiral or oblique fractures with the tibiofibular ligament intact may be fixed by oblique lag screws and/or with a small, one-third tubular plate. Repair to the deltoid ligament avulsion is generally not necessary.[17] Postoperatively, the leg may be treated in a short-leg compression dressing with a plaster or fiberglass splint to control the position of the foot. As soon as the swelling is controlled, at 5 to 7 days, a removable splint can be used and early active motion started. The patient could be weight bearing as tolerated after surgery in the absence of peripheral neuropathy. If the patient is unable to cooperate with the early active range-of-motion protocol or has any degree of peripheral neuropathy, then a short-leg cast is applied for 4 to 6 weeks.[18,19] Weight bearing and strengthening exercises are initiated after 10 to 12 weeks.

iv. **If the tibiofibular syndesmosis is widened**, it is because the distal tibiofibular ligaments are torn. This injury can be associated with a proximal fibula fracture (the Maisonneuve fracture). The recent design of the TightRope (Arthrex) has changed the approach of syndesmosis instability. Its advantages include lack of subsequent surgeries for removal of the device and likely a more physiologic motion of the syndesmosis. The protocol for healing the syndesmosis should not change because of using a different device. If not available, screws should be utilized for fixation of the syndesmosis. Currently, there is no consensus on the number of screws, or number of cortices to purchase, or the timing for screw removal. The authors have seen many more problems following early removal of the syndesmosis screws than from broken screws; therefore, it is recommended to leave them in as weight bearing is progressed. The patient should be advised that the screws may break.

b. **When swelling is already significant**, any gross malalignment should be corrected. Then the leg should be placed in a compression dressing with splints and elevated until the swelling has receded sufficiently for a safe open reduction. To avoid wound healing complications, patients should be seen and surgically treated as soon after the injury as possible.[7] The operative complication rates are four times higher for diabetic[20,21] and obese patients managed operatively.[22]

## E. Complications

1. **Incomplete reduction** is associated with a higher incidence of ankle joint symptoms than are seen when anatomic restitution is achieved. This situation can be improved by osteotomy and internal fixation even years after the fracture occurs.[23] The results after restoring the original anatomy with delayed reconstruction overall are worse than those with early anatomic reduction.[13]

2. **Nonunion, although** rare, can occur and is usually symptomatic. On the medial side, it may be associated with interposition of the posterior tibial tendon or a flap of periosteum. Nonunion of either malleoli should be managed with internal fixation and bone grafting. Deep infection as the cause for the nonunion has to always be evaluated with intraoperative cultures, especially after prior open reduction and internal fixation.

## III. Pilon Fractures

Fractures of the articular surface of the tibia are generally high-energy injuries from axial loads. They occur as a result of high-speed motor vehicle accidents or falls from a height.[24]

A. **Diagnosis** is confirmed by radiographs, as for ankle fractures. The history of high-energy trauma or fall from a significant height should prompt a thorough examination of the heel, foot, and ankle, paying special attention to swelling and tenderness. If the plain radiographs do not sufficiently document the fracture pattern, a computed tomographic (CT) scan is indicated to better delineate the size and location of the bony fragments. This is helpful for planning surgical approaches as well.

B. **Treatment.** Fractures of the joint surface with more than 2 to 3 mm of displacement, either gapping or impaction, are generally managed by open reduction and internal fixation, and in some occasions with bone grafting. Significant swelling of the soft tissues occurs very rapidly with this type of injuries; therefore, operative management must be emergent or otherwise delayed for several days or weeks until the swelling subsides. Plating of an associated fibula fracture, application of an external fixator across the ankle joint, and a calcaneal pin traction on a Bohler frame are valid options in the interim to achieve indirect reduction of the joint fragments and expedite the resolution of the soft-tissue swelling. All those options limit the amount of soft-tissue stripping required in subsequent surgeries that will help to achieve bony consolidation and to decrease the potential complications. Acute compartment syndromes are not uncommon with pilon fractures. If open fasciotomy is performed, the fibula should be plated to restore some stability to the fracture. Because of the high incidence of wound complications and deep infections, there is a trend toward limited fracture exposure, indirect reduction and fixation of the joint surface with lag screws, and complete definitive treatment with an external fixator or percutaneous plates. Bone grafting may not be required if the fracture is not exposed, but it should be carried out if there is any doubt.

C. **Complications.** Deep infection may require multiple debridements, hardware removal, and muscle-flap (often free) coverage.[24] If the problem is identified early, the hardware can be generally left in place while antibiotics are administered. Pilon fractures are associated with a very high rate of complications, and their management should ideally be left to a specialist familiar with this type of injury. In some occasions, the long-term result is a stiff, painful, and chronically swollen ankle that at some point may require an ankle arthrodesis to improve the function and symptoms of the patient.

## IV. Achilles Tendon (Tendo Calcaneus) Ruptures

A. The **history** associated with an Achilles tendon rupture is often diagnostic. The patient profile is a middle-aged individual occasionally involved in recreational sports, also known as "the weekend warrior." Patients with a different profile are worth evaluating for risk factors (i.e., steroid use) because this pathology is fairly unusual in a young healthy individual. It cannot be emphasized enough that a healthy tendon will not rupture during exercise. However, unhealthy tendons do not necessarily cause symptoms. Usually, the patient was running or jumping when a sudden severe pain was felt behind the ankle, almost as if it had been struck by something. Patients will describe the episode as being "… kicked by somebody, I turned around, and there was nobody there …" or being hit by a rock or the opponent's racquet. Afterward, the patient may be able to walk but usually with difficulty.

**B. Examination** is most easily accomplished with the patient prone. By inspection and palpation, the defect in the Achilles tendon can be documented. Squeezing the calf will reproduce plantar flexion of the foot. In the presence of an Achilles tendon rupture, there will be no plantar flexion with squeezing the calf musculature (Thompson test). Even if the plantar flexion is present but decreased, the diagnosis of Achilles tendon rupture can be made. Do not be misled by the patient's ability to plantar-flex the ankle actively because this can be done with the muscles from the deep posterior compartment of the lower leg. Neurovascular examination is normally intact. In case of doubt, depending on the expertise of the radiology department, an ultrasound will be definitive to demonstrate a gap within the tendon fibers. If ultrasound is not available, an MRI will be diagnostic. The treatment guidelines are the same for either a partial or a complete rupture and are more dependent on the patient's profile.

**C. Treatment**

1. Patients with low functional demands may undergo **nonoperative treatment**. The foot is held in equinus for 6 weeks in a short-leg cast. It is extremely important not to force the plantar flexion excessively as the posterior aspect of the most distal part of the lower leg may develop skin necrosis from lack of blood supply. This can be easily demonstrated by the blanching of the skin that takes place with forced plantar flexion. The acute swelling also decreases the tolerance of the skin to plantar flexion. The position chosen for immobilization cannot compromise the posterior skin, and normal color has to be seen along the posterior aspect of the leg. Ambulation using an elevated heel on the shoe for 8 to 12 weeks then follows. Finally, rehabilitation exercises are begun to increase strength and range of motion.

2. **Operative treatment** is often recommended, especially for the young, competitive athlete. The advantages of open treatment are that the proper strength–length relationship of the musculotendinous unit is reestablished, the internal repair probably adds extra strength to the ruptured tendon, and immobilization can be limited. The risk of rerupture of the tendon is lower with operative management.[25] The incision should be made to one side of the tendon (not directly posteriorly) and should not extend distally into the flexor creases posterior to the ankle; this helps minimize adhesions of the tendon to the skin. A careful repair of the tendon sheath also limits these adhesions. The actual type of tendon repair is left to the discretion of the surgeon; numerous materials and patterns of suture repair have been created. The plantaris tendon or the flexor hallucis longus tendon transfer may be used to augment the repair. Postoperatively, the ankle is kept in a slight equinus position with a short-leg cast or boot for 6 weeks. Ambulation and physical therapy are then allowed as tolerated to increase strength and range of motion. Recent publications document no functional outcome differences between operative and nonoperative treatments.[26]

**D. Complications.** The rate of complications with either treatment, conservative or surgical, is similar. The difference is the type of complications that occur. With conservative treatment, the most common complications include rerupture and weakness of the Achilles complex with plantar flexion. The weakness is more noticeable during the practice of sports and very rarely during activities of daily living (ADLs). With surgical treatment, the complications are related to skin dehiscence/necrosis, neurologic damage, and infection. There are no good data to recommend either treatment based on the type of complications (Keating + Will). The final decision must be left to the patient once all the information is presented to him or her in an objective manner.

## REFERENCES

1. Lewis JE, Marymont JV. Ankle arthroscopy and sports-related injuries. In: Mizel MS, Miller RA, Scioli MW, eds. *Orthopaedic Knowledge Update, Foot and Ankle 2*. American Orthopaedic Foot and Ankle Society; 1998:39-54.
2. Jones CB, Gilde A, Sietsma DL. Treatment of syndesmotic injuries of the ankle. *JBJS Rev.* 2015;3:1-15.
3. Dalton GP. Fractures of the talus. In: Mizel MS, Miller RA, Scioli MW, eds. *Orthopaedic Knowledge Update, Foot and Ankle 2*. American Orthopaedic Foot and Ankle Society; 1998:39-54.
4. Bachmann LM, Kolb E, Koller MT, Steurer J, Riet G. Accuracy of Ottawa ankle rules to exclude fractures of the ankle and mid-foot: systematic review. *BMJ.* 2003;326(7386):417.
5. Ebraheim NA, Mekhail AO, Haman SP. External rotation-lateral view of the ankle in the assessment of the posterior malleolus. *Foot Ankle Int.* 1999;20:379-383.
6. Bauer M, Bergström B, Hemborg A, Sandegård J. Malleolar fractures: non-operative versus operative treatment: a controlled study. *Clin Orthop Relat Res.* 1985;(199):17-27.
7. Carragee EJ, Csongradi JJ, Bleck EE. Early complications in the operative treatment of ankle fractures. Influence of delay before operation. *J Bone Joint Surg Br.* 1991;73:79-82.
8. Phillips WA, Schwartz HS, Keller CS, et al. A prospective, randomized study of the management of severe ankle fractures. *J Bone Joint Surg Am.* 1985;67:67-78.
9. Paiement GD, Renaud E, Dagenais G, Gosselin RA. Double-blind randomized prospective study of efficacy of antibiotic prophylaxis for open reduction and internal fixation of closed ankle fractures. *J Orthop Trauma.* 1994;8:64-66.
10. Franklin JL, Johnson KD, Hansen ST Jr. Immediate internal fixation of open ankle fractures. Report of thirty-eight cases treated with a standard protocol. *J Bone Joint Surg Am.* 1984;66:1349-1356.
11. Belcher GL, Radomisli TE, Abate JA, et al. Functional outcome analysis of operatively treated malleolar fractures. *J Orthop Trauma.* 1997;11:106-109.
12. Ponzer S, Nåsell H, Bergman B, Törnkvist H, Stabile LA, Trafton PG. Functional outcome and quality of life in patients with type B ankle fractures: a two year follow-up study. *J Orthop Trauma.* 1999;13:363-368.
13. Donatto KC. Fractures of the ankle. In: Mizel MS, Miller RA, Scioli MW, eds. *Orthopaedic Knowledge Update, Foot and Ankle 2*. American Orthopaedic Foot and Ankle Society; 1998:39-54.
14. Winkler B, Weber BG, Simpson LA. The dorsal antiglide plate in the treatment of Danis-Weber type-B fractures of the distal fibula. *Clin Orthop Relat Res.* 1990;(259):204-209.
15. Böstman OM. Osteoarthritis of the ankle after foreign-body reaction to absorbable pins and screws: a three to nine year follow-up study. *J Bone Joint Surg Br.* 1998;80:333-338.
16. Dijkema AR, van der Elst M, Breederveld RS, Verspui G, Patka P, Haarman HJ. Surgical treatment of fracture-dislocations of the ankle joint with biodegradable implants: a prospective randomized study. *J Trauma.* 1993;34:82-84.
17. Strömsöe K, Höqevold HE, Skjeldal S, Alho A. The repair of a ruptured deltoid ligament is not necessary in ankle fractures. *J Bone Joint Surg Br.* 1995;77:920-921.
18. Hedström M, Ahl T, Dalén N. Early postoperative ankle exercise. A study of postoperative lateral malleolar fractures. *Clin Orthop Relat Res.* 1994;(300):193-196.
19. Søndenaa K, Høigaard U, Smith D, Alho A. Immobilization of operated ankle fractures. *Acta Orthop Scand.* 1986;57:59-61.
20. Flynn JM, Rodriguez-del Rio F, Pizá PA. Closed ankle fractures in the diabetic patient. *Foot Ankle Int.* 2000;21:311-319.
21. McCormack RG, Leith JM. Ankle fractures in diabetics: complications of surgical management. *J Bone Joint Surg Br.* 1998;80:689-692.
22. Böstman OM. Body-weight related to loss of reduction of fractures of the distal tibia and ankle. *J Bone Joint Surg Br.* 1995;77:101-103.
23. Marti RK, Raaymakers EL, Nolte PA. Malunited ankle fractures. The late results of reconstruction. *J Bone Joint Surg Br.* 1990;72:709-713.
24. Pollak AF, McCarthy ML, Shay BR, et al. Outcomes after treatment of high energy tibial plafond fractures. *J Bone Joint Surg Am.* 2003;85:1893-1900.
25. Guss D, Smith JT, Chiodo CP. Acute Achilles tendon rupture. *JBJS Rev.* 2015;4:1-6.
26. Keating JF, Will EM. Operative versus non-operative treatment of acute rupture of tendo-Achilles: a prospective randomised evaluation of functional outcome. *J Bone Joint Surg Br.* 2011;93:1071-1078.

## SELECTED HISTORICAL READINGS

Black HM, Brand RL, Eichelberger MR. An improved technique for the evaluation of ligamentous injury in severe ankle sprains. *Am J Sports Med*. 1978;6:276-282.

Brantigan JW, Pedegana LR, Lippert FG. Instability of the subtalar joints. Diagnosis by stress tomography in three cases. *J Bone Joint Surg Am*. 1977;59:321-324.

Goergen TG, Danzig LA, Resnick D, Owen CA. Roentgenographic evaluation of the tibiotalar joint. *J Bone Joint Surg Am*. 1977;59:874-877.

Jacobs D, Martens M, Van Audekercke R, Mulier JC, Mulier F. Comparison of conservative and operative treatment of Achilles tendon rupture. *Am J Sports Med*. 1978;6:107-111.

Mast JW, Spiegel PG, Pappas JN. Fractures of the tibialpilon. *Clin Orthop Relat Res*. 1988;(230):68-82.

Nistor L. Surgical and non-surgical repair of Achilles tendon rupture. A prospective randomized study. *J Bone Joint Surg Am*. 1981;63:394-399.

Ramsey P, Hamilton W. Changes in tibiotalar area of contact caused by lateral talar shift. *J Bone Joint Surg Am*. 1976;58:356-357.

Yablon IG, Heller FG, Shouse L. The key role of the lateral malleolus in displaced fractures of the ankle. *J Bone Joint Surg Am*. 1977;59:169-173.

# 28 Fractures and Dislocations of the Foot

Jessica M. Downes

## I. Talus Fractures

A. **Background.** Talus fractures are relatively rare; the true incidence is unknown but has been reported to be 0.1% to 2.5% of all fractures.[1]

B. **Mechanism.** These are generally high-energy injuries.[2] Talar neck fractures are believed to occur with hyperdorsiflexion of the ankle. The relatively weak talar neck impinges against the stronger bone of the anterior distal tibia and fractures.[1] Historically, this was called "aviator's astragalus" and was due to upward force of the foot plate when biplanes crashed.

C. **Examination.** In a displaced neck or body fractures, there is frequently significant pain, swelling, and deformity. Skin tenting or traumatic laceration may be present as 20% of talus fractures are open injuries.[1] A thorough neurovascular examination should be performed and documented, especially when deformity is present, both before and after any attempted reduction. Patients should be thoroughly evaluated for any associated injuries.

D. **Imaging.** Anteroposterior (AP), lateral, and mortise views of the ankle and AP, lateral and oblique views of the foot are required to adequately identify talar body, neck, head, and process fractures. A talar neck fracture is further evaluated with a Canale view. Computed tomography (CT) scans are helpful to look at fracture pattern and comminution displacement and to evaluate articular involvement.

E. **Classification.**

1. Orthopaedic Trauma Association (OTA): The talus is anatomically identified as body,[1] neck,[2] and head.[3] Head and body fractures are further classified based on fracture type: avulsion fractures (A), partial articular fractures (B), and complete articular fractures (C). Talus fractures can also be subclassified by location: dome, posterior process, and lateral process, with qualifications for fracture pattern simple versus multifragmentary.[3]

2. **Hawkins classification**[4] (Fig. 28-1). The Hawkins classification is the most popular system for describing talar neck fractures and is as follows:
Type I. Nondisplaced
Type II. Displaced fracture with subtalar subluxation/dislocation
Type III. Displaced fracture with subtalar and ankle subluxations/dislocations
Type IV. Displaced with subtalar, ankle, and talonavicular joint subluxations/dislocations

F. **Treatment.**

1. Urgent Reduction

a. **Fracture dislocations** should be urgently reduced on initial presentation to decrease the risk of skin compromise and osteonecrosis. For closed reduction, the knee of the affected limb should be flexed to relax the gastrocnemius muscle. The foot should be plantar flexed, and the deformity (usually inversion or eversion) should be exaggerated and then reversed to obtain reduction. Avoid repeated forceful reductions.[1] Irreducible injuries, as well as open injuries, should be considered surgical emergencies.

437

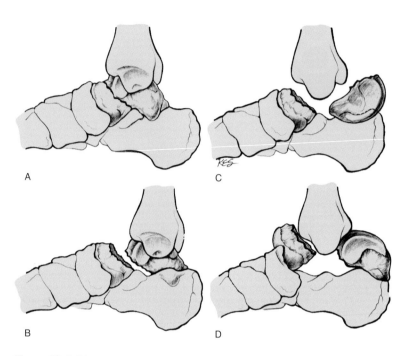

A

B

C

D

**Figure 28-1.** Diagrammatic representation of Hawkins classification of talar neck fractures. **A:** Nondisplaced. **B:** Displaced with associated subtalar joint subluxation. **C:** Talar body dislocated from the ankle mortise. **D:** Talonavicular joint subluxated. (From Hansen ST, Swiontkowski MF. *Orthopaedic Trauma Protocols.* Raven; 1993, with permission.)

  b. Partial **extrusion of the talus** without gross contamination should
     be cleaned with saline and reinserted. Treatment of complete extrusions with or without contamination and partial extrusions with gross
     contamination is controversial. Generally, before reimplantation, a
     5-minute chemical soak with 10% povidone-iodine or 4% chlorhexidine is recommended followed by a saline wash.[3]
        No studies demonstrate a direct correlation between time to reduction and development of avascular necrosis (AVN). However, most surgeons support an "urgent" reduction of displaced talar neck fractures.[2]
2. **Fixation**
   If resources allow, immediate open reduction and internal fixation (ORIF)
   can be performed. Reduction and splinting or temporarily stabilization
   with K wires with delayed definitive fixation, when the soft tissues allow, is also an option. Recent literature shows no significant difference
   in outcomes between emergent and delayed ORIF if the adjacent joints
   are reduced.[3]
   a. **Talar neck fractures** with any displacement require ORIF. This can be
      done through one or preferably two incisions. Fixation can be with either screws or minifragment plates or a combination. Plates are generally used where there is fracture comminution that renders the fracture
      pattern unstable for compression with lag screws.

b. **Talar head, body, and process fractures,** if nondisplaced, can be treated in a non–weight-bearing cast for 6 to 12 weeks or until healing is demonstrated. Displaced fractures (>2 mm) are generally treated with ORIF. Severely comminuted fractures (process or talar head) may also be treated with primary excision if the associated joint (subtalar or talonavicular) is stable.[1,5]

**G. Complications.**

1. **AVN** of the talus is the most devastating complication of talar fractures. The risk of AVN is highest in comminuted body fractures, followed by neck fractures (Type IV with the highest, Type I with the lowest risk).

2. **Posttraumatic arthritis** of the ankle, subtalar, or the talonavicular joint is the *most common* complication of talus fractures, with a 49% to 100% reported incidence rate.[1]

3. **Malunion** has been reported at a rate of 20% to 30%. Varus malunion due to medial fracture comminution is the most common, which predisposes patients to subtalar arthritis.[1]

4. **Nonunion** is rare and reported to occur in 3% to 5% of fractures.

5. **Skin complications and infections** can occur if treatment is delayed, in open injuries, and after surgical management.[1]

**II. Subtalar Dislocation**

A. **Background.** *Subtalar dislocation* is defined as combined dislocation through the talocalcaneal and talonavicular joints. These are uncommon injuries and make up less than 2% of all large joint dislocations. Seventy-five percent of these dislocations are medial, with only 1% to 2% of dislocations being anterior or posterior.[6]

B. **Mechanism.** These injuries generally result from high energy, such as motor vehicle collisions or a fall from a height. Medial dislocations result from a strong inversion force, whereas lateral dislocations result from strong eversion force. Recent literature reports up to 14% of these injuries occur due to sport.[6]

C. **Examination.** There is classic positioning of the foot medially or laterally in reference to the ankle with marked tenting of the skin observed on the side opposite of the foot. A complete neurovascular examination must be completed and documented before and after reduction attempts because the posterior tibial and sural nerves are potentially at risk.

D. **Imaging.** Radiographs to obtain include AP, lateral, and mortise of the ankle and AP, lateral, and oblique of the foot. A CT scan should be obtained postreduction to assess for associated fractures as these occur in 60% of cases.[6]

E. **Classification.** Described by the location of the foot in relation to the talus: medial, lateral, anterior, or posterior.

F. **Treatment.**

1. **Emergent reduction.** This requires adequate anesthesia. The knee should be flexed to take tension off the gastrocnemius muscle. Axial traction on the foot should then be applied. The deformity should be accentuated prior to reversal of the deformity to obtain reduction. If needed, direct pressure can be placed on the prominent talar head or lateral talar body to facilitate reduction.[6] In medial dislocations, reduction may be prevented by interposition of the extensor retinaculum or the extensor digitorum. In lateral dislocations, the posterior tibialis may become entrapped and block reduction.[6-9]

2. **Definitive management.** After reduction of the talus, if the joint is stable and no associated displaced fractures are noted, the patient can be treated in a non–weight-bearing cast or fracture boot for 4 to 6 weeks. Any associated displaced talus fracture should be treated with ORIF if the fragments are large enough to accept implants. In rare cases, the subtalar and talonavicular joints are unstable after reduction. In this setting, temporary

transarticular K wires or external fixation can be used to maintain the reduction. These implants are removed after 3 to 4 weeks.[6]

G. **Complications.** The most feared complication is **AVN**; the incidence is reported at 10% in closed dislocations and up to 50% in open dislocations. **Instability and recurrent dislocation** has been reported, although this is a rare complication and is associated with a duration of immobilization of less than 4 weeks.[6] **Neurovascular injury** is most commonly seen with lateral dislocations and affects the posteromedial neurovascular bundle. These are also seen when soft tissues are entrapped or with open injuries. **Skin necrosis and tendon injuries** have been reported, but these complications are rare. **Post-traumatic subtalar arthritis** is estimated at 40% to 89%. However, only one-third are symptomatic enough to require a fusion.[6]

III. **Calcaneus Fractures**

A. **Background.** Calcaneal fractures are the most common tarsal bone fracture, accounting 1% to 2% of all fractures. These injuries are economically significant, in that 90% of the injuries occur in working people aged 20 to 40 years. These are life-changing injuries, with few patients able to return to their prior level of function.

B. **Mechanism.**

1. **Intraarticular fractures** generally result from high energy, such as a fall from a height or a motor vehicle collision. The mechanism is generally an axial load injury. Associated injuries include compression fractures of the lumbar spine, occasionally fractures about the knee or pelvis, and peroneal tendon subluxation or dislocation.

2. **Avulsion fractures** are typically due to a sudden forceful contraction of the Achilles tendon, which causes a fracture through the posterior tuberosity of the calcaneus rather than a ruptured tendon.

3. **Anterior process** fractures are generally due to inversion of the plantar flexed foot.

C. **Examination.** Generally, the foot is diffusely swollen with lateral and plantar ecchymosis and widening of the heel. There is pain with palpation of the heel and with attempted hindfoot motion. There may also be pain with ankle or foot motion. In open fractures, the wound is most often medial. A complete neurovascular examination is mandatory. Foot compartment syndrome occurs in 2% to 5% of patients; decompression is controversial. Because of the risk of associated injuries, the spine, pelvis, and ipsilateral limb must be thoroughly evaluated.

D. **Imaging.** Initial radiographic evaluation for a suspected calcaneus fracture should include the standard three views of the foot as well as an axial (Harris) heel view. Fractures are identified on radiographs by a line of increased (impaction) or decreased bone density or general distortion of the normal shape of the calcaneus. There are several radiographic measurements that are used to describe calcaneus fractures (Fig. 28-2).

1. **Bohler's angle** is formed by the intersection of two lines: one drawn from the highest point of the anterior process to the highest point of the posterior facet and the second line drawn tangential to the superior aspect of the tuberosity. The angle is normally 25° to 40°. Angulation can also be compared with the uninjured side.

2. **Gissane's angle** is formed by the intersection of a line extending along the posterior facet and a line extending anteriorly to the anterior process. Normal values are 120° to 145°.

3. **Advanced imaging.** A CT scan is then utilized to further clarify the fracture pattern and assess the subtalar joint. Ankle films may be necessary to rule out concomitant injury. Given the association with pelvic and lumbar spine injuries, pelvic and lumbar spine imaging should be considered if there is any concern for injury on physical examination.

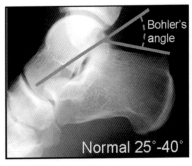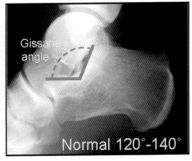

**Figure 28-2.** Bohler's angle and Gissane's angle as seen on the lateral calcaneal view.

**E. Classification.**

1. **Extraarticular fractures** do not involve the subtalar joint. These account for about 25% of all calcaneus fractures and include avulsion fractures (Fig. 28-3), anterior process fractures, and calcaneal body fractures.

2. **Intraarticular fractures** involve the subtalar joint and account for about 75% of all calcaneus fractures. Two main classifications systems for these fractures are as follows:

   a. **Essex-Lopresti** classification is based on radiographs (Fig. 28-4) and includes **tongue-type** fractures, which occur when the tuberosity is

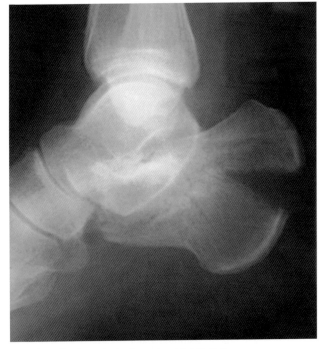

**Figure 28-3.** Lateral radiograph of calcaneal avulsion fracture.

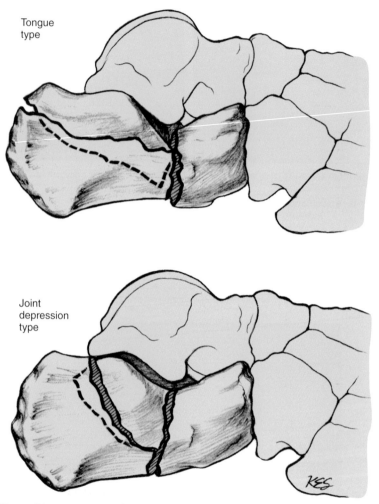

**Figure 28-4.** Diagrammatic representation of tongue-type and joint depression–type calcaneal fractures. (From Hansen ST, Swiontkowski MF. *Orthopaedic Trauma Protocols*. Raven; 1993, with permission.)

continuous with the articular surface. **Joint depression** fractures typically involve a medial sustentaculum fragment, an impacted posterior facet fragment(s), and a displaced lateral wall fragments under the fibula called "lateral wall blowout."

b. The **Sanders** classification is a CT-based classification describing the number and location of fracture lines extending into the posterior facet of the subtalar joint. This is the most commonly used classification because it is both descriptive and prognostic (Fig. 28-5).[10,11]

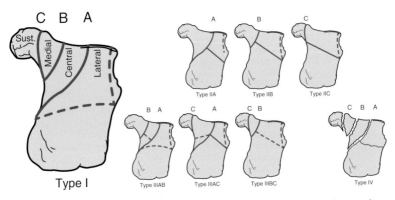

**Figure 28-5.** Schematic depiction of Sanders classification of intraarticular calcaneus fractures. Fracture lines **A-C** describe the position of the primary fracture line in relation to the posterior facet of the subtalar joint. (From Bucholz RW, Heckman JD. *Rockwood & Green's Fractures in Adults*. 5th ed. Lippincott, Williams & Wilkins; 2001, with permission.)

**F. Treatment.**

1. **Surgical urgencies/emergencies** include open fractures and displaced tongue-type and avulsion fractures. If large and displaced, the tuberosity can put pressure on the thin posterior heel skin, leading to skin ulceration and/or necrosis or development of an open fracture. Reduction and fixation is required to reattach the Achilles tendon and take pressure off the skin. This may be done with Steinman pins, screws, or suture anchors depending on the treating surgeon and bone stock. A gastrocnemius recession to take tension off the repair should be considered. Generally, the patient is placed in a well-padded splint postoperatively and transitioned to a cast in slight plantar flexion with non–weight bearing for a period of 6 to 12 weeks.

2. **Nonoperative treatment** is indicated in closed, nondisplaced fractures (all types) and closed, displaced fractures in patients who are poor operative candidates. Nondisplaced avulsion fractures should be splinted in plantar flexion with frequent follow-up and X-rays (XRs) to verify lack of displacement. Initial immobilization is in a well-padded, Robert Jones type splint until the swelling begins to resolve. Once soft tissues allow, transition to a short leg, non–weight-bearing cast for 4 to 6 weeks is allowed, followed by cam boot, range of motion exercises, and continued non–weight bearing for up to 12 weeks depending on fracture type.

3. **Operative treatment** should be considered for all displaced fractures.
   a. **Anterior process fractures**, if displaced and larger in size, may be treated with ORIF. Excision is also an option for comminuted fractures or nonunion.[5]
   b. **Body fractures**, if displaced and associated with heel shortening widening or varus, may be treated with ORIF or percutaneous screw fixation.
   c. **Intraarticular fractures**, reduction and internal fixation is generally recommended for displaced fractures with loss of Bohler's angle. Multiple small studies, including one randomized trial, have suggested better results following operative treatment.[11,12] This also facilitates future subtalar joint fusion if necessary.[13]

   Multiple techniques and approaches can be used to obtain reduction and place fixation, including percutaneous, sinus tarsi, and extensile lateral.

Generally, surgical approach and instrumentation choices are determined by patient and surgeon factors and fracture type. The most common early complication with ORIF is skin breakdown. Soft-tissue swelling must be subsided before surgery is performed, which may take 1 to 2 weeks.

d. **ORIF with primary fusion** combines restoration of calcaneal anatomy with subtalar fusion and may be an option for those fractures that are highly comminuted (Sanders 4), particularly in a patient who wants to limit potential time away from work.

G. **Complications.** There are many complications associated with calcaneus fractures, including fracture blisters, chronic pain related to heel pad injury, peroneal tendonitis, subfibular impingement, and sural neuritis. Peroneal tendon dislocation has a prevalence about 30% and is often missed at the time of injury. Subtalar stiffness and posttraumatic arthritis are the most common complications following calcaneus fractures. Patients who are treated nonoperatively may have increased heel width and difficulty with shoe wear. Wound healing complications and superficial and deep infections, including osteomyelitis, are potential complications for patients who are treated operatively.

IV. **Fractures of the Navicular and Cuboid**

A. **Background.** The navicular is the keystone of the medial longitudinal arch of the foot and articulates with the talus proximally and the cuneiforms distally. The cuboid maintains lateral column length. The cuboid and fourth and fifth metatarsal articulations provide three times the motion as the medial midfoot joints. Fractures of the navicular and cuboid are commonly associated with other midfoot injuries and, if not managed appropriately, can lead to long-term permanent deformity and dysfunction of the foot.[14,15]

B. **Mechanism.** Acute fractures of the navicular body and cuboid body are most commonly due to high-energy trauma. Acute axial load or dorsiflexion forces concentrated on the medial column will fracture the navicular. When the foot is plantar flexed and abducted forcefully, the cuboid can be crushed between the metatarsals and the calcaneus and fractured. Avulsion and tuberosity fractures of the navicular are generally due to low-energy twisting injuries.

C. **Examination.** High-energy injuries generally present with diffuse swelling and ecchymosis. Deformity and fracture blisters may be present. Displaced navicular fractures may cause dorsomedial skin tenting or fracture blisters. Tenderness will be present over the fracture site(s), and it is important to evaluate for associated midfoot injuries and foot compartment syndrome. A complete neurovascular examination is required.

D. **Imaging.** AP, oblique, and lateral views of the foot will identify most fractures. CT scans will help identify subtle injuries and amount of comminution for preoperative planning. Contralateral comparison views can be helpful in cuboid fractures to assess lateral column length.

E. **Classification.**

1. **Acute navicular fractures** are classified by fracture type and include avulsion, tuberosity, and body fractures. Os naviculare may be confused with a navicular fracture and must be differentiated with a careful physical examination (Fig. 28-6).

a. **Navicular** Body fractures have been further classified by Sangeorzan et al.[16] See figure 28-6. Type 1 fractures involve a dorsal fracture fragment that consists of less than 50% of the navicular. Type 2 fractures involve a medial fragment and are usually associated with dorsomedial talonavicular joint subluxation. Type 3 fractures are comminuted and associated with lateral cuneonavicular joint subluxation, cuboid fracture or anterior process of the calcaneus fracture.[16]

2. **Cuboid fractures** do not have a specific classification system; and they are described as intraarticular or extraarticular, displaced or nondisplaced, and avulsion or crush type injury.

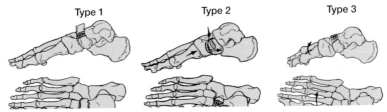

**Figure 28-6.** Diagrammatic representation of navicular body fracture classification. (From Sangeorzan BJ, Benirschke SK, Mosca V, et al. Displaced intra-articular fractures of the tarsal navicular. *J Bone Joint Surg Am.* 1989;71(10):1504-1510, permission pending.) (Left) Type 1, (center) Type 2, (Right) Type 3.

F. **Treatment.**
1. **Nonoperative** is indicated for avulsion fractures with immediate weight bearing in a cam boot. Nondisplaced body fractures are treated with immobilization in short leg cast or cam boot with non–weight bearing for 6 to 8 weeks. Serial radiographs are required to ensure no interval displacement.
2. **Operative treatment** should be considered for navicular or cuboid fractures with more than 2 mm of column shortening, joint line incongruity or displacement of more than 1 to 2 mm, associated midfoot injuries, or irreducible dislocations. Surgical treatment usually consists of ORIF using either screws or minifragment plates. Fractures with severe comminution can be treated with external fixation, transarticular K wires, or bridge plates. Severely comminuted navicular fractures could also be indicated for primary medial column fusion.[14,15]

G. **Complications.** Posttraumatic arthritis and malunion are potential complications. If there is malunion of the navicular, it can lead to medial column shortening and varus foot deformity. Cuboid nonunion can lead to lateral column shortening and pes planovalgus deformity.

V. **Tarsometatarsal Joint Injuries**
A. **Background.** These injuries occur where the metatarsal bones articulate with the cuneiforms and cuboid. Lisfranc is the common term for these injuries, named after a French surgeon in Napoleon's army who amputated the foot at this location. Up to 20% of these injuries may be missed initially, so a high index of suspicion is warranted.[17,18]
B. **Mechanism.** Generally, these are due to high-energy injuries when an axial load is applied to the plantar flexed foot, such as falls from height or motor vehicle accidents. This is increasingly seen in athletes as well. The classic example is a football lineman having someone fall on his planted foot (where the ball of the foot is on the ground and the heel off the ground).
C. **Examination.** The patient is usually point tender or diffusely tender across the tarsometatarsal (TMT) joints. Plantar ecchymosis is classic in this injury. The patient will have pain with forefoot dorsiflexion and abduction, TMT compression, and with the abduction-pronation test.[15]
D. **Imaging.** AP, lateral, and oblique views of the foot are generally diagnostic for widening at the base of the metatarsals, fleck sign (avulsion of the Lisfranc ligament from the base of the second metatarsal), or subluxation of the TMT joint complex. If injury is suspected, but is not obvious on non–weight-bearing films, bilateral weight-bearing AP films can help make the diagnosis. If weight-bearing films are not possible due to pain, stress views may be obtained under anesthesia.

In a normal AP radiograph, the medial border of the second metatarsal lines up with the medial border of the middle cuneiform (Fig. 28-7). On the

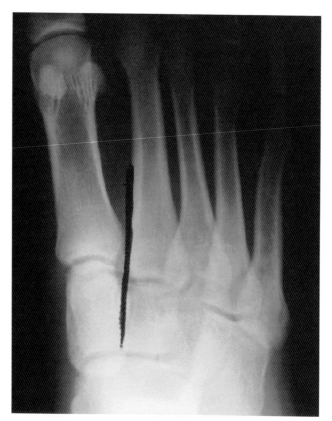

**Figure 28-7.** Anteroposterior radiograph of foot.

oblique, the medial border of the fourth metatarsal lines up with the medial border of the cuboid (Fig. 28-8). For those with a Lisfranc joint injury, the metatarsals most commonly appear displaced to the fibular side of the foot. For a suspected injury with unclear XRs, a CT scan or magnetic resonance imaging (MRI) can be helpful in identifying the injury.

E. **Classification.** This is described based on the type of displacement see (Fig. 28-9).

F. **Treatment.**
  1. **Initial mangement:** Reduction of gross dislocation/displacement should be obtained acutely. If the foot is grossly unstable, pinning may be necessary for temporary reduction until soft tissues allow definitive treatment.
  2. **Definitive management:** Any displaced injuries should be treated with anatomic reduction and fixation. Primary fusion of the involved joints is another alternative and has been shown in one randomized study to give better outcomes in purely ligamentous injuries.[19]

G. **Complications.** Massive swelling, skin necrosis, and foot compartment syndrome can occur in high-energy injuries. Posttraumatic arthritis is common, as well as recurrent instability after nonoperative management or ORIF. Malalignment and deformity can also lead to midfoot arthritis.

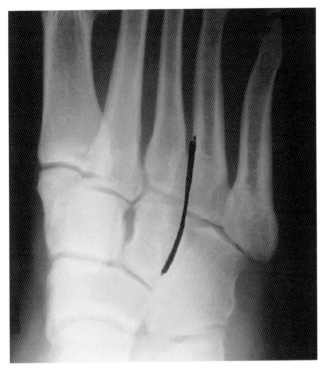

**Figure 28-8.** Oblique radiograph of foot.

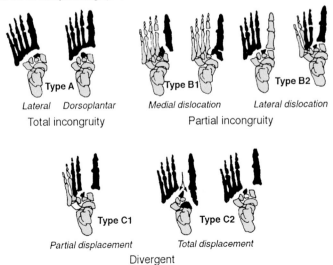

**Figure 28-9.** Myerson classification of Lisfranc fracture–dislocations. (From Myerson MS, Fisher RT, Burgess AR, et al. Fracture-dislocations of the tarsometatarsal joints: end results correlated with pathology and treatment. *Foot Ankle.* 1986;6:225-242, with permission.)

## VI. Metatarsal Fractures

A. **Background.** Metatarsal fractures are very common, accounting 5% of all skeletal fractures and 35% of all foot fractures.[20] The fifth metatarsal is most commonly fractured. Proximal metatarsal fractures are commonly associated with TMT joint injuries. It is useful to divide the forefoot into columns medial (first metatarsal), central, and lateral (fifth metatarsal) when thinking about treatment of metatarsal fractures.

B. **Mechanism.** Metatarsal fractures can be due to direct trauma such as a crush injury or indirect such as rotational injuries or fall from a height. Axial loading and twisting can also lead to metatarsal fracture. Fifth metatarsal avulsion fractures are associated with inversion and plantar flexion injuries resulting from both peroneal contraction and the lateral band of the plantar fascia.

C. **Examination.** The foot is generally point tender and swollen overlying the fracture site. In crush injuries, there will be severe swelling and ecchymosis. Fracture blisters may also be present. Crush injuries can also lead to compartment syndrome.

D. **Imaging.** AP, lateral, and oblique views of the foot diagnose these injuries. CT scans are helpful to evaluate fracture impaction, deformity, and associated injuries.

E. **Classification.** Fractures are described based on their location: head, neck, shaft, or base. Fifth metatarsal fractures are further divided into tuberosity fractures, Jones fractures, and diaphyseal shaft fractures. Tuberosity fractures occur at the very base of the fifth metatarsal and proximal to the fourth to fifth metatarsal articulation. Jones fractures occur at the junction of the metaphysis and diaphysis, which is at the level of the fourth to fifth metatarsal articulation. Diaphyseal shaft fractures occur distal to this.

F. **Treatment.**

1. **First metatarsal fractures**, given their importance in weight bearing, are often treated operatively when any significant angulation, translation, shortening, or instability is present. Operative treatment is generally with buttress plating and screw fixation. Truly nondisplaced first metatarsal fractures can be treated with immobilization and non–weight bearing with serial radiographs. Weight bearing can be initiated when there is radiographic evidence of healing.[20]

2. **Central (second through fourth) metatarsal shaft fractures** that are nondisplaced can generally be treated with a hard-soled shoe and weight bearing as tolerated. If there is significant angulation greater than 10°, plantar displacement, or 3 to 4 mm of translation in any plane, closed or open reduction and fixation should be considered.[20]

3. **Fifth metatarsal fracture** treatment depends on the location within the metatarsal.

   a. **Tuberosity Avulsion fractures** of the fifth metatarsal base can generally be treated nonsurgically with weight bearing as tolerated in a post-op shoe or boot. Tuberosity fractures tend to heal slow and are often asymptomatic before radiographic signs of healing. The ankle should be immobilized to prevent displacing forces of the peroneus brevis tendon on the tuberosity unit radiographic signs of healing or when the patient is asymptomatic.

   If the tuberosity fracture fragment is large and significantly displaced (more than 3 to 4 mm) or involves over 30% of the fifth TMT joint, it may be treated with ORIF.[20]

   b. **Jones fractures** have a high propensity to delayed union and nonunion, given the poor vascular supply to this area of the bone. These can be treated either in a short leg non–weight-bearing cast for 10 to 12 weeks in low-demand patients or with intramedullary screw fixation and early weight bearing in high-demand patients.

    c. **Diaphyseal fractures** can often be treated like central metatarsal fractures with a hard-soled shoe or fracture boot and non–weight bearing for 4 to 5 weeks followed by protected weight bearing for another 4 weeks.[20] If there is displacement greater than 3 to 4 mm and angulation greater than 10°, then ORIF should be performed typically with minifragment plates.

  4. **Metatarsal neck fractures** should be grossly aligned to prevent plantar prominence. If plane films cannot distinguish amount of plantar angulation, a CT scan should be obtained. If multiple fractures are present or significant displacement/angulation is present, percutaneous pinning may be considered.

**G. Complications.** Metatarsalgia can occur with shortening or plantar angulation of shaft or neck fractures. Posttraumatic arthritis can also develop from significant malunion. Nonunion can be seen in Jones fractures. It is rare with other metatarsal fractures. Adjacent nerves in the forefoot can be damaged with metatarsal fractures because of displacement or operative treatment.[20]

**VII. Toe Fractures and Dislocations**

**A. General.** Toe fractures and dislocations are common injuries, with an incidence of 140 cases per 100,000 people per year.[21]

**B. Mechanism.** These injuries frequently occur by "stubbing" the toes against hard objects or axial loading mechanisms. Most commonly, the hallux is affected by a hyperdorsiflexion injury and the fifth toe via an abduction mechanism.

**C. Examination.** Patients usually present with swelling, ecchymosis, and pain over the affected digit. Deformity may be present with dislocations or fracture dislocations. Nail plate, bed, and eponychial injuries can be associated with distal phalanx fractures and, if present, are likely open fractures and should be treated as such.

**D. Imaging.** AP, oblique, and lateral foot views should be obtained to diagnose fractures and dislocations and to evaluate for associated injuries. Isolated lateral XRs of the injured toe may be required to accurately evaluate sagittal plane displacement or deformity.[21]

**E. Treatment.**

  1. **Nondisplaced and minimally displaced phalangeal fractures** are generally treated by taping them to the adjacent toe ("buddy taping"), which acts as a splint. Avoid maceration using dry cotton or Webril between the toes. Buddy tapping for 4 weeks with weight bearing in a hard-soled, wide toe box shoe is adequate treatment for most lesser toe fractures.

  2. Closed reduction is recommended If there is **unacceptable fracture alignment** (significant rotation, angulation, and translation) that will cause impingement or instability with ambulation, closed reduction should be attempted with digital block and typical reduction maneuvers. A pencil in the web space can be useful as a fulcrum to reduce proximal phalanx fractures. **Interphalangeal and metatarsophalangeal joint dislocations** should also have closed reduction under digital block attempted.

  3. **Phalangeal fractures** with unacceptable alignment and **irreducible interphalangeal dislocations and metatarsophalangeal joint dislocations** are indicated for operative treatment, with closed or open reduction and pinning versus ORIF with minifragment screws. Approach for reduction, and fixation type, is dependent on patient- and injury-specific factors. In severely comminuted intraarticular lesser toe phalanx fractures, resection arthroplasty may be a viable treatment option.

  4. **Great toe fractures** are generally treated more aggressively than lesser toe fractures owing to the role of the hallux in gait. Nondisplaced fractures

may be treated with either a boot, cast, or stiff-soled shoe for 6 weeks with serial radiographs. Hallux fractures with displacement more than 1 to 2 mm, angulation more than 5° to 10°, and intraarticular fractures should be considered for ORIF with pins or minifragment screws and plates or a combination, to maintain a plantigrade foot and functional hallux.

5. **Dislocation of the hallux interphalangeal or metatarsophalangeal joints** requires urgent reduction. If irreducible, tendon, capsule, plantar plate, or sesamoid fragment may be interposed and require an open reduction, repair of injured structure, and stabilization with transarticular pins.[21]

## VIII. Sesamoid Fractures

A. **General.** The sesamoids and the capsuloligamentous complex they are encased in is a highly specialized structure. The two sesamoids of the great toe include the medial (tibial) and the lateral (fibular) sesamoids. The sesamoids are bones that are embedded within a capsuloligamentous complex that acts as a pulley to help increase the ability of the tendons to transmit muscles forces.

Injury to the sesamoids and the surrounding soft tissues can lead to significant long-term dysfunction if not treated appropriately. Bipartite sesamoids are present in 10% of the population.[21]

B. **Mechanism.** Acute fractures are usually the result of either a direct force or a forceful hyperextension of the great toe.

C. **Examination.** These injuries usually present with pain on the plantar aspect of the hallux and on palpation of the sesamoids. Patients generally cannot bear weight on the medial ray. Plantar ecchymosis may be present.

D. **Imaging.** AP, medial, and lateral oblique views and an axial view of the sesamoids help identify fractures. Occasionally, advanced imaging with a CT or MRI is indicated in occult fractures or if there is concern for associated soft-tissue injury.

E. **Treatment.** Generally, treatment is symptomatic with protected weight bearing in a stiff-soled shoe or boot until pain free. Metatarsal pad or an orthosis with sesamoid cut-out may help symptoms after an initial period of immobilization. If painful or displaced, these fractures may need bone grafting to promote healing and minifragment screw fixation or partial or complete resection with meticulous soft-tissue reconstruction.[21]

## REFERENCES

1. Buza J, Leucht P. Fractures of the talus: current concepts and new developments. *Foot Ankle Surg.* 2018;24(4):282-290.
2. Ahmad J, Raikin SM. Current concepts review: talus fractures. *Foot Ankle Int.* 2006;27(6):475-482.
3. Grear B. Review of talus fractures and surgical timing. *Orthop Clin North Am.* 2016;47:625-637.
4. Hawkins LG. Fractures of the talus. *J Bone Joint Surg Am.* 1970;52:991-1002.
5. Berkowitz MJ, Kim DH. Process and tubercle fractures of the hindfoot. *J Am Acad Orthop Surg.* 2005;13(8):492-502.
6. Rammelt S, Goronzy J. Subtalar dislocations. *Foot Ankle Clin.* 2015;20(2):253-264.
7. DeLee JC, Curtis R. Subtalar dislocation of the foot. *J Bone Joint Surg Am.* 1982;64:433-437.
8. Monson ST, Ryan JR. Subtalar dislocations. *J Bone Joint Surg Am.* 1981;63:1156-1158.
9. Jungbluth P, Wild M, Hakimi M, et al. Isolated subtalar dislocation. *J Bone Joint Surg Am.* 2010;92:890-894.
10. Sanders R, Fortin P, DiPasquale T, et al. Operative treatment in 120 displaced intraarticular calcaneal fractures. Results using a prognostic computed tomography scan classification. *Clin Orthop Relat Res.* 1993;290:87-95.
11. Sanders R. Current concepts review—displaced intra-articular fractures of the calcaneus. *J Bone Joint Surg Am.* 2000;82:225-250.

12. Thordarson DB, Krieger LE. Operative vs. nonoperative treatment of intra-articular fractures of the calcaneus: a prospective randomized trial. *Foot Ankle Int*. 1996;17:2-9.
13. Radnay CS, Clare MP, Sanders RW. Subtalar fusion after displaced intra-articular calcaneal fractures: does initial operative treatment matter? *J Bone Joint Surg Am*. 2009;91:541-546.
14. Clements JR, Dijour F, Leong W. Surgical management navicular and cuboid fractures. *Clin Podiatr Med Surg*. 2018;35:145-149.
15. Ahmed A, Westrick E. Management of midfoot fractures and dislocations. *Curr Rev Musculoskelet Med*. 2018;11:529-536.
16. Sangeorzan BJ, Benirschke SK, Mosca V, Mayo KA, Hansen ST Jr. Displaced intra-articular fractures of the tarsal navicular. *J Bone Joint Surg Am*. 1989;71(10);1504-1510.
17. Watson TS, Shurnas PS, Denker J. Treatment of Lisfranc joint injury: current concepts. *J Am Acad Orthop Surg*. 2010;18:718-728.
18. Desmond EA, Chou LB. Current concepts review: Lisfranc injuries. *Foot Ankle Int*. 2006;27(8):653-660.
19. Ly TV, Coetzee JC. Treatment of primarily ligamentous Lisfranc joint injuries: primary arthrodesis compared with open reduction and internal fixation. A prospective, randomized study. *J Bone Joint Surg Am*. 2006;88:514-520.
20. Buddecke DE, Polk MA, Barp EA. Metatarsal fractures. *Clin Podiatr Med Surg*. 2010;27:601-624.
21. Mittlmeier T, Haar P. Sesamoid and toe fractures. *Injury*. 2004;35:SB87-SB97.

# 29 Overuse and Miscellaneous Conditions of the Foot and Ankle

Fernando A. Pena and James W. Mazzuca

## I. Achilles Tendinopathy

Achilles tendinopathy encompasses both inflammation and degeneration if present in the peritenon or tendon area.

**A. Insertional** type may be associated with a Haglund's deformity (a bump on the lateral side of the heel) or retrocalcaneal bursitis. This is a typical overuse injury caused by accumulated impact load,[1] which occurs most often in runners and repetitive jumpers. Insertional type occurs more often in an older age group than does noninsertional tendinopathy.

1. **Treatment** will be **nonsurgical** in 95% of cases. Rest, analgesics, cross-training, physiotherapy, orthotics with a heel lift, and, occasionally, casting could all be used. Steroid injections are very seldom indicated.[2,3]

2. **Surgery** is indicated after 6 to 12 months of failed conservative treatment. It should address the following: excise retrocalcaneal bursa, resect superior calcaneal prominence, and debride the diseased or calcified portion of the tendon. Reattach if necessary. The patient should be non–weight bearing for 6 to 8 weeks. Rehabilitation is resumed, but recovery might take up to 1 year. Success rate is 70% to 86%.[4]

**B. Noninsertional** type is very frequently related to the hypovascular zone of the Achilles tendon 2 to 6 cm proximal to its insertion. The most common profile includes repetitive microtrauma, males, older athletes, tight gastrocsoleus complex and hamstrings, and functional overpronation. Extrinsic factors include improper training, improper shoe wear, systemic or injected steroids, and fluoroquinolone antibiotics.[5] There are various classification systems that can be simplified into peritendinitis (sheath only), tendinosis (tendon only), or pantendinitis (sheath and tendon).[6] Diagnosis is primarily by history and clinical evaluation and is confirmed by ultrasound (operator dependent) or magnetic resonance imaging (MRI). Typical signs and symptoms are morning stiffness or pain, start-up pain, postexercise pain, and tendon fullness or the presence of a nodule.

1. **Treatment** in **acute** situations includes pain relief, analgesics, ice, and restriction of activities. A heel lift or boot brace can be used until symptoms subside,[2] followed by a rehabilitation program.[7] Other measures include stretching and strengthening of the Achilles and gastrocsoleus complex, eccentric muscle–tendon strengthening review, modification of training regimens (reduce frequency, duration, and intensity and focus on low-impact activities), correction of structural abnormalities (overpronation), and modifications in footwear. Treatment is 90% to 95% successful, but it usually takes 2 to 6 months to recover from an Achilles tendinopathy.

2. **Treatment** of **chronic** cases (>3 months) depends on severity. Peritendinitis is treated with mechanical "brisement" or surgical debridement followed by an early rehabilitation program.[7] Chronic pantendinitis is treated with debridement, longitudinal tenotomy,[8] or tendon transfer depending on the clinical situation. It appears from the literature that surgical treatment of chronic tendinitis may have better outcomes than nonoperative treatment.

## II. Plantar Heel Pain

Plantar heel pain is a common foot problem. This can be especially true in the athlete. Running and jumping place repetitive stress on the heel and create an overuse syndrome with chronic inflammation. The heel spur seen on plain radiographs is seldom, if ever, the cause of heel pain.

A. **Differential diagnosis.** To differentiate, a thorough history and examination are required. This should include exact location and duration of pain and the relationship to ambulatory/athletic activity. Chronic pain at rest is unusual and might be due to a neoplasm. The differential diagnosis includes the following:

1. Plantar fasciitis—by far the most common reason for plantar heel pain
2. Nerve entrapment
3. Fat pad atrophy
4. Heel bruise
5. Tenosynovitis of flexor hallucis longus or flexor digitorum brevis
6. Stress fracture
7. Tumor

B. **Plantar fasciitis** could be at the insertion into the medial calcaneal tuberosity or midsubstance at the midfoot area and may be due to repetitive traction and microtears. Usually, plantar fasciitis has an insidious onset as an overuse condition in long-distance runners. Midfoot plantar fasciitis is more common in sprinters who run on their toes. Generally speaking, it has a better prognosis.

1. **Symptoms and signs** include pain during the first minutes of walking, especially when first getting out of bed. Pain may subside with low-intensity walking but then recur with prolonged or more vigorous activities.
2. Always evaluate for **leg length discrepancy**. Heel pain is more common in the shorter leg and may be treated with an appropriate lift. Also inquire about a functional short-leg syndrome from running on the same slope of the road. Plantar fasciitis is frequently caused by a shortened Achilles tendon because limited ankle dorsiflexion increases the stress on the plantar fascia. Fasciitis at the insertion has localized deep tenderness. It is usually associated with increased pain with passive dorsiflexion of the toes (windlass mechanism). Midfoot fasciitis has tenderness in midfoot and increased pain with passive dorsiflexion of the toes. Passive dorsiflexion of the big toe aggravates both plantar fasciitis and flexor hallucis longus tendinopathy. Resisted flexion of the big toe is painful only with involvement of the tendon.

C. **Treatment**

1. **Conservative.** The cornerstone of treatment is modification in training, for example, reducing mileage, shortening workouts, and alternating activities such as low-resistance cycling and swimming pool running.[9] There is not a single entity that works for everyone, but conservative measures usually include the following:

   a. A shock-absorbing heel cup for heel pain or a full-length orthotic for midsubstance pain
   b. Although not proven uniquely effective, analgesics, as they do, decrease pain
   c. Physical therapy to include Achilles and plantar fascia stretching, hindfoot taping, contrast baths, and ultrasound treatment.
   d. A night dorsiflexion splint might help to keep the fascia under tension to reduce early morning weight-bearing pain.
   e. Injections may be used in refractory cases. This has historically been done with steroids, although steroids pose a small risk of plantar fascia rupture. Consistent with the fact that this has been noted to be a degenerative rather than an inflammatory process, there are no data demonstrating that the antiinflammatory component of the steroid is necessary. For these reasons, many physicians are moving away from injections.

2. Shockwave therapy, which tries to spur on inflammatory response, has proven to be helpful.[10] The economics of health care have put a limitation on the availability of such treatment modality.

3. **Surgical.** Surgical intervention is rarely required and only for the most recalcitrant of cases, which is usually of 1 year or more duration. When indicated, a partial plantar fascia release is performed, which involves releasing the medial two-thirds of the ligament. A complete release should be avoided because it may increase the compressive forces to the dorsal aspect of the midfoot and decrease flexion forces on the metatarsophalangeal (MTP) joint complex.[11] The patient is allowed to bear weight as tolerated with crutches, and rehabilitation is started after 2 weeks.

D. **Calcaneal fat pad trauma.** The patient complains of diffuse plantar heel pain that is exacerbated with weight bearing and with activities on hard surfaces.

1. **Examination** reveals diffuse tenderness localized to the fat pad. There is no radiation of the pain. The heel pad feels soft and thin, and the underlying calcaneus is palpable.

2. **Treatment** is nonsurgical. A cushioned heel cup and shock-absorbing shoes might help. The patient should reduce activities and avoid running on hard surfaces. Several months may be required to resolve the constellation of symptoms.

E. **Nerve entrapment syndromes**

1. Entrapment of the **first branch of the lateral plantar nerve** is a common cause of chronic heel pain in athletes.[12] The site of compression is between the deep fascia of the abductor hallucis muscle and the medial margin of the quadratus plantae muscle. This injury is more common in athletes who spend a significant amount of time on their toes, such as ballet dancers, figure skaters, and sprinters.

   a. **Diagnosis** is made on clinical grounds. Exclude the more common reasons for heel pain. Early morning pain is less problematic; the pain increases as the day goes on. Tenderness is specific over the area of compression and may radiate down toward the toes (the Tinel's sign).

   b. **Treatment** is similar to that for other causes of heel pain. If conservative treatment fails, a release of the nerve may be done through a medial incision.

2. **Tarsal tunnel syndrome** could also be a source of heel pain. Compression of the posterior tibial nerve within the tarsal tunnel results in tenderness over the area that may shoot down toward the toes on the plantar aspect of the foot. Excessive pronation in long distance runners may place repeated stress on the medial structures of the hindfoot.

   a. On **examination**, there might be burning, pain, or tingling on the plantar aspect of the foot. Pain is more diffuse than with other causes of heel pain. Electromyography studies along with a Tinel's sign (electric shocks down the foot with tapping of the tibial nerve) and a highly suggestive clinical history are critical for the diagnosis of tarsal tunnel syndrome.

   b. **Treatment.** A medial heel wedge or an arch support may decrease the tension on the medial side of the ankle and, therefore, the nerve. Physical therapy can also improve the biomechanics. Steroid injection into the tarsal tunnel might give short-term pain relief. Tarsal tunnel release is helpful in recalcitrant cases.

3. **Metatarsalgia**

   a. Metatarsalgia or pain over the metatarsal heads is the most common forefoot problem. It typically occurs on the second metatarsal head and can have numerous etiologies.

      i. A **tight or shortened Achilles tendon** limits ankle dorsiflexion, which, in turn, increases the forces on the forefoot. A person compensates using the long toe extensors to augment dorsiflexion power, but this pulls the plantar fat pad away from the weight-bearing surface under the metatarsal heads, further aggravating forefoot pain.

ii. Similarly, **idiopathic claw toe deformities** could displace the fat pad and cause metatarsalgia.

iii. **MTP joint capsulitis** may produce pain over the plantar aspect of the joint. This is more common at the second MTP joint and is associated with a long second metatarsal or instability of the first ray.

iv. A **Morton's (or common digital nerve) neuroma** causes pain in the web space as well. It is most common in the third web space (between the third and fourth metatarsals).

b. The differential diagnosis of midfoot to forefoot pain always includes **stress fractures** (see **Section IV**).

c. **Treatment.** The goal is to unload the metatarsal area. Orthotics with metatarsal bars/pads, cushioned shoes, analgesics, and Achilles stretching is the cornerstone of initial management. If conservative management does not help, surgical correction of claw toes or excision of neuroma might be indicated.

### III. Tibialis Posterior Dysfunction Syndrome

Degeneration/rupture of the posterior tibialis tendon (PTT) is a cause of a painful, acquired flatfoot deformity in adults. It is more common in women ages 40 years and older.[13-15] Numerous reports describing the condition have been published over the past 20 years, but it still remains a condition that is not commonly recognized. This could be due to the insidious nature of the condition, usually without a history of acute trauma.[13]

A. **Anatomy.** By virtue of its lever arm length and muscle strength, PTT is the main dynamic stabilizer of the hindfoot against valgus deformity. It also plays a major role in maintaining the medial longitudinal arch. Insufficiency of the PTT results in excessive strain on the static ligament–bone hindfoot and midfoot constraints. The soft tissue gradually elongates, the arch flattens, and the peroneus longus and brevis tendons have an unopposed abduction force on the forefoot.

B. **Etiology of PTT rupture.** To understand the etiology of PTT tears, it is important to remember its function. It resists considerable forces in maintaining the medial longitudinal arch. It also helps locking the midfoot and hindfoot to allow a solid lever arm during the push-off part of the gait cycle. Approximately 20% of PTT ruptures are associated with rheumatic conditions.[13] An estimated 80% of PTT ruptures develop spontaneously. There are several theories to explain this phenomenon.

1. **Mechanical.** The acute angle around the medial malleolus could lead to excessive friction that leads to slow deterioration over many years. This also explains the age predilection of this condition.

2. **Vascular.** Laboratory studies have identified an area of poor blood supply to the tendon behind the medial malleolus. This could lead to a decrease in healing potential after minor trauma.

3. **Achilles tendon contracture.** Either because of gastrocnemius alone or in combination with soleus, a contracture or shortness of the Achilles tendon increases the workload and force on the PTT during the gait cycle.

C. **Clinical presentation.** Contrary to popular belief, PTT rupture or insufficiency is common. A proper history and thorough physical examination are usually all that is needed to make this a straightforward diagnosis.

1. **History.** Onset is insidious, with discomfort reported on the medial side of the foot without any preceding acute trauma. Women are affected more often than men, and persons in their 40s or older are most often affected.

There is not necessarily a relation to activity level. Overweight is also correlated with a higher incidence of PTT pathology.

2. **Symptoms.** Initially, patients complain of only mild-to-moderate pain and of swelling and discomfort on the medial side of the foot and ankle. It is usually not incapacitating; rather, there is a chronic medial weight-bearing ache that limits physical activities. Without treatment, the symptoms typically increase over a variable length of time. In a late stage, the patient might complain of additional weight-bearing pain on the lateral aspect of the ankle, a progressive deformity, and an abnormal gait, which can then become incapacitating.

3. **Signs**
   a. In an early stage, one can see and palpate the swelling behind the medial malleolus and over the course of the PTT to its insertion in the navicular. The tenderness is usually over the same area.
   b. In a more advanced stage, the hallmark deformity becomes apparent. This is a combination of hindfoot valgus, forefoot abduction, and flattening of the medial longitudinal arch.
   c. Much information can be gathered by observing the patient. When viewed from posterior, the amount of heel valgus above the normal neutral to 5° in the weight-bearing position can be noted. The patient is also asked to raise on the toes. A normal PTT locks the hindfoot in varus to give a solid lever for push-off. With an insufficient PTT, the heel does not move into varus, and it is impossible to raise oneself on the toes when performed unilaterally. "Too many toes" are seen when viewed from behind as the hindfoot remains in valgus and the forefoot is in abduction.
   d. Frontal and side views confirm the forefoot abduction and loss of medial arch. An apropulsive, antalgic gait is usually noticed if the patient is asked to walk at a rapid pace.
   e. Physical examination further confirms the clinical suspicion. Tendon and muscle power around the ankle is tested. The PTT is evaluated with the foot in neutral to slight forefoot abduction, and the patient is asked to adduct the forefoot against resistance. Look for recruitment of the tibialis anterior to augment this action to compensate for the weakness or lack of function of the PTT.
   f. The flexibility of the Achilles tendon is tested with the knee first extended to determine the role of the gastrocnemius in possible tightness and then with the knee flexed to isolate the soleus by eliminating the influence of the gastrocsoleus complex.
   g. Range of movement of the ankle, especially the subtalar joint, is evaluated, and any pain is noted. In advanced cases, there might be tenderness on the lateral aspect of the ankle as a result of impingement of the fibula on the calcaneus.

4. **Diagnostic workup.** A thorough history and clinical examination is usually all that is needed to make the diagnosis.
   a. **Plain roentgenographs.** In most cases beyond Stage 1, weight-bearing radiographs show specific changes. The most obvious is the change in the talo–first metatarsal alignment on the anteroposterior (AP) and lateral views. In a normal foot, the talo–first metatarsal alignment is in a straight line. In PTT ruptures, the alignment is altered to varying degrees because of the peritalar subluxation.
   b. **MRI** confirms a tear or degeneration in the PTT and shows the abnormal alignment of the bony elements, but it is costly and usually unnecessary. It is helpful in early, subtle injuries of the tendon and to rule out other causes of medial midfoot pain, such as navicular stress fractures.

c. **Computed tomography** (CT) is not necessary as a primary diagnostic tool, but it can be helpful to determine the integrity of the peritalar joints and, therefore, in **planning** the surgical procedure. It is of great value in the continuing study of the changes in the foot secondary to PTT ruptures.

5. **Classification. Each stage should be regarded as advancement of loss of function to the PTT because of further degeneration of the tendon itself along with greater duration of symptoms.**

a. **Stage 1.** There is swelling and tenderness over the PTT and slight weakness in inversion power, and there is minimal if any hindfoot valgus on weight bearing. This is typically representative of tenosynovitis. No presence of tendon change regarding intrasubstance degeneration or tearing. Typically able to perform unilateral or single-leg heel raise.

b. **Stage 2A.** Progression of pain and weakness associated with PTT representative of some level of intrasubstance degeneration of the tendon itself. There is the presence of flatfoot deformity with heel in valgus but without significant forefoot abduction. The hindfoot is flexible. Unable to perform single-leg heel raise.

c. **Stage 2B.** Only addition to 2A is the presence of "too many toes" sign caused by excessive forefoot abduction related to medial subluxation of the talonavicular joint. Radiographically, >40% uncovering of the talar head medially as seen on anteroposterior view of the foot.

d. **Stage 3.** Progressive dorsolateral peritalar subluxation reaches the point of dislocation in the neglected case. Pain also occurs on the lateral side as a result of impingement of the calcaneus on the distal fibula. The fibula takes an increasing amount of load on weight bearing. It becomes hypertrophic, and stress fractures are not uncommon. The talocalcaneal relation is completely distorted, with minimal actual articular contact. The majority of these deformities are fixed and not passively correctable.

e. **Stage 4: Valgus talus.** The final and more severe stage of PTT dysfunction also includes a valgus alignment of the talus on top of the already mentioned changes present for Stage 3. This valgus alignment of the talus is seen on weight-bearing mortise view of the ankle.

6. **Treatment**

a. Nonsurgical. Other than Grade 1, nonsurgical management of PTT tears is essentially palliative. There has been a great deal of discussion regarding the effectiveness of nonsurgical care regarding Stage 2; however, it has been the author's experience that in most cases, it will result in neither healing of the tendon nor correction of the deformity. Noninvasive means are, therefore, only useful if there are factors present that contraindicate surgical intervention. This includes advanced age, significant medical problems, low activity level, and minimal discomfort. It is still advisable to start most patients on conservative treatment before electing to do surgery. Treatment should be directed to control pain, inflammation, and development of deformity. Options include the use of crutches, minimal weight bearing, or casting in a recent-onset case. Nonsteroidal antiinflammatory drugs (NSAIDs) might help relieve pain and swelling. In more advanced cases, orthotics comes into play. These include heel or sole lifts, inserts, University of California-Berkley Lab (UCBL)-type heel cups, and modified, accommodative shoes. In severe deformities, shoe modifications could be used.

b. **Surgical.** Surgical treatment options include tendon repair, tendon augmentation, and bony stabilization of both nonessential and essential joints.

i. **Stage 1.** A tendon repair is still feasible. The PTT can be augmented with a second tendon. A multitude of augmenting techniques have been described.[13,15] This includes the use of the flexor digitorum longus most frequently, flexor hallucis longus, or peroneus longus that serve as dynamic stabilizers. Free tendon grafts are also used to repair the PTT, although the results are variable. It is of utmost importance to evaluate for tightness of the Achilles tendon and to lengthen it if necessary.

ii. **Stage 2.** In more advanced cases, tendon repair and augmentation are usually not sufficient to relieve pain and prevent deformity. The surgical option is dependent upon the degree and mobility of the deformity. If the peritalar subluxation is still correctable, the improvement of alignment is done primarily by sparing joints. This includes the lateral column distraction fusion that reduces the peritalar subluxation and heel valgus without compromising the important subtalar and talonavicular movement. Other options include a medial calcaneal slide osteotomy or a medial column closing wedge osteotomy to reduce the valgus alignment of the heel.

iii. **Stage 3.** The surgical treatment of peritalar subluxation with a fixed hindfoot deformity usually requires a combination of hindfoot joint fusions. The procedure will have to be tailored to the patient based on the type of deformity.

iv. **Stage 4.** Most cases present with a large degree of osteoarthritis along the ankle and hindfoot. The standard of care will consist of a pantalar arthrodesis.

**IV. Stress Fractures**

   **A. Description.** The foot and ankle are the most common areas for stress fractures. A *stress fracture* is defined as a partial or complete fracture resulting from its inability to withstand repetitive stress applied in a repeated, subthreshold manner. It is, therefore, a series of events causing stress fractures. Ninety-five percent of stress fractures are in the lower extremities, and/or 50% are of the foot and ankle. All the bones of the foot and ankle are susceptible to sustain stress fractures. The metatarsals, although, are involved in 55% of cases, whereas the sesamoids and talus are involved in less than 1%. Stress fractures occur in all sports, but especially in running-based sports.[16] Sedentary people starting a fitness program are more prone to stress fractures. This is a well-demonstrated phenomenon in new military recruits. Stress fractures are more likely to develop in women. Leg length discrepancy, malalignment, prior injury, cavus feet that lack normal pronation, as well as poor physical condition predispose to stress fracture.

   **B. Diagnosis**

   1. The history is fairly typical, with pain being intensified by ongoing training. There might be an association with a recent increase in duration and intensity of training. It is usually insidious, with an increase in pain over a period.

   2. There should always be a high index of suspicion for stress fractures with insidious onset of pain. Physical examination should localize the involved area.

   3. **Standard radiographs** should be the first-line imaging test for evaluation of possible stress fractures. However, one must be aware of their lack of sensitivity. Callus formation is the abnormality seen on plain films and represents the healing of the injury. Plain films will thus be nondiagnostic for the first few weeks. Furthermore, a large percentage will always appear normal on X-rays. Thus, if one's clinical evaluation is suspicious for stress fracture, further imaging is often necessary.[17]

4. **Bone scans.** The gold standard for recognizing a stress reaction in bone is a technetium bone scan. The bone scan becomes positive after a week of ongoing stress reaction in the bone. A negative bone scan effectively rules out a stress fracture.[17]

5. **MRI.** It is useful to list the indication, as special short-tau inversion-recovery (STIR) images may be helpful. It is the most sensitive and specific method of diagnosing and grading stress fractures and is especially helpful in the feet.[18]

6. The combination of a negative roentgenogram and positive bone scan represents an early fracture, and treatment at this stage may prevent long-standing problems. CT scan has a place in diagnosing talus and midfoot fractures because these bones are cancellous in structure and stress fractures are difficult to identify on plain radiographs.

7. The most critical or at-risk stress fractures of the foot are of the navicular, proximal second metatarsal,[19] intraarticular fractures, and the great toe sesamoids. The navicular is particularly difficult to diagnose.[20] Workup should include plain films, MRI, bone scan, and CT scan. Significant disability can result from delayed diagnosis.

### C. Treatment

1. Treatment greatly depends on the location of the stress fracture. For high-risk bones (navicular, talus, etc.), treatment should include 6 weeks of casting followed by verification of union by CT. Resumption of leg-based athletics is at 12 to 18 weeks after initiation of treatment. Custom orthotics should be used when the patient returns to athletics.[17]

2. Noncritical fractures include distal second, third, and fourth metatarsals; the lateral malleolus; and the calcaneus.[21] Treatment should be aimed at keeping the level of activity below that which causes pain. This implies decreasing the level of activity or substituting swimming, biking, circuit training, or other low-impact activities. Shoe orthotics can limit stress in the involved area.[20] Activities can progress as long as they are not painful. There are reasons to try to limit NSAIDs as their antiinflammatory properties can inhibit bone healing and their pain relief properties may give patients a false level of reassurance.[22]

## V. Great Toe Metatarsophalangeal Joint Problems

### A. Turf toe
is defined by some as a sprain of the plantar capsuloligamentous complex. Others use the term to be more encompassing for various injuries around the first MTP joint. Differential diagnosis includes injury to the medial or lateral ligamentous structures, the phalangeal sesamoid ligament, a fractured sesamoid, osteochondral or chondral injury, chondral contusion caused by direct axial impact, and dislocations or injury to the interphalangeal joint.[23] This injury is common in football players but is also seen in basketball and track athletes. Careful history and clinical evaluation are necessary to localize the injury. AP, lateral, oblique, and sesamoid views should be obtained.

1. Initial **conservative treatment** consists of the general approach: rest, ice, compression, and elevation. A postoperative shoe with firm sole to limit movement of the MTP joint helps in ligamentous injuries. The patient's foot is immobilized for 3 weeks, and rehabilitation is started as tolerated. Sesamoid fractures are treated with a cast shoe, with the great toe in 10° of flexion for 8 to 10 weeks.

2. **Surgical treatment** in a case of chondral fracture consists of debridement and drilling of articular surface if pain persists. Partial excision or internal fixation of sesamoid fracture is undertaken when the fracture does not heal.

B. **Hallux rigidus** is degenerative arthritis of the first MTP joint. In most cases, there is no specific predisposing factor.

1. Possible etiologies include congenital flattening of the metatarsal head, metatarsus primus elevatus, osteochondritis of the head, a long hallux, pes planus, and osteochondral injuries (turf toe).

2. Hallux rigidus presents a significant problem for an athlete. Dorsiflexion of the big toe plays an important role in activities such as accelerating and jumping. Compensation by rolling onto the lateral aspect of the foot might cause stress and strain on the ankle, knee, and hip.

3. **Diagnosis.** Enlargement around the MTP joint is usually obvious. This is due to a combination of bony prominences and synovitis. Dorsiflexion is limited and reproduces the patient's pain. Radiographic findings might be minimal in early stages. With time, obvious degenerative changes and osteophytes within the joint become apparent. Sesamoids are generally not involved.

4. Differential diagnosis includes gout or other inflammatory arthritis.

5. **Treatment**
   a. **Conservative.** Pressure against the toe is alleviated by modifying footwear, incorporating a higher and wider toe box, a stiffer sole shoe, a rigid insert, or a rocker bottom sole. NSAIDs or injected steroids might give symptomatic relief.
   b. **Surgical.** Fusion is a good option in older people but would significantly impair athletic performance. In athletes, a cheilectomy (debridement of the MTP joint) with or without a dorsiflexion osteotomy of the proximal phalanges (Moberg procedure) is preferred.[24,25] The patient is permitted to ambulate weight bearing as tolerated in a postoperative shoe. Rehabilitation starts 7 to 10 days after surgery with active and passive range of motion exercises. The patient should wear a soft shoe to allow motion at the MTP joint with walking. Athletes could resume cycling, swimming, and any activity that avoids significant impact against the MTP joint but should avoid running, jumping, and similar activities for 6 to 12 weeks. MTP joint arthroplasties (excision or prosthetic replacement) have very limited application in the young, active population.

## VI. Hallux Valgus (Bunions)

The etiology of hallux valgus is still debated, but there appears to be a significant familial predisposition. Shoe wear has been suggested as an etiologic factor, as a tight toe box and a high heel will place an increased laterally and distally directed force on the great toe. Joint laxity is associated with an increased rate of hallux valgus. Not all hallux valgus deformities are symptomatic. Typically, patients will describe pain over the medial bunion that corresponds to bursal inflammation. In more severe deformities, the main complaint is that of the second and third ray metatarsalgia.

A. **Evaluation**
   1. History
      a. What causes pain?
      b. Shoe wear: Type and any recent changes?
      c. What activities does it affect?
   2. Physical examination
      a. Compare shoe size with foot size. Any change in shoes because of bunions?
      b. Evaluate callus pattern: Lesser metatarsal overload, great toe pronation
      c. Evaluate gait: excessive pronating → more force on the medial rays → increased valgus angulation of the first MTP joint. Evaluate kinetic chain of gait from the pelvis down.
   3. X-rays
      a. Angle of long axis of the first and second metatarsals

### B. Treatment

1. **Conservative**
   a. Shoe modification is the most important. The shoes should be big enough, have a low heel and a wide and deep toe box.
   b. Orthotics to support the medial arch and unload the lesser metatarsal heads might be of benefit.
   c. Bunion pads might help for medial eminence pain.
   d. Silicone spacers could be used between the toes.
   e. Physical therapy if biomechanical factors seem to be resulting in excessive foot pronation.

2. **Surgical**
   a. Surgery should never be for cosmetic reasons, rather for pain and functional reasons
   b. Refer to a surgeon if there is no adequate pain relief after 6 months of appropriate conservative care.

## VII. Claw and Hammer Toes

The claw toe represents a hyperextension deformity of the MTP joint and a flexion deformity of the proximal interphalangeal (PIP) and distal interphalangeal (DIP) joints. This frequently involves multiple toes and is usually an indication of a muscle imbalance between the intrinsic and extrinsic muscles of the toes. The most common complaint is pain and friction over the dorsum of the PIP joint. With time, the plantar fat pad dislocates distally and exposes the metatarsal heads. This results in significant metatarsalgia.

A hammer toe deformity consists of a flexion deformity of the PIP joint; often with this, the MTP joint and the DIP joint are in extension to compensate the excessive flexion. The most common cause of a hammer toe deformity is a result of the toe hitting against the tip of the shoe, resulting in a flexion deformity. These patients typically will have symptoms as a result of a painful corn at the tip of the toe or a callus along the dorsum of the PIP joint of the toe.

### A. Evaluation

1. General
   a. Neurologic abnormalities
   b. Muscle imbalance, specifically gastrocnemius–soleus contracture
   c. Intrinsic muscle imbalance
   d. Diabetes
   e. Vascular compromise
2. Local
   a. Flexible (correctible) deformity: Usually does well with conservative treatment.
   b. Rigid (impossible to passively correct the PIP or DIP deformity)

### B. Conservative treatment

1. Shoe modifications. Should be big enough, low heel, wide and deep toe box. This is especially important for rigid deformities.
2. Orthotics with a metatarsal bar might help to reduce the plantar fat pad and reduce the metatarsal pain.
3. Silicone spacers and sleeves and claw toe splints might be helpful.

### C. Surgical treatment. Only indicated if conservative measures fail.

## REFERENCES

1. Maffulli N, Antonietta F, Leonardo O, Buono AD. Achilles tendinopathy. *JBJS Rev.* 2014;2:1-11.
2. Mohr RN. Achilles tendinitis—rationale for use and application or orthotics. *Foot Ankle Clin.* 1997;2:439-456.
3. Shrier I, Matheson GO, Kohl HW III. Achilles tendinitis: are corticosteroid injections useful or harmful? *Clin J Sport Med.* 1996;6:245-250.

4. McGarvey WC, Palumbo RC, Baxter DE, Leibman BD. Insertional Achilles tendinosis: surgical treatment through a central tendon splitting approach. *Foot Ankle Int.* 2002;23:19-25.
5. McGarvey WC, Singh D, Trevino SG. Partial Achilles tendon rupture associated with fluoroquinolone antibiotics: a case report and literature review. *Foot Ankle Int.* 1996;17:496-498.
6. Maffulli N, Giuseppe LU, Vincenzo D. Novel approaches for the management of tendinopathy. *JBJS.* 2010;92:2604-2613.
7. Johnston E, Scranton P Jr, Pfeffer GB. Chronic disorders of the Achilles tendon: results of conservative and surgical treatments. *Foot Ankle Int.* 1997;18:570-574.
8. Maffulli N, Testa V, Capasso G, Bifulco G, Binfield PM. Results of percutaneous longitudinal tenotomy for Achilles tendinopathy in middle- and long-distance runners. *Am J Sports Med.* 1997;25:835-840.
9. Pfeffer G, Bacchetti P, Deland J, et al. Comparison of custom and prefabricated orthotics in the initial treatment of proximal plantar fasciitis. *Foot Ankle Int.* 1999;20(4):214-221.
10. Gollwitzer H, Amol S, Didomenico L, et al. Clinically relevant effectiveness of focused extra corporeal shock wave treatment in the treatment of plantar fasciitis. *JBJS.* 2015;97:701-708.
11. Daly PJ, Kitaoka HB, Chao EY. Plantar fasciotomy for intractable plantar fasciitis: clinical results and biomechanical evaluation. *Foot Ankle.* 1992;13:188-195.
12. Baxter DE, Pfeffer GB. Treatment of chronic heel pain by surgical release of the first branch of the lateral plantar nerve. *Clin Orthop Relat Res.* 1992;(279):229-236.
13. Johnson KA. Tibialis posterior tendon rupture. *Clin Orthop Relat Res.* 1983;(177):140-147.
14. Sangeorzan BJ, Smith D, Veith R, Hansen ST Jr. Triple arthrodesis using internal fixation in treatment of adult foot disorders. *Clin Orthop Relat Res.* 1993;(294):299-307.
15. Thordarson DB, Schmotzer H, Chon J. Reconstruction with tenodesis in an adult flatfoot model. A biomechanical evaluation of four methods. *J Bone Joint Surg Am.* 1995;77:1557-1564.
16. Ting A, King W, Yocum L, et al. Stress fractures of the tarsal navicular in long distance runners. *Clin Sports Med.* 1988;7:89-101.
17. Santi M, Sartoris DJ. Diagnostic imaging approach to stress fractures of the foot. *J Foot Surg.* 1991;30:85-97.
18. Arendt EA, Griffiths HJ. Use of MR imaging in the assessment and clinical management of stress reactions of bone in high-performance athletes. *Clin Sports Med.* 1997;16:291-306.
19. Micheli LJ, Sohn RS, Solomon R. Stress fractures of the second metatarsal involving Lisfranc's joint in ballet dancers. *J Bone Joint Surg Am.* 1985;67:1372-1375.
20. Schwellnus MP, Jordaan G, Noakes TD. Prevention of common overuse injuries by the use of shock absorbing insoles. *Am J Sports Med.* 1990;18:636-641.
21. Cosman F, Ruffing J, Zion M, et al. Determinants of stress fracture risk in United States Military Academy cadets. *Bone.* 2013;55(2):359-366. doi: 10.1016/j.bone.2013.04.011
22. Dahners LE, Mullis BH. Effects of nonsteroidal anti-inflammatory drugs on bone formation and soft-tissue healing. *J Am Acad Orthop Surg.* 2004;12(3):139-143.
23. Tanner P, Daniel R, Tarakemeh A, Vopat BG, Mulcahey MK. Turf toe. *JBJS Rev.* 2019;7:1-6.
24. Coughlin M, Shurman P. Hallux rigidus. *JBJS.* 2003;85:2072-2088.
25. Mulier T, Steenwerckx A, Thienpont E, et al. Result after cheilectomy in athletes with hallux rigidus. *Foot Ankle Int.* 1999;20(4):232-237.

## SELECTED HISTORICAL READINGS

Anzel SH, Covey KW, Weiner AD, et al. Disruption of muscle and tendons; an analysis of 1,014 cases. *Surgery.* 1959;45:406-414.

Aström M, Gentz CF, Nilsson P, et al. Imaging in chronic Achilles tendinopathy: a comparison of ultrasonography, magnetic resonance imaging and surgical findings in 27 histologically verified cases. *Skeletal Radiol.* 1996;25:615-620.

Bennett GL, Graham CE, Mauldin DM. Triple arthrodesis in adults. *Foot Ankle.* 1991;12(3):138-143.

Bonney G, McNab I. Hallux valgus and hallux rigidus; a critical survey of operative results. *J Bone Joint Surg Br.* 1952;34:366-385.

Dameron TB Jr. Fractures and anatomical variations of the proximal portion of the fifth metatarsal. *J Bone Joint Surg Am.* 1975;57:788-792.

Key JA. Partial rupture of the tendon of the posterior tibial muscle. *J Bone Joint Surg Am.* 1953;35:1006-1008.

Leach RE, Seavey NS, Salter DK. Results of surgery in athletes with plantar fasciitis. *Foot Ankle.* 1986;7:155-161.

Lehman RC, Torg JS, Pavlov H, et al. Fractures of the base of the fifth metatarsal distal to the tuberosity: a review. *Foot Ankle.* 1987;7:245-252.

Lutter LD. Surgical decisions in athletes' subcalcaneal pain. *Am J Sports Med.* 1986;14:481-485.

Puddu G, Ippolito E, Postacchini F. A classification of Achilles tendon disease. *Am J Sports Med.* 1976;4:145-150.

# 30

# Aspiration and Injection of Upper and Lower Extremities

Fernando A. Pena

## I. General Guidelines

A. For any injection, consider infiltrating the subcutaneous skin of the entry site. It will improve the patient's comfort, and it will facilitate several attempts if needed without extra discomfort for the patient. Using an ethyl chloride–based spray is a reasonable alternative to "freeze" the skin in the area of the injection. Pulling the skin taut prior to introducing the needle is also helpful in reducing pain. Accurate placement of intraarticular injections is often based on feel. As the needle penetrates the skin and advances toward the joint, the anesthetic should be injected slowly. When injecting into soft tissue, you will feel resistance to flow on the syringe. Once the needle penetrates the joint, the resistance will dramatically decrease, which confirms intraarticular placement. This is easily reproducible for the knee. In joints with larger soft-tissue coverage, or at risk for neurovascular injury with an injection, guidance with fluoroscopy or ultrasound is recommended.

B. The use of fluoroscopic imaging with radiopaque contrast is a valuable tool to confirm intraarticular placement of therapeutic and diagnostic injections. For example, intraarticular injections and aspirations of the hip can pose a risk of neurovascular injury, and fluoroscopic guidance allows for safe and accurate needle placement. Fluoroscopic guidance is essential for injecting most small joints of the foot that have a very limited joint space for needle entrance. Accurate placement of therapeutic injections can also help diagnostically by determining which joint of the foot and ankle is the pain generator.[1]

C. When using corticosteroids, be aware of the possibility of subcutaneous atrophy or hypopigmentation if the medication is left subcutaneously.

D. In an obese patient, be prepared to use spinal needles.

E. Use larger gauge needles with large syringes (20 mL and above) if an aspiration of a joint is going to be performed as blood or pus presents a thicker texture than synovial fluid.

When trying to rule out a septic joint, avoid having the entry site over the area of cellulitis as this will contaminate the joint and eventually the sample sent to the lab.

## II. The Shoulder Joint

The shoulder joint (i.e., the glenohumeral joint) may be entered either anteriorly or posteriorly as depicted in Fig. 30-1. When using the anterior approach, palpate the medial aspect of the humeral head and enter just medial to this or just lateral to the coracoid process (Fig. 30-1A). In our experience, more physicians now prefer a posterior approach. A posterior aspiration or infiltration of the shoulder is performed with an entry site located approximately 2 cm distal and 1 cm medial to the posterior corner of the acromion (Fig. 30-1B). At this level, the "soft spot" of the shoulder can be felt. The needle will be placed perpendicular to the posterior chest wall and aiming for the coracoid process, which is felt over the anterior aspect of the shoulder with the opposite hand. A "pop" will be felt when the capsule is penetrated with a medium-sized needle. Slight rotation of the arm

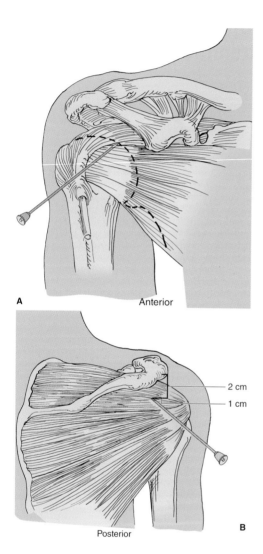

**Figure 30-1.** Shoulder joint and subacromial space.

A Anterior

2 cm

1 cm

Posterior B

may be used to confirm if the needle tip is over the glenoid rim versus the humeral head and the need for any relocation of the needle.

Using the same entry site and with an angle of approximately 30° cephalad, the subacromial space can be reached. Sometimes if the needle is angled too superiorly, or in an obese patient, the needle will hit the posterior margin of the acromion and it will have to be "walked" into the subacromial space.

### III. The Elbow Joint

The elbow (Fig. 30-2) will present a semiflexed position secondary to the pain and increased intraarticular fluid. The entry site will be located at the center of the triangle formed by the lateral epicondyle, the radial head, and the most lateral

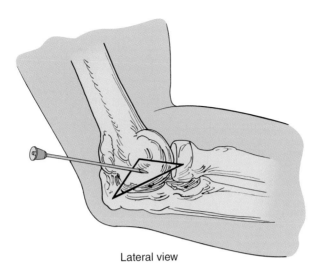

Lateral view

**Figure 30-2.** Elbow joint.

corner of the olecranon. At this level, the "soft spot" of the elbow joint is felt and the elbow joint can be easily reached. A second approach can be done immediately proximal to the superior margin of the olecranon and centered over the middle third of the olecranon through a transtendinous approach for the triceps tendon. This would provide full access to the olecranon fossa.

An injection of the extensor carpi radialis brevis (ECRB) for "tennis elbow" will be performed after identifying the most tender spot. For the most part, it will be located just a few centimeters proximal to the lateral epicondyle. With an angle of 30°, the painful spot is reached with the tip of the needle, and after backing out a few millimeters the medication is injected. Multiple "hits" with the tip of the needle against the lateral cortex of the humerus will be made to "agitate" the attachment site of the ECRB, which will promote healing and pain relief.

### IV. The Wrist Joint

The wrist would be approached from the dorsal aspect (Fig. 30-3). Most commonly, we can access the proximal radiocarpal joint in between the third and fourth extensor tendon compartments. This is located approximately 1 cm distal to the Lister tubercle, which is easily palpable. On the same direction and moving 2 cm distal from the tubercle, we will have access to the intercarpal joint. The joint space in between the carpal bones is quite limited, and most of the time the medication will be placed in between the capsule and bony structures and not in between the carpal bones. The distal radioulnar joint can be approached in between the fourth and fifth extensor tendon compartments. The entry site for the needle is located over a divot, which may be felt radial to the most prominent portion of the ulna.

### V. The Hip Joint

Intraarticular hip injections are safest when done with fluoroscopic or ultrasound guidance.[2] A lateral or anterolateral approach can be recommended to access the hip joint (Fig. 30-4). With any hip aspiration/injection, the femoral pulse must be palpated and marked to get a good sense of the location of the femoral neurovascular bundle to decrease the chances for injury after different maneuvers.

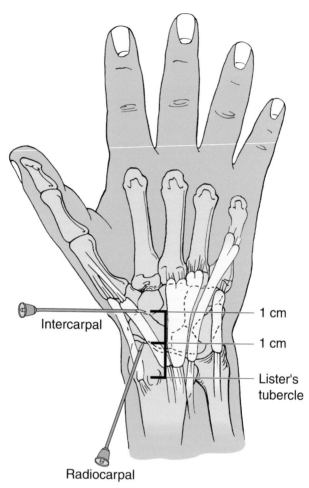

**Figure 30-3.** Wrist joint.

Spinal needles must be used to reach a joint as deep as the hip joint. The antero-lateral approach will have an entry site located approximately over the junction of the lateral third with the middle third of the total distance between the greater trochanter and the inguinal ligament. With this entry site, the needle will be angled approximately 45° cephalad and 45° medially. It is recommended to proceed with imaging intensification to guarantee full access to the hip joint. The lateral approach consists of performing an injection right above the tip of the greater trochanter and aiming straight medial to reach the junction of the femoral head with the femoral neck. The needle will be angled slightly anteriorly in order to correct for the femoral anteversion. An alternative to this is to place the extremity in internal rotation by 15° to 20° and the needle parallel to the coronal plane.

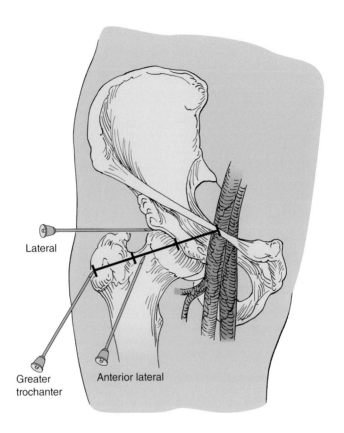

Lateral

Greater
trochanter

Anterior lateral

**Figure 30-4.** Hip joint.

The greater trochanter bursa can be injected easily in the office without any fluoroscopic assistance. The needle is placed slightly distal to the most prominent or painful area and angled 30° to 40° from inferior to superior until the lateral cortex of the femur is touched with the tip of the needle. At this level, pull back a few millimeters and proceed with the injection of the area. The medication should go without much resistance as a confirmation of being in a virtual space (i.e., greater trochanter bursa).

## VI. The Knee Joint

A knee with a moderate to large effusion will present an increased space between the patella and the femur as the patella is translated anteriorly by the increased intraarticular pressure (Fig. 30-5A). Therefore, under those circumstances, the easiest approach is to proceed laterally. The needle will be placed at a 90° angle with the long axis to the limb. The entry site will be located at the level of the proximal pole of the patella. Laterally, a void between the patella and the femur may be felt and the needle will be easily introduced at that level. Aspiration of the joint can be performed at the same time that "milking" of the intraarticular effusion is performed.

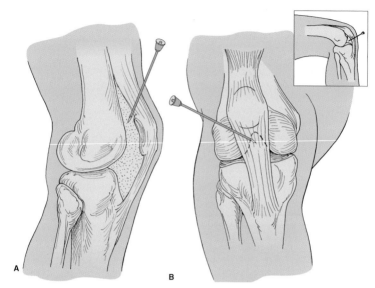

**Figure 30-5.** Knee joint.

An injection of a knee joint without an effusion through this approach is slightly more difficult as there is no virtual space created between the patella and the femoral trochlea. In an attempt to inject the knee joint through the already described lateral approach, the nontrained physician most likely will hit and damage the articular surface of the patella and/or femur. Therefore, the authors prefer to proceed with anterolateral approach, similar to the one performed during knee arthroscopy (Fig. 30-5B). This is located at the level of the inferior pole of the patella and a few millimeters lateral to the border of the patellar tendon. The needle is aimed at 30° caudad and 30° medially toward the trochanteric notch. The knee will be flexed at 90° when this is performed. During the injection of the medication, some resistance may be felt, because of the retropatellar fat pad. This will be avoided by moving the needle either forward or backward until the injection becomes easier to perform. An obvious sign of intraarticular placement is loss of resistance to flow on the syringe or if the needle makes contact with the lateral femoral condyle.

## VII. The Ankle Joint

The safest approach to the ankle joint is through the medial aspect (Fig. 30-6). The needle will be placed at approximately 60° from the sagittal plane with an entry site immediately medial to the anterior tibial tendon. A "soft spot" can be felt, which corresponds to the tibiotalar joint. The "shoulder" of the tibial plafond will be easily identified at that level. Special attention is required to direct the needle to be oblique enough to avoid any scuffing of the cartilage as the ankle joint is a very shallow joint. An alternative approach is to proceed with a lateral aspiration or injection, which will be done lateral to the extensor digitorum longus tendon. Also, 60° of obliquity is recommended. The level for the entry site is similar to the one described for the medial approach. The dorsal cutaneous branch of the superficial peroneal nerve is at risk for an injury with the use of the lateral approach. In most occasions, it can be seen or felt with forced plantar flexion of the foot and the fourth toe, which places the superficial nerve under tension.

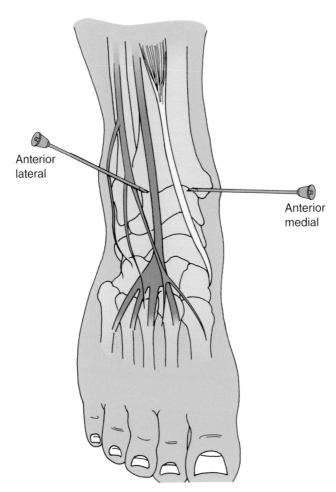

**Figure 30-6.** Ankle joint.

## REFERENCES

1. Cloutier D. Fluoroscopic guided injections in orthopaedic practice: a PA's perspective on a PA-led program. *J Orthop Phys Assist.* 2017;5(2):e9.
2. Balog TP, Rhodehouse BB, Turner EK, et al. Accuracy of ultrasound-guided intra-articular hip injections performed in the orthopedic clinic. *Orthopedics.* 2017;40(2):96-100. doi:10.3928/01477447-20161213-03.

# Index

Note: Page numbers followed by $f$, and $t$ indicate materials in figures, and tables, respectively.